Global Health

Global Health

Ethical Challenges

Edited by

Solomon Benatar
Emeritus Professor of Medicine, University of Cape Town

Gillian Brock
Professor of Philosophy, University of Auckland

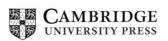

CAMBRIDGE
UNIVERSITY PRESS

University Printing House, Cambridge CB2 8BS, United Kingdom

One Liberty Plaza, 20th Floor, New York, NY 10006, USA

477 Williamstown Road, Port Melbourne, VIC 3207, Australia

314–321, 3rd Floor, Plot 3, Splendor Forum, Jasola District Centre,
New Delhi - 110025, India

79 Anson Road, #06-04/06, Singapore 079906

Cambridge University Press is part of the University of Cambridge.

It furthers the University's mission by disseminating knowledge in the pursuit of
education, learning, and research at the highest international levels of excellence.

www.cambridge.org
Information on this title: www.cambridge.org/9781108728713
DOI: 10.1017/9781108692137

Cambridge University Press © 2011, 2021

First published 2011
Second edition 2021

Printed in the United Kingdom by TJ Books Limited, Padstow Cornwall

A catalogue record for this publication is available from the British Library.

ISBN 978-1-108-72871-3 Paperback

....

Contents

Contents

Contributors

Mariajosé Aguilera
Independent Researcher

Gianna Gayle Herrera Amul
Research Associate, Lee Kuan Yew School of Public Policy, National University of Singapore

Isabella Bakker
Distinguished Research Professor, Department of Political Science, York University, Toronto, ON, Canada

David Benatar
Professor of Philosophy, University of Cape Town, Cape Town, South Africa

Solomon Benatar
Emeritus Professor of Medicine and Senior Scholar, University of Cape Town, Cape Town, South Africa, and Adjunct Professor, Dalla Lana School of Public Health, University of Toronto, Toronto, ON, Canada

Anne-Emanuelle Birn
Professor of Social and Behavioral Health Sciences, Dalla Lana School of Public Health, University of Toronto, Toronto, ON, Canada

David E. Bloom
Clarence James Gamble Professor of Economics and Demography, Harvard T.H. Chan School of Public Health, and Department of Global Health and Population, Harvard University, Cambridge, Massachusetts, USA

Gillian Brock
Professor of Philosophy, Humanities, University of Auckland, New Zealand

Allen Buchanan
Professor, Duke University, Durham, North Carolina, USA, and The Dickson Poon School of Law, King's College, London, United Kingdom

Colin D. Butler
Honorary Professor, National Centre for Epidemiology and Population Health, The Australian National University, Canberra, Australia

Daniel Cadarette
Research Assistant, Harvard T.H. Chan School of Public Health, and Department of Global Health and Population, Harvard University, Cambridge, Massachusetts, USA

Carlos Caceres
Professor, Interdisciplinary Research Center on Sexuality, AIDS, and Society, Cayetano Heredia University, Lima, Peru

Donald C Cole
Professor Emeritus, Dalla Lana School of Public Health, University of Toronto, Toronto, ON, Canada

Ibrahim Daibes
Former Program Manager, Global Health Research Initiative, Ottawa, ON, Canada

Denis Daneman
Chair Emeritus, Department of Pediatrics, University of Toronto, and Pediatrician-in-Chief Emeritus, The Hospital for Sick Children, Toronto, ON, Canada

Angus J. Dawson
Professor of Bioethics and Director of Sydney Health Ethics, Sydney University School of Public Health, Sydney, NSW, Australia

Matthew DeCamp
Associate Professor, University of Colorado, Boulder, Colorado, USA

Avram Ezra Denburg
Assistant Professor, Institute of Health Policy, Management and Evaluation, University of Toronto Staff Oncologist, and Clinician Scientist, Department

of Hematology/Oncology, The Hospital for Sick Children, Toronto, ON, Canada

James Dwyer
Professor of Bioethics and Humanities, Center for Bioethics and the Humanities, SUNY Upstate Medical University, Syracuse, New York, USA

Alie Eleveld
Safe Water and AIDS Project, Kisumu, Kenya

Sarah Elton
Assistant Professor, Department of Sociology, Ryerson University, Toronto, ON, Canada

Agata Ferretti
Professor, Swiss Federal Institute of Technology (ETH), Zürich, Switzerland

Ruth P. Fitzgerald
Professor, Department of Social Anthropology, School of Social Sciences, University of Otago, Dunedin, New Zealand

Lisa Forman
Associate Professor, Dalla Lana School of Public Health, University of Toronto, Toronto, ON, Canada

Joseph Gafton
Department of History, Queen Mary University of London, London, United Kingdom

Stephen Gill
Distinguished Research Professor. Department of Politics, York University, Toronto, ON, Canada

Eduardo J. Gómez
Associate Professor College of Health Lehigh University Bethlehem, Pennsylvania

Nicole Hassoun
Department of Philosophy, Cornell University, Ithaca, New York, USA, and Department of Philosophy, Binghamton University, Binghamton, New York, USA

Mark D. Hathaway
Sessional Lecturer, School of the Environment, University of Toronto.

Henk ten Have
Professor of Healthcare Ethics, Center for Healthcare Ethics, Duquesne University, Pittsburgh, Pennsylvania, USA

David Hunter
University of Adelaide, Adelaide, SA, Australia

Samia Hurst
Professor, Institute for Ethics, History, and the Humanities, Faculty of Medicine, University of Geneva, Switzerland

Melanie Jansen
Paediatric Intensive Care Unit and Centre for Children's Health Ethics and Law, Children's Health Queensland Australia

Jonathan Kennedy
Senior Lecturer, Queen Mary University of London, London, United Kingdom

Meri Koivusalo
Professor, Department of Global Health and Development, Tampere University, Tampere, Finland

Ramya Kumar
Lecturer, Department of Community and Family Medicine, Faculty of Medicine, University of Jaffna, Jaffna, Sri Lanka

Ronald Labonté
Professor and Distinguished Research Chair, Department of Globalization and Health Equity, School of Epidemiology and Public Health, University of Ottawa, Ottawa, ON, Canada

Alex John London
Clara L. West Professor of Ethics and Philosophy, Carnegie Mellon University, Pittsburgh, Pennsylvania, USA

Jenevieve Mannell
Centre for Gender and Global Health, Institute for Global Health, University College, London, United Kingdom

Angela Mashford-Pringle
Assistant Professor, Dalla Lana School of Public Health, University of Toronto, Toronto, ON, Canada

Alex Mauron
Institute for Ethics, History, and the Humanities, Faculty of Medicine, University of Geneva, Switzerland

David McCoy
Professor of Global Public Health, Queen Mary University of London, London, United Kingdom

Martin McKee
Professor of European Public Health, London School of Hygiene and Tropical Medicine, London, United Kingdom

Nathalie Mezger
MSF, Switzerland

Angelica Motta
Interdisciplinary Research Center on Sexuality, AIDS, and Society, Cayetano Heredia University, Lima, Peru

Jing-Bao Nie
Professor, Bioethics Centre, Otago Medical School University of Otago, Dunedin, New Zealand

Aloyce Odhiambo
Safe Water and AIDS Project, Kisumu, Kenya

Tikki Pang
Visiting Professor, Lee Kuan Yew School of Public Policy, National University of Singapore, Singapore

Thomas Pogge
Leitner Professor of Philosophy and International Affairs, Yale University, New Haven, Connecticut, USA

Blake Poland
Associate Professor, Dalla Lana School of Public Health, University of Toronto, Toronto, ON, Canada

David B. Resnik
National Institute of Environmental Health Sciences, National Institutes of Health, Bethesda, Maryland, USA

Jeff Rudin
Research Associate, Alternative Information and Development Centre, Cape Town, South Africa

Erica Di Ruggiero
Associate Professor, Office of Global Public Health Education and Training, Dalla Lana School of Public Health, University of Toronto, Toronto, ON, Canada

David Sanders
Emeritus Professor of Public Health, University of the Western Cape, Cape Town, South Africa

Ted Schrecker
Professor of Global Health Policy, Population Health Sciences Institute, Newcastle University, Newcastle upon Tyne, United Kingdom

Geordan Shannon
Centre for Gender and Global Health, Institute for Global Health, University College London, London, United Kingdom

Christine Straehle
Professor of Practical Philosophy, University of Hamburg, Hamburg, Germany

Godfrey B. Tangwa
Professor of Philosophy, University of Yaoundé 1, Yaoundé, Cameroon

Sandra Tomsons
Senior Scholar, University of Winnipeg, Winnipeg, MB, Canada

Ross Upshur
Professor, Dalla Lana School of Public Health, University of Toronto, Toronto, ON, Canada

Effy Vayena
Professor, Swiss Federal Institute of Technology (ETH), Zürich, Switzerland

Dillon Wamsley
PhD student, Department of Politics, York University, Toronto, ON, Canada

Kate Williams
Marie Stopes International, London, United Kingdom

James Wilson
Professor, Department of Philosophy, University College London, United Kingdom

Jonathan Wolff
Professor, Blavatnik School of Government, University of Oxford, Oxford, United Kingdom

Anthony B. Zwi
Professor of Global Health and Development, School of Social Sciences, Faculty of Arts and Social Sciences, University of New South Wales, Sydney, NSW, Australia

Introduction

Improving and promoting global health continues to be one of the largest and most important challenges facing humanity in the twenty-first century. The task has become even more difficult since our first edition appeared almost a decade ago, given the accelerated destruction of the planet and the associated compounded threats to health that now present themselves. The emergence and spread of COVID-19 and the implications of this pandemic for life, health, and our planet exemplify how the world can change so rapidly and profoundly. The domino effects of the pandemic in an unstable global system are triggering multiple tipping points with implied radical alterations to the trajectory of life as we have known it. This is a stark reminder that despite all the major advances in science, healthcare, health, and longevity since the Enlightenment, and despite all the promises of genetic medicine and artificial intelligence, the long-term health and survival of our species are now, more than ever, intensely threatened.

This second edition, which was largely completed before COVID-19 and therefore cannot include a comprehensive review of its effects and ramifications, aims to showcase some of these new and escalating threats, along with illuminating some of the many other obstacles we now face in partnering globally to solve these formidable challenges.

By *global health*, we mean the health of all people globally within sustainable and healthy living (local and global) conditions. In order to achieve this ambitious goal, we need to understand, among other things, the value systems, modes of reasoning, and power structures that have driven and shaped the world over the past century. We also need to appreciate the unsustainability of many of our current consumption patterns (and here we include the escalating appetite for eating meat with all its implications for the live-animal ("wet") food markets and intensive animal farming that enable the transmission of zoonotic infections from animals to humans, as well as the severely adverse effects of meat production on the environment) and the driving forces that lie behind them, before we can address threats to the health and lives of current and particularly future generations.

The world and how we live in it have been changing dramatically over many centuries, but in the past 60 years, change has been more rapid and profound than ever in the past. Many positive changes have been associated with impressive economic growth and advances in science and medicine and in social policies regarding access to health promotion. These include greater focus on a primary healthcare approach with more equitable access, expansion of social programs to improve living conditions, and a welcome increasing emphasis on the rights of all individuals to be equally respected.

Sadly, emphasis on the exaggerated expectations of the most privileged people has resulted in neglect of a large proportion of the world's population with consequent widening disparities in wealth and health and exacerbation of the social and societal determinants of health. To give just one example, increases in air pollution caused major reductions in intelligence amounting to the equivalent of losing one year or more of education and killed 7 million people in 2015 – 16% of all deaths globally.[1] This is three times the annual deaths from HIV/AIDS, tuberculosis, and malaria combined. In addition, many of the world's healthcare "systems" have increasingly become *distorted*, *dysfunctional*, and *unsustainable*. By *distorted*, we mean that healthcare services are not designed to meet equitably the range of local demands posed by changing burdens of disease in aging and more ethnically diverse populations with multiple chronic noncommunicable diseases.

---

[1] Zhang, X., Chen, X., & Zhang, X. (2018). The impact of exposure to air pollution on cognitive performance. *Proceedings of the National Academy of Sciences of the United States of America* 115(37), 9193–9197. https://doi.org/10.1073/pnas.1809474115.

Dysfunctionality arises from health services being driven more by powerful adverse market forces and the escalating requirements of bureaucracy than by emphasis on serving patients optimally and sustaining the professionalism required of healthcare workers in the care of patients and the training of new generations of professionals. Increasing commodification of healthcare services and a much-expanded bureaucracy are among other complex forces contributing to physician burnout and patient dissatisfaction with the services they receive. Finally, marginal benefits for a few (driven by the self-interest of segments of the health machine, for example, the pharmaceutical industry, and the pressure to raise research funds and publish) are often prioritized while other cost-effective activities of potentially great benefit to many more people are ignored. The introduction of new, effective, but expensive therapies further strains resources and contributes to disproportionate rising costs of healthcare that are becoming *unsustainable*.

The stresses imposed on health systems globally by emergencies such as the COVID-19 pandemic reveal the "rescue" emphasis of biomedicine, with neglect of the public health and pandemic planning required to face such threats when they arise. COVID-19 has also been a stark reminder of the many millions of deaths and social devastation caused by the 1918 flu pandemic. The deaths of many front-line health workers and the inadequate provision of protective equipment highlight the personal risks resulting from weak commitments to public health, and remind us of the ethical challenges that healthcare professionals face with dedication and courage.

Disparities in health and access to healthcare thus continue to widen globally. Such disparities, combined with population growth, unsustainable consumption patterns, the emergence of many new infectious diseases (and multidrug resistance), accelerating catastrophic anthropogenic climate change, escalating ecological degradation, numerous local and regional wars, a stockpile of nuclear weapons, and massive dislocations of people and new terrorist threats, including cyber attacks (to list just some relevant factors), have severe implications for individuals' and populations' health.[2]

Deeper understanding of the urgency of the challenges we face and the feasible changes that could be made to address them is a necessary first step toward expressing better commitment to genuine respect for the dignity of all people (and showing respect for everyone's dignity is an ideal our international agreements increasingly claim to embrace).

Adequate understanding of ethical issues concerning health requires that we extend our focus from the micro level of individual health and the ethics of interpersonal relationships to include ethical considerations regarding public and population health and justice concerns more generally, including environmental justice and stewardship for future generations. The domain of global health ethics provides a context within which the many relevant disciplines that have valuable insights to offer can usefully engage to promote better understanding of the extensive changes that are needed to assist in developing a global state of mind about the world and our place in it. Arguably this is more relevant than ever to making many of the necessary progressive changes required for survival on a wounded planet.

After noting the poor state of global health, there are *three main issues* covered by almost all contributing authors. They *direct our attention to ways in which we exacerbate poor global health* and *what we should do to remedy the factors identified* and *offer reasons why we ought to do something* about the highlighted problems, thereby connecting global health issues more strongly with the domains of social and intergenerational justice. Many of the chapters in this volume provide constructive suggestions about how national and global policy and institutional changes could function differently to make significant improvements. Together they contribute to a deeper understanding of the challenges we face in trying to improve global health and provide much practical and theoretical guidance toward building a case for our ability and motivation to make a real difference.

In what follows, we give a brief description of some key themes discussed in the chapters. A note

---

[2] We note here that the topics covered in this volume are by no means fully inclusive of the numerous problems that undermine and aggravate conditions for overcoming global health challenges. For example, we have not included chapters on such issues as global mental health, illicit trade in

human organs, child labor, use of children as soldiers, trade in sex and drugs, cultural practices that have serious adverse health effects, pervasive corruption in business and healthcare, and widespread Mafia-like organizations that increasingly influence (even control) the lives of many. All these factors contribute to global injustices as well. Several chapters from the first edition of this book (11, 21, 22, 23, 26, and 27) have not been updated and included – yet remain of great relevance.

about structure might be important here. Because almost all the authors cover the issue of responsibilities and global health, it has been difficult to impose a rigid structure on these chapters and the subsections of the book. Like the subject matter under investigation, several issues are intimately linked. Our subsections are meant to guide the reader to some ways in which we might group the various chapters to highlight certain core issues, even though there are many possible pathways through this innovative collection. Indeed, most of the chapters tackle several key themes, presenting some important empirical information helpful in understanding why there is so much poor health, providing ethical analysis and argument, along with offering constructive ideas about how we should shape the future in efforts to improve global health.

The chapters in Section 5 perhaps diverge from this general pattern. They focus on an issue that we see as increasingly important to address, namely developing helpful insights into and guidelines regarding how we can better communicate with each other about global health issues across differences in ways of seeing ourselves and the world. The need for constructive cross-cultural dialogue in partnering to address global health issues has, in our view, been a neglected issue that deserves a much greater focus. Diverse perspectives, which rely on contrasting metaphysical, epistemological, cultural, political, and religious assumptions (to name just a few sources of widespread difference), inform the range of orienting normative frameworks adopted by people across the planet. In tackling our global health challenges, we need to take this diversity more seriously and develop stronger tools for meaningful communication to traverse divides that threaten the global solidarity required for peaceful progress. In short, we must improve our interphilosophies dialogue – a challenge requiring humility and tolerance. We hope that our highlighting this important need will encourage more theorists and practitioners to develop well-reasoned work in this crucial area.

Global Health: Definitions, Descriptions, and Some Central Relationships

Probably the most striking feature about the current state of global health is that it is characterized by such radical inequalities. Here are some examples of the more widely noticed and documented kinds: (1) maternal mortality in 2015 ranged from 7 per 100,000 pregnancies in Canada to 134 in South Africa, 789 in southern Sudan, and 1,360 in Sierra Leone,[3] (2) the death rate under five years of age ranges from 5 per 1,000 live births in Canada to 137 per 1,000 live births in Somalia, where the average fertility rate is 6.6 children per woman and 1 of every 12 Somalian women dies from pregnancy-related causes, (3) life expectancy at birth spans the wide range of 49 years to over 80 years, (4) annual per capita healthcare expenditure in 2014 extended from a low of less than $50 in many poor countries to over $9,000 in the United States, and (5) the number of physicians per 100,000 people ranges from 2 in Malawi to 351 in the United States, 328 in Sweden, and 591 in Cuba.[4] Within most countries, these patterns of difference also persist with dramatic (although typically smaller) differences in life expectancy and other key metrics of health between the highest and lowest socio-economic groups and across population groups.

Ted Schrecker and Ronald Labonte argue that a largely accurate explanation for these types of differences involves potentially avoidable poverty and material deprivation (Chapter 1). However, these authors remind us that we should resist the inference that policies that promote economic growth are therefore the best way to achieve good population health. There is a threshold level (at annual per capita income of about US$5,000) beyond which the relationship between life expectancy at birth and per capita incomes breaks down. In addition, we see many countries with very good life expectancies at birth despite quite low per capita incomes. For example, in Costa Rica, with a per capita income of about US$10,500 per year, life expectancy is 79 years, notably more than the 78 years those who reside in the United States can expect to live, where per capita income is greater than US$45,000.[5] Other social changes besides economic growth can have significant consequences for health. For example, improved female literacy and

---

[3] Of all the maternal deaths worldwide, 88% occur in two regions, Sub-Saharan Africa and South Asia (Roser, M., & Ritchie, H. [2013]. Maternal mortality. Available at https://ourworldindata.org/maternal-mortality).

[4] Gill, S. R., & Benatar, S. R. (2019). Reflections on the political economy of planetary health. *Review of International Political Economy* 27(1). https://doi.org/10.1080/09692290.2019.1607769

[5] However, it should not be forgotten that economic growth remains important in countries with very low per capita incomes (e.g., <$2,000–$3,000) and that the extent of income disparities within countries is also important.

commitment to health as a social goal in Kerala (in India) have resulted in low infant and maternal mortality despite very low income (annual per capita income of about US$3,000). Another example is how increased urbanization and globalization have allowed the consolidation of power over food systems, which can lead to detrimental consumption patterns. Consider, for instance, how Mexicans now consume 50% more Coca-Cola products per person than those who reside in the United States.

Some gains in the state of world health have been achieved through improved vaccination coverage and access to affordable antiretroviral therapies, but much work remains to amplify these meager gains. Providing extra resources for healthcare is at least part of what is needed. Jeffrey Sachs has calculated that a tax of 1 cent in every $10 earned by the wealthiest 1 billion people in the world could provide the $35 billion required per year to give the poorest 1 billion people a $50 annual per capita healthcare package.[6]

However, we must be careful not to assume that health inequalities will resolve themselves as more resources are devoted to addressing deprivations in health directly. Many other factors are relevant. For instance, economic globalization is contributing to rising inequalities, which are likely to affect health inequalities through both direct and indirect channels, notably by affecting the distribution of political power and influence. Power asymmetries associated with globalization create and sustain harmful outcomes on many levels.

Indeed, the distribution of power and social, political, and economic resources is crucial in influencing and explaining population health. In Chapter 2, Anne-Emanuelle Birn and Ramya Kumar analyze the societal determinants of health: factors that shape health at various levels, including household, community, national, and global levels. Living conditions both at the household and at community levels can cause numerous ailments including respiratory, gastrointestinal, and metabolic diseases. Availability of potable water and adequate sanitation is a key factor. Though water is essential for life, more than a billion people (one-sixth of the world's population) have an inadequate supply. The facts about access to adequate sanitation are even more striking – almost half the world's population has inadequate access to basic sanitation facilities, which can result in soil contamination and increased rates of communicable diseases. The impact of other factors analyzed includes nutrition and food security (over 50% of child deaths are attributable to poor nutrition), housing conditions, public health and healthcare services, and transportation. Social policies and government regulation (or the lack thereof) can also affect health in dramatic ways through, for example, the domains of education, taxation, labor, and environmental regulations. Patterns of unequal resource distribution and political power thus play a fundamental role as the societal determinants of health. To address radical health inequalities effectively, we must adopt a societal determinants of health approach.

Infectious diseases are one of the most important areas for global concern. Historically, these have caused more morbidity and mortality than any other cause, including wars. Tuberculosis alone has killed a billion people during the last two centuries. The evolving global health system has done much to protect and promote human health. However, the world continues to be confronted by long-standing, emerging, and reemerging infectious disease threats. These threats differ widely in terms of severity and probability. They also have varying consequences for morbidity and mortality, as well as for a complex set of social and economic outcomes. To various degrees, they are also amenable to alternative responses, ranging from clean water provision to regulation to biomedical countermeasures. Whether the global health system as currently constituted can provide effective protection against a dynamic array of infectious disease threats has been called into question by recent outbreaks of Ebola, Zika, dengue, Middle East respiratory syndrome, severe acute respiratory syndrome, influenza, and most recently and spectacularly COVID-19 and by the looming threat of rising antimicrobial resistance. The concern is magnified by rapid population growth in areas with weak health systems, urbanization, globalization, climate change, civil conflict, and the changing nature of pathogen transmission between human and animal populations. There is also potential for human-originated outbreaks emanating from laboratory accidents or intentional biological attacks.

In Chapter 3, David Bloom and Daniel Cadarette discuss these issues, along with the need for a (possibly self-standing) multidisciplinary "Global Technical

---

[6] Jeffrey Sachs during a video conference presentation at the Canadian Conference on International Health, Ottawa, October 2009.

Council on Infectious Disease Threats" to address emerging global challenges with regard to infectious disease and associated social and economic risks. They suggest that such a council could strengthen the global health system by improving collaboration and coordination across organizations (e.g., the World Health Organization [WHO], Gavi [the Vaccine Alliance], the Coalition for Epidemic Preparedness Innovations [CEPI], national centers for disease control, and pharmaceutical manufacturers); filling in knowledge gaps with respect to (for example) infectious disease surveillance, research and development needs, financing models, supply chain logistics, and the social and economic impacts of potential threats; and making high-level, evidence-based recommendations for managing global risks associated with infectious disease. It has been argued elsewhere that without new forms of governance that transcend the current dominant paradigm, which has been causally implicated in current global health threats, insufficient progress is likely.[7]

Gender equality in medicine, global health, and science could potentially lead to substantial health, economic, and social gains. In Chapter 4, Geordan Shannon, Melanie Jansen, Kate Williams, Carlos Caceres, Angelica Motta, Aloyce Odhiambo, Alie Eleveld, and Jenevieve Mannell highlight both missed and future opportunities. They suggest that to understand these potential opportunities, gender analyses should be situated in the context of political influences and structural inequalities and draw on contemporary social movements. They outline some important differences between male and female patterns of health and illness and the care different health practitioners might offer. They argue for endeavors that go beyond quantitative gender equality and include striving for a cultural transformation that allows for the inclusion of values of transparency, honesty, fairness, and justice. They conclude that achieving gender equality is not simply instrumental for health and development but rather that its impact could have wide-ranging benefits as a matter of fairness and social justice for everyone.

Martin McKee presents an account of how health, well-structured and well-integrated healthcare systems, and economic growth can all coexist and be mutually supporting (Chapter 5). Healthcare, when appropriately delivered, can yield substantial gains in population health which further reduce the demand for healthcare. Better population health can result in faster economic growth through enhanced productivity. The additional economic growth can increase resources available for healthcare, and further investment in healthcare can also contribute to economic growth. None of this necessarily follows, however. Concerted action by governments is needed to ensure that these relationships are mutually supportive and beneficial.

Global Health Ethics, Responsibilities, and Justice: Some Central Issues

David Hunter and Angus J. Dawson explore the question of whether there is a need for global health ethics (Chapter 6). They begin by examining different ways of understanding the term *global health ethics* and proceed to examine arguments that could be used either to support or rebut more substantive accounts of global health ethics, including those based on beneficence, justice, and harm, and more cosmopolitan accounts. Some of the arguments they explore that are used to resist more substantive global health ethics include those concerning the moral relevance of distance, property rights, and duties to prioritize the interests of compatriots. They argue that we need not necessarily take a stand on any of these arguments to make a convincing case for the various global obligations we have with respect to health. Sometimes a case for global responsibilities pertaining to health can be marshaled via more self-interested concerns, such as with infectious diseases or with the public goods nature of many global health issues (again, as is the case with infectious diseases). It is gratifying that interest in global health ethics has expanded in the past decade.[8]

Jonathan Wolff makes a case for the strategic value of a human rights approach in contributing to positive global health outcomes (Chapter 7). Whatever concerns one might have about the philosophical or

---

[7] Gill, S., & Benatar, S. R. (2016). Global health governance and global power: a critical commentary on the Lancet–University of Oslo Commission Report. *International Journal of Health Services* **46**(2). https://doi.org/10.1177/0020731416631734.

[8] See, for example, Robson, G., Gibson, N., Thompson, A., et al. (2019). Global health ethics: critical reflections on the contours of an emerging field, 1977–2015. *BMC Medical Ethics* (2019) **20**:53. https://doi.org/10.1186/s12910-019-03 91-9; Lowry, C. & Schüklenk, U. (2009). Two models in global health ethics. *Public Health Ethics* 2(3), 276–284; Stapleton, G., Schröder-Bäck, P., Laaser, U., et al. (2014). Global health ethics: an introduction to prominent theories and relevant topics. *Global Health Action* 7(23569), 1– 7.

theoretical grounds for the approach, it does have an important advantage, namely that in many cases because human rights are objects of actual international agreements, there are some powerful mechanisms of potential enforcement available for protecting health in certain cases. Illustrating the approach with reference to case law, Wolff shows how and when the approach might prove especially effective.

While global health policy increasingly locates the imperative to advance the social determinants of health within a human rights framework, it is unclear what this actually means in law and practice. Lisa Forman explores the extent to which international human rights law addresses the social determinants of health within its protections of the right to health (Chapter 8). She considers the practical impact of such laws, given that many are skeptical of such an approach, concerned, for instance, that the right to health is vague, ineffective, or damaging to population health outcomes.[9]

The idea of who is responsible for doing what with respect to global health is a key issue and one touched on by most of the contributors to this volume. Allen Buchanan and Mathew DeCamp offer some useful guidelines in translating our shared obligation to "do something" to improve global health into a more determinate set of obligations (Chapter 9). They argue that states in particular have more extensive and specific responsibilities than is typically assumed to be the case because they are the current primary agents of distributive justice, influential actors in the burden of disease, and indeed have the greatest impact on the health of individuals in our world. But nonstate actors (such as the World Trade Organization [WTO] and global corporations) have important responsibilities as well, which are discussed. Furthermore, institutional innovation is needed to enable distribution of responsibilities more fairly and comprehensively and to ensure accountability. Some of the determinate obligations Buchanan and DeCamp identify for states include avoidance of committing injustice that has health-harming effects, for example, not fighting unjust wars abroad or assisting in training military personnel of states likely to use force unjustly. In supporting

unjust governments and upholding the state system, we contribute to upholding unjust regimes that have health-harming effects, not least through displacement and migration of people desperate to escape unlivable conditions. Simply refraining from such activities could do much to improve global health. As one example, they point out that between 2000 and 2006, 3.9 million people died in the Congo from war and that every violent death in that war zone was accompanied by no less than 62 "nonviolent" deaths in the region – from starvation, disease, and associated events.

Avram Ezra Denburg and Denis Daneman are concerned with global child health in Chapter 10. As they note, wide and remediable disparities persist in the health and well-being of children worldwide that warrant sustained ethical inquiry if we are to identify collective obligations to address them. This chapter is an effort to highlight some of the differentiating biological and normative dimensions of childhood to arrive at a more nuanced conception of how prevailing bioethical principles apply to children in a global context. Denburg and Daneman focus on three sentinel overlapping ideas that have fundamentally changed societal views on the status of children: the best interests of the child, children's autonomy, and the rights of the child. They then examine the role of current child rights law and scholarship in establishing and defending international responsibilities for the promotion and protection of child health globally. Finally, they consider a set of core principles for global health ethics – equity, freedom, and solidarity – and their specific application to child health, exploring potential synergies between global health ethics and child rights through the lens of early childhood development. Their analysis suggests that the moral language for addressing children's health and well-being globally remains underdeveloped – particularly in regard to collective responsibilities for policy and action.

Analyzing Some Reasons for Poor Health

In Chapter 11, Meri Koivusalo traces the many ways in which trade can and does affect health, and vice versa. It is clear that robust interests in trade can undermine health-related priorities and practice. For instance, trade liberalization policies in agricultural products can affect price, availability, and access to basic food commodities that result in less healthy diets

---

[9] Several other authors discuss the issue of human rights and health – the pitfalls and possibilities. Some are more skeptical about its current usefulness and draw attention to the fact that failure to meet human rights on a grand scale is predominantly the outcome of defects in global legal and economic structural arrangements (see Chapters 18 and 38).

for local populations and related issues of food security. Furthermore, trade liberalization has made available more hazardous substances such as tobacco and alcohol, leading to unhealthy consumption patterns. Poor, developing countries may be more vulnerable to adverse effects of trade liberalization than wealthier ones. We need improved global governance concerning health and trade that better acknowledges and tackles the wide-ranging effects of trade on health. The call for better global governance in a variety of domains is one that is made by many other authors.

Jeff Rudin and David Sanders explore the origins and factors that perpetuate the crippling debt that poor countries owe to the wealthy, focusing especially on structural adjustment programs (Chapter 12). They also explore the connection between debt and health and note that the magnitude of the debt owed by poor countries is frequently unpayable, especially in the case of Africa (the poorest continent) and not least because of the ongoing extraction of resources from such countries that intensifies their poverty and reduces their ability to repay debt.

The link between armed conflict, violence, international arms trading, and detrimental effects on global health is easy to appreciate. These adverse impacts include death, injury, and maiming from weapons use in conflict. There are massive opportunity costs to health, economic development, and human well-being when there is large-scale diversion of resources from health and human services to weapons expenditure. The impact of conflict can be far-reaching and includes important effects on children, such as psychological damage, loss of educational opportunities, destruction of families and nurturing environments, abuse, and the conscription of child soldiers. With trade in weapons growing fast and currently constituting one of the largest economies in the world, the effects on human health and well-being are worrisome.

Given these facts, it is no surprise that the World Health Assembly affirmed that "the role of physicians and other health professionals in the preservation and promotion of peace is the most significant factor for the attainment of health for all."[10] In their contribution to this volume (Chapter 13), Jonathan Kennedy, David McCoy, and Joseph Gafton analyze how the

international arms trade affects global health. They begin by analyzing recent trends in the prevalence and nature of armed conflict. They then move on to investigate the nature of the international arms industry and its patterns of military expenditure and trade in weapons, threats to health from weapons of mass destruction, and efforts to prevent war. They also discuss how artificial intelligence might influence the nature of armed conflict in the future and the implications of these developments for health. The indirect effects of war on health are often unappreciated, and protracted health crises are often a festering feature of war-torn countries.

Samia A. Hurst, Nathalie Mezger, and Alex Mauron discuss many of the complex issues involved when our duties to rescue bump up against significant resource shortages (Chapter 14). They describe the ethical challenges that face such organizations as Doctors Without Borders with humanitarian agendas that are driven by a rights-based view of international health. Both in the initial phases of many humanitarian disasters and in their aftermath, there are difficult issues concerning fair allocation. An increasing number of humanitarian situations are protracted rather than acute, and here it is particularly difficult to honor rights-based claims to healthcare. Hurst, Mezger, and Mauron illustrate how the challenges extend beyond meeting emergency needs to dealing with more protracted crises and the implications these have for "propping up repressive and irresponsible governments." They focus on how resources could be fairly allocated when it is not possible to meet all needs, and they offer a variant of the Daniels and Sabin account of procedural fairness as a plausible option.

The high media profile of humanitarian crises in recent years has attracted resources from wealthy countries. Whereas some of these resources are new, others represent shifts in allocations within only minimally increased official development aid (ODA) budgets. Indeed, there have been significant shifts away from projects that may contribute to structural developments with the potential to advance the economies of poor countries toward humanitarian emergencies and specific health problems – for example, HIV/AIDS. Whether or not such aid is effective has been a topic of great controversy in recent years. Overlapping and contesting views have been offered.[11] Although it is clear

---

[10] World Health Assembly, The Role of Physicians and Other Health Professionals in the Preservation and Promotion of Peace Is the Most Significant Factor for the Attainment of Health for All. Available at https://apps.who.int/iris/handle/10665/160590.

[11] See, for instance, William Easterly (2006), *The White Man's Burden: Why the West's Efforts to Aid the Rest Have Done So Much Ill and So Little Good* (New York: Penguin Press); Paul Collier (2007), *The Bottom Billion: Why the*

that some impressive short-term gains have been achieved in focused areas (such as HIV/AIDS), it is generally agreed that, for a variety of reasons, disappointingly little development of infrastructure or economies has resulted from ODA.

Anthony B. Zwi begins by describing the marked changes in patterns of health-related development assistance in recent years (Chapter 15). He provides an overview of both the value and the underpinning values that shape development assistance for health (DAH) in a chapter structured around four key elements: (1) motivations and influences on development assistance, (2) trends in development assistance for health, (3) debates and critiques of "aid" structures and approaches, and (4) ongoing challenges around more meaningful and equitable DAH. He also reviews some controversial aspects of ODA, such as trends in the magnitude of such aid, the intentions that lie behind it, possible shortcomings (in particular as ODA relates to global health), and some emerging issues that require attention. He does so by considering the "seven deadly sins" associated with ODA described by Nancy Birdsall. These constitute impatience with institution building, envy among competing donors, ignorance as evidenced by failure to evaluate impact, pride (failure to exit), sloth (using participation to justify ownership), greed (stingy transfers), and foolishness (underfunding of public goods). He focuses his discussion on how these sins impact on health and concludes with some recommendations for new approaches. Some new references update the metrics in this chapter.

Eduardo Gomez draws attention to an international consensus that has emerged in recent years that emphasizes the need for nations to combine the two previously separate areas of healthcare and foreign policy (Chapter 16). This has led to a movement toward global health diplomacy. Global health diplomacy certainly has an important role to play in sharing critical healthcare information and avoiding the spread of pandemic diseases. However, we should be mindful of important challenges related to inequality that this move presents; for instance, in the quest to

Poorest Countries Are Failing and What Can Be Done About It (New York: Oxford University Press); Jeffrey Sachs (2005), *The End of Poverty: Economic Possibilities for Our Time* (New York: Penguin Press); and Dambisa Moyo (2009), *Dead Aid: Why Aid Is Not Working and How There Is a Better Way for Africa* (New York: Farrar, Straus & Giroux), for some of this debate.

increase a nation's international influence, it might underinvest in domestic healthcare systems or focus on particular diseases of international concern to the detriment of local populations' other health needs. The recent withdrawal of US funding for the WHO illustrates the potential adverse impact of unilateral decision making on global health.

Solomon Benatar, Ross Upshur, and Stephen Gill draw attention to the fact that scientific and technological progress and diverse socioeconomic systems contributing to fostering great "accelerations" in the scale of production, consumption, communication, and transportation, particularly since 1945, have improved the duration and quality of life for many people (Chapter 17). Yet disparities in health have been sustained and even increased. They argue that lying at the heart of many of these upstream causes of poor health is the way in which the global economy operates without any ethical underpinnings. They note that while spectacular progress, both intellectual and material, has been achieved through the Enlightenment notion of the centrality of the individual and the supremacy of science and technology in advancing health and healthcare practices, such progress, achieved through transformations driven principally by the power structures, geopolitical arrangements, and patterns of social and economic organization of world capitalism, in which the profit motive and the drive to consume today (often frivolous) are without concern for the well-being of future generations, negates the human rights and dignity of many today at costs that will also be borne by future generations.

In the past 30 years, an extreme form of capitalist and hypermaterialistic thinking and practice (neoliberalism) has come to pervasively dominate the practices and principles of healthcare systems and almost all aspects of social life, including education and the governance of nature and the biosphere. Accelerating the transformation of aspects of each into salable commodities has distorted some of the cherished key Enlightenment principles. It is the ethical, material, political, health, and ecological nature and consequences of this perspective that they critically address in this chapter. Developing alternatives to enhance the health of people on a finite planet would need to begin by acknowledging how value distortions have shaped and governed how we currently live within a structurally violent global political economy, in which crises of ethics, economy, social development, health, and ecology have led to dehumanizing core/periphery disparities. Benatar, Upshur, and Gill suggest that use of our creative intellect and imagination could help a shift toward a global frame of mind capable of sociopolitical innovation to reconceptualize the idea and promotion of a more sustainable good society.

It is worth signaling here the as yet unknown but potentially serious and long-lasting implications of the COVID-19 pandemic for the airline, tourist, restaurant, and other business industries. In the short term, negative effects include loss of many jobs, and positive effects include radical reductions in pollution that are improving visibility and reducing deaths from pollution in many major cities and allowing some natural habitats to regenerate. The ideas for a more sustainable society are further developed by Stephen Gill, Isabella Bakker, and Dillon Wamsley, who remind us that it has been more than 10 years since the 2008 global financial crisis, and yet intensifying inequalities, global austerity, and ecological degradation continue to shape global health in profound ways (Chapter 18). Their chapter places these developments in the context of a wider *global organic crisis* – a fundamental crisis that has deep social, economic, and ecological dimensions in ways that are significantly reshaping communities, livelihoods, and the biosphere. To help clarify what is at issue, Gill, Bakker, and Wamsley outline several concepts to understand the current conjuncture of global capitalism and its various effects on health, illustrating these concepts by examining current crises in global food production and consumption and the social and political forces that challenge dominant models. Finally, they illustrate how fiscal pressures exerted on governments over the past several decades have undermined the provisioning of global health and contributed to the *enclosure of the social commons*, which threatens the livelihood and well-being of the majority of the world's population, some alternative solutions to which are highlighted in the final chapter (Chapter 38) by these same authors.

Ted Schrecker, Anne-Emaneulle Birn, and Mariajosé Aguilera make the case that extraction industries severely compromise global health justice in several ways (Chapter 19). Examining a range of resource-based economic activities organized around what Saskia Sassen calls "logics of extraction," they describe a *global extractive order* in which benefits and negative health implications are asymmetrically experienced.

They first identify five generic pathways from extraction to health outcomes and summarize the case for considering the extractive order's impact on health as a matter of global justice. They analyze arguments that extraction can be managed to benefit health through expansion of resources available for social provision and poverty reduction. They also examine land and water grabs, a relatively new form of cross-border resource appropriation with potentially far-reaching effects on health. Finally, they suggest some prerequisites and challenges for transforming the extractive order to meet the requirements of global justice.

Environmental Considerations

One core issue that this second edition aims to emphasize is that planetary health is integrally enmeshed with global health issues. Failure to acknowledge the importance of planetary health omits a key component of how we should address our health challenges and neglects its increasing significance to many of the salient issues. The relationship between human health and the physical, biological, and social environment raises important issues that extend far beyond clinical medicine to encompass interactions between human beings and nonhuman species, habitats, ecosystems, the atmosphere, oceans, and the biosphere. These issues often have local, national, and international components with implications for public health, global health, social justice, international justice, intergenerational justice, climate justice, and more.

In Chapter 20, David B. Resnik provides an overview of environmental health ethics and explores some of the issues that arise in this area of study, including pollution control, waste management, chemical regulation, agricultural practices, the built environment, and climate change.

Colin D. Butler continues the exploration of these themes in Chapter 21 on ecological ethics, planetary sustainability, and global health. He argues that adverse global environmental change is the stepchild of inequality, population size, resource consumption, limited human ingenuity, and cooperation failures. Civilization, and therefore population health, is in grave danger, though we seem to fail to appreciate this. Climate-damaging carbon emissions are still subsidized in many countries. Recognition by health workers that climate change and other aspects of "planetary overload" constitute an existential risk remains grossly inadequate, especially among researchers, funders, and policymakers. Encouragingly, younger generations are much better at sensing the danger and are advocating for solutions that could promote a wiser, fairer, and more sustainable civilization.

The Anthropocene epoch is characterized by changes in weather and climate that may make human life in some parts of the world difficult or impossible. This is expected to lead to massively increased migratory movements. In Chapter 22, Christine Straehle describes the challenges faced by migrants and the countries to which they migrate in increasing numbers because of climate change. She defines specific risks that climate-induced migrants face, and she explores relocation adaptation strategies taken by affected countries. She points out that from a health perspective, relocation may improve the social determinants of health but poses possible problems for individual autonomy and collective self-determination. She also addresses the call to identify climate-induced migrants as climate refugees and argues against their equivalence to those fleeing from abusive political regimes. She concludes that mass migration in the Anthropocene epoch demands new tools to protect individual basic needs and reveals the need for a dramatic change in the environmental policy and migration regimes of rich countries. Rich countries have the highest ecological footprint and therefore have remedial responsibilities to assist countries that have contributed least to climate change but suffer the greatest impact. Against this background, she regards current policies of nonentrée as moral failures. It should be noted too that the COVID-19 pandemic with its isolating preventive measures is having a profound immediate effect on migratory flows and the immediate health of migrants in transit, which further challenges humanitarian organizations.

David Benatar reminds us that concern with global health ethics is invariably limited to ethical issues that pertain to global *human* health rather than a more expansive notion of global health that includes other species (Chapter 23). He argues that this focus is unfortunate and that we do have duties (whether direct or indirect) concerning nonhuman animals and the environment. He draws attention to the ways in which human and animal interests coincide and also the ways in which environmental degradation from our mass breeding and consumption of animal products threatens human health. Whereas there is widespread awareness of how destruction of the environment can affect human well-being and health (through processes such as global warming, ozone depletion, and desertification), there is much less awareness of how connected animal and human interests are and of the extent of cruelty to sentient creatures in the meat and dairy industries. Many infectious viral diseases have animal origins, including some of the most recent high-profile ones, such as SARS, HIV, "swine influenza," and COVID-19. Although some animal-to-human transmission of diseases is probably inevitable, much could be avoided through better treatment of animals, especially keeping them in less crowded, more sanitary conditions. Of course, if humans did not eat them in the first place, fewer animals would be bred for human consumption, and the risks would reduce. Significant advantages could be accrued through an increasing shift away from eating meat to vegetarian diets, because about 20% of the warming the planet has experienced can be attributed to the methane produced by cows.

Henk ten Have draws attention to some of these planetary considerations with a key emphasis on environmental degradation (Chapter 24). Social media have made possible much inspirational global activism and social movements focused on health justice, environmental justice, food justice, and water justice, to name only a few. There is an important role for sociological and moral imagination in driving movements to overcoming injustice. Imagining is a creative way of knowing, as well as seeing things differently. It provides resistance against dehumanizing tendencies and can help to overcome experiences of disrespect and humiliation.

The Importance of Including Cross-Cultural Perspectives and the Need for Dialogue

As signaled, developing helpful models of how we talk about global health issues across lines of difference is a key need that deserves far more attention. This section includes some attempts to do just that.

Jing-Bao Nie and Ruth P. Fitzgerald point out that prominent bioethical debates, on such issues as the notion of common morality and a distinctive "Asian" bioethics in contrast to a "Western" one, reveal some deeply rooted and still popular but seriously problematic methodological habits in approaching cultural differences, most notably dealing with radically dichotomized East/West and local/universal conceptions. In Chapter 25, a "transcultural" approach to bioethics and cultural studies is proposed. It takes seriously the challenges offered by social sciences, particularly in anthropology, toward the development of new methodologies for comparative and global bioethics. The key methodological complexities of addressing "ethical transculturalism" include acknowledging the great internal plurality within every culture, highlighting the complexity of cultural differences, upholding the primacy of morality, and incorporating a reflexive theory of social power.

Godfrey B. Tangwa reflects on the virtual absence of an African voice and perspective in global discourses of medical research ethics, especially considering the high burden of diseases and epidemics on the African continent and the fact that the continent is actually the scene of numerous medical research studies (Chapter 26). He considers some reasons for this state of affairs, as well as how the situation might be redressed. Using examples from the HIV/AIDS and Ebola epidemics, he argues that the marginalization of Africa in medical research and medical research ethics can be traced to a Eurocentric hegemony derived from colonialism and colonial indoctrination. As we consider how to improve our attempts to improve cross-cultural dialogue and action in medical research ethics, Tangwa suggests that we critically reflect on some key ideas.

In Chapter 27, Solomon Benatar, Ibrahim Daibes, and Sandra Tomsons note that with the growth in multijurisdictional and multicultural global health partnerships, the adequacy of the prevailing bioethical paradigm guiding the conduct of global health research and practices is being increasingly challenged. In response to the challenges and conflicts that decision makers in global health research and practice face, Benatar, Daibes, and Tomsons propose an innovative methodology that could be developed to bridge the gap between polarized systems of ideas and values concerning metaphysical, moral, and political issues. Their interphilosophies methodology provides the potential to construct a new, shared paradigm for global health ethics, thereby increasing the capacity for solidarity and shared decision making in global health research and practice. This approach calls for

greater humility and willingness to learn from others, for example, that our dominant ontological and epistemological perspectives encourage detachment from nature through a fundamental misunderstanding of the human/nature relationship and that our individualistic moral values and competitive political values reduce the potential for achieving intra- and intergenerational solidarity. The dialogical approach encourages the avoidance of adversarial attitudes toward polarized extremes of different worldviews and seeks their overlapping common ground identifiable at the convergence of their respective metaphysical, epistemological, and axiological spectra. Achieving this requires a measure of epistemological humility and respect for the dignity of others.

Mark D. Hathaway, Blake Poland, and Angela Mashford-Pringle explore the ethical challenge posed by ecocide – the destruction of Earth's life-sustaining systems – employing a variety of lenses that go beyond the traditional purview of Western ethics (Chapter 28). Using ecopsychology, the relationship between separative consciousness and exploitation is considered. The chapter proposes that addressing the ecological crisis will entail not only technological, political, and economic changes but also moving away from a worldview rooted in separative consciousness, instrumental thinking, hierarchy, exploitation, and a focus on competition. This transformation can also be understood in terms of changing our collective story toward a narrative that emphasizes interconnection, cooperation, meaning, community, and the flourishing of life. Drawing on insights from Indigenous traditions (sumak kaysay/buen vivir and the good life/mino-bimaadiziwin) as well as global South perspectives (Bhutan's gross domestic happiness and the Earth Charter), the nature of living well as a basis for health ethics is explored. Finally, key facets of pathways toward integral health are examined, including decolonization and reindigenization, reconnection and reinhabitation with the land, drawing on insights from animistic and ecophenomenological perspectives, and movements for regenerative sustainability such as the permaculture and transition movements.

Shaping the Future

Tikki Pang and Gianna Gayle Herrera Amul note that global health research remains critical in the development and implementation of inclusive, equitable, and sustainable policies and interventions (Chapter 29). Given the developments in global health research, particularly in monitoring, financing, partnerships, and setting guidelines, several challenges remain to be addressed not only by the global health research community but also by research funders, governments, and the private sector. There is a need to prioritize the ethical dimensions of global health research, particularly in addressing the "parachutes and parasites" in global health research, cross-cultural communication issues, capacity building, predatory publishing, accessibility and benefit sharing, the role of corporations, and waste in global health research. With this in mind, the new global health research agenda needs to push for research influencing policy and advocacy, making the case for greater returns on investments for health research, promoting local and national health research systems, and innovating toward research methodologies for effective policy implementation.

An issue that troubles many in developed countries concerned with global health ethics is the way in which clinical research is being increasingly "outsourced" to poor countries with vulnerable populations. Does the severe deprivation in these countries render such activities exploitative? Or, alternatively, by providing some benefits (albeit sometimes small ones) to these people, are we assisting them? Under what conditions is research in developing countries morally defensible? Alex John London addresses these questions in Chapter 30. By outlining his "human development approach" to international research, he argues for a position in which basic social institutions can be expected to advance the interests of all community members. Moreover, on this approach, there are obligations to ensure that the results of the research are translatable into sustainable benefits for its population. This entails obligations either to build alliances with those able to translate the research into sustainable benefits or to "locate the research within a community with similar health priorities and more appropriate health infrastructure." Instructive examples of research that passes and fails the test are discussed.

As Thomas Pogge notes in Chapter 31, about a third of annual human deaths are traceable to poverty, and these are easily preventable through such measures as safe drinking water, vaccines, antibiotics, better nutrition, and cheap rehydration packs. Is there an obligation to alleviate world poverty and to prevent such deaths? Pogge argues that whatever the merits of the case that we should help more, there is much more clearly an obligation to harm less. How do we currently harm the poor? In multiple ways, he argues. One can challenge the legitimacy of our currently highly uneven global distributive patterns concerning income and wealth, which have emerged from a single historical process pervaded by injustices (such as slavery and colonialism). One might also criticize the dense web of institutional arrangements that we have created, and now fail to reform, that foreseeably and avoidably perpetuate poverty. Pogge argues that the way in which we fail to reform these various institutional arrangements, which foreseeably and avoidably perpetuate massive global poverty, is morally culpable. There are many institutional arrangements that ought to be reformed on these grounds. The long list would include upholding grossly unjust intellectual property regimes that require all members of the WTO to grant 20-year product patents that effectively make new medicines unaffordable for most of the world's population. Pogge argues that small changes to the rules incentivizing pharmaceutical research and development would produce large health gains in poor and affluent countries – gains that, over time, would easily cover the economic cost of the scheme. With this example, he shows how the present rules governing the world economy, designed and imposed to serve powerful corporate and political interests, could be adjusted in minor but highly effective ways to better serve the interests of all.

Nicole Hassoun emphasizes that understanding the impact of key technologies on the global burden of disease is essential to policymakers' ability to extend access to important medicines to achieve UN Sustainable Development Goal 3 and fulfill everyone's human right to health (Chapter 32). Hassoun discusses a comprehensive new model of the global health impact of medicines on morbidity and mortality. Measuring impact is important for evaluating performance, setting targets, guiding the distribution of scarce health resources, and advancing access to affordable medicines. The global health impact model currently evaluates the global impact of medicines for HIV/AIDS, malaria, tuberculosis, and neglected tropical diseases (NTDs) and aggregates this information by company, drug, and disease as well as country. It estimates disease impact in the absence of treatment using data on drug effectiveness (or, barring that, efficacy), disease incidence, patient treatment coverage, and the global burden of disease that remains after treatment. Making the new model and data on medicines' global health impact available to researchers, policymakers, consumers, companies, and other key stakeholders increases their ability to promote global health. It can help states, nongovernmental organizations, and companies promote new market strategies as well as innovative health policies that aim to provide worldwide equal access to medicine.

James Wilson examines the ethics of philanthro-capitalism, especially concerning its operation in the domain of global health (Chapter 33). Philanthrocapitalism involves individuals who have become massively wealthy in capitalist systems applying the very same skills and techniques they used to create their wealth to the project of giving their fortunes away. Philanthrocapitalism has become a vital topic in global health above all because of the Bill & Melinda Gates Foundation (BMGF), which through the sheer scale of its grant giving holds more influence over the direction of global health policy than any actor other than the United States. Philanthropy on the scale of the BMGF is possible only in circumstances of extreme wealth inequality, so any celebration of the good done by the BMGF needs to be tempered by a sober assessment of the justice of a system that allows such extreme wealth accumulation. The chapter examines whether giving by the super-wealthy should be thought of as a duty or a matter of discretion and the extent to which givers assume it to be their prerogative to choose causes that maximize the good done. It concludes with an ethical analysis of the effects of the BMGF on global health, examining both the BMGF's effects on global health governance and its gradual broadening of focus from technocratic isolationism toward international consensus building and an increasing focus on women's empowerment.

Effy Vayena and Agata Ferretti argue that big data and artificial intelligence (AI) enabling tools are set to transform the healthcare landscape not only in high-income countries but also in low- and middle-income countries (Chapter 34). New digital technologies bring the potential to extend access to healthcare and improve public health surveillance and global health. However, the digital revolution also raises several ethical challenges, such as privacy, bias in AI-based application, harm mitigation, fair benefit

distribution, and accountability. If these challenges are not addressed adequately, they can undermine the goal of bringing healthcare benefits to those most in need. To date, the scholarly literature has paid limited attention to the implications of these issues for global health. Although a number of global initiatives aim to determine the ethical principles that should guide the further development of digital technologies and especially AI, there is no parallel activity in the specific domain of digital health. It is important that many stakeholders participate in conversations concerning digital health. As Vayena and Ferretti argue, stakeholders should agree to an ethical framework that enables the kind of digital technologies that will promote global health and serve the health needs of all.

Erica Di Ruggiero reviews rising global challenges to the health of populations and to the planet and calls for innovative strategies and "solutions" that aspire to contribute to developing sustainability globally (Chapter 35). In addition, health has become highly vulnerable in a global policy context dominated by growing interests in national security and economic competitiveness. It should perhaps come as no surprise that health is by far the most extensively discussed topic of governance globally, with a wide array of institutions seeking to contribute to its development or attainment. Governance is realized when a collective of individuals or institutional arrangements come together to accomplish an agreed end, which can and should involve the participation of state and nonstate actors. In this chapter, Di Ruggiero examines some of the conceptual and analytical issues related to global health and its governance. She reflects on the global policy context with particular attention to the UN Millennium Development Goals and Sustainable Development Goals and the implications for governance. She explores several issues, such as power, competing priorities, and actor dynamics and partnerships, and makes several suggestions for further scholarly inquiry and action.

James Dwyer engagingly reflects on his experiences teaching global health ethics (Chapter 36). He reviews some of the content of his syllabus, the students' reactions to it, and his own reflections on those experiences. In a particularly useful section, he explores a notion of responsiveness to global health injustices and offers guidelines for assisting students in thinking about morally appropriate responses to problems of global health. He formulates eight questions for students to consider when reflecting on whether to work abroad in low-income countries because often that engagement is of questionable value for destination countries.

Sarah Elton and Donald C. Cole also offer helpful advice to educators, given the many ethical issues involved with teaching global health in the Anthropocene (Chapter 37). They describe three theoretical perspectives that inform their teaching: post-humanism, political ecology, and ecological determinants of health. They share examples of applying these frameworks in course design and ethical explorations around topics as diverse as the meat production and consumption industries, resource extraction and artisanal mining, and the Sustainable Development Goals. Advice is offered concerning mainstreaming ecological perspectives in global health ethics training and pushing educational institutions to better embrace ecological perspectives in dialogue, teaching, and actions.

In the final chapter in this volume (Chapter 38), Isabella Bakker, Stephen Gill, and Dillon Wamsley offer a vision of a new "common sense" given all the many health challenges we have been discussing in this volume. They offer a set of alternative modes of thinking and forms of political praxis associated with ecological sustainability, democratic governance, social provisioning, and the care economy, as well as issues of global health inequity. New financing and enhanced public provisions to restore and extend the social commons, plus more sustainable, socially just, and equitable redistributive policies, should help better socialize the risks of a global majority. This requires confronting and reforming the complexities of local and global taxation. Bakker, Gill, and Wamsley also outline the need for a new epistemological framework, one that is capable of engaging with ongoing social struggles and new modes of thinking. It should generate a new common sense concerning people and the planet that could help promote political action to reverse deepening crises and offer real and sustainable alternative visions of society and the biosphere.

To improve people's health globally and pursue the goals described in this book will require a considerable amount of collaborative transdisciplinary research and pervasive community engagement at many levels. It is arguable that this challenge for social innovation is as great as, if not greater than, the scientific and technological innovation for developing an HIV vaccine. If equivalent research resources and intellectual attention were to be allocated to cross-disciplinary, socially innovative research, significant progress is entirely possible. Though we have significant intellectual and material resources to improve global health, there is little reason to expect that major new initiatives such as those envisioned in this volume will be implemented without a great deal of effort in mobilizing the political will to do so. We continue to be cautiously optimistic that well-constructed arguments can, on occasion and in the right circumstances, play a significant role in influencing the future. It is therefore particularly gratifying to see that on learning how destruction of the planet is likely to affect them, younger generations are signaling their growing impatience with older generations' continued apathy. Their sense of urgency is putting pressure on policymakers to take immediate action. And, in time, they will become the policymakers and, it is hoped, be in positions to enact the progressive changes we need. Perhaps they will draw inspiration from some of our courageous global leaders, such as Nelson Mandela, who famously said: "It always seems impossible until it's done."[12]

---

[12] Inaugural address, 1994.

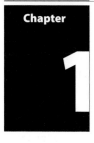

State of Global Health in a Radically Unequal World

Patterns and Prospects

Ted Schrecker and Ronald Labonté

Introduction: "If Living Were a Thing That Money Could Buy"

Imagine for a moment a series of disasters that kills more than 800 women every day for a year: the equivalent of two or three daily crashes of crowded long-distance airliners or the equivalent of the direct death toll from the attack on the World Trade Center and the Pentagon every four days. There is little question that such a situation would quickly be regarded as a humanitarian emergency, as the stuff of headlines, especially if ways of preventing the events were well known and widely practiced (as is the case with avoiding crashes in civil aviation). However, remarkably little attention is paid outside the global health and human rights domains to complications of pregnancy and childbirth that kill more than 300,000 women every year – a cause of death now almost unheard of in high-income countries (HICs), although this would not have been the case a century ago. A Canadian woman's lifetime risk of dying from complications of pregnancy or childbirth is 1 in 8,800 for a woman in Sub-Saharan Africa, the world's poorest region, it is 1 in 37 (World Health Organization et al., 2019).

This is one example among many of the health contrasts between rich and poor worlds. Average life expectancy at birth (LEB) worldwide has been estimated at 28.5 years in 1800, much of the short average lifespan caused by high rates of death in the early years of life. By the end of the twentieth century, worldwide average LEB had increased to roughly 67 years (Riley, 2005), due in large measure to reductions in infant and child mortality. However, global progress conceals large variations between countries. For example, Canadians born today can expect to live to the age of 82, a figure that is among the world's highest. In the world's least-developed countries, as classified by the United Nations, where nearly a billion of the world's

people live, estimated LEB averages 64 years (World Bank, 2017).[1]

Differences in the prevalence of specific diseases are even more dramatic. Although the acquired immune deficiency syndrome (AIDS) was first identified in HICs, more than 95% of new HIV infections now occur outside those countries, with the highest prevalence rates in Sub-Saharan Africa, accounting for more than two-thirds of the world's infected population and an estimated 660,000 of the estimated 940,000 annual deaths from AIDS (UNAIDS, 2018a). Importantly, the number of AIDS-related deaths has declined sharply from a high of approximately 2 million in 2005 because of the rapid increase in access to antiretroviral therapy (discussed later in this chapter), but a slow decline in the number of new infections means that the number of people living with human immunodeficiency virus (HIV) worldwide continues to rise. Malaria and tuberculosis have been almost entirely vanquished in HICs. Elsewhere in the world, malaria kills an estimated 435,000 people per year and tuberculosis 1.6 million (World Health Organization [WHO], 2018, 2019), despite the demonstrated effectiveness of relatively low-cost solutions.[2] Health disparities between rich and poor countries involve not only differences in the kinds of illnesses that affect their populations but also the ages at which illness and death occur. Of the estimated 5.4 million deaths of children age five years or under that occurred worldwide in 2017, just 60,000 occurred in HICs, but 2.75 million occurred in Sub-Saharan Africa (GBD 2017 Mortality Collaborators,

---

[1] World Bank, https://data.worldbank.org/indicator/SP
.DYN.LE00.IN?view=chart (accessed April 4, 2019).
[2] An exception involves increasingly prevalent drug-resistant strains of tuberculosis worldwide. However, the spread of those strains is itself largely attributable to a history of inadequate provision of the resources necessary to vaccinate against tuberculosis and treat it using first-line drugs in low-income countries (Coker, 2004).

2018). And although the worldwide risk of child death declined steadily through the last decades of the twentieth century, far more substantial gains could have been achieved because it has long been recognized that most child deaths outside the high-income world result from causes that are either extremely uncommon in those countries or rarely result in death there (Hug, Sharrow, & You, 2017)

Deprivation and Economic Gradients

The intuitive and largely accurate explanation for many of these differences involves poverty and material deprivation. An estimated 897 million people worldwide in 2012 were living on US$1.90 a day or less[3] on the World Bank's contentious definition of extreme poverty (World Bank & International Monetary Fund [IMF], 2016: 29–35). More than 800 million people worldwide were undernourished in 2016, reversing a long-standing if gradual decline according to the United Nations Food and Agriculture Organization (FAO et al., 2017). These are risibly inadequate indicators of the prevalence of material deprivation with consequences for health. "In Zambia, for example, a person on the poverty line can afford a daily diet of two–three plates of *nshima* (a maize staple known as mealie meal), a sweet potato, a few spoonfuls of oil, a couple of teaspoons of sugar, a handful of peanuts and twice a week, a banana or mango and a small serving of meat. Such a person would have just 28% of his budget left over for other things," including of course such basics as housing (*The Economist*, 2016). The FAO undernourishment figures capture only continuous insufficiency of caloric intake over a period of at least a year. Thus, on more realistic indicators, material deprivation is far more widespread than the World Bank and other international agencies acknowledge in their optimistic self-reports (Hickel, 2016; Reddy & Lahoti, 2016).

Economic deprivation creates situations in which the daily routines of living are themselves hazardous. Charcoal, crop residue, and dung smoke from cooking fires are major contributors to respiratory disease among the world's poor, mainly in rural areas (Perez-Padilla, Schilmann, & Riojas-Rodriguez, 2010). In the fast-growing cities of the developing world, almost 900 million people were estimated to live in slums, as defined by UN Habitat, in 2014 – a number that

was projected to rise to 2 billion by 2030, with associated exposure to multiple hazardous living and working conditions (Ezeh et al., 2017). Lack of access to clean water, for example, is a major contributor to infectious diarrhea and a variety of parasitic diseases (Prüss-Ustün et al., 2014), yet an estimated 660 million people lack access to clean water, and 2.4 billion people have no access to basic sanitation (UNICEF & World Health Organization [WHO], 2015); it is, of course, primarily the poorest people and regions in the countries in question that continue to lack access (WHO & UNICEF, 2017). A further dimension of the role of material deprivation involves the lack of resources to access healthcare. At the individual level, the need to pay for healthcare and the loss of livelihoods associated with illness push an estimated 150 million people into poverty every year (WHO, 2010) – a problem that historically was often worsened by health sector "reforms" actively promoted by HICs through such agencies as the World Bank (Lister & Labonté, 2009; Stubbs et al., 2017; Yates, 2009).[4]

In many respects, then, the words of the folk song "All My Trials" (made famous by Joan Baez) ring true: living is a thing that money can buy; the rich do live, and the poor do die, much earlier and from different causes. In addition to differences among countries, socioeconomic gradients in health status – inverse correlations between health status and various indicators of socioeconomic status – are almost universal within national and subnational boundaries, in countries rich and poor alike. Figure 1.1 shows such gradients in mortality among children under age five (U5MR): children in the poorest fifth of the population in six largely dissimilar low- and middle-income countries (LMICs) are at least twice as likely to die before their fifth birthday, and sometimes three times as likely, as children in the richest fifth. In India alone, a WHO commission estimated in 2008 that 1.4 million child deaths would be prevented each year if the U5MR for the entire Indian population were reduced to the level characteristic of its richest quintile (Commission on Social Determinants of Health, 2008: 29).

---

[4] We recognize the importance of poor governance (including corruption) in many LMICs, but these dynamics cannot be isolated from the actions of the rich world, notably in supporting corrupt but convenient regimes and offering a hospitable environment for flight capital and tax avoidance (see e.g. Baker, Cardamone et al., 2015; Organisation for Economic Co-operation and Development, 2014; Valencia, 2013, among many other sources).

---

[3] In 2011 US dollars, converted using a purchasing power parity (PPP) calculation that is itself dubious in terms of its relation to the actual needs of poor people.

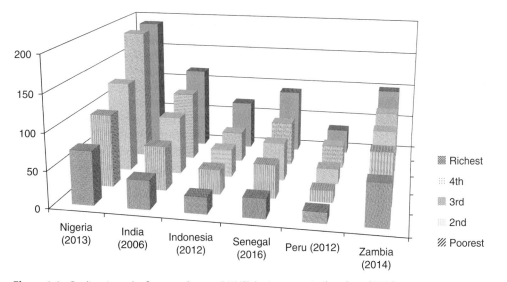

Figure 1.1. Gradient in under-five mortality rate (U5MR), by income quintile, selected LMICs

Source: Data from World Bank Health Nutrition and Population Statistics, http://databank.worldbank.org/data/reports.aspx?source=health-nutrition-and-population-statistics-by-wealth-quintile.

Socioeconomic gradients reflect not only daily conditions of life and work but also economic influences on access to health services. For example, socioeconomic gradients are pronounced in access to key health system interventions such as antenatal care and attendance by skilled health personnel at birth that improve maternal, newborn, and child health (WHO, 2015b). Importantly, "world scale" socioeconomic gradients in health are widespread in HICs as well. The Eight Americas Study in the USA, where racial and economic inequalities tend to be superimposed on one another, found that the life expectancy of African Americans in "high risk" urban counties was almost nine years shorter than that of the mostly white residents of Middle America (Murray et al., 2006). In the words of the authors, "tens of millions of Americans are experiencing levels of health that are more typical of middle-income or low-income developing countries" (Murray et al., 2006: 9). A decade later, Shaefer, Wu, & Edin (2017) pointed out that African-American men with limited education had a life expectancy at birth in 2008 comparable with the national averages for Pakistan, Bhutan, and Mongolia; the infant mortality rate among African Americans in 2011 was higher than the national averages for Tonga and Grenada; and high-poverty US cities had a homicide rate that made them almost as dangerous as Colombia and Brazil. And *circa* 2015, the difference in male LEB between the most and least economically deprived wards of the small English postindustrial city of Stockton-on-Tees, where one of us (TS) lived and worked until recently, was larger than the difference in national average male life expectancy between the United Kingdom and Tanzania (Schrecker, 2018).

Growth (and Wealth) Are Not Enough

Discussions of global health ethics must avoid the simplistic leap from this set of observations to the conclusion that greater wealth through economic growth is the surest route to better health – and, therefore, that improvements in population health are best achieved by policies that promote economic growth. Superficial support for the growth → wealth → health causal pathway comes from a widely cited graph known as the *Preston curve*, after the demographer who first drew it. Figure 1.2 shows the Preston curves for the years 2015 and 1960. The graph represents most of the world's countries with a circle, the area of which is proportional to the size of the country's population. The vertical axis shows average life expectancy at birth, and the horizontal axis shows the country's gross domestic product (GDP) per capita, adjusted for purchasing power. The dotted trend lines on the graph show the national average life expectancy that would be anticipated at a given level of GDP per capita based on a population-weighted average of all

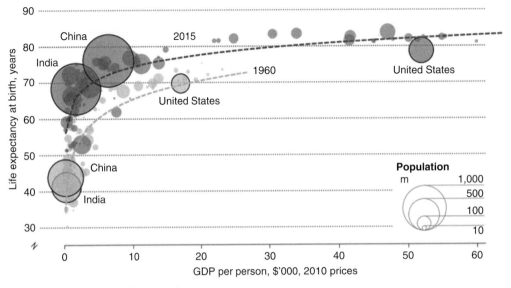

Figure 1.2. Preston curves for 1960 and 2015

Source: J. McDermott, An affordable necessity: Special report on universal health care, *The Economist*, April 28, 2018. Copyright © *The Economist*, London, 2018.

the national data. The graph shows strong returns to economic growth in terms of LEB at low per capita incomes, up to about US$7.40 per day, which is seen by many as the minimum level at which one could not be considered materially very poor (Labonté & Ruckert, 2019: 149–150). Above that point, a weaker but still positive relation between LEB and per capita income is evident.[5]

Wide variations exist in LEB among countries with comparable GDP per capita figures, which are not fully evident in this version of the graph. For example, in 2016, LEB in the USA, with a GDP per capita of $59,531, was 79 years, but it was 80 years in Chile and Costa Rica, countries with GDP per capita levels of $24,635 and $17,073, respectively (in 2017, again after adjustment for purchasing power). Conversely, some countries do far less well in terms of LEB than one might expect given their income levels. The United States in fact is one of these underperformers, quite probably because of a continuing failure to provide access to healthcare to millions of its people (Barnett & Berchick, 2017) and an emerging epidemic of "deaths of despair" among

a subpopulation trapped by stagnating economic prospects (Case & Deaton, 2017). Indeed, one of Preston's original conclusions was that "[f]actors exogenous to a country's level of income probably account for 75%–90% of the growth in life expectancy for the world as a whole between the 1930s and the 1960s. Income growth per se accounts for only 10%–25%" (Preston, 2007: 486; original publication 1975). In the recent past, the most conspicuous outliers in this respect were countries in Sub-Saharan Africa, where life expectancy was drastically reduced by the AIDS epidemic (see Figure 1.3 and a version of the Preston curve for the year 2000 in Deaton [2003: 116]).

Two sets of factors are relevant to explaining such variations. The first set comprises advances in medical treatment and preventive health measures such as antibiotics, immunization, and antiretroviral therapy for HIV/AIDS. The upward movement of the dotted trend line in the Preston curve over time can be thought of as the treatment and prevention dividend, examples of which are cited in this chapter's concluding section. The second set of factors involves the extent to which countries use their available resources in ways that result in widely shared improvements in health status for their populations – including access to advances in treatment and prevention. The underperformance of the United States has already been noted. Conversely, Sri Lanka, Costa Rica, and the

---

[5] The same is not necessarily true for more nuanced indicators of health status, such as chronic disease prevalence or limited functioning as a result of disability (to give but two examples); mortality-based indicators are intrinsically crude.

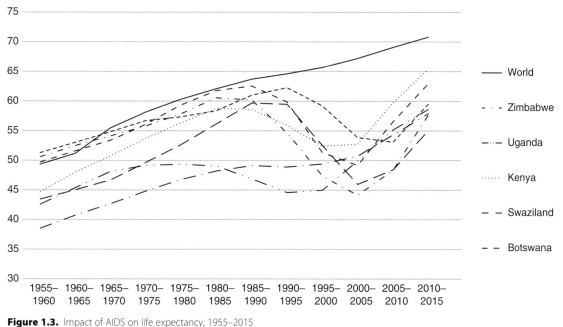

Figure 1.3. Impact of AIDS on life expectancy, 1955–2015
Source: Data from United Nations Department of Economic and Social Affairs, *World Population Prospects: The 2017 Revision*, DVD edition.

Indian state of Kerala are often cited as overperformers in population health status despite low GDP per capita, attributed to their attention to accessible primary healthcare and other social protection measures – what Riley (2008) refers to as "social growth" (see also Balabanova et al., 2013).

Based on such examples, Angus Deaton (2006: 3), who was later to win a Nobel Prize in economics, concluded: "Economic growth is much to be desired because it relieves the grinding material poverty of much of the world's population. But economic growth, by itself, will not be enough to improve population health, at least in any acceptable time. . ... As far as health is concerned, the market, by itself, is not a substitute for collective action." This collective action pertains not only to the second set of factors (how countries allocate resource priorities and distribution) but also to the first set of factors (publicly financed or supported innovations in health knowledge, technology, and global diffusion). Deaton points out that most health innovations that contributed to the global convergence in health in the last half of the last century, which has now been replaced by divergence (Moser, Shkolnikov, & Leon, 2007), originated in wealthier countries. "In this sense, the first world has been responsible for producing the global public goods of medical and health-related

research and development from which everyone has benefited, in poor and now-rich countries alike" (Deaton, 2004: 99). In the last 20 years, however, companies in HICs have led a push for worldwide expansion of intellectual property protection, notably in knowledge-based industries such as information technology and pharmaceuticals. This has led to the emergence of one of the most contentious issues in contemporary global health: that of access to essential medicines and other health technologies (Muzaka, 2014). There is also the vexing, more basic question of whether such a profit-driven regime of innovation priorities can effectively support research into diseases that afflict mainly people who are too poor to represent a commercially attractive market (Pedrique et al., 2013).

How Health Risks Are Distributed

A further complication of the relation between economic growth and health involves how growth influences the nature and distribution of risks to health. It was once argued that countries experienced a relatively standardized *epidemiological transition* as they grew richer, in which infectious or communicable diseases (disproportionately affecting children) declined while chronic diseases (disproportionately affecting adults) increased (Omran, 1971). Although still useful, the concept only partially captures a pattern in which LMICs are increasingly affected by a "double burden of disease," as persistent or resurgent communicable diseases coexist with rapid increases in noncommunicable diseases such as cardiovascular disease, diabetes, and cancer (see Agyei-Mensah & de-Graft Aikins, [2010] for an important case study). Figure 1.4 shows that the age-adjusted death rates from such noncommunicable diseases as cardiovascular diseases and cancer in LMICs in some regions are actually higher than in the high-income world, although their *proportional* contribution to mortality in some regions is lower because of the toll taken by other causes of death.

It was estimated at the start of this century that 100 million men in China alone would die from smoking-related diseases between 2000 and 2050 (Zhang & Cai, 2003). Additionally, road traffic accidents kill an estimated 1.2 million people a year, disproportionately in LMICs (WHO, 2015a). Ironically, those most likely to be injured are the poor, who are least likely to own a vehicle – a distribution of risks that is sometimes exacerbated by planning practices that favour high-speed roads for the emerging middle classes. In many cases, additional hazards are associated with exposures to industrial or motor vehicle pollution and dangers in the industrial or agricultural workplace. In a standard text on global health, Birn, Pillay, & Holtz (2017: 231–284) have suggested that it may be useful to replace the familiar categories of communicable and noncommunicable diseases with a threefold typology: diseases of marginalization and deprivation, such as diarrhea, neglected tropical diseases, malaria, and respiratory infections; diseases of modernization and work, such as cardiovascular disease, cancer, and road traffic injuries; and diseases of marginalization and modernization, such as diabetes, chronic obstructive pulmonary disease (COPD), tuberculosis, and HIV/ AIDS. Socioeconomic gradients are observable with respect to all three categories of disease, including those widely if mistakenly regarded as "diseases of affluence" (Ezzati et al., 2005).

The significance of the double burden of disease concept is illustrated by the coexistence of undernutrition with rapid growth of overweight and obesity in LMICs – indeed, in some instances, of undernutrition and overweight in the same household (Black et al., 2013). Reflecting a *nutrition transition* involving a rapid shift to diets higher in ultraprocessed foods

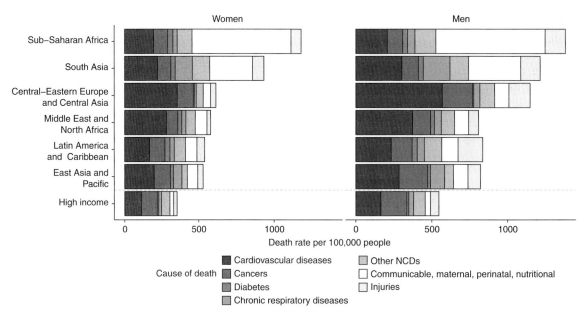

Figure 1.4. Age-adjusted death rates from various causes, 2010

Source: Data from R. Lozano et al., Global and regional mortality from 235 causes of death for 20 age groups in 1990 and 2010: a systematic analysis for the Global Burden of Disease Study 2010. *Lancet* **380** (2012), 2095–2128. Death rates are for all ages and were standardized with the WHO standard population: O. Ahmad et al., Age standardization of rates: a new WHO standard (GPE Discussion Paper Series No. 31). Geneva: WHO, 2001. Reprinted from M. Di Cesare et al., Inequalities in non-communicable diseases and effective responses. *Lancet*, **381** (2013), 585–597. Copyright © 2013, with permission from Elsevier.

(Monteiro et al., 2013) coupled with reductions in physical activity, overweight and obesity in several middle-income countries are approaching the levels seen in countries such as the USA. An especially striking study involves a sample of women in regions that account for more than 70% of Brazil's population. In 1975, almost twice as many Brazilian women were underweight as were obese; by 1997, the proportions had reversed, with the increases in obesity concentrated among low-income women (Monteiro, Conde, & Popkin, 2004; see also Mendez, Monteiro, & Popkin, 2005). The emergence of this socioeconomic gradient is a broader trend once a certain income threshold is passed (Malik, Willett, & Hu, 2013), and the connection with aggressive marketing of ultraprocessed foods appears to be worldwide (Baraldi et al., 2018; Louzada et al., 2018; Martínez Steele et al., 2017; Monteiro et al., 2018; Moodie et al., 2013). Further, the prevalence of overweight and obesity in many cases is increasing far more rapidly than it did in the HICs decades earlier (Popkin, 2006), setting the stage for increases in cardiovascular disease and diabetes that will widen existing health disparities and challenge the ability of health systems to respond.

Globalization, Markets, and Health in an Unequal World

Globalization, defined here as "[a] pattern of transnational economic integration animated by the ideal of creating self-regulating global markets for goods, services, capital, technology, and skills" (Eyoh & Sandbrook, 2003: 252), presents broader challenges as well. Perhaps most fundamentally, as the editor of *Le Monde Diplomatique* has put it, globalization is an "inequality machine [that] is reshaping the planet" (Halimi, 2013), as bidding wars of all kinds become transnational in scope. As just two examples, production is now organized in commodity chains that routinely cross multiple national borders, with the hunt for lower-cost labor – facilitated by a legal infrastructure of trade and investment agreements and dramatic reductions in the cost of transport and communication – being a major driver of that organizational pattern. Conversely, "the prime resources of the city are increasingly appropriated by the affluent. And globalization is inflationary as the new rich are able to pay more for a range of key goods, especially land" (United Nations Human Settlements Programme, 2003: 52) – hence such paradoxes as

Luanda, the capital city of oil-rich Angola, where poverty is endemic, appearing in some league tables as the most expensive city in the world (Ngugi, 2017). One can find graphic illustrations of many such metropolitan juxtapositions of wealth and poverty in Johnny Miller's remarkable aerial photographs (www.unequalscenes.com).

The academic literature suggests that while inequality among countries may be decreasing, notably because of rapid growth in some emerging economies, within-country economic inequality is increasing, sometimes rapidly, as is the worldwide concentration of wealth at the pinnacle of the global distribution (Milanovic, 2016; Zucman, 2019). In a synthesis of evidence drawing mainly on the *Forbes* billionaires list and on research for Swiss wealth manager Credit Suisse (Shorrocks, Davies, & Lluberas, 2018), Oxfam International notes that "in 2017, 43 billionaires held as much wealth as the bottom 50% of the world population; in 2018, this figure decreased to 26 billionaires" (Revollo et al., 2019: 7). Further, the (predivorce) wealth of one person, Amazon founder Jeff Bezos, *circa* 2018 amounted to 100 times the total annual health budget of Ethiopia, Africa's second-largest country and as of 2019 one of the least-developed countries (LDCs) as ranked by the United Nations (Revollo et al., 2019: 5). Such comparisons actually understate the extent of concentration because "there are many more individuals who own $5 million, $20 million, or $100 million than there are billionaires, and the former command a potentially much larger fraction of world wealth than the latter" (Zucman, 2019: 22). Such figures must be viewed against a background of minimal progress, outside China, in reducing the number of people living in extreme poverty after 1990 on the World Bank's definition (*The Economist*, 2016), during a period in which the inflation-adjusted value of the world's economic product more than doubled.

Why does this matter for global health justice? An accumulating body of evidence – so far largely from the high-income world, where data are more abundant and reliable – indicates that high levels of inequality increase the prevalence of adverse health outcomes and a variety of other social problems across an entire jurisdiction (county, metropolitan area, or country): the *Spirit Level argument* (Wilkinson & Pickett, 2010; for an updated review of extensive additional evidence, see Pickett & Wilkinson, 2015). This evidence is, of course, far from convincing in political terms because rising inequality means that the wealthy are increasingly able to isolate themselves from problems outside their epidemiologic worlds, living in gated communities; paying privately for almost all services, including security; and in the extreme, commuting by helicopter and completely avoiding ground-level transit (Phillips, 2008). Concentration of income and wealth is likely to translate into concentration of political influence; an expanding body of recent political science research corroborates the conclusion of earlier analyses ranging across a spectrum from mainstream to Marxist that policymakers disproportionately respond to the preferences of the rich, even under conditions of formal democracy (Bartels, 2004, 2017; Gilens, 2012; Page & Bartels, 2013), conditions that are increasingly under siege (Freedom House, 2018).

Conclusion and Prospects for the Future: Money and Power Matter

It can always be argued that the longer-term benefits of integration into the global marketplace have yet to materialize; growth should eventually generate resources to improve health for all. Whereas growth *may* of course do so, recall Deaton's skepticism about what might be called the *waiting for Godot approach* to population health. This approach was articulated with unusual frankness by a team of World Bank economists writing about the former Soviet Union and its Eastern European satellites: "In the long run, the transition towards a market economy and adoption of democratic forms of government should ultimately lead to improvements in health status. ... In the short run, however, one could expect that health status would deteriorate" (Adeyi et al., 1997: 133). Anticipation of long-term gains is better understood as an expression of faith than as an evidence-based assessment. Nobel Prize–winning economist Joseph Stiglitz, formerly of the World Bank, has described the consequences of the post-1980 promotion of a particular market-focused vision of globalization by the governments of major G7 powers, acting on their own and through multilateral institutions such as the World Bank and the IMF, as "a lost quarter-century in Africa, a lost decade in Latin America, and a transition from communism to the market economy in the former Soviet Union and eastern Europe that was, to say the least, a disappointment" (Stiglitz, 2016). This point is especially important because of

philosopher Thomas Pogge's complex and nuanced argument (1) that a basic "negative obligation" exists to avoid doing harm and that obligation extends across national borders, (2) that the contemporary global economic order systematically neglects that obligation, and (3) that the neglect is avoidable; it is not difficult to envision alternative sets of economic and political institutions and underlying distributions of power that would not demand long periods of pain and widespread persistence of ill-health in anticipation of health gains at some indeterminate point in the future (Pogge, 2001, 2004, 2007).

More immediately, rising inequality and wealth concentration have important implications for progress toward such objectives as universal health coverage (UHC) – a target of the United Nations' Sustainable Development Goals (SDGs) and a programmatic priority of the WHO, although uncertainty remains about how UHC will be interpreted with respect to the mix of public/private provision and financing (Sengupta, 2013). The most fine-grained estimate of the cost of achieving this target available at the time of writing is that an "ambitious" scenario would require additional spending of US$134 billion (at 2014 currency values) initially, rising to US$371 billion in 2026–2030 (Stenberg et al., 2017). Many middle-income countries could mobilize these resources domestically, but substantial and sustained external assistance would be required in the case of many low-income countries (Sachs, 2012). Even low-income countries have substantial opportunities to expand health spending that are arithmetically, if not politically, feasible (McIntyre, Meheus, & Røttingen, 2017; Meheus & McIntyre, 2017). Increasing inequality is likely to complicate these questions of political feasibility, as is the ability of the wealthy to avoid taxation by shifting resources to tax havens (Harrington, 2016) – a topic that merits a chapter of its own (Brock, 2011). The global arithmetic is that an annual levy of 0.5% on the wealth of the richest 1% would suffice to finance this level of expenditure (Revollo et al., 2019: 18–19). Indeed, a global financial transaction tax of 0.05% on all currency exchanges (including speculative "shadow banking" and derivative markets) is estimated to be sufficient to fund implementation of all 17 SDGs and their 169 targets (Labonté & Ruckert, 2019: 396).

Despite the uncertainties created by globalization, many efforts to improve the health status of people outside the metaphorical castle walls have succeeded in recent years. The drop in measles mortality is one of the great global health success stories (Perry et al., 2014), and crucially, the number of people living with HIV/AIDS who are receiving antiretroviral therapy increased from fewer than 1 million at the turn of the millennium to more than 20 million in 2017 (UNAIDS, 2018b) – still far from universal access, and the bitterly contested political economy of this transition again would merit a chapter of its own (but see 't Hoen et al., 2011; UNAIDS, 2015: 78–95). Such success stories depended on effective and sustained mobilization of financial and other resources, both domestically and internationally. They are also consistent with a biomedical perspective shaped by experience with communicable diseases, a necessary condition for which is exposure to a particular pathogen; the complexities of dealing with a rising burden of noncommunicable diseases, which may have multiple sufficient causes, are conceptually more challenging for many health professionals quite apart from the politics of mobilizing an expanding quantum of resources and, more fundamentally, addressing the "power asymmetries" (Ottersen et al., 2014: 631) that generate and perpetuate health inequalities on multiple scales. The global reach of transnational corporate promotion of ultraprocessed foods is just one example among many. Moreover, as the 2015 *Lancet* Commission on Planetary Health noted, aggregate human health has been improving (if inequitably so) at the same time as our ecological boundaries that support life are being broached. The stark conclusion was that "we have been mortgaging the health of future generations to realise economic and development gains in the present" (Whitmee et al., 2015: 1973).

We make two points by way of conclusion. First, money matters, and global health ethics must start from the position that rhetoric is no substitute for commitments of resources to protect health on a much larger scale than at present. This can serve as a point of agreement even among researchers and practitioners who disagree about the relative value of improving social determinants of health and those who emphasize the "upstream" social determinants of health, usually with a focus on poverty and economic inequality, and those who dismiss interventions to address these factors as "romantic but impracticable notions" (Jha et al., 2005: 1539), arguing instead for a focus on biomedical innovations and scaling up health systems. In fact, all of these are

necessary, with the relative importance depending on context. No investment in health systems will undo the damage caused by indoor air pollution from cooking smoke, and health systems are only one among many influences on the incidence of HIV infection; no investment in social determinants of health will substitute for effective immunization programs or antiretroviral therapies; and neither problem can be addressed without real resources.

Second, in today's global environment, a preoccupation with setting priorities in resource-poor settings is a diversion or worse (Schrecker, 2013). The questions of far greater importance, as suggested by the work of Pogge and many others, is why some settings are resource poor and others not, and how to change that. The fact that resource scarcities condemn millions every year to premature and avoidable deaths and millions more to shorter and less healthy lives than most readers of this volume take for granted must be understood as policy-generated, resulting from particular power asymmetries, choices that could have been made differently, and institutions that can function differently. "If living were a thing that money could buy," indeed.

Acknowledgment

Research for the original version of this chapter was partially supported by the Canadian Institutes of Health (Research Grant No. 79153).

References

Adeyi, O., Chellaraj, G., Goldstein, E., Preker, A. S., & Ringold, D. (1997). Health status during the transition in Central and Eastern Europe: development in reverse? *Health Policy and Planning* **12**, 132–145.

Agyei-Mensah, S., & de-Graft Aikins, A. (2010). Epidemiological transition and the double burden of disease in Accra, Ghana. *Journal of Urban Health* **87**, 879–897.

Baker, R., Cardamone, T., Kar, D., Pogge, T., & Solheim, E. (2015). *Illicit Financial Flows: The Most Damaging Economic Condition Facing the Developing World*. Washington, DC: Global Financial Integrity. Retrieved from www.gfintegrity.org/wp-content/uploads/2015/09/Ford-Book-Final.pdf.

Balabanova, D., Mills, A., Conteh, L., et al. (2013). Good health at low cost 25 years on: lessons for the future of health systems strengthening. *Lancet* **381**, 2118–2133.

Baraldi, L. G., Martinez Steele, E., Canella, D. S., & Monteiro, C. A. (2018). Consumption of ultra-processed foods and associated sociodemographic factors in the USA between 2007 and 2012: evidence from a nationally representative cross-sectional study. *BMJ Open* **8**, E020574.

Barnett, J. C., & Berchick, E. R. (2017). *Health Insurance Coverage in the United States: 2016*. Washington, DC: US Census Bureau. Retrieved from www.census.gov/content/dam/Census/library/publications/2017/demo/p60-260.pdf.

Bartels, L. M. (2004). *Economic Inequality and Political Representation*. Syracuse, NY: Maxwell School of Citizenship and Public Affairs, Syracuse University.

Bartels, L. M. (2017). *Political Inequality in Affluent Democracies* (CSDI Working Paper No. 5–2017). Nashville, TN: Center for the Study of Democratic Institutions, Vanderbilt University. Retrieved from www.vanderbilt.edu/csdi/research/Working_Paper_5_2017.pdf.

Birn, A.-E., Pillay, Y., & Holtz, T. (2017). *Textbook of Global Health*, 4th ed. New York: Oxford University Press.

Black, R. E., Victora, C. G., Walker, S. P., et al. (2013). Maternal and child undernutrition and overweight in low-income and middle-income countries. *Lancet* **382**, 427–451.

Brock, G. (2011). International taxation, in Benatar S., & Brock G. (eds.), *Global Health and Global Health Ethics*. Cambridge, UK: Cambridge University Press, pp. 274–288.

Case, A., & Deaton, A. (2017). Mortality and morbidity in the 21st century. *Brookings Papers on Economic Activity* **2017**, 397–476.

Coker, R. J. (2004). Review: Multidrug-resistant tuberculosis: public health challenges. *Tropical Medicine & International Health* **9**, 25–40.

Commission on Social Determinants of Health (2008). *Closing the Gap in a Generation: Health Equity Through Action on the Social Determinants of Health (Final Report)*. Geneva: WHO. Retrieved from http://whqlibdoc.who.int/publications/2008/9789241563703_eng.pdf.

Deaton, A. (2003). Health, inequality, and economic development. *Journal of Economic Literature* **41**, 113–158.

Deaton, A. (2004). Health in an age of globalization. *Brookings Trade Forum* **2004**, 83–130.

Deaton, A. (2006). Global patterns of income and health. *Wider Angle* **2006**(2), 1–3.

The Economist (2016). How the other tenth lives (October 6), www.economist.com/finance-and-economics/2016/10/06/how-the-other-tenth-lives.

Eyoh, D., & Sandbrook, R. (2003). Pragmatic neo-liberalism and just development in Africa, in Kohli A., Moon C., & Sørensen G. (eds.), *States, Markets, and Just Growth: Development in the Twenty-first Century*. Tokyo: United Nations University Press, pp. 227–257.

Ezeh, A., Oyebode, O., Satterthwaite, D., et al. (2017). The history, geography, and sociology of slums and the health problems of people who live in slums. *Lancet* **389**, 547–558.

Ezzati, M., Vander Hoorn, S., Lawes, C. M., et al. (2005). Rethinking the "diseases of affluence" paradigm: global patterns of nutritional risks in relation to economic development. *Public Library of Science Medicine* **2**, e133.

Food and Agriculture Organization of the United Nations (FAO), International Fund for Agricultural Development, UNICEF, World Food Program, & WHO (2017). *The State of Food Security and Nutrition in the World 2017*. Rome: FAO. Retrieved from www.fao.org/3/a-I7695e.pdf.

Freedom House (2018). *Freedom in the World 2018*. Washington, DC: Freedom House.

GBD 2017 Mortality Collaborators (2018). Global, regional, and national age-sex-specific mortality and life expectancy, 1950–2013; 2017: a systematic analysis for the Global Burden of Disease Study 2017. *Lancet* **392**, 1684–1735.

Gilens, M. (2012). *Affluence and Influence: Economic Inequality and Political Power in America*. Princeton, NJ: Russell Sage Foundation and Princeton University Press.

Halimi, S. (2013, May). Tyranny of the one per cent. *Le Monde Diplomatique*, English edition.

Harrington, B. (2016). *Capital Without Borders: Wealth Managers and the One Percent*. Cambridge, MA: Harvard University Press.

Hickel, J. (2016). The true extent of global poverty and hunger: questioning the good news narrative of the Millennium Development Goals. *Third World Quarterly* **37**, 749–767.

Hug, L., Sharrow, D., & You, D. (2017). *Levels and Trends in Child Mortality: Report 2017: Estimates Developed by the UN Inter-agency Group for Child Mortality Estimation*. New York: UNICEF. Retrieved from www.childmortality.org/files_v21/download/IGME%20report%202017%20child%20mortality%20final.pdf.

Jha, P., Brown, D., Nagelkerke, N., Slutsky, A. S., & Jamison, D. T. (2005). Global IDEA: Five members of the Global IDEA Scientific Advisory Committee respond to Dr. Moore and Colleagues. *Canadian Medical Association Journal* **172**, 1538–1539.

Labonté, R., & Ruckert, A. (2019). *Health Equity in a Globalizing Era: Past Challenges, Future Prospects*. Oxford, UK: Oxford University Press.

Lister, J., & Labonté, R. (2009). Globalization and health systems change, in Labonté R., et al. (eds.), *Globalization and Health: Pathways, Evidence and Policy*. New York: Routledge, pp. 181–212.

Louzada, M., Ricardo, C. Z., Steele, E. M., Levy, R. B., Cannon, G., & Monteiro, C. A. (2018). The share of ultra-processed foods determines the overall nutritional quality of diets in Brazil. *Public Health Nutrition* **21**, 94–102.

Malik, V. S., Willett, W. C., & Hu, F. B. (2013). Global obesity: trends, risk factors and policy implications. *Nature Reviews Endocrinology* **9**, 13–27.

Martínez Steele, E., Popkin, B. M., Swinburn, B., & Monteiro, C. A. (2017). The share of ultra-processed foods and the overall nutritional quality of diets in the US: evidence from a nationally representative cross-sectional study. *Population Health Metrics* **15**, 6.

McIntyre, D., Meheus, F., & Røttingen, J. A. (2017). What level of domestic government health expenditure should we aspire to for universal health coverage? *Health Economics, Policy and Law* **12**, 125–137.

Meheus, F., & McIntyre, D. (2017). Fiscal space for domestic funding of health and other social services. *Health Economics, Policy and Law* **12**, 159–177.

Mendez, M. A., Monteiro, C. A., & Popkin, B. M. (2005). Overweight exceeds underweight among women in most developing countries. *American Journal of Clinical Nutrition* **81**, 714–721.

Milanovic, B. (2016). *Global Inequality: A New Approach for the Age of Globalization*. Cambridge, MA: Belknap Press of Harvard University Press.

Monteiro, C. A., Moubarac, J. C., Cannon, G., Ng, S. W., & Popkin, B. (2013). Ultra-processed products are becoming dominant in the global food system. *Obesity Reviews* **14**, 21–28.

Monteiro, C. A., Conde, W. L., & Popkin, B. M. (2004). The burden of disease from undernutrition and overnutrition in countries undergoing rapid nutrition transition: a view from Brazil. *American Journal of Public Health* **94**, 433–434.

Monteiro, C. A., Moubarac, J. C., Levy, R. B., et al. (2018). Household availability of ultra-processed foods and obesity in nineteen European countries. *Public Health Nutrition* **21**, 18–26.

Moodie, R., Stuckler, D., Monteiro, C., et al. (2013). Profits and pandemics: prevention of harmful effects of tobacco, alcohol, and ultra-processed food and drink industries. *Lancet* **381**, 670–679.

Moser, K., Shkolnikov, V., & Leon, D. (2007). World mortality 1950–2000: divergence replaces convergence from the late 1980s, in Caraël M., & Glynn J. R. (eds.), *HIV, Resurgent Infections and Population Change in Africa*. Dordrecht, Netherlands: Springer Netherlands, pp. 11–25. DOI:10.1007/978-1-4020-6174-5_1.

Murray, C. J. L., Kulkarni, S. C., Michaud, C., et al. (2006). Eight Americas: investigating mortality disparities across races, counties, and race-counties in the United States. *PLoS Medicine* **3**, e260.

Muzaka, V. (2014). Trade rules and intellectual property protection for pharmaceuticals, in Brown G., Yamey G., & Wamala S. (eds.) *The Handbook of Global Health Policy*. New York: Wiley, pp. 409–424.

Ngugi, F. (2017). What makes Luanda most expensive city in the world? Face2Face Africa, https://face2faceafrica.com/article/luanda-expensive-2.

Omran, A. R. (1971). The epidemiologic transition: a theory of the epidemiology of population change. *Milbank Memorial Fund Quarterly* **49**, 509–538.

Organisation for Economic Co-operation and Development (2014). *Illicit Flows from Developing Countries: Measuring OECD Responses*. Paris: OECD. Retrieved from www.oecd.org/dac/governance-development/IFF_R5_13mars14.pdf.

Ottersen, O. P., Dasgupta, J., Blouin, C., et al. (2014). The political origins of health inequity: prospects for change. *Lancet* **383**, 630–667.

Page, B. I. & Bartels, L. M. (2013). Democracy and the policy preferences of wealthy Americans. *Perspectives on Politics* **11**, 51–73.

Pedrique, B., Strub-Wourgaft, N., Some, C., et al. (2013). The drug and vaccine landscape for neglected diseases (2000–2011): a systematic assessment. *Lancet Global Health* **1**, e371–e379.

Perez-Padilla, R., Schilmann, A., & Riojas-Rodriguez, H. (2010). Respiratory health effects of indoor air pollution (Review article). *International Journal of Tuberculosis and Lung Disease* **14**, 1079–1086.

Perry, R. T., Gacic-Dobo, M., Dabbagh, A., et al. (2014). Global control and regional elimination of measles, 2000–2012. *Morbidity and Mortality Weekly Report* **63**, 103–107.

Phillips, T. (2008, June 20). High above Sao Paulo's choked streets, the rich cruise a new highway. *The Guardian*. Retrieved from www.guardian.co.uk/world/2008/jun/20/brazil.

Pickett, K. E., & Wilkinson, R. G. (2015). Income inequality and health: a causal review. *Social Science & Medicine* **128**, 316–326.

Pogge, T. (2001). Priorities of global justice. *Metaphilosophy* **32**, 6–24.

Pogge, T. (2004). Relational conceptions of justice: responsibilities for health outcomes, in Anand S., Peter F., & Sen A. (eds.), *Public Health, Ethics and Equity*. Oxford, UK: Clarendon Press, pp. 135–161.

Pogge, T. (2007). Severe poverty as a human rights violation, in Pogge T. (ed.), *Freedom from Poverty as a Human Right: Who Owes What to the Very Poor?* Oxford, UK: Oxford University Press, pp. 11–53.

Popkin, B. M. (2006). Global nutrition dynamics: the world is shifting rapidly toward a diet linked with noncommunicable diseases. *American Journal of Clinical Nutrition* **84**, 289–298.

Preston, S. H. (2007). The changing relation between mortality and level of economic development. *International Journal of Epidemiology* **36**, 484–490.

Prüss-Ustün, A., Bartram, J., Clasen, T., et al. (2014). Burden of disease from inadequate water, sanitation and hygiene in low- and middle-income settings: a retrospective analysis of data from 145 countries. *Tropical Medicine & International Health* **19**, 894–905.

Reddy, S., & Lahoti, R. (2016). $1.90 per day: what does it say? The new international poverty line. *New Left Review*, **new series** (97), 106–127.

Revollo, P. E., Mariotti, C., Mager, F., & Jacobs, D. (2019). *Public Good or Private Wealth? Methodology Note.* Oxford, UK: Oxfam International. Retrieved from https://oxfamili brary.openrepository.com/bitstream/handle/10546/620599 /tb-public-good-or-private-wealth-methodology-note-2101 19-en.pdf.

Riley, J. C. (2005). Estimates of regional and global life expectancy, 1800–2001. *Population and Development Review* **31**, 537–543.

Riley, J. C. (2008). *Low Income, Social Growth and Good Health: A History of Twelve Countries.* Berkeley: University of California Press.

Sachs, J. D. (2012). Achieving universal health coverage in low-income settings. *Lancet* **380**, 944–947.

Schrecker, T. (2013). Interrogating scarcity: how to think about "resource-scarce settings." *Health Policy and Planning* **28**, 400–409.

Schrecker, T. (2018). On health inequalities, Davos, and deadly neoliberalism. Policies for Equitable Access to Health, www.peah.it/2018/01/on-health-inequalities-davos -and-deadly-neoliberalism/

Sengupta, A. (2013). Universal health coverage: beyond rhetoric (Occasional Paper No. 20), Municipal Services Project, Kingston, Ontario, Canada. Retrieved from www .municipalservicesproject.org/sites/municipalservicespro ject.org/files/publications/OccasionalPaper20_Sengupta_ Universal_Health_Coverage_Beyond_Rhetoric_No v2013_0.pdf.

Shaefer, H. L., Wu, P., & Edin, K. (2017). Can poverty in America be compared to conditions in the world's poorest countries? *American Journal of Medical Research* **4**, 84–92.

Shorrocks, A., Davies, J., & Lluberas, R. (2018). *Global Wealth Report 2018.* Zurich: Credit Suisse Research Institute. Retrieved from www.credit-suisse.com/media/ass ets/corporate/docs/publications/research-institute/global- wealth-report-2018-en.pdf.

Stenberg, K., Hanssen, O., Edejer, T. T.-T., et al. (2017). Financing transformative health systems towards achievement of the health Sustainable Development Goals: a model for projected resource needs in 67 low-income and middle-income countries. *Lancet Global Health* **5**, e875–e887.

Stiglitz, J. (2016, August 10). The problem with Europe is the euro. *The Guardian.* Retrieved from www .theguardian.com/business/2016/aug/10/joseph-stiglitz- the-problem-with-europe-is-the-euro.

Stubbs, T., Kentikelenis, A., Stuckler, D., McKee, M., & King, L. (2017). The impact of IMF conditionality on government health expenditure: a cross-national analysis of 16 West African nations. *Social Science & Medicine* **174**, 220–227.

't Hoen, E., Berger, J., Calmy, A., & Moon, S. (2011). Driving a decade of change: HIV/AIDS, patents and access to medicines for all. *Journal of the International AIDS Society* **14**, 15.

UNAIDS (2015). *How AIDS Changed Everything – MDG6: 15 Years, 15 Lessons of Hope from the AIDS Response.* Geneva: UNAIDS. Retrieved from www.unaids.org/sites/ default/files/media_asset/MDG6Report_en.pdf.

UNAIDS (2018a). *Fact Sheet: World AIDS Day 2018.* Geneva: UNAIDS. Retrieved from www.unaids.org/sites/ default/files/media_asset/UNAIDS_FactSheet_en.pdf.

UNAIDS (2018b). *Miles to Go: Closing Gaps, Breaking Barriers, Righting Injustices.* Geneva: UNAIDS. Retrieved from www.unaids.org/sites/default/files/media_asset/miles- to-go_en.pdf.

UNICEF & WHO (2015). *Progress on Sanitation and Drinking Water: 2015 Update and MDG Assessment.* Geneva: WHO.

United Nations Human Settlements Programme (2003). *The Challenge of Slums.* London: Earthscan. Retrieved from www.unhabitat.org/pmss/getPage.asp? page=bookView&book=1156.

Valencia, M. (2013, February 16). Storm survivors: a special report on offshore finance. *The Economist.* Retrieved from www.economist.com/special-report/2013/02/16/storm- survivors.

Whitmee, S., Haines, A., Beyrer, C., et al. (2015). Safeguarding human health in the Anthropocene epoch: report of the Rockefeller Foundation–Lancet Commission on planetary health. *Lancet* **386**, 1973–2028.

Wilkinson, R. & Pickett, K. (2010). *The Spirit Level: Why Equality is Better for Everyone.* London: Penguin.

World Bank & IMF (2016). *Global Monitoring Report 2015/ 16: Development Goals in an Era of Demographic Change.* Washington, DC: World Bank. Retrieved from http://pub docs.worldbank.org/pubdocs/publicdoc/2015/10/50300144 4058224597/Global-Monitoring-Report-2015.pdf.

World Health Organization (WHO) (2010). *World Health Report 2010: Health Systems Financing – The Path to Universal Coverage.* Geneva: WHO. Retrieved from www .who.int/whr/2010/en/index.html.

World Health Organization (WHO) (2015a). *Global Status Report on Road Safety 2015.* Geneva: WHO. Retrieved from http://apps.who.int/iris/bitstream/10665/189242/1/978924 1565066_eng.pdf?ua=1.

World Health Organization (WHO) (2015b). *State of Inequality: Reproductive, Maternal, Newborn and Child Health.* Geneva: WHO. Retrieved from http://apps.who.int

/iris/bitstream/10665/164590/1/9789241564908_eng.pdf?
ua=1&ua=1.

World Health Organization (WHO) (2018). Tuberculosis
(Fact Sheet), www.who.int/news-room/fact-sheets/detail/
tuberculosis.

World Health Organization (WHO) (2019). Malaria (Fact
Sheet), www.who.int/news-room/fact-sheets/detail/
malaria.

World Health Organization & UNICEF (2017). *Progress on
Drinking Water, Sanitation and Hygiene: 2017 Update and
SDG Baselines*. Geneva: WHO. Retrieved from www.who.int
/entity/mediacentre/news/releases/2017/launch-version-
report-jmp-water-sanitation-hygiene.pdf?ua=1.

World Health Organization, UNICEF, UNFPA, World
Bank Group & United Nations Population Division (2019).
Trends in Maternal Mortality 2000 to 2017. Geneva: WHO.
Retrieved from: http://www.unfpa.org/sites/default/files/pu
b-pdf/Maternal_mortality_report.pdf.

Yates, R. (2009). Universal health care and the removal of
user fees. *Lancet* **373**, 2078–2081.

Zhang, H., & Cai, B. (2003). The impact of tobacco on lung
health in China. *Respirology* **8**, 17–21.

Zucman, G. (2019). *Global Wealth Inequality* (NBER
Working Paper No. 25462). Cambridge, MA: National
Bureau of Economic Research. Retrieved from http://
gabriel-zucman.eu/files/Zucman2019.pdf.

Societal Determinants and Determination of Health*

Anne-Emanuelle Birn and Ramya Kumar

Introduction

In 2017, Cubans lived, on average, to the age of 79 years – the same as in the United States (World Bank, 2019a). Yet US per capita income is approximately eight times that of Cuba (World Bank, 2019b). Similarly, Sri Lankans – earning US$4,060 per capita annually – had a life expectancy of 77 years (World Bank, 2019a, 2019b), 2 years more than in the state of Mississippi (USA), where annual per capita income is more than fivefold this level at US$22,500 (National Geographic, 2018; United States Census Bureau, n.d.). What makes Cubans and Sri Lankans live as long as or longer than those in significantly richer countries like the United States?

Consider another remarkable set of comparisons *within* countries. In Australia, Indigenous persons live, on average, nine years less than nonindigenous counterparts (Australian Institute of Health and Welfare, 2019). In Canada, too, there is a 10-year life-expectancy gap between residents of Nunavut, a largely Inuit territory, and those living in British Columbia (Canadian Institute for Health Information, 2019). Meanwhile, life expectancy among Indian women varies markedly by state, from 65 years in Assam to 79 years in Kerala (Singh et al., 2017). What explains such variations in life expectancy within countries?

The answer to these questions has far less to do with the *specific individuals* living in these settings than with the *structure of their societies* and their corresponding position in the global economy. Recognizing that such health differences are neither inevitable nor natural, this chapter explores health inequities – health status differences between socially defined groups that are unjust, unfair, and avoidable – and their underlying and interacting societal determinants.

---

* This chapter has been adapted and updated, with permission, from Chapter 7 of Anne-Emanuelle Birn, Yogan Pillay, and Timothy H. Holtz, *Textbook of Global Health*, 4th ed, Oxford University Press, New York, USA, 2017.

How Health Is Societally Determined

Each of us experiences ill-health individually, yet virtually every bout of illness or injury can also be understood in societal terms. People are exposed, susceptible, and resistant to different diseases in particular ways: pesticide plant workers or people residing near toxic waste dumps have a higher cancer incidence linked to their exposure to dangerous chemicals; homicides are higher in populations wracked by poverty and (state-sanctioned) violence; narcotic drug use, while certainly personally addictive, is heavily mediated by economic insecurity, social exclusion, and organized crime; and infants living in dwellings without potable water are more likely to get diarrhea, with susceptibility exacerbated by poor nutritional status. Relatedly, in 2020, patterns of COVID-19 cases and deaths in North America, the United Kingdom, and elsewhere are mediated by class/classism and race/racism, with working-class and racialized populations subject to greater occupational exposures and worse outcomes because of a series of factors discussed in this chapter, including structural inequalities and poorer healthcare access (Bailey & Moon, 2020).

Put differently, diseases may be distributed by chance among individuals (not everyone is exposed and not everyone exposed becomes ill), but at a population level, these same chances are "structured" by "historically contingent causal processes" that shape a range of existing, albeit dynamic determinants of health (Krieger, 2014a: 660). Who works in dangerous occupations or lives in hazardous conditions is not randomly decided but rather reflects societal arrangements along different axes of power, including wealth, social class, race and ethnicity, gender, geographic location, political structure, and so on.

The term *social determinants of health*, widely used especially following its explication by the World

Health Organization (WHO) Commission on Social Determinants of Health, refers to concrete factors related to resources and interactions among people and communities. Here, action targets improving conditions of daily life, tackling inequitable distribution of resources, and measuring health effects using data-driven evidence (WHO, 2008). By contrast, we employ *societal determinants of health* (SDOH) to refer more emphatically to the structural forces that affect health. We maintain that these determinants emphasize a broader array of factors and processes that, in effect, determine the rules regarding access to resources and relationships between and among societal groups. What is more, we believe that these determinants are dynamic and amenable to change by human agency and specific policies that unfold within and across societies.

A further conceptual dimension relates to the mechanisms of power through which SDOH operate. The Latin American concept of social (or societal) *determination* of health shifts emphasis from *what* (factors) to *who* (i.e., which groups and political and economic forces) is determining both the factors and the processes that produce and reproduce health/illness (Breilh, 2013). Thus, instead of simply identifying housing as a key determinant of health, a societal determination approach demands accounting for how real estate and other business interests and government actors drive land policies, housing markets, maintenance of housing stock, tenant, lending, and ownership policies, municipal services, neighborhood quality (i.e., parks, transport access, schools, food stores, recreation, etc.), water and sanitary conditions, and waste and pollution, as well as zoning, class and racial discrimination, and so on. Thus, housing is not a static category that independently shapes health but one that is influenced by and interacts with a host of historical and contextual political, economic, environmental, geographic, and social factors.

In other words, if SDOH are the "causes of the causes" of health and disease (Marmot, 2005), societal determinants are "the causes of the causes of the causes" or the political economy forces driving the determinants (Birn, 2009). As such, societal determination of health reflects health and disease as processes, with perpetrating and nameable forces that lead to the physical embodiment (experiences, behaviors, exposures expressed on human bodies) of health, illness, and premature death.

Understanding Health and Health Inequities

SDOH approaches offer essential ingredients for explaining the existence of health inequities, but how can we explain the ways in which health/illness inequities are expressed in populations? Viewed via a *biomedical lens*, health derives from a combination of one's genetic heritage and individual biology and lifelong health and disease experiences (and behavior). Health differences among individuals and groups thus result from natural variation, inherent differences that have evolved over time, individual "risk factors," and different opportunities accorded by genetics and biology. A *behavioral/lifestyle model* views health as a function of choices around how one lives in terms of diet, exercise, occupation, residence, and aspects of personal behavior, such as substance use or safe sex. From this perspective, health "disparities" are seen as a function of health behaviors, in turn, shaped by individual choice.

Both of these models are based on individualized and decontextualized understandings of how health and health inequity are produced. Just as the biomedical model sidesteps the societal influences shaping every occurrence of disease, death, or injury, the lifestyle model overlooks the day-to-day constraints of, for example, what foods are affordable and accessible, the presence/absence of parks and safe spaces, job possibilities, daily and long-term family responsibilities, and stressful work and living conditions.

Psychosocial theory explains the social patterning of ill-health by considering the health impact of individual perceptions and responses to the social environment within the family, community, school, workplace, and wider society. These contexts and social interactions, combined with one's social status, shape experiences of psychological stress and associated responses (e.g., depression), mediated by coping skills, social support, and sense of control (Kubzansky, Winning, & Kawachi, 2014).

Here an individual's position in the social hierarchy acts as the prime psychological stressor/buffer. Not only are working-class persons exposed to greater stress, but they also may have fewer personal and social resources to manage stressful circumstances. Among postulated mechanisms, physiologic responses of distress and resentment over the life course have been linked to endocrinologic, nervous system, and other regulatory imbalances, for example, raising blood pressure and negatively affecting cardio-vascular health (Berkman & Kawachi, 2014).

Unlike biomedical and lifestyle explanations, psychosocial theory does not focus solely on individual biology and behavior or overlook the role of social context. However, it deemphasizes *who* and *what* cause the differential exposures and capacities of resistance to stress in the first place and how political, social, and economic agendas, values, power, and practices shape societal hierarchies and the nature and distribution of stress exposures.

A *critical political economy approach*, by contrast, elucidates the role of political and economic systems and key actors – and their accompanying values and priorities – in structuring patterns of health and health inequity. From this perspective, social structures (namely observable, patterned relationships among groups), and the asymmetries of power perpetuated through these structures, are largely (although not entirely) determined by political and economic forces. These structural forces shape but do not negate human agency and biology, although political economy may not elaborate the mechanisms that connect the political to the biological.

Employing the notion of embodiment, or "how we literally embody, biologically, our lived experience, in societal and ecological context" (Krieger, 2014b: 48), *ecosocial theory* helps explain how SDOH are biologically expressed in individuals and populations. Individuals (and communities) embody their living conditions, including social relations and structures of power, over the life course and across generations. Paying particular heed to race, class, and gender, ecosocial theory addresses the "cumulative interplay among exposure, susceptibility, and resistance" – whereby past and ongoing biological incorporation of social relations of power are integrated into present health and disease experience (Krieger, 2008: 225). Together, critical political economy and ecosocial theory inform societal determination, enabling an understanding of who and what is responsible for power asymmetries and, in turn, inequities in health (Figure 2.1).

Operationalizing the Political Economy of Health through SDOH

The above-reviewed roster of societal determination frameworks helps to concretize how injustice is embodied in health outcomes and inequity and lays out the dimensions of injustice that need to be considered to address health inequity. Here we apply a societal determination lens to a case to illustrate how determinants at multiple levels converge on health.

Imagine Lee – a migrant laborer working in construction in a rapidly growing metropolis – who falls 10 stories from a scaffolding and dies. At the *broadest (macro) level*, Lee's fall may be linked to the free-market economic system, in which profits come before worker safety and well-being. A building boom driven by global financial interests and facilitated by trade treaties signed by governments – many under austerity pressures, and representing elite interests – gives investors and transnational corporations (TNCs) enormous power to evade taxes and flout labor laws. As such, working-class efforts to organize for social security benefits and workplace safety are constrained by restrictions on unionization and threats of job loss and repression.

At an *intermediate (macro-meso) level* linked to government policies, Lee's low earnings derive from minimum wage levels that are inadequate and poorly enforced, which help the country attract foreign direct investment; because his position as a migrant worker is precarious, he has little recourse. What is more, the company's meager safety training and low-grade scaffolding materials are aided by scant regulations and oversight, within increasingly fragmented production processes that outsource activities at various levels.

At the *individual level*, Lee may have been inattentive and insufficiently conscious of safety, or just unlucky (as the word *accident* implies), and thus slipped to his death. If we examine Lee's living conditions (*meso-local level*), however, we learn that he is chronically sleep deprived because of his long and stressful commute to work – he can only afford to reside in a distant slum. Moreover, his flimsy dwelling cannot keep out disease-bearing rodents and insects, whose bites provoke an itchy rash. Perhaps in his exhaustion, he scratched his arm, inopportunely letting go of the scaffolding. Lee's fall – whether in Dubai or Dublin – may be construed as one person's misfortune, but viewed through a lens of SDOH, it can be understood as the result of an interdependent set of political, economic, and social forces operating at multiple levels.

In the remainder of this chapter, we flesh out a comprehensive and structured, if condensed, array of factors that influence health, paying particular attention to *how* SDOH are translated into health inequities that unjustly and avoidably cut short millions of lives and cause enormous suffering. While we retain

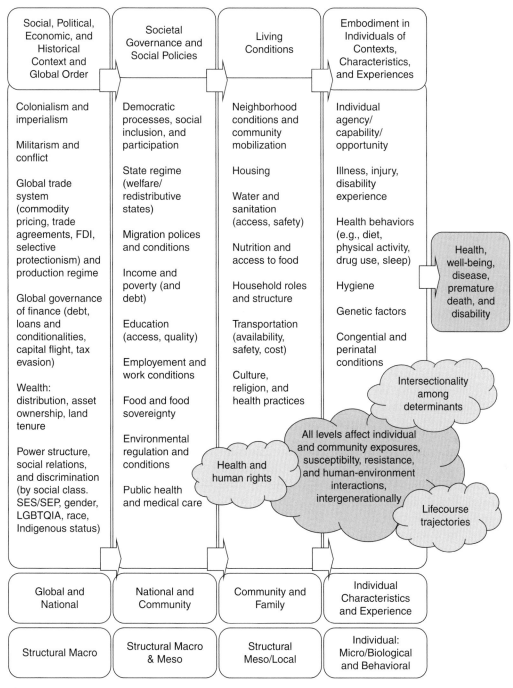

Social, Political, Economic, and Historical Context and Global Order	Societal Governance and Social Policies	Living Conditions	Embodiment in Individuals of Contexts, Characteristics, and Experiences
Colonialism and imperialism Militarism and conflict Global trade system (commodity pricing, trade agreements, FDI, selective protectionism) and production regime Global governance of finance (debt, loans and conditionalities, capital flight, tax evasion) Wealth: distribution, asset ownership, land tenure Power structure, social relations, and discrimination (by social class. SES/SEP, gender, LGBTQIA, race, Indigenous status)	Democratic processes, social inclusion, and participation State regime (welfare/ redistributive states) Migration polices and conditions Income and poverty (and debt) Education (access, quality) Employement and work conditions Food and food sovereignty Environmental regulation and conditions Public health and medical care	Neighborhood conditions and community mobilization Housing Water and sanitation (access, safety) Nutrition and access to food Household roles and structure Transportation (availability, safety, cost) Culture, religion, and health practices	Individual agency/ capability/ opportunity Illness, injury, disability experience Health behaviors (e.g., diet, physical activity, drug use, sleep) Hygiene Genetic factors Congential and perinatal conditions

Health, well-being, disease, premature death, and disability

Intersectionality among determinants

All levels affect individual and community exposures, susceptibilty, resistance, and human-environment interactions, intergenerationally

Health and human rights

Lifecourse trajectories

Global and National	National and Community	Community and Family	Individual Characteristics and Experience

Structural Macro	Structural Macro & Meso	Structural Meso/Local	Individual: Micro/Biological and Behavioral

Figure 2.1. Political economy of global health framework.
Source: Extensively adapted with permission from Gloyd (1987).

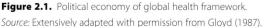

a determinant-by-determinant organization for purposes of clarity, we recognize the effects of concurrent and synergistic forms of oppression and privilege posited by intersectionality (Crenshaw, 1991; Kapilashrami, Hill, & Meer, 2015) and endorse a life-course understanding of health and health inequities, acknowledging the long-term effects of physical and social exposures in later life (Braveman, 2014; Jacob et al., n.d.).

From Past to Present: The Political, Economic, and Social Forces Shaping Health and Health Inequities

At the broadest level, SDOH can be understood in relation to social, political, economic, and historical forces that play out in global and national arenas. At the global level, these forces include colonialism, imperialism, militarism, nationalism, wealth and ownership concentration, and unfair production, financial, and commercial arrangements (Ng & Muntaner, 2014). They are also made visible at the national level through current power configurations reflecting discriminatory social structures around class, race, and gender relations.

(Neo)Colonialism, Imperialism, Militarism/ Nationalism, and Violence

The rules and social arrangements that govern the contemporary world order derive from long historical processes of accumulation and exploitation under prefeudal and feudalistic societies, accelerating under imperialism and capitalism. Although few colonies remain, the current global political structure reflects geopolitical relations that have been in place for centuries (Czyzewski, 2011). Commodity pricing, debt regimes, and international organizations, to name but a few forces, largely maintain and reproduce historical asymmetries between colonial powers and colonized countries. From slavery to tithing of peasant agricultural output, colonial military occupation and resource extraction, and current global finance mechanisms that protect corporate profitmaking over virtually all other social values, these systems influence health across intersecting pathways such as infringement of sovereignty and self-determination, limited control over resources, repressive social policies, ongoing conflict, and so on.

The field of global health is rife with examples of the ways in which colonial power structures influenced– and still influence– the health of those living on the margins. A horrifying example from the 1940s is the gross violation of ethics by US Public Health Service doctors carrying out treatment efficacy research that involved inoculating sex workers, military personnel, prisoners, and the mentally infirm with sexually transmitted infections in Guatemala (Reverby, 2012). While such dehumanizing acts were made possible by the racist underpinnings of imperial medicine, neocolonial aspirations still drive global health activity, whether pharmaceutical profiteering enabled by the Global Fund or health-damaging austerity reforms sanctioned by international development agencies in debt-ridden low- and middle-income countries (LMICs; Stubbs et al., 2017).

To explore another avenue, war remains a much-used tool to consolidate power and ensure access to mineral resources. During the twentieth century, almost 200 million people lost their lives directly or indirectly as a result of war, with civilians constituting over half of the casualties. Militarism, the precursor to war, escalates all forms of violence within and between countries. In 2016, at least 560,000 people lost their lives violently, mostly in conflict or by homicide (McEvoy & Hideg, 2017). As military spending and arms trade rise across the world (Stockholm International Peace Research Institute, 2019), scarce resources are channeled away from social and infrastructural endeavors – parks, quality schools, good housing, safe employment, and so on – all of which are of critical importance to health.

Wars are fought in the name of the nation, with nationalism fostering ethnoreligious tension and anti-immigrant sentiment. Whether the 2016 Trump victory in the United States, the 2016 UK referendum in support of Brexit, the triumphant far right across Europe and in Brazil, or Modi's 2019 victory in India, renewed nationalism has unleashed levels of racist violence not witnessed in many decades.

Financialization, Governance, Trade, and Production Regimes under Contemporary Global Capitalism

A host of global arrangements, including rule-making bodies, international financial institutions (IFIs), financialization processes, and trade treaties, have direct and indirect health effects (Schrecker & Bambra, 2015; Stubbs et al., 2017). The current phase of capitalism, *neoliberal globalization*, jump-started with the 1980s debt crisis in LMICs (and accelerated worldwide amid the 2008–2012 global financial crisis), when IFI loans and accompanying conditionalities originally known as *structural adjustment programs* (SAPs) denuded government capacity and stripped resources away from the social sectors, reorienting regulation to favor capitalist interests over public need (Harvey, 2010). LMIC populations, and later high-income country (HIC) populations, especially the most marginalized groups, faced the effects of unemployment, malnutrition, hazardous exposures, cuts to public spending, and increased poverty. Among other effects, SAPs played a devastating role in the inadequate initial response to the HIV pandemic in Sub-Saharan Africa (Baker, 2010), and for decades, austerity regimes have promoted privatization and have channeled funds away from social provisioning, resulting in deficient resources for preventing and treating tuberculosis in LMICs (Austin, DeSciscolo, & Samuelsen, 2016).

Financialization, referring to the dominance of "financial motives," markets, actors, and institutions "in the operation of the domestic and international economies" (Epstein, 2005: 3) and in all aspects of life (from household and small farmer debt to the role of insurance conglomerates in elections), has been a critical dimension of neoliberal globalization (Harvey, 2010). In recent decades, financialization has infiltrated multiple domains of social reproduction, including healthcare, education, and welfare (Fine, 2012). In this context, universal health coverage (UHC) – a UN Sustainable Development Goal (SDG) target embraced by state and nonstate actors alike – has facilitated the entry of global finance capital into the health sector, allowing limitless profits to be made as governments increasingly outsource provisioning to the private healthcare industry. This has deepened financialization (Hunter & Murray, 2019) even though many dominant actors do not acknowledge this and instead emphasize UHC's equity aspirations, which are jeopardized by these very financialization processes.

The global trade system, governed by the World Trade Organization (WTO) and a myriad of bilateral and regional trade and investment agreements, exemplifies how unequal power relations are created and sustained and manifest in inequitable health outcomes. In the education sector, trade agreements have enabled multinational giants to influence national education policy. Bridge International Academies, for instance, lobbies for and promotes a hugely profitable form of low-resource, standardized, technology-based schooling in parts of Africa and Asia. Employing a *public-private partnership model*, many such initiatives outsource provision of education to an unaccountable and weakly regulated private sector, lowering quality and widening inequity (Spreen & Kamat, 2018; Oxfam, 2019).

Trade agreements also protect big businesses from "impediments to competition," such as subsidies for local industries and regulations, at the expense of small-scale producers and laborers in HICs and LMICs alike. Exemplifying the concentration of power (and profits) enabled by such trade arrangements, world food production and trade are now controlled by a small number of megacompanies. In fact, just 50 food manufacturers account for 50% of food sales worldwide (Oxfam, 2018).

Wealth and Health: Distribution, Assets, and Land Tenure

Wealth and Income Distribution

Wealth and its distribution shape and are shaped by access to power and resources across countries and institutions, in many ways setting the basic political, economic, and social institutions and rules that govern society. Wealth (and its distribution) influences health *both* by determining the material circumstances that affect health – including via livelihoods and social conditions – *and* through its relation to societal power structures that shape broader social relations and policies, from economic security and social protections via welfare/redistributive states, to employment and workplace conditions, to political social justice struggles affecting those relations and structures (de Andrade et al., 2015).

Wealth inequality, which captures property and nonincome financial assets, is far larger than income inequality, and, thus, decreases in income inequality may leave maldistribution of wealth (e.g., between men and women or by race/ethnicity, class, region), and corresponding political influence/power largely intact (Thrasher, 2015). Yet income or even wealth inequality alone cannot explain the effects of discrimination along racial, gender, or other lines or how unequal power structures and relations manifest and affect patterns of health and health (in)equity (Coburn, 2011).

Land Tenure and Property Ownership

Property ownership and land tenure are fundamental dimensions of wealth and economic security in both rural and urban settings. Holding and farming land are the prime rural livelihood source, involving

400 million subsistence or small-scale farms that support approximately one-third of the world's population. In the mid-twentieth century, land reform was a key feature of social movements from Bolivia to Taiwan, improving the lot of millions of smallholders. In more recent decades, productive land has become increasingly concentrated in the hands not just of domestic elites but also of large agribusinesses, enabled by deregulation, trade agreements, and the penetration of TNCs. Reflecting this trend, just 1% of the world's farms are over 50 hectares in size but represent 65% of the world's agricultural lands (Oxfam, 2018). In India, millions of small farmers have lost their livelihoods in recent decades, unable to survive against large competitors; hundreds of thousands of farmers have committed suicide in the context of bankruptcy, indebtedness, and crop failure (Holla & Ittyerah, 2018; Reddy & Mishra, 2010).

Worldwide, agribusiness takeovers by Monsanto and other multinational corporations have had drastic effects on local producers, provoking marked reductions in the number of small farms, jeopardizing livelihoods, and creating export-oriented monocultures. Landless farmers are among the world's most disenfranchised populations, even as they organize politically, demanding food justice through, for example, La Via Campesina and Brazil's Landless Workers' Movement.

Meanwhile, in cities, where 55% of the world's population now lives (United Nations Department of Economic and Social Affairs [UN-DESA], 2018), inequitable property ownership influences health and well-being via the effects of real estate speculation, gentrification, and redevelopment policies. Past and present, urban poor and working classes (joined by rural populations dispossessed of their land) have engaged in intense struggles over public space and private property (Harvey, 2006).

A nefarious accompanying trend in this era of financialization is predatory lending, whereby bankers encourage working-class populations – often racial and ethnic minorities – to purchase property beyond their means, strangling them with debt and eventual bankruptcy in a context of economic precariousness. In the United States, the 2008 housing crash led to a racialized geography of foreclosure, home abandonment, and bank repossession in the worst-hit places (Bond & Browder, 2019; Dorling, 2015). Similarly, slum clearance policies, euphemized as urban renewal, have forced the poorest groups out of central urban locations, breaking up communities and jeopardizing social ties, livelihoods, and access to social services, all with negative health effects including rising mortality (Ezeh et al., 2017).

Power Structure, Social Relations, and Discrimination

Social Class, Socioeconomic Status, and Socioeconomic Position

Crucial to understanding health inequities is the role of social class, theorized by Karl Marx as people's relation to ownership of assets and the production process. Social class explains health outcomes above and beyond income, reflecting class oppression – the deprivation, exclusion from control, and appropriation of the exploited group's productivity and assets – and resistance in the form of class struggle. Social class operates synergistically with other forms of oppression, including racism and patriarchy/gender oppression.

Although social class is well theorized, using it systematically poses a significant challenge because most governments do not routinely collect data by class. The United Kingdom is a notable exception,[1] making possible the landmark 1980 "Black Report," which tracked mortality and life expectancy differentials by five occupational classes from the 1930s through the 1970s. Revealing widening class differentials in mortality despite the 1948 establishment of the UK's National Health Service, the report argued that these differences derived from inequities in living and working conditions, not healthcare access and utilization, and were thus amenable to change through social and economic policies (Black et al., 1980).

Evidenced by numerous studies in HICs, socioeconomic status (SES) helps explain how assets and characteristics intertwine to create social differences (Glymour, Avendano, & Kawachi, 2014). The UK's Whitehall Studies of tens of thousands of civil servants starting in the late 1960s employed occupational grade as a measure of SES, uncovering a "social gradient in health" even in the absence of poverty or

---

[1] From 1911 to 2001, the United Kingdom's registrar-general collected routine mortality data by social class, as measured by occupational category. It was then replaced with a larger socioeconomic classification based on employment relations and occupational conditions (Glymour, Avendano, & Kawachi, 2014).

material deprivation. Men in the lowest of four occupational grades were found to have the highest death rate from coronary heart disease, with mortality decreasing stepwise from the lowest to the highest occupational class (Rose & Marmot, 1981). Social gradient in health findings was replicated for women (Marmot & Brunner, 2005) and shown to be compounded by racism, sexism, and ableism (Braveman et al., 2015; Potente & Monden, 2018).

Gender Inequality, Patriarchy, and Sexuality

Gender refers to social conceptions, roles, and identities rather than biology. Gendered health differences may result from differing (unequal) household responsibilities, decision-making power, occupational roles, or legal rights and entitlements. Health outcomes linked to sex-based differences in biology may not be gendered per se, and the distinction between gender and sex is contested (Butler, 1990).

Gender does matter for health outcomes that involve "sex"-linked biology. For instance, in Sierra Leone, where maternal mortality is the world's highest at 1,360 deaths per 100,000 live births (WHO, 2019a), preventable causes – hemorrhage, sepsis, and abortion – account for over 50% of maternal deaths. Similarly, across the world, restrictions on access to abortion result in 25 million unsafe abortions per year (Ganatra et al., 2017), accounting for an estimated 13% of global maternal mortality, or 47,000 maternal deaths per year (WHO, 2012), many of them preventable.

Gender-based violence (GBV), experienced by over a third of women and girls globally, results from patriarchal norms around authority; gender stereotyping; tolerance of domestic violence; laws and practices limiting women's access to land, property, and other economic resources; and limited female education and wage earning. The control and regulation of women's bodies to conform to hegemonic standards of beauty, through cosmetic surgery, pharmaceuticals, and other technologies, are also a form of GBV.

Gendered norms affect men's health at multiple levels (Benatar, 2012). Gendered divisions of labor lead to differential health outcomes, with men more likely to work in dangerous or high-stress jobs outside the home, and women, children, and the elderly – especially in LMICs – more exposed to strenuous and potentially hazardous household activities such as field work, water collection, and cooking with inadequate ventilation (Sehgal & Krishnan, 2013). However, these roles are changing, with women taking on the responsibility for income generation alongside growing male unemployment. (See Chapter 4 for further details.)

Health concerns related to gender and sexual identity stem from pervasive societal prejudice against LGBTQ people, occurring through institutionalized oppression via law, policing, health provider ignorance, and/or limited services (Raifman, 2018). Other forms of discrimination manifest through social policies around housing, schooling, and employment, as well as threats, bullying, and violence, which cause physical harm or death as well as mental health problems (Gnan et al., 2019). Ultimately, gender interacts and intersects with class, race, and other axes of difference and discrimination in shaping access to education, employment, healthcare, and social services (Connell, 2012).

Race and Racism

Race is a social construction developed to classify groups according to arbitrary, usually "visible" characteristics. Historically, dominant societal groups have elaborated racial distinctions to establish or preserve power and privilege at the expense of oppressed groups, for example, justifying slavery or colonial expansion. These historical and contemporary patterns of power asymmetries have ongoing repercussions, generating worse health for "racialized" groups compared with dominant groups.

Racism – distinguished from race – is the enactment of structural and systematic forms of oppression and discrimination against particular racial groups by institutions and individuals, with racial definitions themselves arising from oppressive systems of race relations. Although the state plays a critical legal and enforcement role that either permits or prohibits racism, dominance and oppression are institutionalized in multifarious extralegal ways through practices that maintain the privilege enjoyed by dominant groups (Krieger, 2014a).

Descendants of Africans enslaved in North America, Brazil, the Caribbean, and elsewhere have experienced unspeakable loss of freedom, and centuries of social disruption, death, illness, disability, and physical and psychological abuse. Yet the legacy is not uniform across regions (Bergad, 2007): descendants of enslaved persons comprise the majority population in some countries and have realized important sociopolitical gains (e.g., in Barbados), whereas in other settings (e.g., the United States), there is ongoing racial discrimination and persistent "embodied" oppression. Institutionalized racism often manifests in a racialized division of labor, particularly in HICs. In Canada, immigration policies guide the selection of highly skilled workers, but, on arrival, racialized immigrants encounter under-employment, because their preimmigration qualifications and work experience are often not recognized by employers (Mawani, 2019).

Racism negatively affects health through concurrent pathways, with historical context determining their relative significance. Embodied manifestations of discrimination are evidenced by health inequities in self-rated health, physical health (e.g., obesity, blood pressure, preterm delivery), mental health, and health behaviors, such as substance use, or utilization of healthcare services (Paradies et al., 2015). Moreover, racialized children often experience the effects of deprivation into adulthood even if their life circumstances improve (Krieger, 2011).

Race-based health differences go beyond SES explanations and universal measures: in New Zealand, racism experienced by Māori-descended populations is associated with adverse health outcomes irrespective of economic deprivation levels (Harris et al., 2012). Similar findings are reported from Brazil, where Afro-descendant women are less likely than others to receive adequate prenatal care through the universal national health system (Domingues et al., 2015).

Clearly, policies matter in addressing the health effects of racism. In the United States, the 1964 Civil Rights Act's overturning of "Jim Crow laws" (legalized segregation and racial discrimination enforced across a band of Southern states) resulted in a convergence of infant mortality rates between the African-American population in states with and without Jim Crow laws (Krieger et al., 2013). However, infant mortality rates still remain twice as high for African-American versus white Americans (Mathews, MacDorman, & Thoma, 2015), and maternal mortality rates among non-Hispanic African-American women are triple those of non-Hispanic white women (Roeder, 2019). In response, African-American women are organizing, demanding health and justice on their own terms (Villarosa, 2018).

Racial and ethnic discrimination has likewise worsened health outcomes in other settings. In South Africa, the legacy of the apartheid system of state-sanctioned segregation and discrimination – which endured into the 1990s – is evidenced in under-five mortality rates that are five times higher among Africans than among whites. In Europe, the Roma ethnic minority, disenfranchised across the region, has a life expectancy up to 20 years lower than non-Roma populations (European Commission, 2014).

At present in the United States and worldwide, powerful struggles against police brutality and systemic racism have gained widespread traction and solidarity, building on years of groundwork by the Black Lives Matter movement (Taylor, 2016).

Indigenous Status and (Neo-)Colonial Oppression

The colonization process and ongoing discrimination against Indigenous peoples – involving violence, forcible removal from ancestral lands, denial of heritage, loss of livelihood, and absence of social protections – has denigrated traditional ways of life, kinship structures, and spiritual beliefs while generating near-universal patterns of racial and cultural discrimination and government paternalism (Walters et al., 2011). This is illustrated by Australian and Canadian experiences, where for almost a century these governments forcibly removed thousands of Indigenous children from their families and communities, placing them in residential schools where they faced violence, overcrowding, malnutrition, and forced labor.

Canada's Truth and Reconciliation Commission's 2015 report on the century-long residential school system linked it to "cultural genocide" seeking to "eliminate Aboriginal governments; ignore Aboriginal rights; terminate the Treaties; and, through a process of assimilation, cause Aboriginal peoples to cease to exist as distinct legal, social, cultural, religious, and racial entities in Canada" (Truth and Reconciliation Commission of Canada, 2015: 1). The schools' dilapidated, unsanitary, and hazardous conditions led to up to 30,000 deaths (of a total of at least 150,000 Indigenous children forced into these schools over more than a century) from tuberculosis, influenza, pneumonia, and fires.[2] School staff tormented students with rampant physical and sexual abuse, which also created the conditions for student-to-student abuse. Adding to this mistreatment, in the 1960s, large numbers of Indigenous children were removed without cause from their families and placed into

---

[2] Documentation of these patterns began as far back as 1907 in Canada (Bryce, 1922; Sproule-Jones, 1996).

foster care. These experiences have affected the health and well-being not only of survivors but also of their families and broader communities, many of whom suffer mental health, narcotics addictions, and abuse problems. Into the present, a recent national inquiry concluded that violence amounting to "a race-based genocide" targeting women, girls, and gender diverse and nonbinary people in Canada had resulted in "increased rates of violence, death and suicide in Indigenous populations" (National Inquiry into Murdered and Missing Indigenous Women and Girls, 2019: 1–2).

Historical and contemporary oppression of Indigenous peoples worldwide is reflected in alarmingly high poverty rates, limited access to potable water, poor-quality housing stock, inadequate healthcare access, disproportionate incarceration and foster care rates, and high levels of exposure to environmental toxins, all jeopardizing health (UN-DESA, 2015). Across the Americas, Indigenous populations experience extreme poverty rates of up to 90%, more than twice the rates of nonindigenous groups, as well as high rates of chronic and infectious diseases and suicide. In Mato Grosso do Sul, Brazil, for example, Indigenous people account for 3% of the population but 20% of suicide deaths (Economic Commission for Latin America and the Caribbean, 2014).

Long-standing and (re-)emerging Indigenous resistance movements, such as Canada's grassroots Idle No More, have mobilized to protect Indigenous rights to water and traditional ways of life, garnering notable support transnationally from Indigenous movements as well as from unions, students, and other groups.

Societal Governance and Social Policies

Governments employ a range of policies that shape health through their effects on: poverty, inequality, and discrimination; access to and quality of education; employment and work conditions; food sovereignty; environmental conditions and industrial regulations; public health and medical care; and social security benefits. Societal measures are often constrained and intertwined with determinants at the global level, namely trade agreements, debt and financial obligations, and the enduring effects of colonialism. Other state-level factors include democratic processes, transparency/corruption, social inclusion/exclusion, migration policies

and conditions, and policing and justice systems. These policies are inherently linked to the ways (and extent to which) governments respect, protect, and fulfill human rights obligations.

Democratic Processes, Social Inclusion, and Participation

The ability to participate fully in community and political life appears to engender well-being (Crammond & Carey, 2016). Social exclusion – the inability of certain marginalized groups (e.g., people who are homeless or poor, racial/ethnic and sexual minorities, persons with disabilities, and undocumented workers) to fully participate in civic life – is often the result of structural inequalities, lack of access to resources, prejudice, and/or stigma (Ruckert & Labonté, 2014). In many societies, persons with disabilities are unable to find steady employment (Bambra, 2011). Such social exclusion may lead to poor physical and mental health, increased levels of societal violence, and premature mortality. Conversely, social inclusion provides access to resources and social support networks and adequate housing, education, and transportation (Ruckert & Labonté, 2014).

Incarceration is a literal form of social exclusion. The United States has the largest number of people in prison (more than 2.1 million) and the world's highest incarceration rate at 655 per 100,000 population (Walmsley, 2018), disproportionately harming low-income groups and racial/ethnic minorities. Discriminatory policing and justice systems, such as heavy-handed police monitoring of racialized and low-income areas, and mandatory minimum sentencing for small crimes (e.g., not paying fines), generate soaring incarceration rates and disenfranchisement as well as perpetuate poverty, unemployment, and attendant higher illness and premature death rates among racialized and low-income populations (Travis, Western, & Redburn, 2014).

Welfare/Redistributive States as SDOH

A product of working-class and other struggles against brutal working and living conditions in industrializing countries in the late nineteenth and early twentieth centuries, the welfare state has been recognized as a key determinant of population health and health equity because of its central functions of ensuring income redistribution; protecting against immiseration, unemployment, and ill-health; providing universal public healthcare and education; and improving occupational health and safety standards. Less acknowledged, however, is that such social benefits and entitlements in HICs both reflect and are supported through colonial and continued postcolonial extraction and exploitation (Bhambra & Holmwood, 2018).

The pivotal welfare-state mechanism enhancing population health and health equity is redistribution. This entails fair, progressive, and adequate income, property, and corporate taxation, and the reallocation (transfer) of income and/or services back to the population through either universal or targeted measures. State revenues may be directly channeled to individual or family income (e.g., family allowances, child/maternity benefits, paid parental leave, and disability or retirement pensions) or may involve services (e.g., daycare and healthcare spending; Beckfield et al., 2015), both of which significantly curb inequality and poverty. For instance, before taxes and transfers, the 2012 poverty rate was 29.2% in the United States and 35.6% in France. After redistribution, US poverty dropped by over 11 points to 17.9%, while in France, poverty plunged by a far more dramatic 27.5 points to 8.1% (Organisation for Economic Co-operation and Development [OECD], 2015). Indeed, the limits to universality and redistribution in the United States (notwithstanding sizable government spending) has led to its underperformance in social welfare (and health) relative to its level of economic development.

The most successful welfare states – in terms of positive aggregate health outcomes (e.g., life expectancy) – have been characterized by strong labor movements and socialist or social democratic political parties; high corporate taxes; progressive income taxes; high expenditures on social security; high levels of employment, particularly in the public sector, and decent unemployment compensation; (near) universal and publicly provided health and social services coverage; low rates of poverty and wage disparities; and policies that support women's labor market participation and enforce shared responsibility of unpaid caregiving (dual-earner models) and adequate subsidies to single mothers and divorced women (Borrell et al., 2013). Although social democratic societies with universal, public, and comprehensive social security systems and strong unions, such as Sweden, experience less poverty and better health than less redistributive societies, class-based and other inequalities persist. Yet even those in the lowest economic stratum in social democratic countries fare better than those in

higher economic stratums in less redistributive societies (Mackenbach, 2015).

Though there is limited systematic research on these questions outside HICs, the experience of Cuba, Costa Rica, the state of Kerala (India), and Sri Lanka, among others, demonstrates links between welfare-state redistribution and equitable and favorable health outcomes. Debt-ridden LMICs face challenges in sustaining welfare states because of a combination of austerity policies, relatively few formal sector jobs (and large informal sectors contributing minimally to the tax base), weak internal revenue collection systems, and tax evasion by domestic and foreign businesses and wealthy individuals. Economies reliant on exports of primary products, for example through resource extraction – tied to the constraints of the global economic order – reinforce these patterns, underscoring the difficulties of sustaining universal welfare provisions in many LMICs (Martínez Franzoni & Sánchez-Ancochea, 2013).

Migration

In 2015, 244 million people – 3% of the global population – were international migrants, and another 740 million were internal migrants (International Organization for Migration, 2017). From Mexico to the Mediterranean, tens of thousands die along migrant routes every year (Migration Data Portal, 2019; United Nations High Commissioner for Refugees, 2019). In destination settings, many migrants experience racial and cultural discrimination, psychological stress, poor working conditions, underemployment, loss of family and social support, incarceration under inhumane conditions, and lack of political representation and social benefits, all translating into adverse health effects. In 2019, there were almost 80 million refugees and internally displaced persons forcibly uprooted by armed conflict, political persecution, livelihood loss, famine, and ecological disasters, leading to negative health outcomes, from physical and psychological trauma to nutritional deficiencies and waterborne diseases (Lori & Boyle, 2015; see also Chapter 22).

Poverty

Extreme poverty is characterized by very low income and lack of access to basic necessities – food, shelter, and water/sanitation. The World Bank (2019c) estimates that in 2015 10% of the world's population lived below the poverty line, which it defines as having under purchasing power parity (PPP)$1.9/day. This level is so low that it prevents satisfaction of the most basic needs of survival. A higher cutoff of PPP$10/day or more depending on the cost of living would better measure, and reveal much higher, destitution levels (Samman et al., 2013) and lend support to minimum/living-wage movements across the world.

Poverty affects health through multiple channels, including: material deprivation and lack of access to life necessities and opportunities; discrimination, social exclusion, and stress; and unhealthy coping behaviors (e.g., narcotics use). The relationship between income inequality and adverse health outcomes, including violence and homicide, is well established (Pickett & Wilkinson, 2015).

Although poverty is often gauged by low income, improving income does not directly address power inequities in terms of wealth distribution. For example, many governments implement cash transfer programs to raise the incomes of the poorest groups, helping lift people out of absolute poverty. However, oppressive structures of power often remain largely intact. As such, universal social policies – which are themselves both the result and the makings of greater equality in political power and wealth – are likely to have a far greater impact on health than income redistribution per se (Starfield & Birn, 2007).

Education

Education is associated with better health through channels that go beyond income effects. Social epidemiologists have shown that education: offers access to a greater range of employment possibilities at better pay (with higher likelihood of benefits, protection from workplace hazards, job security, and room for advancement); supports development of cognitive, coping, and emotional skills for decision making and the ability to take, or advocate for, health-promoting measures; enables young people to spend more time in school; and fosters social connections that confer health advantages via professional networks, neighborhood ties, political engagement, and other factors (Glymour, Avendano, & Kawachi, 2014).

Crucially, education can also help expand "democratic public life" (Giroux, 2010: 715) through its emancipatory potential – as Paulo Freire (2012 [1970]) puts it, education as the practice of freedom. But long-term underfunding of public education systems across the world has constrained realization of these goals. In many settings, austerity policies plague education budgets and promote privatization, limiting access to education and denying individuals and communities from attaining their fullest (health) potential.

Over 250 million children are deprived of education globally (United Nations Children's Fund [UNICEF], 2019). Widely enforced enrollment and school supply fees exclude millions of children and youth, especially girls and young women, from accessing education, whether public or private. For instance, Nigeria's public education system is in shambles, with 10.5 million children lacking access to basic education (UNICEF, 2017), while a flourishing private education sector caters to children from wealthier and privileged backgrounds (Imoka, 2019).

Employment and Work Conditions

The nature of work, its physical and psychosocial dimensions, structures of authority and control, and level of compensation and stability make work a key SDOH. Globally, in 2015, there were an estimated 374 million occupational injuries and more than 2.4 million occupational deaths from work-related injuries and diseases (Hamalainen, Takala, & Kiat, 2017). An additional 160 million cases of nonfatal job-related diseases add to the massive yearly occupational-related disease burden (International Labour Organization [ILO], 2015a). Dangerous sectors such as farming, construction, and coal mining (ILO, 2015b) have the least workers' compensation benefits and protection under occupational health and safety laws, further imperiling workers' health (Lucchini & London, 2014).

TNCs critically affect health both directly – through marketing of harmful products (e.g., unhealthy food/beverages), hazardous production processes, prohibitive pricing of health-enhancing products (e.g., pharmaceuticals) – and indirectly – through their impact on (lowering) tax revenues and (weakening) government regulations on worker, environmental, and consumer safety (Baum et al., 2016; Freudenberg, 2014).

In LMICs, special economic zones present a unique set of occupational hazards where workers are exposed to harmful ergonomic conditions (e.g., repetitive work and prolonged standing), noise pollution, excessive heat or cold, and/or toxic chemicals, dust, and fumes (De Neve & Prentice, 2017), exacerbated by booming export-led chemical, electronics, and biotechnology industries exposing workers to solvents, glues, and heavy metals without adequate safety measures or supervision. Such occupational exposures are associated with a rising incidence of diabetes, heart disease, cancer, and neurologic, endocrinologic, and mental disorders, as well as job-related disabilities (Berkman, Kawachi, & Theorell, 2014).

In addition to income, employment confers social protections such as health benefits, sickness and unemployment coverage, pensions, education, and training for advancement, as well as social networks and labor solidarity. Despite labor- and social movement–driven improvements in work conditions in some countries, across others there has been considerable deterioration in recent decades, with austerity crackdowns on unions and the constant threat of relocatation to lower-wage settings generating miserable pay, long hours, hazardous exposures, and few safety protections (Benach et al., 2014). Deleterious health effects are compounded where mechanisms are not in place to address gender-based, racial, ageist, ableist, and other forms of discrimination (Bambra, 2011).

Environmental Conditions

Environmental problems and their health consequences derive from two key processes: depletion and contamination. Depletion of water, forests, soil, and flora and fauna affects human health by reducing availability of and access to basic necessities such as drinking water and arable land and impeding livelihoods. Contamination of air, water, and soil, which occurs through industrial extraction, production, transport, and consumption, leads to exposure to a variety of harmful chemical, biological, and physical agents. Environmental changes are critically shaped by economic, social, and military activities (McNeill, 2000) and by climate change (Klein, 2014), with multifarious health consequences of environmental degradation (Perera & Nagaraj, 2017; see also Chapters 19 and 21).

Public Health and Medical Care

Public health activities span clean water provision, sanitation, safe refuse disposal, disease surveillance, housing regulations and inspection, maternal and child health programs, food safety, environmental and occupational protections, school health, and road safety, among others. Because public health's role in preventing adverse effects is most noticeable

when it falters, its visibility as a health determinant may be muted, even though, past and present, public health activities have contributed significantly to reductions in mortality. Indeed, primary healthcare and public health, integrated with and influenced by other determinants, have played a key role in up to half of infant mortality reductions over time (Macinko, Starfield, & Erinosho, 2009).

Curative medicine has also contributed, albeit less so, to mortality reductions, particularly through surgical interventions, antibiotics, and injury and emergency care. The healthcare system itself can promote (or jeopardize) health, depending on its accessibility and quality, how equitably it is financed and delivered, whether it inflicts harm or discriminates, how it interacts with local healers and healing beliefs, and the extent to which it prioritizes preventive services and public health over curative services (Loewenson & Gilson, 2012).

A misguided *over*emphasis on curative care runs the risk of channeling much-needed funds away from other social realms such as education, nutrition, housing, water, and sanitation to the multi-trillion-dollar healthcare industry. Indeed, this is one among many critiques of the SDG's UHC target, which aims to expand access to essential healthcare services of high quality to all without financial hardship (WHO, 2019b) but may well squeeze out investment in other key SDOH. Public health and medical care organizations and access are strongly affected by both national regulations, social protection policies, and global trade and investment rules (e.g., pharmaceuticals), as well as IFI and health and development agency pressures.

From Living Conditions to Embodied Influences

Living conditions encompass housing and neighborhoods, availability of potable water and safe sanitation, food quality and safety, access to social services, good-quality transportation, household roles, and related social stress (and its mitigators, including leisure). Various cultural and religious aspects of health, or other ways of being or living, intertwine with and affect health at household and community levels.

Housing and Neighborhoods

The features of people's immediate surroundings are among the most evident determinants of health. For instance, without adequate housing and access to clean water and plumbing, maintaining personal hygiene is extremely difficult. Availability of neighborhood resources for well-being is also key: day-care centers, schools, health and social services, parks/green spaces for safe physical activity, stores with affordable, healthy foods, transport, and recreation and community spaces.

Overcrowding and inadequate ventilation, food storage, and sanitation facilitate the spread of airborne, food- and waterborne, and skin ailments, including tuberculosis, diarrhea, lice, and scabies, as witnessed with persistent housing deficiencies in Canada's Inuit and First Nations communities (Webster, 2015). Flimsy housing structures provide little or no protection from storms, fires, and earthquakes, and recycled industrial materials and lead paint can cause fatal poisonings and severe neurologic and cognitive problems. These aspects also affect psychological well-being, health behaviors, and sleep, as well as school and work capacity.

Up to 1.6 billion people across the world are estimated to suffer from inadequate or unstable housing (Habitat for Humanity, 2015). Informal settlements (or "slums") have spread rapidly in the context of unplanned urbanization. In 2015–2016, an estimated 1 billion people, or one in eight people, lived in informal settlements, mostly on the outskirts of cities in Africa, Asia, Latin America, and the Pacific. Slum dwellers have little or no access to clean water, sanitation, and other public services, as well as, importantly, no security of land tenure (UN-Habitat, 2016). At press, COVID-19 is spreading rapidly across slums in India, where preventive measures such as hand washing and maintaining physical distance mean little because of limited access to water and cramped living conditions; the population density exceeds 250,000 persons per square kilometer in Mumbai's Dharavi, India's biggest slum (Yashoda, 2020).

An extreme housing concern, homelessness affects an estimated 100 million people globally (Habitat for Humanity, 2015). Homelessness "guesstimates" in LMICs go from less than 1% of the population in Paraguay to nearly 20% in Laos (United Nations Development Program, 2014). The problem is not confined to LMICs: in 2018, an estimated 550,000 persons were homeless in the United States, although the proportion of homeless people at any given time is far lower in HICs than in most LMICs (Organisation for Economic Co-operation and Development, 2020).

Even societies with extensive social services for the homeless – including free healthcare, accessible shelters, food banks, and employment training programs – cannot compensate for the health effects of not having a permanent home (Hwang et al., 2011). In many locales, homeless people are jailed or abused by the police. Children who live on the streets are subject to violence by shopkeepers, gangs, or government authorities. The desperate conditions of homelessness may lead to drug use, sex work, and deterioration of mental health, leading to death rates among homeless people up to 13 times higher than for others (Vuillermoz et al., 2014).

Beyond housing, neighborhoods and communities also shape health and health behaviors. Unhealthy activities, namely smoking, narcotics use, alcohol consumption, and poor diet, are influenced by people's surroundings, particularly marketing of/access to these substances, peer pressure, family and community behavior, the media, and absence of local resources to relieve stress and boredom, as well as broader SDOH. Other less tangible neighborhood features such as unemployment rates; crime; community solidarity; social, racial, and cultural tolerance; political empowerment; and civic engagement also critically affect health (Roux & Mair, 2010).

Water and Sanitation

Water is fundamental to life, yet over one-sixth of the world's population lives without an adequate supply of safe water. A third of the world's population (2.4 billion people, mostly in rural areas) lacks access to even the most basic sanitation and must resort to using pit latrines, fields, and ditches (UNICEF & WHO, 2015). Water- and sanitation-related illnesses kill at least 1.4 million people each year and are among the leading causes of preventable mortality and morbidity (Forouzanfar et al., 2015). Diarrheal disease alone accounts for 842,000 deaths annually, about half of them among children under five (UNICEF, 2018).

Women and girls, particularly within refugee or internally displaced populations, are disproportionately affected by poor water supply and sanitation. They typically bear responsibility for collecting water, often over great distances, and are subjected to injury from heavy loads and assault, jeopardizing school attendance and other activities. Girls are also more likely to stay away from school, particularly during menstruation, because of a lack of sanitation facilities (WaterAid, 2018).

Nutrition and Access to Food

A healthy diet is essential to child development and growth and to overall human flourishing. Feeding is foremost a family/household/community responsibility, yet it is profoundly shaped by national policies as well as global factors affecting land tenure and food production processes. While the idea of food security – as a means of addressing LMIC famines often through food aid that displaces local agricultural production – emerged in the 1970s, it refrained from addressing asymmetrical power and unfair global trade rules that jeopardize smallholders. The more recent concept and practice of food sovereignty, championed by La Via Campesina, stresses "the right of peoples to healthy and culturally appropriate food produced through ecologically sound and sustainable methods, and their right to define their own food and agriculture systems" (Declaration of Nyeleni, 2007: 1).

Today, nearly one-ninth of all people (roughly 820 million) are undernourished, with over double that number hungry (Food and Agriculture Organization, 2018; Hickel, 2016). In parallel, malnutrition is increasingly associated with chemically processed foods with high sugar and fat content, or "empty calories." These foods, because of agricultural subsidies and mass production predominantly in HICs, are widely available, cheaper than fresh produce and nutritional foods, and heavily marketed, including in LMICs (Rao et al., 2013).

Healthy food selection in stores is often limited and expensive in poor urban neighborhoods in HICs, whereas high-calorie and refined "junk food" is widely available and targeted at low-income communities with attendant problems of obesity, cardiovascular disease (CVD), certain cancers, dental caries, low-birth-weight babies, diabetes, and vitamin deficiencies (WHO, 2015). In the United States, increasing consumption of fruits and vegetables through reforms to improve access to nutritious foods, such as investments in grocery stores and farmers' markets, would prevent an estimated 120,000 deaths per year from CVD alone and save US$17 billion annually in medical costs (O'Hara, 2013).

Transport

Transport influences health through multiple mechanisms: road injuries and fatalities, poor air quality and related respiratory illness, interpersonal security, noise, cost, commuting time, and overall quality of life (Nieuwenhuijsen et al., 2016). Inadequate or unaffordable transport can affect school and work attendance and healthcare access, among other issues.

Most directly, road traffic collisions are a leading cause of death among young people (WHO, 2013). Traffic fatality and injury rates vary by SES and geography, with poor and working classes disproportionately affected especially in LMICs, where pedestrians constitute the bulk of those harmed. HICs have seen a steady decline in traffic fatalities since the 1970s – due to a combination of improved road and automobile safety, legal restrictions and sanctions, and trauma care – but LMICs have experienced significant increases. Much of the difference relates to safety measures, reflecting poor vehicle and road regulation in many LMICs.

Inadequate public transport systems have given rise to a constellation of other health problems in LMICs. Unplanned urbanization combined with increased vehicle ownership across South and Southeast Asian cities have resulted in severe traffic, lengthened commutes, and excessive air pollution (Verma & Kulshrestha, 2018).

Culture, Religion, and Health Practices

Culture is an oft-invoked determinant of health that is enormously complex (and thus necessarily oversimplified here). Referring to socially transmitted frameworks of meaning, culture is the basis for how people interpret and engage with the world (e.g., through day-to-day customs and dietary and sanitary rituals) through personal and collective experience. This may include specific ways in which health and illness are defined, understood, and addressed.

In some cultures, pregnancy is medicalized and treated as though it were a disease; in others, it is understood in spiritual or kinship terms. Among the Maya, a fever may be considered an ailment rather than a symptom; in wine-loving France, general malaise is frequently referred to as a "liver crisis"; and in the United States, chronic fatigue syndrome is characterized as afflicting young urban professionals working long hours. Even within a single cultural context, ways of viewing and addressing sickness and health may differ (Das, 2015).

Religion, which intersects with culture, also shapes health behavior, utilization of medical care, and understandings of well-being. Many religions call on prayer as a treatment, while others eschew medical care; Muslims and Jews practice circumcision; and Jehovah's Witnesses refuse blood transfusions. Practices of hygiene, diet, and end-of-life care also vary among Hindus, Buddhists, Christians, and adherents to other religions, with attendant health effects.

However, cultural and religious influences on health are often overemphasized or sensationalized by dominant actors, particularly when the illness and/or treatments are considered "exotic." For example, most HIV prevention work in Sub-Saharan Africa focuses on sexual practices, to the neglect of major structural issues such as poverty, migration, poor nutrition and housing, unsafe employment, and inadequate social services.

Embodiment (in Individual People) of Contexts, Characteristics, and Experiences

To recapitulate how these SDOH are intertwined, we next consider the convergence of various SDOH to make diabetes Mexico's leading cause of death and examine the influence of factors at multiple levels – from global trade to government policies, food sovereignty, and living and household conditions.

Two Faces of Malnutrition Driving Mexican Mortality

In a tragic twist, just a generation ago, Mexico's leading cause of death was malnutrition-related infant mortality. Since 2000, type 2 diabetes (linked to a different variant of malnutrition) has been Mexico's primary cause of death, soaring to over 100,000 fatalities per year. With one of the highest population prevalences in the world (Barquera et al., 2018), diabetes in Mexico is driven by widespread consumption of junk food, including soft drinks, fast food, and prepackaged energy-dense, low-nutrition foods.

Mexico's 1994 entry with the United States and Canada into the North American Free Trade Agreement (NAFTA) – liberalizing trade and investment – shepherded this transformation with the "opening" of Mexico's agriculture and food markets. Corn subsidies in the United States artificially lowered prices (and expanded the US share of the global market), while simultaneously in Mexico, NAFTA-driven export-oriented agribusiness massively displaced small farms unable to compete with cheap imports. This created a new dependency on imported maize, wheat, and other essential foodstuffs (Otero, 2011). As a result, the traditional (and nutritionally ideal) Aztec/Nahuatl diet of corn tortillas, beans, chilies, and other fresh vegetables and fruits became less accessible, violating principles of food sovereignty even as food insecurity was addressed at some level among Indigenous and low-income populations, as processed foods became more available and affordable.

NAFTA's removal of domestic agriculture protections caused the agricultural labor force in Mexico to fall by 1.8 million people between 1998 and 2007. Failure to absorb this labor force into other sectors accelerated rural-urban migration (initially to deregulated factory work in border areas) and undocumented migration to the United States, causing Mexico to increasingly rely on migrant remittances and thereby lose its "labor sovereignty" (Otero, 2011: 391).

As small farmers went out of business and traditional foods became more expensive, "Big Food" foreign direct investment (FDI) poured into Mexico by the billions. By the early 2000s, processed foods accounted for about three-quarters of total FDI. Massive food retailing and marketing expanded distribution of (and demand for) these unhealthy foods through chain supermarkets and small convenience stores (or *tiendas*), easing Big Food's infiltration of Mexico's small towns and outskirt communities. Consequently, consumption of processed foods and beverages soared (Hawkes, 2006). Migration also played a role, because remittances enabled the purchase of TNC-marketed foods, leading to higher obesity rates (Riosmena et al., 2012).

To add insult to injury (or disease, in terms of diabetes), the continued poor quality of the water supply, despite official figures to the contrary (Stigler-Granados et al., 2014), has made sugar-laden soft drinks a cheaper, more accessible (and addictive), and safer option in the short run (at least relating to bacterial content) than piped water in much of Mexico. Not only are sweeteners (ironically largely corn based and grown in the United States) in soft drinks symbolic of the displacement of local crops and diet, but they are also a key factor leading to diabetes, as are sugars, independent of overweight and obesity (Basu et al., 2013).

Clearly, the diabetes crisis in Mexico is neither solely a function of biomedical factors nor simply attributable to unhealthy food and beverage choices, as per the behavioral model. Based on the psychosocial model, unhealthy behaviors are triggered by the environment of many low-income Mexicans: increasing violence, economic insecurity, and deteriorating living conditions. Accordingly, cheap and widely available junk food (not requiring time and resources of fuel, a kitchen, etc. for food preparation) and soft drinks became both attractive and convenient.

A critical political economy model highlights how the needs of the majority of Mexicans have been politically trumped by domestic elites and foreign interests, with NAFTA opening the floodgates to FDI penetration by food and beverage TNCs into Mexican markets. To this analysis, ecosocial theory adds an understanding of how diabetes has become metabolically and physiologically inscribed on the bodies of tens of millions of Mexicans, not abstractly, but concretely and intergenerationally, under historical and contemporary social relations of power.

Conclusion: What Is to Be Done?

Viewed through a lens of SDOH, health and illness result from an interdependent set of political, economic, and social forces operating at multiple levels. Despite this reality, health promotion policies mostly emphasize behavior change at the individual level, presuming that better knowledge influences attitudes and motivates behavioral change. Indeed, carried out in a vacuum, without understanding and addressing the interlinked "causes of the causes of the causes," a behavioral policy approach can yield very little (Mackenzie et al., 2016).

In bringing critical political economy and ecosocial theories to fruition, various generic and global strategies merit attention. At the micro level, people and communities could be mobilized to advocate for social spending *as* health spending. Healthcare providers could be trained to see beyond a person's presenting problem to consider the conditions in which they live, love, work, and play. Public health efforts could emphasize a range of collective protections, with favorable SDOH serving as a gauge of healthy societies. Government policy, at the fulcrum of SDOH, could be held to account to alleviate poverty through broad tax redistribution and social welfare policies and profoundly addressing discrimination (Krieger, 2007). At the global level, struggles around equitable systems of trade, investment, environmental protection, taxation, and other forms of socially just governance must take precedence over business interests, focusing on fair distribution of political and economic power.

Notwithstanding ample and growing evidence about health inequities and their link to SDOH, too few societies use this knowledge to shape social and economic policies. Whether this is because the evidence is not credible to policymakers or because the evidence that "counts" simply does not delve into these questions, changing the status quo challenges deeply entrenched interests and ideological positions: those wielding power remain unwilling to seriously consider changing societal patterns of distribution. These are fundamentally *political* issues: whether societies adopt solidarity or retain skewed power arrangements as an organizing principle has repercussions for virtually every aspect of life. Social movements that battle for healthy and just social policies and against power asymmetries at local, national, and global levels can play a meaningful role in pushing governments and other societal institutions to reduce health inequity, but responsibility and accountability also rest with elected officials and international agencies.

References

Austin, K. F., DeSciscicolo, C., and Samuelsen, L. (2016). The failures of privatization: a comparative investigation of tuberculosis rates and the structure of healthcare in less-developed nations, 1995–2010. *World Development*, **78**, 450–460.

Australian Institute of Health and Welfare (AIHW). (2019). *Deaths in Australia*. AIHW, July 17 (online). Available at www.aihw.gov.au/reports/life-expectancy-death/deaths-in-australia/contents/life-expectancy.

Bailey, Z. D., & Moon, J. R. (2020). Racism and the political economy of COVID-19: will we continue to resurrect the past? *Journal of Health Politics, Policy and Law*. DOI:https://doi.org/10.1215/03616878-8641481 (accessed June 22, 2020).

Baker, B. K. (2010). The impact of the International Monetary Fund's macroeconomic policies on the AIDS pandemic. *International Journal of Health Services*, **40**(2), 347–363.

Bambra, C. (2011). *Work, Worklessness, and the Political Economy of Health*. New York: Oxford University Press.

Barquera, S., Schillinger, D., Aguilar-Salinas, C.A., et al. (2018). Collaborative research and actions on both sides of the US-Mexico border to counteract type 2 diabetes in people of Mexican origin. *Global Public Health*, **14**(1), 84.

Basu, S., Yoffe, P., Hills, N., et al. (2013). The relationship of sugar to population-level diabetes prevalence: an econometric analysis of repeated cross-sectional data. *PLoS One*, **8**(2), e57873.

Baum, F. E., Sanders, D. M., Fisher, M., et al. (2016). Assessing the health impact of transnational corporations: its importance and a framework. *Globalization and Health*, **12**(27), 1–7.

Beckfield, J., Bambra, C., Eikemo, T. A., et al. (2015). An institutional theory of welfare state effects on the distribution of population health. *Social Theory and Health*, **13**(3), 227–244.

Benach, J., Vives, A., Amable, M., et al. (2014). Precarious employment: understanding an emerging social determinant of health. *Annual Review of Public Health*, **35**, 229–253.

Benatar, D. (2012). *The Second Sexism: Discrimination against Men and Boys*. Chichester, UK: Wiley.

Bergad, L. (2007). *The Comparative Histories of Slavery in Brazil, Cuba, and the United States*. Cambridge, UK: Cambridge University Press.

Berkman, L. F., & Kawachi, I. (2014). A historical framework for social epidemiology: social determinants of population health, in Berkman, L. F., Kawachi, I., & Glymour, M. M. (eds.), *Social Epidemiology*, 2nd ed. New York: Oxford University Press, pp. 1–16.

Berkman, L. F., Kawachi, I., & Theorell, T. (2014). Working conditions and health, in Berkman, L. F., Kawachi, I., and Glymour, M. M. (eds.), *Social Epidemiology*, 2nd ed. New York: Oxford University Press, pp. 153–181.

Bhambra, G. K., & Holmwood, J. (2018). Colonialism, postcolonialism and the liberal welfare state. *New Political Economy*, **23**(5), 574–587.

Birn, A. E. (2009). Making it politic(al): Closing the Gap in a Feneration – health equity through action on the social determinants of health. *Social Medicine*, **4**(3), 166–182.

Black, S. D., & Research Working Group (Morris, J. N., Smith, C., & Townsend, P.) (1980). *Inequalities in Health: Report of a Research Working Group*. London: Department of Health and Social Security.

Bond, P., & Browder, L. (2019). Deracialized nostalgia, reracialized community, and truncated gentrification: capital and cultural flows in Richmond, Virginia, and Durban, South Africa. *Journal of Cultural Geography*, **36**(2), 211–245.

Borrell, C., Palència, L., Muntaner, C., et al. (2013). Influence of macrosocial policies on women's health and gender inequalities in health. *Epidemiologic Reviews*, **36**, 31–48.

Braveman, P. (2014). What is health equity: and how does a life-course approach take us further toward it? *Maternal and Child Health Journal*, **18**(2), 366–372.

Braveman, P., Heck, K., Egerter, S., et al. (2015). The role of socioeconomic factors in black–white disparities in preterm birth. *American Journal of Public Health*, **105**(4), 694–702.

Breilh, J.(2013). La determinación social de la salud como herramienta de transformación hacia una nueva salud pública (salud colectiva). *Revista Facultad Nacional de Salud Pública*, **31**(suppl. 1), 13–27.

Bryce, P. (1922). *The Story of a National Crime, Being an Appeal for Justice to the Indians of Canada: The Wards of the Nation, Our Allies in the Revolutionary War, Our Brothers-in-Arms in the Great War*. Ottawa: J. Hope.

Butler, J. (1990). *Gender Trouble: Feminism and the Subversion of Identity*. New York: Routledge.

Canadian Institute for Health Information (2019). *Life Expectancy at Birth* (online). Available at https://your healthsystem.cihi.ca/hsp/inbrief?lang=en#!/indicators/011/life-expectancy-at-birth/;mapC1;mapLevel2;/.

Coburn, D. (2011). Global health: a political economy of historical trends and contemporary inequalities, in Teeple, G., & McBride, S. (eds.), *Relations of Global Power: Neoliberal Order and Disorder*. Toronto: University of Toronto Press, pp. 118–151.

Connell, R. (2012). Gender, health and theory: conceptualizing the issue, in local and world perspective. *Social Science and Medicine*, **74**(11), 1675–1683.

Crammond, B. R., & Carey, G. (2016). Policy change for the social determinants of health: the strange irrelevance of social epidemiology. *Evidence and Policy: A Journal of Research, Debate and Practice* (epub ahead of publication).

Crenshaw, K. (1991). Mapping the margins: intersectionality, identity politics, and violence against women of color. *Stanford Law Review*, **43**(6), 1241–1299.

Czyzewski, K. (2011). Colonialism as a broader social determinant of health. *The International Indigenous Policy Journal*, **2**(1).

Das, V. (2015). *Affliction: Health, Disease, Poverty*. New York: Fordham University Press.

de Andrade, L. O. M., Pellegrini, A., Solar, O., et al. (2015). Social determinants of health, universal health coverage, and sustainable development: case studies from Latin American countries. *Lancet*, **385**(9975), 1343–1351.

Declaration of Nyeleni (2007). Available at https://nyeleni.org/IMG/pdf/DeclNyeleni-en.pdf.

De Neve, G., & Prentice, R. (2017). Introduction: rethinking garment workers' health and safety, in Prentice, R., & De Neve, G. (eds.), *Unmaking the Global Sweatshop: Health and Safety of the Worlds' Garment Workers*. Philadelphia: University of Pennsylvania Press, pp. 1–25.

Domingues, R., Viellas, E. F., Dias, M. A. B., et al. (2015). Adequacy of prenatal care according to maternal characteristics in Brazil. *Revista Panamericana de Salud Pública*, **37**(3), 140–147.

Dorling, D. (2015). *All That Is Solid. How the Great Housing Disaster Defines Our Times, and What We Can Do About It*. London: Penguin UK.

Economic Commission for Latin America and the Caribbean (2014). *Guaranteeing Indigenous People's Rights in Latin America: Progress in the Past Decade and Remaining Challenges (English Summary)*. Santiago, Chile: ECLAC.

Epstein, G. (2005). *Financialization and the World Economy*. Cheltenham, UK: Edward Elgar Publishing.

European Commission (2014). *Roma Health Report: Health Status of the Roma Population. Data Collection in the Member States of the European Union*. Brussels: European Commission.

Ezeh, A., Oyebode, O., Satterthwaite, D., et al. (2017). The history, geography, and sociology of slums and the health problems of people who live in slums. *Lancet*, **389**(10068), 547–558.

Fine, B. (2012). Financialization and social policy, in Utting, P., Razavi, S., & Buchholz, R. V. (eds.), *The Global Crisis and Transformative Social Change*. London: Palgrave Macmillan, pp. 103–122.

Food and Agriculture Organization (2018). *The State of Food Security and Nutrition in the World: Building Climate Resilience for Food Security and Nutrition*. Rome: FAO.

Forouzanfar, M. H., Alexander, L., Anderson, H. R., et al. (2015). Global, regional, and national comparative risk assessment of 79 behavioural, environmental and occupational, and metabolic risks or clusters of risks in 188 countries, 1990–2013: a systematic analysis for the Global Burden of Disease Study 2013. *Lancet*, **386**(10010), 2287–2323.

Freire, P. (2012 [1970]). *Pedagogy of the Oppressed*. New York: Bloomsbury Academic.

Freudenberg, N. (2014). *Lethal but Legal: Corporations, Consumption, and Protecting Public Health*. New York: Oxford University Press.

Ganatra, D., Gerdts, C., Rossier, C., et al. (2017). Global, regional, and subregional classification of abortions by safety, 2010–2014: estimates from a Bayesian hierarchical model. *Lancet*, **390**(10110), 2372–2381.

Giroux, H. (2010). Rethinking education as the practice of freedom: Paulo Freire and the promise of critical pedagogy, *Policy Futures in Education*, **8**(6), 715–721.

Glymour, M. M., Avendano, M., & Kawachi, I. (2014). Socioeconomic status and health, in Berkman, L. F., Kawachi, I., & Glymour, M. M. (eds.), *Social Epidemiology*, 2nd ed. New York: Oxford University Press, pp. 17–62.

Gloyd, S. (1987). Child survival and resource scarcity. Paper presented at the International Congress of the World Federation of Public Health Associations, Mexico City. March 1987.

Gnan, G. H., Rahman, Q., Ussher, G., et al. (2019). General and LGBTQ-specific factors associated with mental health and suicide risk among LGBTQ students. *Journal of Youth Studies* **22**(10), 1393–1408.

Habitat for Humanity (2015). *World Habitat Day 2015 Key Housing Facts* (online). Available at www.habitat.org/getinv/events/world-habitat-day/housing-facts.

Hamalainen, P., Takala, J., & Kiat, T. B. (2017). *Global Estimates of Occupational Accidents and Work-Related Illness 2017*. Singapore: Workplace Safety and Health Institute (online). Available at www.icohweb.org/site/images/news/pdf/Report%20Global%20Estimates%20of%20Occupational%20Accidents%20and%20Work-related%20Illnesses%202017%20rev1.pdf.

Harris, R., Cormack, D., Tobias, M., et al. (2012). The pervasive effects of racism: experiences of racial discrimination in New Zealand over time and associations with multiple health domains. *Social Science and Medicine*, **74**(3), 408–415.

Harvey, D. (2006). *Spaces of Global Capitalism: Towards a Theory of Uneven Geographical Development*. London: Verso.

Harvey, D. (2010). *The Enigma of Capital*. New York: Oxford University Press.

Hawkes, C. (2006). Uneven dietary development: linking the policies and processes of globalization with the nutrition transition, obesity and diet-related chronic diseases. *Globalization and Health*, **2**(1), 4.

Hickel, J. (2016). The true extent of global poverty and hunger: questioning the good news narrative of the Millennium Development Goals. *Third World Quarterly*, **37**(5), 749–767.

Holla, R., & Ittyerah, A. (2018). Agricultural crisis in India and its impact on nutrition. *World Nutrition*, **9**(3), 292–313.

Hunter, B. M., & Murray, S. F., 2019. Deconstructing the financialization of healthcare. *Development and Change*, **50**(5), 1263–1287.

Hwang, S. W., Gogosis, E., Chambers, C., et al. (2011). Health status, quality of life, residential stability, substance use, and healthcare utilization among adults applying to a supportive housing program. *Journal of Urban Health*, **88**(6), 1076–1090.

Imoka, C. (2019). A decolonial analysis of student success in Nigerian secondary schools. PhD dissertation, University of Toronto.

International Labour Organization (2015a). *Global Trends on Occupational Accidents and Diseases*. World Day for Safety and Health at Work, April 28 (online). Available at www.ilo.org/legacy/english/osh/en/story_content/external_files/fs_st_1-ILO_5_en.pdf.

International Labour Organization (2015b). *Hazardous work* (online). Available at www.ilo.org/safework/areasofwork/hazardous-work/lang–en/index.htm.

International Organization for Migration. (2017). *World Migration Report 2018*. Available at www.iom.int/sites/default/files/country/docs/china/r5_world_migration_report_2018_en.pdf.

Jacob, C., Baird, J., Barker, M., et al. (n.d). *The Importance of a Life Course Approach to Health: Chronic Disease Risk from Preconception through Adolescence and Adulthood* (online). Available at www.who.int/life-course/publications/life-course-approach-to-health.pdf.

Kapilashrami, A., Hill, S., & Meer, N. (2015). What can health inequalities researchers learn from an intersectionality perspective? Understanding social dynamics with an inter-categorical approach? *Social Theory and Health* 13, 288–307.

Klein, N. (2014). *This Changes Everything: Capitalism vs. the Climate*. New York: Simon & Schuster.

Krieger, N. (2007). Why epidemiologists cannot afford to ignore poverty. *Epidemiology*, **18**(6), 658–663.

Krieger, N. (2008). Proximal, distal, and the politics of causation: what's level got to do with it? *American Journal of Public Health*, **98**(2), 221–230.

Krieger, N. (2011). *Epidemiology and the People's Health: Theory and Context*. New York: Oxford University Press.

Krieger, N., Chen, J. T., Coull, B., et al. (2013). The unique impact of abolition of Jim Crow laws on reducing inequities in infant death rates and implications for choice of comparison groups in analyzing societal determinants of health. *American Journal of Public Health*, **103**(12), 2234–2244.

Krieger, N. (2014a). Discrimination and health inequities. *International Journal of Health Services*, **44**(4), 643–710.

Krieger, N. (2014b). Got theory? On the 21st c. CE rise of explicit use of epidemiologic theories of disease distribution: a review and ecosocial analysis. *Current Epidemiology Reports* 1(1), 45–56.

Kubzansky, L.D., Winning, A., & Kawachi, I. (2014). Affective states and health, in Berkman, L. F., Kawachi, I., & Glymour, M. M. (eds.), *Social Epidemiology*, 2nd ed. New York: Oxford University Press, pp. 320–364.

Loewenson, R., & Gilson, L. (2012). The health system and wider social determinants of health, in Smith, R. D., & Hanson, K. (eds.), *Health Systems in Low-and Middle-Income Countries: An Economic and Policy Perspective*. New York: Oxford University Press, pp. 219–242.

Lori, J. R., & Boyle, J. S. (2015). Forced migration: health and human rights issues among refugee populations. *Nursing Outlook*, 63(1):68–76.

Lucchini, R. G., & London, L. (2014). Global occupational health: current challenges and the need for urgent action. *Annals of Global Health*, 80(4):251–256.

Macinko, J., Starfield, B., & Erinosho, T. (2009). The impact of primary healthcare on population health in low- and middle-income countries. *Journal of Ambulatory Care Management*, 32(2), 150–171.

Mackenbach, J. P. (2015). Socioeconomic inequalities in health in high-income countries: the facts and the options, in Detels, R., Gulliford, M., Karim, Q. A., & Tan, C. C. (eds), *Oxford Textbook of Global Public Health*. New York: Oxford University Press.

Mackenzie, M., Collins, C., Connolly, J., et al. (2017). Working-class discourses of politics, policy and health: "I don't smoke; I don't drink. The only thing wrong with me is my health." *Policy & Politics*, **45**(2), 231–249.

Marmot, M. G. (2005). The social determinants of health inequalities. *Lancet*, **365**(9464), 1099–1104.

Marmot, M., & Brunner, E. (2005). Cohort profile: the Whitehall II study. *International Journal of Epidemiology*, **34**(2), 251–256.

Martínez Franzoni, J., & Sánchez-Ancochea, D. (2013). Can Latin American production regimes complement universalistic welfare regimes? Implications from the Costa Rican case. *Latin American Research Review*, **48**(2):148–173.

Mathews, T. J., MacDorman, M. F., & Thoma, M. E. (2015). Infant mortality statistics from the 2013 period linked birth/infant death data set. *National Vital Statistics Reports*, **64**(9):1–30.

Mawani, F. (2019). Conceptualization, measurement, and association of underemployment to mental health inequities between immigrant and Canadian-born labour force participants. PhD dissertation, University of Toronto.

McEvoy, C., & Hide, G. (2017). *Global Violent Deaths 2017: Time to Decide*. Geneva: Small Arms Survey (online). Available at www.smallarmssurvey.org/fileadmin/docs/U-Reports/SAS-Report-GVD2017.pdf.

McNeill, J. R. (2000). *Something New Under the Sun: An Environmental History of the Twentieth-Century World* (The Global Century Series). New York: W.W. Norton.

Migration Data Portal (2019). *Migration Deaths and Disappearances* (online). Available at www.unhcr.org/desperatejourneys/.

National Geographic (2018). If you're an average American, you'll live to be 78.6 years old (online). Available at www.nationalgeographic.com/culture/2018/12/life-expectancy-united-states/.

National Inquiry into Murdered and Missing Indigenous Women and Girls (2019). Executive Summary of the Final Report: National Inquiry into Missing and Murdered Indigenous Women and Girls (online). Available at www.mmiwg-ffada.ca/wp-content/uploads/2019/06/Executive_Summary.pdf.

Ng, E., & Muntaner, C. (2014). A critical approach to macrosocial determinants of population health: engaging scientific realism and incorporating social conflict. *Current Epidemiology Reports*, 1(1), 27–37.

Nieuwenhuijsen, M. J., Khreis, H., Verlinghieri, E., & Rojas-Rueda, D. (2016). Transport and health: a marriage of convenience or an absolute necessity. *Environment International* 88, 150–152.

O'Hara, J. (2013). *The $11 Trillion Reward: How Simple Dietary Changes Can Save Lives and Money, and How We Get There.* Cambridge, UK: Union of Concerned Scientists.

Organisation for Economic Co-operation and Development (2015). *OECD Income Distribution Database (IDD): Gini, Poverty, Income, Methods and Concepts* (online). Available at www.oecd.org/social/income-distribution-database.htm (accessed July 16, 2015).

Organisation for Economic Co-operation and Development (2020). *Homeless Population* (online). Available at www.oecd.org/els/family/HC3-1-Homeless-population.pdf.

Otero, G. (2011). Neoliberal globalization, NAFTA, and migration: Mexico's loss of food and labor sovereignty. *Journal of Poverty*, **15**(4), 384–402.

Oxfam (2018). *Ripe for Change: Ending Human Suffering in Supermarket Supply Chains.* Oxfam GB, Oxford, UK (online). Available at www-cdn.oxfam.org/s3fs-public/file_attachments/cr-ripe-for-change-supermarket-supply-chains-210618-en.pdf.

Oxfam. (2019). *False Promises.* Oxfam GB, Oxford, UK (online). Available at https://oxfamilibrary.openrepository.com/bitstream/handle/10546/620720/bp-world-bank-education-ppps-090419-summ-en.pdf.

Paradies, Y., Ben, J., Denson, N., et al. (2015). Racism as a determinant of health: a systematic review and meta-analysis. *PLoS One*, **10**(9), e0138511.

Perera, I., & Nagaraj, V. (2017). The Meethotamulla tragedy: the face, not failure, of development. Groundviews, April 18 (online). Available at https://groundviews.org/2017/04/18/the-meethotamulla-tragedy-the-face-not-failure-of-development/.

Pickett, K. E., & Wilkinson, R. G. (2015). Income inequality and health: a causal review. *Social Science & Medicine*, **128**, 316–326.

Potente, C., & Monden, C. (2018). Disability pathways preceding death in England by socio-economic status. *Population Studies*, **72**(2), 175–190.

Raifman, J. (2018). Sanctioned stigma in health care settings and harm to LGBT youth. *JAMA Pediatr*, **172**(8), 713–714.

Rao, M., Afshin, A., Singh, G., et al. (2013). Do healthier foods and diet patterns cost more than less healthy options? A systematic review and meta-analysis. *BMJ Open*, **3**(12), e004277.

Reddy, D. N., and Mishra, S. (eds.) (2010). *Agrarian Crisis in India.* New Delhi: Oxford University Press.

Reverby, S. (2012). Ethical failures and history lessons: the US Public Health Service research studies in Tuskegee and Guatemala. *Public Health Reviews*, **34**(1), 1–18.

Riosmena, F., Frank, R., Akresh, I. R., & Kroeger, R. A. (2012). US migration, translocality, and the acceleration of the nutrition transition in Mexico. *Annals of the Association of American Geographers*, **102**(5), 1209–1218.

Roeder, A. (2019). America is failing black mothers. *Harvard Public Health* (Winter) (online). Available at www.hsph.harvard.edu/magazine/magazine_article/america-is-failing-its-black-mothers/.

Rose, G., & Marmot, M. G. (1981). Social class and coronary heart disease. *British Heart Journal*, **45**(1), 13–19.

Roux, A. V., & Mair, C. (2010). Neighborhoods and health. *Annals of the New York Academy of Sciences*, **1186**(1), 125–145.

Ruckert, A., & Labonté, R. (2014). The social determinants of health, in Brown, G. W., Yamey, G., & Wamala, S. (eds.), *The Handbook of Global Health Policy.* Hoboken, NJ: Wiley, pp. 267–285.

Samman, E., Ravallion, M., Pritchett, L., et al. (2013). Eradicating global poverty: a noble goal, but how do we measure it?. ODI Working Paper No. 2, Overseas Development Institute, London (online). Available at www.odi.org/sites/odi.org.uk/files/odi-assets/publications-opinion-files/8440.pdf.

Schrecker, T., & Bambra, C. (2015). *How Politics Makes Us Sick: Neoliberal Epidemics.* London: Palgrave Macmillan.

Sehgal, M., & Krishnan, A. (2013). *Indoor Air Pollution and Child Health in India: Child Poverty Insights.* New York: UNICEF.

Singh, A., Shukla, A., Ram, F., et al. (2017). Trends in inequality in length of life in India: a decomposition analysis by age and causes of death. *Genus*, **73**(1), 5.

Spreen, A., & Kamat, S. (2018). From billionaires to the bottom billion: who's making education policy for the poor in emerging economies?, in Steiner-Khamsi, G., & Draxler, A. (eds.), *The State, Business and Education: Public Private Partnerships Revised.* Cheltenham, UK: Edward Elgar Publishing, pp. 106–130.

Sproule-Jones, M. (1996). Crusading for the forgotten: Dr. Peter Bryce, public health, and prairie Native residential schools. *Canadian Bulletin of Medical History*, **13**, 199–224.

Starfield, B., & Birn, A.-E. (2007). Income redistribution is not enough: income inequality, social welfare programs, and achieving equity in health. *Journal of Epidemiology and Community Health*, **61**(12), 1038–1041.

Stigler-Granados, P., Quintana, P. J., Gersberg, R., et al. (2014). Comparing health outcomes and point-of-use water quality in two rural Indigenous communities of Baja California, Mexico before and after receiving new potable water infrastructure. *Journal of Water Sanitation and Hygiene for Development*, **4**(4), 672–680.

Stockholm International Peace Research Institute (2019). *World Military Expenditure Grows to $1.8 Trillion in 2018.* April 29 (online). Available at www.sipri.org/media/press-release/2019/world-military-expenditure-grows-18-trillion-2018.

Stubbs T., Kentikelenis, A., Stuckler, D., et al. (2017). The impact of IMF conditionality on government health expenditure: a cross-national analysis of 16 West African nations. *Social Science and Medicine*, **174**, 220–227.

Taylor, K.-Y. (2016). *From #Black Lives Matter to Black Liberation*. Chicago: Haymarket Books.

Thrasher, S. W. (2015). Income inequality happens by design: we can't fix it by tweaking capitalism. *The Guardian*, December 5. Available at www .theguardian.com/commentisfree/2015/dec/05/income-inequality-policy-capitalism.

Travis, J., Western, B., & Redburn, S. (2014). *The Growth of Incarceration in the United States: Exploring Causes and Consequences*. Washington, DC: National Research Council.

Truth and Reconciliation Commission of Canada (2015). *Honouring the Truth, Reconciling for the Future: Summary of the Final Report of the Truth and Reconciliation Commission of Canada*. Winnipeg: Truth and Reconciliation Commission.

United Nations Children's Fund (2017). *Education*. (online). Available at www.unicef.org/nigeria/education.

United Nations Children's Fund (2018). *Diarrhoeal Disease*. (online). Available at https://data.unicef.org/topic/child-health/diarrhoeal-disease/#more–1517.

United Nations Children's Fund (2019). *Annual Report 2018* (online). Available at www.unicef.org/media/55486/file/UNICEF-annual-report-2018%20revised%201.pdf.

United Nations Children's Fund (UNICEF) & World Health Organization (WHO) (2015). *Progress on Sanitation and Drinking Water: 2015 Update and MDG Assessment*. Geneva: WHO.

United Nations Department of Social and Economic Affairs (UN-DESA) (2015). *State of the World's Indigenous Peoples, 2015*, Vol. 2, *Indigenous Peoples' Access to Health Services*. New York: Department of Economic and Social Affairs of the United Nations.

United Nations Department of Social and Economic Affairs (UN-DESA) (2018). *2018 Revision of World Urbanization Prospects*, May 16 (online). Available at www.un.org/development/desa/publications/2018-revision-of-world-urbanization-prospects.html.

United Nations Development Program (2014). *Human Development Report 2014. Sustaining Human Progress: Reducing Vulnerabilities and Building Resilience*. New York: United Nations Development Program.

UN-Habitat (2016). *Urbanization and Development: Emerging Futures World Cities Report 2016* (online). Available at https://new.unhabitat.org/sites/default/files/download-manager-files/WCR-2016-WEB.pdf.

United Nations High Commissioner for Refugees. (2019). *Desperate Journeys: Refugees and migrants arriving in Europe and at Europe's borders* (online). Available at www .unhcr.org/desperatejourneys/.

United States Census Bureau (n.d.). *Quick Facts: Mississippi*. Washington, DC: US Department of Commerce (online). Available at www.census.gov/quickfacts/fact/table/MS/BZA115216.

Verma, K., & Kulshrestha, U. (2018). Feasible mitigation options for air pollution and traffic congestion in metro cities. *Journal of Indian Geophysical Union*, **22**, 212–218.

Villarosa, L. (2018). Why America's black mothers and babies are in a life-or-death crisis. *New York Times Magazine*, April 11 (online). Available at www.nytimes.com/2018/04/11/magazine/black-mothers-babies-death-maternal-mortality.html.

Vuillermoz, C., Aouba, A., Grout, L., et al. (2014). Estimating the number of homeless deaths in France, 2008–2010. *BMC Public Health*, **14**(1), 690.

Walmsley, R. (2018). *World Prison Population List*, 12th ed. London: Institute for Criminal Policy Research.

Walters, K. L., Mohammed, S. A., Evans-Campbell, T., et al. (2011). Bodies don't just tell stories, they tell histories. *Du Bois Review: Social Science Research on Race*, **8**(1), 179–189.

WaterAid (2018). *Better Toilets, Accurate Information about Periods Crucial to Keeping Girls in School*, May 23 (online). Available at www.wateraid.org/au/articles/better-toilets-accurate-information-about-periods-crucial-to-keeping-girls-in-school.

Webster, P. C. (2015). Housing triggers health problems for Canada's First Nations. *Lancet* **385**(9967):495–496.

World Health Organization (WHO) (2012). *Unsafe Abortion Incidence and Mortality*. (online). Available at https://apps.who.int/iris/bitstream/handle/10665/75173/WHO_RHR_12.01_eng.pdf;jsessionid=BA2671ABBA1C0891FD5223EC89359E07?sequence=1.

World Health Organization (WHO) (2013). *Global Status Report on Road Safety 2013: Supporting a Decade of Action*. Geneva: World Health Organization.

World Health Organization (WHO) (2015). *Healthy Diet: Fact Sheet* (online). Available at www.who.int/mediacentre/factsheets/fs394/en/.

World Health Organization (WHO) (2019a). *World Health Statistics 2019* (online). Available at https://apps.who.int/iris/bitstream/handle/10665/324835/9789241565707-eng.pdf?ua=1.

World Health Organization (WHO) (2019b). *SDG 3: Ensure Healthy Lives and Promote Wellbeing for All at All Ages*. Sustainable Development Goals (online). Available at www .who.int/sdg/targets/en/.

World Health Organization Commission on Social Determinants of Health (2008). *Closing the Gap in a Generation* (online). Available at https://apps.who.int/iris/bitstream/handle/10665/43943/9789241563703_eng.pdf;jsessionid=80E4AAFACD619BC0CCA550B9B1FFB62D?sequence=1.

World Bank (2019a). *Life Expectancy at Birth, Total (Years)* (online). Available at https://data.worldbank.org/indicator/sp.dyn.le00.in.

World Bank (2019b). *GNI per Capita, Atlas Method (Current US$)* (online). Available at https://data.worldbank.org/indicator/ny.gnp.pcap.cd.

World Bank (2019c). *Poverty* (online). Available at www.worldbank.org/en/topic/poverty/overview.

Yashoda, V (2020). COVID-19 comes to Asia's most densely populated slum (online). Available at https://thediplomat.com/2020/04/covid-19-comes-to-asias-most-densely-populated-slum/.

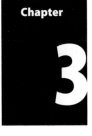

Strengthening the Global Response to Infectious Disease Threats in the Twenty-First Century, with a COVID-19 Epilogue*

David E. Bloom and Daniel Cadarette

Introduction

In 1918, as the First World War was winding to a close, a mysterious disease that left victims blue in the face and gasping for air tore through the trenches crisscrossing Europe and traversed the oceans, stowed away on warships. By the time the so-called Spanish flu had run its course in 1920, the pandemic had infected more than a quarter of the world's population and resulted in some 30 million to 100 million deaths (Patterson & Pyle, 1991; Johnson & Mueller, 2002). In comparison, the two world wars are estimated to have killed roughly 77 million combined (*The Economist*, 2018). By any measure, the 1918 flu pandemic was one of the worst catastrophes of the twentieth century.

In the 100 years that have passed since the Spanish flu first besieged the world, no pandemic has approached its magnitude of fatality over such a short period. Humanity's relative good fortune with respect to infectious disease can be attributed, in part, to the elaborate global health system the world has gradually developed as an attempted bulwark against infectious disease threats, both known and unknown. This system consists of various formal and informal networks of organizations that serve different stakeholders; have varying goals, modalities, resources, and accountability; operate at different territorial levels (i.e., local, national, regional, or global);

and cut across the public, private-for-profit, and private-not-for-profit sectors.

Despite its track record, whether the global health system as currently constituted can provide effective protection against an expanding and evolving array of infectious disease threats has been called into question by recent outbreaks of Ebola, Zika, dengue, Middle East respiratory syndrome (MERS), severe acute respiratory syndrome (SARS), influenza, and COVID-19, as well as the looming specter of rising antimicrobial resistance (AMR). These diseases – along with a slew of other known and unknown pathogens – jeopardize not only human health but also various forms of social and economic well-being. Of particular concern is the lack of a single entity that has a sufficiently high-level and comprehensive view of the full range of potential threats – whether naturally occurring, accidental, or due to intentional biological attack – and of the network of organizations tasked with their surveillance, prevention, and mitigation.

To address emerging global challenges with regard to infectious disease and associated social and economic risks, we propose the formation of a multidisciplinary *global technical council on infectious disease threats*. This council, which may be self-standing or housed within an existing organization, would strengthen the global health system by doing the following: (1) improving collaboration and coordination across relevant organizations; (2) filling in knowledge gaps with respect to (for example) infectious disease surveillance, research and development (R&D) needs, financing models, supply-chain logistics, and the social and economic impacts of potential threats; and (3) making high-level evidence-based recommendations for managing global risks associated with infectious disease.

---

* This chapter was originally written in the fall of 2019, before reports emerged of a pneumonia outbreak caused by an unidentified pathogen in Wuhan, China. In light of the ongoing COVID-19 pandemic, we have made several minor updates to the main text of this chapter, such as adding relevant entries to Tables 3.1 and 3.2. We have also added an epilogue on some preliminary lessons learned from the pandemic.

Background

Increased longevity is among the most remarkable aspects of human progress. Global life expectancy has increased by 27 years since 1950 (United Nations Department of Economic and Social Affairs, 2019). Large numbers of people are now living into their eighth and ninth decades (United Nations Department of Economic and Social Affairs, 2019), and life expectancy is projected to exceed 85 years in several countries (and 80 years in many more) in the second half of this century (Foreman et al., 2018). These advances reflect precipitous declines in infectious disease mortality, for which we can thank improvements in sanitation, hygiene, the availability of clean water, nutrition, vaccination, antibiotics, medical practices, and health systems, as well as income growth.

While infectious diseases and associated mortality have abated, they remain a significant threat throughout the world. In the twenty-first century, we continue to fight both old pathogens – such as the plague – that have afflicted humanity for millennia and new pathogens – such as human immunodeficiency virus (HIV) – that have mutated or have spilled over from animal reservoirs. Some infectious diseases – such as tuberculosis (TB) and malaria – are endemic to many areas, imposing substantial but steady burdens. Others – such as influenza – fluctuate in pervasiveness and intensity, wreaking havoc in the developing and developed worlds alike when an outbreak (a sharp increase in prevalence in a relatively limited area or population), an epidemic (a sharp increase covering a larger area or population), or a pandemic (an epidemic covering multiple countries or continents) occurs. Table 3.1 details some of these most prominent cases of the last hundred years.

Perhaps the greatest challenge of anticipating and responding to epidemics is the vast array of possible causes, including pathogens that are currently unknown. In May 2016, the World Health Organization (WHO) published a list of epidemic-potential disease priorities requiring urgent R&D attention (WHO, 2016). That list has since been updated three times, most recently in early 2020 (see Table 3.2; WHO, 2020b). The Blueprint list of priority diseases "focuses on severe emerging diseases with potential to generate a public health emergency, and for which no, or insufficient, preventive and curative solutions exist" (WHO, 2017c: 1). It was developed through expert consultation involving both the Delphi method and multicriteria decision analysis. The top prioritization criteria considered were (in order) potential for human transmission, availability of medical countermeasures, severity or case-fatality rate, human/animal interface, other factors (not defined), the public health context of the affected area, potential societal impacts, and evolutionary potential. The list's inclusion of "Disease X," which is intended to represent the potential for an unknown pathogen to spread through the population, is particularly noteworthy in the context of COVID-19.

Beyond the included pathogens, diseases that are currently endemic in some areas but could spread without proper control to others represent another category of threat. Tuberculosis, malaria, HIV infection, and dengue are examples. Pandemic influenza also merits special attention; indeed, the WHO has developed a separate Pandemic Influenza Preparedness Framework (WHO, 2011).

Meanwhile, the very drugs that helped produce miraculous declines in infectious disease mortality over the second half of the twentieth century are now beginning to lose their effectiveness. AMR is on the rise throughout much of the world, and widespread panresistant "superbugs" could pose yet another threat if we fail to act (Review on Antimicrobial Resistance, 2014). While rapid transmission of resistant pathogens is unlikely to occur in the same way that it may with pandemic threats, the proliferation of superbugs is making the world an increasingly risky place. AMR threats also differ from epidemic threats in a number of other respects: Most of the top AMR threats are bacterial, and many are typically contracted as nosocomial infections; pathogens of epidemic potential tend to be viral and often emerge from zoonotic reservoirs to cause outbreaks in human populations.

Table 3.3 documents the WHO's list of priority pathogens for R&D of new antibiotics (Tacconelli et al., 2017). The list was selected through a multicriteria decision analysis incorporating both quantifiable evidence and the input of 70 experts with different backgrounds and from a variety of geographies. Notably, the list was not developed to prioritize the top public health threats with respect to AMR but rather to identify the pathogens for which R&D needs are greatest, considering both health burden and availability of treatment. The WHO explicitly excluded TB from the list and included only bacterial pathogens.

Table 3.1 Prominent Outbreaks, Epidemics, and Pandemics of the Last Century

Year(s)	Pathogen/ disease	Geographic location	Cases/ mortality	Other notes	Sources
1918–1920	Influenza (Spanish flu)	Worldwide	500 million cases and 30–100 million deaths	The Spanish flu claimed the lives of 2%–5% of world's population, far exceeding the death toll of World War I.	Patterson & Pyle, 1991; Johnson & Mueller, 2002; Taubenberger & Morens, 2006
1957–1958	Influenza (Asian flu)	Worldwide	1–2 million deaths	Accelerated development of a vaccine limited the spread of the responsible influenza strain.	Saunders-Hastings & Krewski, 2016
1968–1969	Influenza (Hong Kong flu)	Worldwide	500,000–2 million deaths	The Hong Kong flu was the first virus to spread extensively as a result of air travel.	Saunders-Hastings & Krewski, 2016
1960–2019	HIV/AIDS	Worldwide, primarily Africa	70 million cases and 35 million deaths	HIV was first identified in 1983. The earliest known case came from a blood sample collected in 1959.	Barré-Sinoussi et al., 1983; Zhu et al., 1998; WHO, 2019c
1961–2019	Cholera	Worldwide	1.4–4 million annual cases and 21,000–143,000 annual deaths	The seventh cholera pandemic began in South Asia in 1961. Recent notable outbreaks include those in Zimbabwe in 2008–2009, Haiti from 2010 to the present, and Yemen from 2016 to the present.	Camacho et al., 2018; WHO, 2019a
1974	Smallpox	India	130,000 cases and 26,000 deaths	One of the worst smallpox epidemics of the twentieth century occurred just three years before the disease was eradicated.	Weinraub, 1974
1994	Plague	India	693 suspected cases and 56 deaths	The outbreak originated in Surat, India. Within days, hundreds of thousands of the city's 1.6 million residents fled, spreading the disease across five states.	CDC, 1994; Post & Clifton, 1994
2002–2003	SARS	Originated in China, spread to 37 countries	8,098 cases and 774 deaths	International business travel allowed the SARS virus to spread quickly across continents.	Olsen et al., 2003; CDC, 2012

Table 3.1 (cont.)

Year(s)	Pathogen/ disease	Geographic location	Cases/ mortality	Other notes	Sources
2009	Influenza (swine flu)	Worldwide	284,000 deaths	Many public and private facilities in Mexico closed in an attempt to prevent the spread of the "swine flu" during the early days of the epidemic. The pork industry also suffered losses, even though eating pork products posed no risk.	Carroll & Tuckman, 2009; Welch, 2009; Dawood et al., 2012
2014–2016	Ebola	West Africa, primarily Guinea, Liberia, and Sierra Leone	28,600 cases and 11,325 deaths reported (likely underestimates)	300,000 doses of an experimental Ebola vaccine were subsequently stockpiled.	Gavi, 2016; CDC, 2017
2015–2019	Zika	The Americas, primarily Brazil	Unknown number of cases and no deaths reported	The Zika epidemic has resulted in few, if any, deaths. However, birth defects resulting from infection in pregnant women occurred frequently, which prompted some governments to encourage delaying pregnancy for as long as two years.	Partlow, 2016
2016	Dengue	Worldwide	100 million cases and 38,000 deaths	Dengue outbreaks occur periodically in affected regions. The year 2016 was notable for the unusual scale of outbreaks across the globe.	Institute for Health Metrics and Evaluation, 2019
2017	Plague	Madagascar	2,417 cases and 209 deaths	Plague is endemic in Madagascar, but an increase in pneumonic plague, which can be transmitted from human to human, was associated with the recent spike in cases.	WHO, 2017e
2018–2020	Ebola	Democratic Republic of the Congo (DRC)	3,481 cases and 2,299 deaths[a]	The Ebola epidemic in the DRC was the second-largest Ebola outbreak/ epidemic on record. A ring vaccination strategy was being used in an effort to protect the contacts	WHO, 2018a, 2019b

Table 3.1 (cont.)

Year(s)	Pathogen/ disease	Geographic location	Cases/ mortality	Other notes	Sources
				of people known to be infected.	
2018–2019	Measles	Worldwide	10 million cases and 140,000 deaths in 2018	Measles cases have surged in both developing and developed settings because of inadequate vaccination coverage. For example, there were more than 5,000 measles deaths in the DRC in 2019, whereas the United States is in jeopardy of losing its measles elimination status.	CDC, 2019; Patel et al., 2019; UNICEF, 2019
2019–2020	COVID-19	Worldwide	Global documented cases and deaths exceeded 23 million and 800,000, respectively, as of August 24, 2020	Experts project that on the order of 70% of the world's population could be infected before the pandemic ends and that the global (in the absence of vaccination) economy will suffer its greatest losses since the Great Depression.	Axelrod, 2020; D'Souza & Dowdy, 2020; Gopinath, 2020; *New York Times*, 2020

[a] As of November 5, 2019.

Table 3.2 WHO's Blueprint List of Priority Diseases Requiring Urgent R&D Attention, 2020

Disease	Description	Availability of biomedical countermeasures	Sources
COVID-19 (SARS-CoV-2)	Highly transmissible disease caused by a coronavirus that can lead to a wide range of serious complications, including pneumonia, acute respiratory failure, multiple organ system failure, heart injury, and stroke	Numerous treatments and vaccine candidates (some funded by the Coalition for Epidemic Preparedness Innovations [CEPI]) under research or in clinical trials as of May 2020	Bangalore et al., 2020; CDC, 2020b; Oxley et al., 2020
Crimean-Congo hemorrhagic fever (CCHF)	Hemorrhagic fever caused by virus transmitted primarily through ticks and livestock, with a case-fatality rate of up to 40%; human-to-human transmission possible	No vaccine available; ribavirin (antiviral) provides some treatment benefit	WHO, 2013
Ebola virus disease	Hemorrhagic fever caused by virus transmitted from wild animals, with a case-fatality rate of up to 90% (50% is average); human-to-human transmission possible	Experimental vaccine and treatments available	WHO, 2018b

Table 3.2 (cont.)

Disease	Description	Availability of biomedical countermeasures	Sources
Marburg virus disease	Hemorrhagic fever caused by virus transmitted by fruit bats, with a case-fatality rate of up to 88% (50% is average); human-to-human transmission possible	No vaccine available	WHO, 2017b
Lassa fever	Hemorrhagic fever caused by virus transmitted from items that have contacted rodent urine or feces, with a case-fatality rate of 15% in severe cases (1% overall); human-to-human transmission possible	No vaccine available; vaccine development funded by CEPI	WHO, 2017a; CEPI, 2019b
Middle East respiratory syndrome coronavirus (MERS-CoV)	Respiratory disease caused by a coronavirus transmitted by camels and humans, with a case-fatality rate of 35%	No vaccine available; vaccine development funded by CEPI	CEPI, 2019b; WHO, 2019e
Severe acute respiratory syndrome (SARS)	Respiratory disease caused by a coronavirus transmitted from human to human and from an unknown animal reservoir (possibly bats), with a case-fatality rate of 10%	No vaccine available; experimental vaccines are under development	WHO, 2003, 2019f
Nipah and henipaviral diseases	Disease caused by a virus transmitted by fruit bats, pigs, and humans; can manifest as an acute respiratory syndrome or encephalitis; the case-fatality rate is estimated at 40%–75% and depends on local capabilities	Vaccine development funded by CEPI	WHO, 2018d; CEPI, 2019b
Rift Valley fever	Disease caused by a virus transmitted by contact with the blood or organs of infected animals or by mosquitos; in severe cases, can manifest in an ocular infection, as meningoencephalitis, or as a hemorrhagic fever; up to 50% case-fatality rate in patients with hemorrhagic fever; no human-to-human transmission reported	An experimental, unlicensed vaccine exists but is not commercially available; vaccine development funded by CEPI	WHO, 2018e; CEPI, 2019b
Zika	Disease caused by a flavivirus transmitted by *Aedes aegypti* mosquitoes; can result in microcephaly in infants born to infected mothers and in Guillain-Barré syndrome; human-to-human transmission possible	No vaccine available	WHO, 2018g

Table 3.2 (cont.)

Disease	Description	Availability of biomedical countermeasures	Sources
Disease X	"Disease X" represents pathogens currently unknown to cause human disease, requiring cross-cutting preparedness.	CEPI is funding the development of institutional and technical platforms that allow for rapid R&D in response to outbreaks of any number of pathogens for which vaccines do not yet exist.	WHO, 2018c; CEPI, 2019a

Note: In addition to the vaccines under development noted in this table, CEPI is also funding the development of a vaccine for Chikungunya virus, which is not currently included on the WHO's Blueprint list of priority diseases.

Table 3.3 WHO Priority Pathogens List for R&D of New Antibiotics

Pathogen	Resistance
Priority 1: Critical	
Acinetobacter baumannii	Carbapenem resistant
Pseudomonas aeruginosa	Carbapenem resistant
Enterobacteriaceae	Carbapenem resistant, third-generation cephalosporin-resistant
Priority 2: High	
Enterococcus faecium	Vancomycin resistant
Staphylococcus aureus	Methicillin resistant, vancomycin intermediate and resistant
Helicobacter pylori	Clarithromycin resistant
Campylobacter	Fluoroquinolone resistant
Salmonella species	Fluoroquinolone resistant
Neisseria gonorrhoeae	Third-generation cephalosporin resistant, fluoroquinolone resistant
Priority 3: Medium	
Streptococcus pneumoniae	Penicillin nonsusceptible
Haemophilus influenzae	Ampicillin resistant
Shigella species	Fluoroquinolone resistant

Source: Tacconelli et al., 2017.

Beyond the pathogens on this list, mounting resistance against the drugs used to treat TB, HIV infection, malaria, and *Candida auris* infection is especially concerning. Resistant TB, for instance, is already responsible for 240,000 deaths globally per year (out of 700,000 total AMR-related deaths, which is likely an underestimate; Review on Antimicrobial Resistance, 2014; WHO, 2017d).

Finally, the global health community must also acknowledge the real threat posed by the possibility of a human-caused infectious disease outbreak, whether from the accidental release of infectious agents from a research facility or from an intentional biological attack. Over the past half-century, several alarming (but thankfully contained) events of this sort have occurred. In 1993, the Japanese doomsday cult Aum Shinrikyo sprayed anthrax spores from the top of a cooling tower in Tokyo in a failed attempt to start an epidemic (Takahashi et al., 2004). (In 1995, the same group used a chemical weapon similar to sarin in an attack on the Tokyo subway system that caused 13 deaths and many injuries [Ramzy, 2018].) In 2001, an attacker with unknown motives caused terror and chaos in the United States by mailing letters laced with anthrax to the offices of two senators and multiple members of the news media, resulting in five deaths (Shane, 2010). And in 2014, an accident involving live anthrax bacteria at the US Centers for Disease Control and Prevention (CDC) potentially exposed dozens of workers to the pathogen (McNeil, 2014). As long as stores of dangerous pathogens, such as anthrax and smallpox, are maintained (for research purposes), the potential for a damaging accident or intentional attack will remain. Advancements in gene editing and the end of a US government–imposed moratorium on funding potentially risky research involving the editing of deadly viruses may amplify the threat. As early as 2002, researchers demonstrated the feasibility of chemically synthesizing highly infectious agents such as poliovirus (Cello, Paul, & Wimmer, 2002). More recently, another team of researchers synthesized horsepox, a relative of smallpox not known to harm humans (Noyce, Lederman, & Evans, 2018). The success of this latter experiment suggests that with rudimentary scientific knowledge and a relatively small amount of money, a group with nefarious intent could synthesize smallpox without significant difficulty and in a short amount of time (Kupferschmidt, 2017).

Infectious Disease Threats Pose Economic and Social Risks

Infectious disease threats – and the fear and panic that may accompany them – map to various economic and social risks. With respect to outbreaks and epidemics (whether naturally occurring or human initiated), there are obvious costs to the health system in terms of medical treatment and outbreak control. A sizable outbreak can overwhelm the health system, limiting the capacity to deal with other routine health issues and thereby compounding the stress on the system. Beyond shocks to the health sector, epidemics force those who are ill and their caretakers to miss work or be less effective at their jobs, disrupting productivity. When critical human resources such as engineers, policymakers, healthcare professionals, public safety officers, and other difficult-to-replace frontline workers are affected, productivity impacts can be magnified.

Fear of infection can result in social distancing or the closing of schools, enterprises, commercial establishments, transportation, and public services – all of which disrupt economic and other socially valuable activities. Concern over the spread of even a relatively contained outbreak can lead to decreased trade. For example, a ban imposed by the European Union on the export of British beef lasted for 10 years following the identification of a mad cow disease outbreak in the United Kingdom despite relatively low (hypothesized) transmission to humans (BBC News, 2006; CDC, National Center for Emerging and Zoonotic Infectious Diseases (NCEZID), 2018). Travel and tourism to regions affected by outbreaks are also likely to decline, as has happened in Brazil and several Southeast Asian countries when dengue incidence spiked (Mavalankar et al., 2009; Bärnighausen et al., 2013a, 2013b; Constenla, Garcia, & Lefcourt, 2015). During the COVID-19 pandemic, tourism has essentially come to a halt, imposing a substantial short- and long-run financial burden on related industries (Chokshi, 2020; Molla, 2020). In the case of some long-running epidemics, such as HIV infection and malaria, foreign direct investment can be deterred as well (Alsan, Bloom, & Canning, 2006; Asiedu, Jin, & Kanyama, 2015).

As demonstrated by the COVID-19 pandemic, the economic risks of epidemics are not trivial. China's economy shrank by 6.8%, South Korea's by 1.4%, and the United States' by 4.8% in the first quarter of 2020 (Bureau of Economic Analysis, 2020; He, 2020; Nagarajan, 2020). At the global scale, the International Monetary Fund (IMF) projects a contraction of 3% over the full year (International Monetary Fund, 2020b); this would represent the worst economic downturn since the Great Depression (Gopinath, 2020). A recent study estimated the expected per annum cost of pandemic influenza at roughly $500 billion (0.6% of global income), inclusive of both the cost of lost income and the intrinsic cost of elevated mortality (Fan, Jamison, & Summers, 2018). The World Bank similarly estimated that a flu pandemic causing 28 million or more excess deaths could result in a loss of as much as 5% of global gross domestic product (GDP; Burns, van der Mensbrugghe & Timmer, 2008; Jonas, 2013). The large projected economic impacts of COVID-19 and an influenza pandemic stem substantially from anticipated high mortality and morbidity. However, even when the health impact of an outbreak is relatively limited, its economic consequences can quickly become magnified. Liberia, for example, saw GDP growth decline eight percentage points from 2013 to 2014 during the recent Ebola outbreak in West Africa, even as the country's overall death rate fell over the same period (World Bank, 2018; United Nations, Department of Economic and Social Affairs, 2019).

As with outbreaks and epidemics, the economic risks of AMR begin with increased costs to the health system. Resistant infections demand the use of more expensive second- and third-line treatments and are sometimes associated with prolonged hospital stays (Pooran et al., 2013; Friedman, Temkin, & Carmeli, 2016; Thorpe, Joski, & Johnston, 2018). As the incidence of resistant infections grows, the cumulative magnitude of these costs will grow as well.

Perhaps the biggest fear with AMR is that it will progress to the point where a significant number of infections are entirely untreatable. Absent such a calamity, we can nonetheless envision a world in which contracting infectious diseases will carry an increased risk of mortality or severe morbidity. As broad-spectrum antibiotics lose their effectiveness, certain procedures (including some common surgeries) that rely on prophylactic antibiotic use may be deemed too risky to administer, resulting in additional morbidity. Some level of decreased productivity is almost certain to be a consequence of AMR's health impact because excess morbidity and mortality will remove people from the labor force or otherwise diminish their capacity to work. In some economies, reductions in livestock output resulting from the spread of disease in animal populations could have major repercussions. In a high-impact scenario, AMR may also lead to notable reductions in international trade.

Projections of AMR's potential economic impact vary significantly because the magnitude of AMR's eventual health burden is difficult to predict for a variety of reasons. The upper bounds of existing estimates are alarming. According to the World Bank, AMR could reduce global GDP by 3.8% by 2050 in a worst-case scenario, with developing economies bearing a disproportionate burden

(Adeyi et al., 2017). And a 2014 report by the Review on Antimicrobial Resistance, which was commissioned by David Cameron and chaired by Jim O'Neill, projected a cumulative cost of $100 trillion by the midcentury mark if resistance in a number of pathogens, including TB, malaria, and HIV, were to progress unchecked (Review on Antimicrobial Resistance, 2014). While the likelihood of these extreme scenarios is debatable, it is certain that AMR poses a sizable economic risk.

Infectious disease threats pose additional social risks beyond those that are strictly economic. Outbreaks and epidemics have the potential to induce geopolitical instability. Fear of an outbreak could lead people to flee their homes (as occurred following an outbreak of plague in Surat, India, in 1994 [Post & Clifton, 1994]), potentially causing an international migration crisis. Epidemics could also increase the vulnerability of a weak government – especially one with an accompanying weak health system – leading to state fragility.

The social risks associated with infectious disease threats raise many ethical questions related to balancing the common good with individual well-being (Dawson, 2011; Selgelid, 2011; Smith et al., 2019). National and international policymakers and the societies they represent must determine, for example, if and when imposition of quarantines, travel restrictions, and mandatory vaccination is justified.

Challenges

There are a number of complicating factors when it comes to managing the risk of infectious disease. Several ongoing demographic trends point toward an increased potential for transmission of pathogens. Whereas the populations of many developed countries are stabilizing or even declining in size, rapid population growth continues in regions where infectious disease outbreaks are likely to originate and where many countries have weak health systems that may struggle to cope with epidemics. The population of Sub-Saharan Africa, for instance, is increasing at a rate of 2.65% per year – more than twice the highest rate of population growth experienced by high-income countries since the 1950s (United Nations, Department of Economic and Social Affairs, 2019). The year 2007 marked the first time in history in which a greater proportion of the world's population lived in urban than in rural areas (United Nations, Department of Economic and Social Affairs,

2018). Urbanization means more humans living in close quarters with each other, amplifying the transmissibility of contagious disease. In areas experiencing rapid urbanization, housing shortages can lead to the growth of slums, which force more people to live in conditions with substandard sanitation, poor access to clean water, and severe crowding, compounding the problem. Finally, with the share of older adults increasing in every country (United Nations, Department of Economic and Social Affairs, 2019), global population aging could further exacerbate the potential for widespread transmission of infectious disease, because immunosenescence leaves the elderly more vulnerable to infection (Aw, Silva, & Palmer, 2007).

Climate change may also play a role in driving pathogen transmission as the habitats of various common disease-carrying vectors – such as the *Aedes aegypti* mosquito, which can spread dengue, Chikungunya, Zika, and yellow fever, among other pathogens – expand (Ebi & Nealon, 2016). Human interactions with animal populations have always carried a risk of producing pathogen spillovers (Garrett, 1995; Wolfe, Dunavan, & Diamond, 2007), and the changing nature of these interactions – as factory farming increases to meet food demand and humans continue to encroach on natural habitats, for example – could promote additional zoonoses. Indeed, billions of people currently live in impoverished situations in close association with animals conducive to transmission (from animals to humans) of pathogens, many of which are unknown. Civil conflict often results in new disease outbreaks or the exacerbation of ongoing ones, especially when populations are displaced, public health infrastructure is affected, or the provision of basic care and immunizations is interrupted (Reuters, 2018; Bonner, 1994; Coutts & Fouad, 2014; Fox, 2018). In general, socioeconomic factors – especially poverty and associated deprivation of access to safe and salubrious living conditions – have a large role in determining the risks and outcomes of outbreaks and epidemics (Benatar, 2015).

The phenomenon of globalization compounds the risks posed by the aforementioned challenges. Many diseases with epidemic potential can be transmitted rapidly, both within and across countries. The proliferation and ease of international air travel and trade increase the difficulty and importance of containing outbreaks in their early phases. Globalization also has implications for AMR: the movement of people makes populations with low rates of circulating resistance

vulnerable to importation of resistant strains from other areas of the globe.

Perhaps the chief challenge for managing AMR is that the use of antimicrobials constitutes its most powerful driver, with each consumed dose placing evolutionary pressure on target and bystander pathogen populations to develop and proliferate mechanisms of resistance. The baked-in nature of the problem is compounded by the fact that there is currently tremendous need for increased access to antimicrobials in low- and middle-income countries (LMICs), where many people continue to die every year from infectious diseases that are easily treated in the developed world (Laxminarayan et al., 2016). As the international community strives to close this access gap, national and global AMR response plans should be carefully designed to avoid exacerbating the unmet need for antimicrobials in LMICs and its consequences for human health.

Several factors complicate management of the risk for biological accidents and attacks. With respect to accidents, there is a complicated tradeoff between enabling socially valuable research on dangerous pathogens (in order to better understand their spread or contribute to the development of countermeasures, for example) and imposing necessary safeguards to limit any potential danger. Removing barriers to research on deadly pathogens (including through the manipulation of their genetic makeup) may allow us to be better prepared for naturally occurring outbreaks and attacks, but some specialists worry about the possibility of human error leading to catastrophe (Lipsitch & Galvani, 2014). Experts cite the relative ease and low cost of producing certain biological agents as a concern when it comes to intentional biological attack, which could come at the hands of a terrorist organization (Riedel, 2004; Goel, 2015). In addition, some biological agents that may be used in an attack (such as anthrax) have lengthy incubation periods, which could make it difficult for national governments to locate and apprehend attackers or otherwise organize a response (National Academies & US Department of Homeland Security, 2004).

There are numerous economic and political challenges to implementing the measures needed to prepare for and respond to infectious disease threats. First, the likelihood of any single infectious agent sparking an epidemic (including via an accident or attack) is relatively low, even if the aggregate risk is high. The diffuse nature of these threats can make it difficult to both prioritize available responses and summon the necessary political will to invest in prevention and preparedness, although this may change following the COVID-19 pandemic. Similarly, the magnitude of AMR's consequences is not immediately obvious to many policymakers or to the general public. Currently, AMR is a slow-burning problem that directly affects the lives of a relatively small portion of the global population. If left unchecked, however, that problem could grow exponentially.

Another political challenge involves the lack of a reliable mechanism for incentivizing international collaboration in the development of new biomedical countermeasures. Manufacturers from high-income countries must sometimes rely on LMICs to provide biological samples needed for R&D, but LMICs have legitimate concerns that they may not receive an equitable share of any benefits resulting from their contributions, including access to vaccines, drugs, and other products. In 2007, these concerns prompted Indonesia to refuse sharing influenza samples needed for vaccine development with the WHO (Fidler, 2010). The Nagoya Protocol, which came into effect in 92 countries in 2010, was intended to help address this problem by creating an enforceable system to ensure the sharing of benefits resulting from research based on genetic resources shared between countries. However, some people feel that the requirements imposed by the Nagoya Protocol are too cumbersome and that potential jail sentences for scientists who are found to be in violation of its provisions could suppress important research (Cressey, 2014). The global community must continue working to find the right balance between ensuring that manufacturers intent on developing critical products for global health can access needed resources expeditiously and promoting an equitable distribution of benefits resulting from those products.

There are established financing issues for global public goods, such as vaccines to fight epidemics. Whereas the social value of these vaccines and similar products may be very high, the expected private value to the companies most likely to manufacture them is often quite low (Rappuoli, Black, & Bloom, 2018). For-profit pharmaceutical companies are unlikely to invest in R&D of a product unless it promises a substantial return on investment. Social investment has also suffered, at times, when no immediate crisis spurs public and political interest. For example, prior to the COVID-19 pandemic, US government investments to contend with outbreaks had fallen 50% from their level during the 2014 Ebola outbreak (Monaco & Gupta, 2018). This cycle of panic and neglect makes it difficult for the global health community to make long-term commitments to necessary epidemic preparedness programs.

There are also scientific and economic barriers specific to the development of effective responses to AMR. Scientifically, bacteria have developed numerous mechanisms for evading antibiotics, and finding new points of attack is becoming increasingly challenging. Economically, there is a misalignment of interests between society (which has an interest in limiting the use of novel antimicrobials as much as possible to protect their effectiveness while ensuring their availability at low cost to those who most need them) and pharmaceutical companies (which have an interest in producing products that will be used widely and yield substantial profits). These barriers have conspired to produce no truly novel class of antibiotics in over three decades (Rappuoli, Bloom, & Black, 2017).

Beyond the demographic, social, and economic challenges we have enumerated, the world faces a number of organizational challenges to its ability to manage infectious disease threats. The global system for monitoring, preventing, and responding to infectious diseases is massively complex. Key elements of this system include local and national governments, supranational governmental organizations (e.g., the United Nations and WHO), international legal agreements (e.g., the International Health Regulations and the Nagoya Protocol), international coalitions and alliances (e.g., the Global Health Security Agenda and CEPI), financing facilities (e.g., the Pandemic Emergency Financing Facility), donors (e.g., the Bill & Melinda Gates Foundation and the Wellcome Trust), and nongovernmental organizations (e.g., Gavi, The Vaccine Alliance; the Red Cross; and Médecins Sans Frontières).

The good news is that a number of organizations and entities are in place to help protect the world from calamity. The bad news is that deficiencies exist within this complex system, especially when it comes to coordinating activities among all the players. The 2014 Ebola crisis in West Africa highlighted significant gaps between the WHO's intended functions and its real-world effectiveness as a protector of global health security, as well as more general gaps within the global health system (Garrett, 2015; Heymann

61

et al., 2015; WHO, 2015; National Academy of Medicine, 2016; United Nations General Assembly, 2016). Multiple postmortem reports on the crisis explicitly called for the establishment of a new Center for Health Emergency Preparedness and Response within the WHO to ensure that the organization would better manage epidemic risks moving forward (Moon et al., 2015; WHO, 2015; National Academy of Medicine, 2016; United Nations General Assembly, 2016). The WHO answered these calls by instituting a new Health Emergencies Program in 2016 to streamline its activities related to health emergencies and create better internal alignment. While the establishment of this program represents a step in the right direction, a vacuum still remains when it comes to the critical role of coordination.

The establishment in 2018 of the Global Preparedness Monitoring Board (GPMB), which is coconvened by the WHO and the World Bank, represents another positive step in terms of bolstering the WHO's reach and effectiveness in the area of outbreak and epidemic preparedness and response (WHO, 2018). Whereas the GPMB is intended to take on some portion of the coordinating role that is dearly needed, the board has an initial term of only five years without expectation of continuation, and members meet only twice per year. This lack of a sustainable organizational plan and lack of dedicated resources (especially human resources) call into question whether creation of the GPMB represents sufficient change.

National governments have also taken it upon themselves to address the shortcomings revealed by the 2014 Ebola crisis. The Global Health Security Agenda (GHSA), which was started by the United States and launched in 2014, is now a partnership of over 70 countries, international organizations, and nongovernmental stakeholders. The GHSA has similar aims to the International Health Regulations (IHR), with a focus on helping participating countries build core capacities for outbreak detection, preparedness, and response. The GHSA is a welcome addition to the global health landscape. However, the GHSA is yet another entity focused only on a portion of epidemic disease management, neglecting, for example, R&D of relevant biomedical countermeasures. It also adds another layer of complexity to the global health system because its responsibilities overlap with those assigned to the WHO under the IHR. Finally, the GHSA, GPMB, and Health Emergencies Program all appear to ignore the challenge of AMR.

In addition to improved coordination, more organizational support for funding R&D of technologies to deal with infectious disease threats is dearly needed. For example, whereas the CEPI is, in principle, filling an important gap by supporting the early development of vaccines for diseases of epidemic potential, there are reasons to question whether current levels of investment are adequate. CEPI's initial business plan proposed investing $600 million to $1 billion in vaccine R&D (CEPI, 2016). However, a subsequent analysis conducted by the organization determined that funding the early development of vaccine candidates against all 11 diseases originally included on the WHO's R&D Blueprint priority list in 2015 would likely cost between $2.8 billion and $3.7 billion (Gouglas et al., 2018). This does not account for the cost of scaling up vaccine production and delivery in the event of an outbreak, nor does it cover nearly all potential epidemic threats.

The recently launched Combating Antibiotic-Resistant Bacteria Biopharmaceutical Accelerator (CARB-X) is fulfilling a similar role to CEPI with respect to promoting early R&D of biomedical countermeasures for resistant pathogens (CARB-X, 2019a). CARB-X provides financial, scientific, and business support for antibiotics, vaccines, rapid diagnostics, and other products for resistant bacterial infections. As with CEPI, there is reason to question whether CARB-X, which plans to invest up to $500 million between 2016 and 2021, has enough funding to have a meaningful impact on the anticipated global AMR burden. In addition, CARB-X may be unnecessarily excluding potential high-impact AMR interventions from consideration for financial support. To qualify for funding through CARB-X, research must target pathogens on the AMR priority pathogen lists established by the WHO and the US CDC. Based on this criterion, some products that could have a significant AMR impact, such as a universal (or improved seasonal) influenza vaccine, are ineligible. In general, CARB-X may do well to diversify its investment portfolio, which currently contains only four vaccines (CARB-X, 2020).

In the wake of Ebola, the world reactively added several new elements to an already complex global system for managing infectious disease threats. There is reasonable justification for each of these elements and a role for them to play. However, given the massive risks associated with infectious disease threats in terms of human health and other

Table 3.4 Selected Approaches to Infectious Disease Threats

- Health systems strengthening
- Improved (sustainable) urban infrastructure
- Improved public health infrastructure, including clean water and sanitation
- Increased routine immunization
- Mass vaccination following the detection of outbreak-prone diseases (e.g., yellow fever)
- Surveillance of infectious disease in human and animal populations, including rates of resistance

  o Building local (laboratory and epidemiologic) capacity to diagnose and report cases of infectious disease
  o Leveraging opportunities for informal surveillance (e.g., Google Flu Trends [no longer operating publicly], ProMED)

- Surveillance of possible terrorist organizations and activities
- Monitoring of biocontainment procedures and capabilities in microbiology laboratories
- Regular monitoring of preparedness for outbreaks and biosecurity incidents at national and supranational levels (e.g., joint external evaluations)
- Regulation of access to antimicrobials for both humans and livestock
- Investment in R&D of biomedical countermeasures

  o Vaccines
  o Antimicrobials
  o Diagnostics
  o Monoclonal antibodies and other novel treatments
  o Platform technologies

- Supply-chain strengthening and diversification
- Improved systems for rapid, appropriately targeted distribution of countermeasures in the event of an emergency
- Coordination of efforts across countries and institutions, including surveillance efforts, information sharing, and stockpiling of relevant health technologies

forms of social and economic well-being, more resources and proactive reforms are needed. Having evolved in a piecemeal, somewhat ad hoc fashion over the course of more than half a century, the current global system lacks coherence. Insufficient coordination among stakeholder organizations leads to inefficiency and missed opportunities. Many responses are available and required to proactively reduce the risk posed by infectious disease threats and prepare for inevitable outbreaks (see Table 3.4). While many organizations are currently engaging in one or more of these activities to tackle a piece of the problem, the world remains in need of a reliable, well-staffed, and well-resourced global entity to put all the pieces together.

Toward a Unified Approach

In order to better protect the world from infectious disease and the myriad attendant social and economic consequences, we propose the formation of a standing multidisciplinary Global Technical Council on Infectious Disease Threats. This council would focus explicitly on volatile infectious disease threats as opposed to more stable and predictable global health challenges (e.g., endemic disease). Its mission would be to reduce the health, social, and economic risks

emanating from diseases of epidemic potential, AMR, and biosecurity threats. The council would have three principal aims: (1) to improve collaboration and coordination within the global health system, (2) to fill in critical knowledge gaps, and (3) to advise existing organizations. The council could be either freestanding or subsumed within another entity. The council is intended to support and enhance efforts already being made by the WHO, the World Bank, CEPI, Gavi, the GHSA, national governments, global nonprofits, and other organizations.

As indicated by its name, the focus of the Global Technical Council on Infectious Disease Threats would be technical. In other words, the council's outputs would be based on rigorous reviews of the available evidence, and it would operate apolitically. To that end, it would be staffed by a multidisciplinary team of experts working full time. Although it would likely be beneficial to keep the size of the council relatively small, it should encompass – at a minimum – the following areas of expertise: epidemiology, economics, finance, outbreak response, public health, health systems science, R&D, international law, politics, biostatistics and modeling, supply-chain management, and clinical trial design.

In service of its mission and to fulfill its aims, the council would take on a variety of activities. It would identify gaps in disease surveillance, outbreak readiness, basic research on pathogens, R&D of biomedical countermeasures, supply-chain and delivery systems, and financing. Council experts would fill in knowledge gaps in these areas, where possible, through active research and solicit and sometimes fund additional needed research from external experts and entities. The council would also make high-level, evidence-based recommendations to organizations operating in the domain of infectious disease threats; these recommendations would be based on the technical knowledge of its experts and literature reviews. For example, the council would regularly carry out health technology assessments, considering the full health, social, and economic benefits of potential interventions for responding to priority infectious disease threats (Bloom, Fan, & Sevilla, 2018; WHO Initiative for Vaccine Research, 2019), as well as the degree to which alternative interventions may be complementary or substitutable (Sevilla et al., 2018). Economic evaluations of potential investments in interventions for specific infectious disease risks (e.g., a vaccine against Marburg virus) would be conducted in such a way as to account for the opportunity cost of foregoing a similar level of investment in horizontal programs such as health systems strengthening and improved infectious disease surveillance. The council would issue technical communications through a public forum such as an online bulletin, and it would publish an annual report.

The council would also foster coordination and collaboration among existing organizations – seeking to reduce duplication of effort, promote integration of ongoing activities, encourage partnerships (including between the public and private sectors), and discourage the use of public funds for the R&D of products for which there are already reasonable market incentives. This coordinating role may be especially impactful with regard to an established but fragmented network of pandemic preparedness funds that appear to overlap in remit, while leaving substantial funding gaps unaddressed (Glassman, Datema, & McClelland, 2018).[1]

The council may advocate for innovative financing collaborations such as the recently established partnership between CEPI, Gavi, the government of Norway, and the International Finance Facility for Immunisation to help fund CEPI's vaccine-development portfolio (Gavi, The Vaccine Alliance, 2018). The council would also seek to develop innovative mechanisms for facilitating the sharing between countries of biological samples critical to the development of novel biomedical countermeasures.

The council would function much like an independent think tank, and its authority would derive from the credibility of its experts and the evidence and advice they produce. Funding could come from national governments and major donors (similar to the CEPI model). Accountability would come, principally, from the transparent nature of the council's activities and the publicity of its results. In addition, oversight could be provided by an external review board composed of the leadership from organizations such as the WHO, CEPI, Gavi, Médecins Sans Frontières, and the World Bank. This review board would operate in consultation with representatives of other interested parties, such as private industry, national governments, and patient advocacy groups.

The formation and operation of the council would result in greater efficiency within the global health system; increased mitigation of health, social, and economic risks due to infectious disease; and the improved protection of at-risk populations.

The preceding enumeration of council activities and attributes is not intended to be exhaustive. Ideally, before the council's formation, a rigorous landscape analysis of existing global health organizations and the activities they perform would be conducted in order to (1) identify the most significant shortcomings of the current system, including redundancies, (2) confirm the need for the technical council, and (3) establish a comprehensive strategy for the council's funding, structure, and initial plan of action.

As stated earlier, the proposed council could potentially be housed within the WHO (or another body), or it could be established as a free-standing entity. If housed within the WHO, the purely technical and apolitical nature of the body would bolster the legitimacy of WHO recommendations and activities with regard to infectious disease threats. In this vein, it would be important for council experts to be

---

[1] In particular, there has been some controversy regarding the World Bank's Pandemic Emergency Financing Facility in terms of the structure of its payouts and returns to investors (Jonas, 2019). The council could potentially help address such controversies by providing guidance on the sustainability of pandemic funding and the nature of

equitable criteria for triggering the transfer of funds to countries during outbreaks.

granted the autonomy to make their assessments and recommendations independently of any political influence from WHO leadership. At the same time, the council would work collaboratively with existing WHO programs and advisory committees, such as the Health Emergencies Programme and the Strategic Advisory Group of Experts on Immunization. It may be possible to essentially convert the GPMB into the technical council by dedicating sufficient resources to employ a full-time expert staff and ensuring that the GPMB/council will remain in existence beyond five years. It would likely also make sense for the council to be given oversight of other WHO programs and activities, such as the Global Outbreak Alert Response Network (GOARN).

Indeed, the proposed technical council overlaps in some of its capacities with the GOARN (WHO, 2019d). Established in 2000, the GOARN has three stated aims: "combating the international spread of outbreaks, ensuring appropriate technical assistance reaches affected states rapidly and contributing to long-term epidemic preparedness and capacity building" (WHO in South-East Asia, 2020). The GOARN is intended to coordinate outbreak-response activities among disparate entities such as national ministries of health and public health institutions, research institutions, laboratories and surveillance initiatives, and international organizations. While both the Council and GOARN have coordination at their hearts, the council would stand apart in several meaningful ways. First, the GOARN does not maintain a dedicated technical workforce, employing only an operational support team of eight staff members (Global Outbreak and Response Network, 2019). Second, while the GOARN may, in principle, include outbreaks resulting from laboratory accidents or biological attacks within its remit, it does not appear to address AMR. Third, the council would take a more proactive and comprehensive approach to addressing volatile infectious disease threats than the GOARN currently does. Whereas the GOARN has taken on some capacity-building responsibilities, such as establishing a standard training package for urgent responders to outbreaks (Global Outbreak and Response Network, 2017), it does not engage in many important elements of epidemic prevention and preparedness. As explained earlier, the council would have a wider lens, taking on – in addition to outbreak response – R&D needs, surveillance, basic infectious disease

research, legal frameworks, epidemic-related financing, and supply-chain management, for example.

If the council were established as an entity separate from the WHO, any resulting competition that emerged between the council and the WHO would likely represent a boon for the global community because it would force both the council and the WHO to step up their games in order to remain relevant in the space of infectious disease threats. Indeed, experts have previously cited the benefits of competition in other domains of global health and international development (Bergsten, 2015; Rudan & Chan, 2015; Stiglitz, 2015; Wang, 2017).

Conclusion

Uncertainty abounds with respect to infectious disease threats and their consequences. Nevertheless, outbreaks and epidemics are virtually guaranteed to continue (Garrett, 1994; Gates, 2015), AMR will remain a threat as long as we rely on standard antimicrobial therapies, and biosecurity risks are an inherent consequence of pathogen research and human conflict. Fortunately, responses exist to all these forms of infectious disease threats. The world currently lacks a unified system for developing and implementing these responses in an efficient, coordinated fashion. The establishment of a multidisciplinary global technical council on infectious disease threats would go a long way toward reducing unnecessary waste within the global health system, redirect resources where needed, and mitigate the risks posed by infectious disease.

Epilogue: COVID-19

The COVID-19 pandemic (see Table 3.1) has shed new light on many of the topics covered in this chapter. For the most part, the pandemic has served to validate what we had previously written and reinforces its importance: Infectious disease threats pose a serious risk to global health, that risk is increasing for a variety of reasons, epidemics can lead to severe social and economic fallout, and global health governance as currently constituted is ill-equipped to protect the international community.

The COVID-19 pandemic also has drawn our attention to a number of previously un- or under-recognized realities worthy of documentation and reflection. Here are 14 of our biggest takeaways from COVID-19 to date, in no particular order:

1. The social effects of pandemics are more profound and potentially more devastating than even we had appreciated. In some countries, the necessary imposition of social distancing measures has resulted in mass isolation and loneliness, which pose risks to mental and physical health (Ducharme, 2020; Kanter & Manbeck, 2020). School closures and confinement to stressful home environments will likely disrupt many children's socioemotional development (Moroni, Nicoletti, & Tominey, 2020). Many families and individuals have had to forego once-in-a-lifetime events such as weddings and graduations, whereas others have been forced to grieve the deaths of loved ones alone (Bettiza, 2020). Racism, scapegoating, and jingoism have been especially ugly features of the global crisis (Margolin, 2020). It is difficult to quantify these impacts, but they are substantial and could have domino effects.

2. In addition to diminishing the capacity of the health system to deal with routine ailments, outbreaks may cause people to refrain from seeking critical care, exacerbating the damage. In areas with the heaviest burden of COVID-19, such as New York City, people seem to have avoided hospitals, even for life-threatening conditions such as heart attacks and strokes (Krumholz, 2020; Stone & Yu, 2020). Furthermore, in health systems that are either purely or partly private, epidemic-related disruptions have the potential to generate sector-specific downward spirals. Loss of income from the deferral or cancellation of elective procedures during the pandemic is likely to lead to decreased staffing, which could constrain capacity moving forward (Fadel et al., 2020; Sainato, 2020).

3. Even in developed settings, outbreaks and epidemics can trigger a cascade of infectious diseases because routine vaccination is disrupted. In the United States, orders for routine childhood vaccines have so far declined by roughly 2.5 million doses, including 250,000 doses of measles-containing vaccine (Branswell, 2020; Santoli et al., 2020). For a country already struggling to maintain its measles elimination status, this could amount to a second public health catastrophe lumped on top of the pandemic (Kuehn, 2019). By contrast, over the longer term, it is conceivable that the pandemic will spur greater support for and uptake of vaccination and other preventive measures, with concomitant health benefits.

4. The potential need to ration ventilators, personal protective equipment (PPE), and diagnostic testing during the pandemic, as well as vaccines and treatments once available, has been widely recognized, and a number of reasonably thoughtful plans for equitable provision have been devised by clinicians, bioethicists, and other experts (Bloom et al., 2020; Emanuel et al., 2020; Members of Harvard Medical School Center for Bioethics, 2020; Vergano et al., 2020; Yamey et al., 2020). Moving forward, it is advisable to establish and agree to such plans during "peace times" to avoid rushed or ad hoc decision making that may be needlessly inefficient or ethically indefensible. Processes for drafting prioritization plans should be transparent and involve public participation, including hearing from those who may be adversely affected by approaches that deviate from established societal standards (e.g., rationing based on prognosis as opposed to a first-come, first-served approach).

5. Similar preplanning should take place with respect to identifying facilities that could be used as temporary hospitals or isolation facilities during an outbreak. Around the world, stadiums, convention and recreation centers, hotels, and university residences have all been converted to support outbreak response (BBC, 2020a; Chen et al., 2020; Enos, 2020). Governments should create standing plans for such adaptation in the event of major outbreaks and practice their implementation through simulation-based exercises (Pearce, 2019; WHO, 2020a).

6. Although the recent establishment of CEPI has positioned us to move quickly through early R&D of vaccines for epidemic diseases, we also need new institutional structures and innovative mechanisms to accelerate late development (i.e., phase III trials) and the scale-up of manufacturing. Without dramatically shortening the normal timeline for these processes, several years could elapse between identification of a viable COVID-19 vaccine candidate and population access (Thompson, 2020). On a related note, consensus should also be sought for ethical guidance on the potential implementation of human challenge vaccine trials in the context of epidemics.

7. We had previously written about the potential for outbreaks and epidemics to disrupt supply chains. The COVID-19 pandemic has emphasized the importance of strengthening and diversifying the supply chain for pharmaceuticals and other health technologies in particular. The United States, for example, relies heavily on China for the provision of pharmaceutical ingredients, medical devices, and PPE, arousing concern that it will be unable to secure sufficient supply of these goods if the Chinese economy is locked down or if the Chinese government reserves them for its own population (Lupkin, 2020; Sutter, Sutherland, & Schwarzenberg, 2020). In addition to shoring up supply chains, the international community would do well to generously fund and maintain shareable stockpiles of essential emergency countermeasures, such as PPE, ventilators, and select vaccines. Rules governing the administration of stockpiles must be carefully delineated and codified in international law to prevent potential manipulation by self-interested national governments.

8. The pandemic has highlighted the importance of public trust in government, institutions, and society during times of crisis. Certain elements (e.g., eschewing or relaxing full lockdowns) of the so-far successful responses to COVID-19 in countries such as Germany, South Korea, Singapore, and Taiwan have proven difficult to enact in others such as the United States, Italy, and France, where trust in government is lower (Aron, 2020; Archer & Ron-Levey, 2020; Campbell, 2020). The pandemic also highlights the importance of civic awareness and a sense of civic duty in controlling infectious diseases and cushioning their impact.

9. Better mechanisms are still needed to promote rapid information sharing within and across countries during outbreaks. Local Chinese officials appear to have concealed the COVID-19 outbreak in its early days, costing the international community precious time to mount a response (as the national Chinese government did during the 2002–2003 SARS epidemic) (Kahn, 2003; Yang, 2020).

10. Existing networks for routine infectious disease surveillance are woefully inadequate, even in high-income settings. Public health agencies have determined that COVID-19 was likely circulating in Europe and the United States weeks before it was officially detected in either location (BBC, 2020b, 2020c; Sommer, 2020).

11. Clear public health communication is of paramount importance during outbreaks and epidemics. For example, confusion over apparently inconsistent recommendations regarding the use of facemasks could have been avoided if officials had more openly and consistently explained why they were advocating against public use of medical-grade PPE early in the pandemic and emphasized that guidance may change as more evidence came to light (Devlin & Campbell, 2020; McNamara, 2020). Clear and consistent messaging may also serve as an antidote to misinformation spread online and through social networks.

12. Better coordination and communication between health and economic policymakers are dearly needed. Inconsistencies in policy objectives, responses, and messaging between these groups have fueled popular misunderstanding that the health and economic impacts of the pandemic are fundamentally at odds with each other. In reality, in some settings (e.g., high-income countries), good economic performance may be promoted most effectively by first protecting population health (Associated Press & Wiseman, 2020), whereas in others (e.g., low-income countries where the risk of extreme poverty is high), population health may be best protected by ensuring economic continuity (Cash & Patel, 2020).

13. It is not surprising that members of marginalized communities and those with underlying health conditions – two groups that often overlap – are suffering disproportionately from COVID-19, particularly in the United States (Dorn, Cooney, & Sabin, 2020). However, the degree to which the effects of the pandemic are being felt differentially is harrowing. In New York City, the COVID-19 mortality rate was more than twice as high in black people as in white people through mid-April 2020 (CDC, 2020a). COVID-19-related job losses are also higher among black people, as well as Hispanics and women (Aratani & Rushe, 2020; Jones, 2020; Montenovo et al., 2020). Among children, students from low-income families (which are disproportionately of color) are more likely to struggle to keep up with distanced education and may altogether lack access to the technology required for participation in online schooling; some children may also struggle to obtain

adequate nutrition without access to school meals (Dunn et al., 2020; Meckler, Strauss, & Heim, 2020; Strauss, 2020). In sum, the present situation highlights disparities in access to health care, education, and economic opportunity and their potential to lead to extremely detrimental effects.

14. Dramatically different policy responses to epidemics may be called for in different development settings, according to variations in underlying health burdens, the availability of healthcare resources, and relevant tradeoffs between health and other forms of well-being. The documented death toll of the COVID-19 pandemic has been greatest in high- and upper-middle-income countries to date, but developing regions remain extremely vulnerable (IMF, 2020a; *New York Times*, 2020). Notwithstanding the significant health threat COVID-19 poses for low- and middle-income populations, it may not always be wise for these countries to pursue the same policies as high-income countries (e.g., strict social distancing measures) because they may be difficult to implement, and the risk of increased poverty precipitated by economic shutdown and its implications for nutrition and other diseases could represent an even greater threat (Cash and Patel, 2020; Glassman, Chalkidou, and Sullivan, 2020).

There is much uncertainty with respect to the future course of the COVID-19 pandemic. The ultimate global toll – including loss of life, long-term disability, economic damage, and social effects – is not yet known but is already devastating in some locales. Unfortunately, as we have pointed out, there are many reasons to believe that major outbreaks and epidemics will become more common moving forward. While there is still a massive amount of work to be done in responding to the current situation (to say the least), we have already learned many valuable lessons that can be applied to reduce the risk of future catastrophes. The global population would be well served to get to work on preparing for the next outbreak as soon as humanly possible.

Authors' Note

This chapter is a revised and updated version of an article that appeared in *Frontiers in Immunology* on March 28, 2019 with the title "Infectious Disease Threats in the 21st Century: Strengthening the Global Response" and under the research topic "A Global Perspective on Vaccines: Priorities, Challenges and Online Information." Prior versions of Tables 3.1, 3.2, and 3.3, along with small portions of this article, also appeared in an earlier article titled, "Epidemics and Economics," coauthored by DEB, DC, and J. P. Sevilla and published as a short commentary in *Finance & Development* in June 2018.

Acknowledgments

The authors thank Solomon Benatar, Gillian Brock, and Aldo Tagliabue for offering valuable comments and editorial support. DEB and DC received general support for their work on this article from the Bill & Melinda Gates Foundation through the Value of Vaccination Research Network.

References

Adeyi, O. O., Baris, E., Jonas, O. B., et al. (2017). *Drug-Resistant Infections: A Threat to Our Economic Future*, Vol. 2 (Final Report 114679). Washington, DC: World Bank.

Alsan, M., Bloom, D. E., & Canning, D. (2006). The effect of population health on foreign direct investment inflows to low- and middle-income countries. *World Development* **34** (4), 613–630. https://doi.org/10.1016/j.worlddev.2005.09.006.

Aratani, L., & Rushe, D. (2020). African Americans bear the brunt of COVID-19's economic impact. *The Guardian*, April 28. Available at www.theguardian.com/us-news/2020/apr/28/african-americans-unemployment-covid-19-economic-impact.

Archer, K., & Ron-Levey, I. (2020). Trust in government lacking on COVID-19's frontlines. Gallup Blog, March 20. Available at https://news.gallup.com/opinion/gallup/296594/trust-government-lacking-frontlines-covid.aspx.

Aron, R. (2020). Combating COVID-19: lessons from Singapore, South Korea and Taiwan. Knowledge@Wharton, April 21. Available at https://knowledge.wharton.upenn.edu/article/singapore-south_korea-taiwan-used-technology-combat-covid-19/.

Asiedu, E., Jin, Y., & Kanyama, I. K. (2015). The impact of HIV/AIDS on foreign direct investment: evidence from sub-Saharan Africa. *Journal of African Trade* **2**(1), 1–17. https://doi.org/10.1016/j.joat.2015.01.001.

Associated Press & Wiseman, P. (2020). Reopening the US economy too soon could cause a "double-dip" recession. *Fortune*, May 11. Available at https://fortune.com/2020/05/11/us-economy-reopen/.

Aw, D., Silva, A. B., & Palmer, D. B. (2007). Immunosenescence: emerging challenges for an ageing population. *Immunology* **120**(4), 435–446. https://doi.org/10.1111/j.1365-2567.2007.02555.x.

Axelrod, J. (2020). Coronavirus may infect up to 70% of world's population, expert warns. *CBS News*, March 2. Available at www.cbsnews.com/news/coronavirus-infection-outbreak-worldwide-virus-expert-warning-today-2020-03-02/.

Bangalore, S., Sharma, A., Slotwiner, A. et al. (2020). ST-segment elevation in patients with COVID-19: a case series. *New England Journal of Medicine* **382**(25), 2478-2480. https://doi.org/10.1056/NEJMc2009020.

Bärnighausen, T., Bloom, D. E., Cafiero, E. T., & O'Brien, J. C. (2013a). The impact of dengue on tourism in Brazil: an empirical study. Working paper.

Bärnighausen, T., Bloom, D. E., Cafiero, E. T., & O'Brien, J. C. (2013b). Valuing the broader benefits of dengue vaccination, with a preliminary application to Brazil. *Seminars in Immunology* **25**(2), 104–113. https://doi.org/10.1016/j.smim.2013.04.010.

Barré-Sinoussi, F., Chermann, J. C., Rey, F. et al. (1983). Isolation of a T-lymphotropic retrovirus from a patient at risk for acquired immune deficiency syndrome (AIDS). *Science* **220**(4599), 868–871. Available at www.jstor.org.ezpprod1.hul.harvard.edu/stable/1690359.

BBC (2006). End to 10-year British beef ban. *BBC News*, May 3. Available at http://news.bbc.co.uk/2/hi/4967480.stm.

BBC (2020a). Coronavirus: field hospitals treating patients around world. *BBC News*, March 30. Available at www.bbc.com/news/world-52089337.

BBC (2020b). Coronavirus: first US deaths weeks earlier than thought. *BBC News*, April aa. Available at www.bbc.com/news/world-us-canada-52385558.

BBC (2020c). Coronavirus: France's first known case "was in December." *BBC News*, May 5. Available at www.bbc.com/news/world-europe-52526554.

Benatar, S. (2015). Explaining and responding to the Ebola epidemic. *Philosophy, Ethics, and Humanities in Medicine* **10**, 5. https://doi.org/10.1186/s13010-015-0027-8.

Bergsten, F. (2015). US should work with the Asian Infrastructure Investment Bank. *Financial Times*, March 15. Available at www.ft.com/content/4937bbde-c9a8-11e4-a2d9-00144feab7de.

Bettiza, S. (2020). Coronavirus: how COVID-19 is denying dignity to the dead in Italy. *BBC News*, March 25. Available at www.bbc.com/news/health-52031539.

Bloom, D. E., Cadarette, D., Ferranna, M., & Seligman, B. (2020). A matter of life and death. *Finance & Development*, April.

Bloom, D. E., Fan, V. Y., & Sevilla, J. P. (2018). The broad socioeconomic benefits of vaccination. *Science Translational Medicine* **10**(441), eaaj2345. https://doi.org/10.1126/scitranslmed.aaj2345.

Bonner, R. (1994). The Rwanda disaster: the scene; cholera stalks the Rwandan refugees. *New York Times*, July 22, p. A00001.

Branswell, H. (2020). Routine vaccinations for US children have plummeted during the COVID-19 pandemic. *Stat*, May 8. Available at www.statnews.com/2020/05/08/childhood-vaccinations-decline-coronavirus-pandemic/.

Bureau of Economic Analysis (2020). Gross domestic product, 1st quarter 2020 (advance estimate). Available at www.bea.gov/news/2020/gross-domestic-product-1st-quarter-2020-advance-estimate.

Burns, A., van der Mensbrugghe, D., & Timmer, H. (2008). Evaluating the economic consequences of avian influenza (Report No. 47417), World Bank, Washington, DC.

Camacho, A., Bouhenia, M., Alyusfi, R. et al. (2018). Cholera epidemic in Yemen, 2016–18: an analysis of surveillance data. *Lancet Global Health* **6**(6), e680–e690. https://doi.org/10.1016/S2214-109X(18)30230-4.

Campbell, C. (2020). South Korea's health minister on how his country is beating coronavirus without a lockdown. *Time*, April 30. Available at https://time.com/5830594/south-korea-covid19-coronavirus/.

CARB-X (2019a) *About CARB-X*. Available at https://carb-x.org/about/overview/ (accessed February 8, 2019).

CARB-X (2020) *Portfolio-Product Developers*. Available at https://carb-x.org/portfolio/gallery/ (accessed August 24, 2020).

Carroll, R., & Tuckman, J. (2009). Swine flu: Mexico braces for unprecedented lockdown. *The Guardian*, April 30. Available at www.theguardian.com/world/2009/apr/30/swine-flu-mexico-government-lockdown.

Cash, R., & Patel, V. (2020). Has COVID-19 subverted global health? *Lancet* **395**(10238), 1687-1688. https://doi.org/10.1016/S0140-6736(20)31089-8.

Cello, J., Paul, A. V., & Wimmer, E. (2002). Chemical synthesis of poliovirus cDNA: generation of infectious virus in the absence of natural template. *Science* **297**(5583), 1016LP–1018. https://doi.org/10.1126/science.1072266.

Centers for Disease Control and Prevention (CDC), National Center for Emerging and Zoonotic Infectious Diseases (NCEZID), Division of High Consequence Pathogens and Pathology (DHCPP) (2018). *Variant Creutzfeldt-Jakob Disease (vCJD): Risk for Travelers*. Available at www.cdc.gov/prions/vcjd/risk-travelers.html (accessed December 5, 2018).

Centers for Disease Control and Prevention (CDC) (1994). International notes update: human plague – India, 1994. *MMWR Morbidity and Mortality Weekly Report* **43**(41), 761–762.

Centers for Disease Control and Prevention (CDC) (2012). *Frequently Asked Questions about SARS.* Atlanta: CDC.

Centers for Disease Control and Prevention(CDC) (2017). *2014–2016 Ebola Outbreak in West Africa.* Atlanta: CDC.

Centers for Disease Control and Prevention (CDC) (2019). Measles cases and outbreaks. Available at www.cdc.gov/measles/cases-outbreaks.html.

Centers for Disease Control and Prevention (CDC) (2020a). *COVID-19 in Racial and Ethnic Minority Groups.* Available at www.cdc.gov/coronavirus/2019-ncov/need-extra-precautions/racial-ethnic-minorities.html (accessed May 11, 2020).

Centers for Disease Control and Prevention (CDC) (2020b). *Interim Clinical Guidance for Management of Patients with Confirmed Coronavirus Disease (COVID-19).* Atlanta: CDC Available at www.cdc.gov/coronavirus/2019-ncov/hcp/clinical-guidance-management-patients.html (accessed May 11, 2020).

Chen, S., Zhang, Z., Yang, J. et al. (2020). Fangcang shelter hospitals: a novel concept for responding to public health emergencies. *Lancet,* **395**(10232), 1305–1314. https://doi.org/10.1016/S0140-6736(20)30744-3.

Chokshi, N. (2020). The airline business is terrible: it will probably get even worse. *New York Times,* May 10. Available at www.nytimes.com/2020/05/10/business/airlines-coronavirus-bleak-future.html.

Gavi, The Vaccine Alliance (2018). Coalition for Epidemic Preparedness Innovation turns to IFFIm to accelerate funding for new vaccine development. Press release, December 12. Available at www.gavi.org.

Coalition for Epidemic Preparedness Innovations (CEPI) (2016). *Preliminary Business Plan,* 2017–2021. Oslo, Norway.

Coalition for Epidemic Preparedness Innovations (CEPI) (2019a). *Our Platform Technology.* Available at https://cepi.net/research_dev/technology/ (accessed February 7, 2019).

Coalition for Epidemic Preparedness Innovations (CEPI) (2019b). *Priority Diseases.* Available at https://cepi.net/research_dev/priority-diseases/ (accessed February 7, 2019).

Constenla, D., Garcia, C., & Lefcourt, N. (2015). Assessing the economics of dengue: results from a systematic review of the literature and expert survey. *Pharmacoeconomics* **33**(11), 1107–1135. https://doi.org/10.1007/s40273-015-0294-7.

Coutts, A. P., & Fouad, F. M. (2014). Syria's raging health crisis. *New York Times,* January 1. Available at www.nytimes.com/2014/01/02/opinion/syrias-raging-health-crisis.html.

Cressey, D. (2014). Biopiracy ban stirs red-tape fears. *Nature,* **514** (7524), 14–15. Available at www.nature.com/news/biopiracy-ban-stirs-red-tape-fears-1.16028.

Dawood, F. S., Iuliano, A. D., Reed, C. et al. (2012). Estimated global mortality associated with the first 12 months of 2009 pandemic influenza A H1N1 virus circulation: a modelling study. *Lancet Infectious Diseases* **12**(9), 687–695. https://doi.org/10.1016/S1473-3099(12)70121-4.

Dawson, A. (ed.) (2011). *Public Health Ethics: Key Concepts and Issues in Policy and Practice.* Cambridge, UK: Cambridge University Press. https://doi.org/10.1017/CBO9780511862670.

Devlin, H., & Campbell, D. (2020). WHO considers changing guidance on wearing face masks. *The Guardian,* April 1. Available at www.theguardian.com/world/2020/apr/01/all-uk-hospital-staff-and-patients-should-wear-masks-says-doctors-group.

D'Souza, G., & Dowdy, D. (2020). *What Is Herd Immunity and How Can We Achieve It with COVID-19?* Available at www.jhsph.edu/covid-19/articles/achieving-herd-immunity-with-covid19.html.

Ducharme, J. (2020). COVID-19 is making America's loneliness epidemic even worse. *Time,* May 8. Available at https://time.com/5833681/loneliness-covid-19/.

Dunn, C. G., Kenney, E., Fleischhacker, S. E., & Bleich, S. N. (2020). Feeding low-income children during the COVID-19 pandemic. *New England Journal of Medicine,* **382**(18), e40. https://doi.org/10.1056/NEJMp2005638.

Ebi, K. L., & Nealon, J. (2016). Dengue in a changing climate. *Environmental Research* **151**, 115–123. https://doi.org/10.1016/j.envres.2016.07.026.

The Economist (2018). A deadly touch of flu. *The Economist* **428**(9111), 75–77.

Emanuel, E. J., Persad, G., Upshur, R. et al. (2020). Fair allocation of scarce medical resources in the time of COVID-19. *New England Journal of Medicine* **382**(21), 2049–2055. https://doi.org/10.1056/NEJMsb2005114.

Enos, C. (2020). Universities in Boston area to house health care workers, first responders during the COVID-19 crisis. *Boston Globe,* April 9. Available at www.bostonglobe.com/2020/04/09/metro/universities-boston-area-house-health-care-workers-first-responders-during-covid-19-crisis/.

Fadel, L., Stone, W., Anderson, M., & Benincasa, R. (2020). As hospitals lose revenue, more than a million health care workers lose jobs. National Public Radio (NPR), May 8. Available at www.npr.org/2020/05/08/852435761/as-hospitals-lose-revenue-thousands-of-health-care-workers-face-furloughs-layoff.

Fan, V. Y., Jamison, D. T., & Summers, L. H. (2018). Pandemic risk: how large are the expected losses? *Bulletin of the World Health Organization* **96**(2), 129–134. https://doi.org/10.2471/BLT.17.199588.

Fidler, D. P. (2010). Negotiating equitable access to influenza vaccines: global health diplomacy and the controversies surrounding avian influenza H5N1 and pandemic influenza H1N1. *PLoS Medicine* **7**(5), e1000247–e1000247. https://doi.org/10.1371/journal.pmed.1000247.

Foreman, K. J., Marquez, N., Dolgert, A. et al. (2018). Forecasting life expectancy, years of life lost, and all-cause and cause-specific mortality for 250 causes of death: reference and alternative scenarios for 2016–40 for 195 countries and territories. *Lancet* **392**(10159), 2052–2090. https://doi.org/10.1016/S0140-6736(18)31694-5.

Fox, M. (2018). "Perfect storm" of conflict threatens Ebola fight in Congo. *NBC News*, September 25. Available at www.nbcnews.com/storyline/ebola-virus-outbreak/perfect-storm-conflict-threatens-ebola-fight-congo-n912856.

Friedman, N. D., Temkin, E., & Carmeli, Y. (2016). The negative impact of antibiotic resistance. *Clinical Microbiology and Infection* **22**(5), 416–422. https://doi.org/10.1016/j.cmi.2015.12.002.

Garrett, L. (1994). *The Coming Plague: Newly Emerging Diseases in a World Out of Balance*. New York: Penguin.

Garrett, L. (2015). Ebola's lessons: how the WHO mishandled the crisis. *Foreign Affairs* **94**(5), 80–107.

Gates, B. (2015). The next epidemic: lessons from Ebola. *New England Journal of Medicine* **372**(15), 1381–1384. https://doi.org/10.1056/NEJMp1502918.

Gavi,The Vaccine Alliance (2016). Ebola vaccine purchasing commitment from Gavi to prepare for future outbreaks. Available at www.gavi.org/library/news/press-releases/2016/ebola-vaccine-purchasing-commitment-from-gavi-to-prepare-for-future-outbreaks/.

Glassman, A., Chalkidou, K., & Sullivan, R. (2020). Does one size fit all? Realistic alternatives for COVID-19 response in low-income countries. Center for Global Development, April 2. Available at www.cgdev.org/blog/does-one-size-fit-all-realistic-alternatives-covid-19-response-low-income-countries.

Glassman, A., Datema, B., & McClelland, A. (2018). Financing outbreak preparedness: where are we and what next? Center for Global Development, November 9. Available at www.cgdev.org/blog/financing-outbreak-preparedness-where-are-we-and-what-next.

Global Outbreak and Response Network (2017). Leading public health institutions define guidance for emergency responders to respond to future disease outbreaks. London. Available at https://extranet.who.int/goarn/content/leading-public-health-institutions-define-guidance-emergency-responders-respond-future.

Global Outbreak and Response Network (2019). Global Outbreak and Response Network. Available at https://extranet.who.int/goarn/.

Goel, A. K. (2015). Anthrax: a disease of biowarfare and public health importance. *World Journal of Clinical Cases* **3**(1), 20–33. https://doi.org/10.12998/wjcc.v3.i1.20.

Gopinath, G. (2020). The great lockdown: worst economic downturn since the Great Depression. IMF Blog, April 14. Available at https://blogs.imf.org/2020/04/14/the-great-lockdown-worst-economic-downturn-since-the-great-depression/.

Gouglas, D., Thanh Le, T., Henderson, K. et al. (2018). Estimating the cost of vaccine development against epidemic infectious diseases: a cost minimisation study. *Lancet Global Health* **6**(12), e1386–e1396. https://doi.org/10.1016/S2214-109X(18)30346-2.

He, L. (2020). South Korea's economy just recorded its worst contraction since the Great Recession because of the coronavirus pandemic. *CNN Business*, April 22. Available at www.cnn.com/2020/04/22/economy/south-korea-economy-coronavirus/index.html.

Heymann, D. L., Chen, L., Takemi, K. et al. (2015). Global health security: the wider lessons from the West African Ebola virus disease epidemic. *Lancet* **385**(9980), 1884–1901. https://doi.org/10.1016/S0140-6736(15)60858-3.

Institute for Health Metrics and Evaluation (2019). *GBD Results Tool*. Available at http://ghdx.healthdata.org/gbd-results-tool (accessed February 12, 2019).

International Monetary Fund (IMF) (2020a). Six charts show how COVID-19 is an unprecedented threat to development in sub-Saharan Africa. *IMF News*, April 15. Available at www.imf.org/en/News/Articles/2020/04/13/na0413202-six-charts-show-how-covid-19-is-an-unprecedented-threat-to.

International Monetary Fund (IMF) (2020b). *World Economic Outlook: The Great Lockdown*. Washington, DC.

Johnson, N. P. A. S., & Mueller, J. (2002). Updating the accounts: global mortality of the 1918–1920 "Spanish" influenza pandemic. *Bulletin of the History of Medicine* **76**(1), 105–115. https://doi.org/10.1353/bhm.2002.0022.

Jonas, O. B. (2013). *Pandemic Risk*. Washington, DC: World Bank.

Jonas, O. B. (2019). Pandemic bonds: designed to fail in Ebola. *Nature* **572**(7769), 285. https://doi.org/10.1038/d41586-019-02415-9.

Jones, C. (2020). Historic layoffs take biggest toll on blacks, Latinos, women and the young. *USA Today*, May 8. Available at www.usatoday.com/story/money/2020/05/08/covid-19-layoffs-take-toll-women-people-color-and-young/3094964001/.

Kahn, J. (2003). China discovers secrecy is expensive. *New York Times*, April 13. Available at www.nytimes.com/2003/04/13/weekinreview/china-discovers-secrecy-is-expensive.html.

Kanter, J., & Manbeck, K. (2020). Rates of depression are expected to rise in the wake of coronavirus, as isolation and financial woes multiply. COVID-19 could lead to an epidemic of clinical depression, and the health care system isn't ready for. *The Conversation*, April 1. Available at https://theconversation.com/covid-19-could-lead-to-an-epidemic-of-clinical-depression-and-the-health-care-system-isnt-ready-for-that-either-134528.

Krumholz, H. M. (2020). Where have all the heart attacks gone? *New York Times*, April 6. Available at www .nytimes.com/2020/04/06/well/live/coronavirus-doctors-hospitals-emergency-care-heart-attack-stroke.html.

Kuehn, B. (2019). US narrowly preserves measles elimination status. *Journal of the American Medican Association* **322**(20), 1949. https://doi.org/10.1001/jama.2019.18901.

Kupferschmidt, K. (2017). How Canadian researchers reconstituted an extinct poxvirus for $100,000 using mail-order DNA. July 6. Available at ScienceMag.org.

Laxminarayan, R., Matsoso, P., Pant, S. et al. (2016). Access to effective antimicrobials: a worldwide challenge. *Lancet* **387**(10014), 168–175. https://doi.org/10.1016/S0140-6736(15)00474-2.

Lipsitch, M., & Galvani, A. P. (2014). Ethical alternatives to experiments with novel potential pandemic pathogens. *PLOS Medicine* **11**(5), e1001646. https://doi.org/10.1371/journal.pmed.1001646.

Lupkin, S. (2020). What would it take to bring more pharmaceutical manufacturing back to the US? NPR, April 24. Available at www.npr.org/sections/health-shots/2020/04/24/843379899/pandemic-underscores-u-s-dependence-on-overseas-factories-for-medicines.

Margolin, J. (2020). FBI warns of potential surge in hate crimes against Asian Americans amid coronavirus. *ABC News*, March 27. Available at https://abcnews.go.com/US/fbi-warns-potential-surge-hate-crimes-asian-americans/story?id=69831920.

Mavalankar, D. V., Puwar, T. I., Murtola, T. M., & Vasan, S. S. (2009) *Quantifying the Impact of Chikungunya and Dengue on Tourism Revenues* (Working Paper No. 2009-02-03). ResearchGate, Ahmedabad, India.

McNamara, A. (2020). Should the public wear face masks? Experts are weighing new guidance. *CBS News*, April 3. Available at www.cbsnews.com/news/wear-face-masks-coronavirus-public-experts/.

McNeil, Jr., D. G. (2014). CDC shuts labs after accidents with pathogens. *New York Times*, July 12, p. A1. Available at www.nytimes.com/2014/07/12/science/cdc-closes-anthrax-and-flu-labs-after-accidents.html.

Meckler, L., Strauss, V., & Heim, J. (2020). Millions of public school students will suffer from school closures, education leaders have concluded. *Washington Post*, April 13. Available at www.washingtonpost.com/local/education/online-learning-summer-school-coronavirus/2020/04/11/de11c278-7adc-11ea-a130-df573469f094_story.html.

Members of Harvard Medical School Center for Bioethics (2020). A message to the public from Mass. doctors, nurses, and ethicists about the coronavirus. *Boston Globe*, March 30. Available at www.bostonglobe.com/2020/03/30/opinion/message-public-mass-doctors-nurses-ethicists-about-coronavirus/.

Molla, R. (2020). How the coronavirus has affected airlines, hotels, and cruises in one chart, *Vox*, March 4.

Monaco, L., & Gupta, V. (2018). The next pandemic will be arriving shortly. Foreign Policy, September 28. Available at https://foreignpolicy.com/2018/09/28/the-next-pandemic-will-be-arriving-shortly-global-health-infectious-avian-flu-ebola-zoonotic-diseases-trump/.

Montenovo, L., Jiang, X., Rojas, F. L. et al. (2020). Determinants of disparities in COVID-19 job losses (NBER Working Paper No. 27132). National Bureau of Economic Research, Cambridge, MA. https://doi.org/10.3386/w27132.

Moon, S., Sridhar, D., Pate, M. A. et al. (2015). Will Ebola change the game? Ten essential reforms before the next pandemic. Report of the Harvard-LSHTM Independent Panel on the Global Response to Ebola. *Lancet* **386**(10009), 2204–2221. https://doi.org/10.1016/S0140-6736(15)00946-0.

Moroni, G., Nicoletti, C., & Tominey, E. (2020). Children's socio-emotional skills and the home environment during the COVID-19 crisis. *VoxEU*, April 9. Available at https://voxeu.org/article/children-s-socio-emotional-skills-and-home-environment-during-covid-19-crisis.

Nagarajan, S. (2020). China's economy suffers its first contraction in 28 years, shrinking 6.8% in an "extraordinary shock" to the global economy. *Business Insider*, April 17. Available at markets.businesseinsider.com.

National Academy of Medicine (2016) *The Neglected Dimension of Global Security: A Framework to Counter Infectious Disease Crises*. Washington, DC: National Academies Press. https://doi.org/10.17226/21891.

National Academy of Medicine & US Department of Homeland Security (2004). *Biological Attack: Human Pathogens, Biotoxins, and Agricultural Threats*. Available at www.dhs.gov/sites/default/files/publications/prep_biological_fact_sheet.pdf.

New York Times (2020). Coronavirus map: tracking the global outbreak, *New York Times* August 24. Available at www.nytimes.com/interactive/2020/world/coronavirus-maps.html (accessed August 24, 2020).

Noyce, R. S., Lederman, S., & Evans, D. H. (2018). Construction of an infectious horsepox virus vaccine from chemically synthesized DNA fragments. *PLoS ONE* **13**(1), e0188453. https://doi.org/10.1371/journal.pone.0188453.

Olsen, S. J., Chang, H., Cheung, T. Y. et al. (2003). Transmission of the severe acute respiratory syndrome on aircraft. *New England Journal of Medicine* **349**(25), 2416–2422. https://doi.org/10.1056/NEJMoa031349.

Oxley, T. J., Mocco, J., Majidi, S. et al. (2020). Large-vessel stroke as a presenting feature of COVID-19 in the young. *New England Journal of Medicine* **382**(20), e60. https://doi.org/10.1056/NEJMc2009787.

Partlow, J. (2016). As Zika virus spreads, El Salvador asks women not to get pregnant until 2018. *Washington Post*, January 22.

Patel, M. K., Dumolard, L., Nedelec, Y. et al. (2019). Progress toward regional measles elimination: worldwide, 2000–2018. *MMWR Morbidity and Mortality Weekly Report*, **68**(48), 1105–1111. https://doi.org/10.15585/mmwr.mm6848a1.

Patterson, K. D., & Pyle, G. F. (1991). The geography and mortality of the 1918 influenza pandemic. *Bulletin of the History of Medicine* **65**(1), 4–21.

Pearce, K. (2019). Pandemic simulation exercise spotlights massive preparedness gap. Johns Hopkins University Hub, November 6. Available at https://hub.jhu.edu/2019/11/06/event-201-health-security/.

Pooran, A., Pieterson, E., Davids, M. et al. (2013). What is the cost of diagnosis and management of drug resistant tuberculosis in South Africa? *PloS ONE* **8**(1), e54587–e54587. https://doi.org/10.1371/journal.pone.0054587.

Post, T., & Clifton, T. (1994). The plague of panic. *Newsweek* **124**(15), 40–42.

Ramzy, A. (2018). Japan hangs cult leader for 1995 subway attack. *New York Times*, July 6, p. A6. Available at www.nytimes.com/2018/07/05/world/asia/japan-cult-execute-sarin.html.

Rappuoli, R., Black, S., & Bloom, D. E. (2019). Vaccines and global health: in search of a sustainable model for vaccine development and delivery. *Science Translational Medicine* **11**(497), eaaw2888. https://doi.org/10.1126/scitranslmed.aaw2888.

Rappuoli, R., Bloom, D. E., & Black, S. (2017). Deploy vaccines to fight superbugs. *Nature* **552**, 165–167.

Reuters (2018). Yemen cholera outbreak accelerates to 10,000+ cases per week: WHO. October 2. Available at www.reuters.com/article/us-yemen-security-cholera/yemen-cholera-outbreak-accelerates-to-10000-cases-per-week-who-idUSKCN1MC23J.

Review on Antimicrobial Resistance (2014). *Antimicrobial Resistance: Tackling a Crisis for the Health and Wealth of Nations*. London: HM Government and Wellcome Trust.

Riedel, S. (2004). Biological warfare and bioterrorism: a historical review. *Proceedings (Baylor University Medical Center)* **17**(4), 400–406. Available at www.ncbi.nlm.nih.gov/pubmed/16200127.

Rudan, I., & Chan, K. Y. (2015). Global health metrics needs collaboration and competition. *Lancet* **385**(9963), 92–94. https://doi.org/10.1016/S0140-6736(14)62006-7.

Sainato, M. (2020). US for-profit healthcare sector cuts thousands of jobs as pandemic rages. *The Guardian*, April 14. Available at www.theguardian.com/us-news/2020/apr/14/healthcare-job-cuts-coronavirus-worker-layoffs.

Santoli, J. M., Lindley, M. C., DeSilva, M. B. et al. (2020). Effects of the COVID-19 pandemic on routine pediatric vaccine ordering and administration – United States, 2020. *MMWR Morbidity and Mortality Weekly Report*, May 8. Available at http://dx.doi.org/10.15585/mmwr.mm6919e2externalicon.

Saunders-Hastings, P. R., & Krewski, D. (2016). Reviewing the history of pandemic influenza: understanding patterns of emergence and transmission. *Pathogens (Basel, Switzerland)* **5**(4), 66. http://dx.doi.org/10.3390/pathogens5040066.

Selgelid, M. J. (2011). Justice, infectious diseases and globalization, in Brock, G., & Benatar, S. (eds.), *Global Health and Global Health Ethics*. Cambridge, UK: Cambridge University Press, pp. 89–96. http://dx.doi.org/10.1017/CBO9780511984792.008.

Sevilla, J. P., Bloom, D. E., Cadarette, D. et al. (2018). Toward economic evaluation of the value of vaccines and other health technologies in addressing AMR. *Proceedings of the National Academy of Sciences USA* **115**(51), 12911 LP–12919. http://dx.doi.org/10.1073/pnas.1717161115.

Shane, S. (2010). After 8 years, F.B.I. shuts book on anthrax case. *New York Times*, February 20, p. A1. Available at www.nytimes.com/2010/02/20/us/20anthrax.html.

Smith, M. J., Nixon, S., Upshur, R. et al. (2019). Public health ethics, in Bailey, T., Sheldon, C. T., & Shelley, J. J. (eds.), *Public Health Law and Policy in Canada*, 4th ed. Toronto: LexisNexis Canada.

Sommer, L. (2020). Why the warning that coronavirus was on the move in US cities came so late. NPR, April 24. Available at www.npr.org/sections/health-shots/2020/04/24/842025982/why-the-warning-that-coronavirus-was-on-the-move-in-u-s-cities-came-so-late.

Stiglitz, J. (2015). In defence of the Asian Infrastructure Investment Bank. *The Guardian*, April 14. Available at www.theguardian.com/business/2015/apr/14/in-defence-of-the-asian-infrastructure-investment-bank.

Stone, W., & Yu, E. (2020). Eerie emptiness of ERs worries doctors: where are the heart attacks and strokes? NPR, May 6. Available at www.npr.org/sections/health-shots/2020/05/06/850454989/eerie-emptiness-of-ers-worries-doctors-where-are-the-heart-attacks-and-strokes.

Strauss, V. (2020). Why covid-19 will "explode" academic achievement gaps. *Washington Post*, 17 April. Available at: www.washingtonpost.com/education/2020/04/17/why-covid-19-will-explode-existing-academic-achievement-gaps/.

Sutter, K. M., Sutherland, M. D., & Schwarzenberg, A. B. (2020). *COVID-19: China Medical Supply Chains and Broader Trade Issues*. Available at https://crsreports.congress.gov/product/pdf/R/R46304.

Tacconelli, E., Magrini, N., Carmeli, Y. et al. (2017). *Global Priority List of Antibiotic-Resistant Bacteria To Guide Research, Discovery, and Development of New Antibiotics*. Geneva: WHO.

Takahashi, H., Keim, P., Kaufmann, A. F. et al. (2004). *Bacillus anthracis* incident, Kameido, Tokyo, 1993. *Emerging Infectious Diseases* **10**(1), 117–120. http://dx.doi.org/10.3201/eid1001.030238.

Taubenberger, J. K., & Morens, D. M. (2006). 1918 influenza: the mother of all pandemics. *Emerging Infectious Diseases* **12**(1), 15–22. http://dx.doi.org/10.3201/eid1201.050979.

Thompson, S. A. (2020). How long will a vaccine really take? *New York Times*, April 30. Available at www.nytimes.com/interactive/2020/04/30/opinion/coronavirus-covid-vaccine.html.

Thorpe, K. E., Joski, P., & Johnston, K. J. (2018). Antibiotic-resistant infection treatment costs have doubled since 2002, now exceeding $2 billion annually., *Health Affairs (Project Hope)* **37**(4), 662–669. http://dx.doi.org/10.1377/hlthaff.2017.1153.

United Nations Children's Fund (UNICEF) (2019). 4,500 children under the age of five died from measles in the Democratic Republic of the Congo so far this year. November 27. Available at www.unicef.org/press-releases/4500-children-under-age-five-died-measles-democratic-republic-congo-so-far-year.

United Nations, Department of Economic and Social Affairs/Population Division (2018). *World Urbanization Prospects: The 2018 Revision* (online edition). Available at http://esa.un.org/unpd/wup/Methodology/WUP2018-Methodology.pdf.

United Nations Department of Economic and Social Affairs/Population Division (2019). *World Population Prospects: The 2019 Revision* (online edition). Available at https://population.un.org/wpp/.

United Nations General Assembly (2016). Protecting humanity from future health crises: report of the High-level Panel on the Global Response to Health Crises. Available at https://digitallibrary.un.org/record/822489?ln=en.

Van Dorn, A., Cooney, R. E., & Sabin, M. L. (2020). COVID-19 exacerbating inequalities in the US. *Lancet* **395** (10232), 1243–1244. https://doi.org/10.1016/S0140-6736(20)30893-X.

Vergano, M., Bertolini, G., Giannini, A. et al. (2020) *Raccomandazioni di Etica Clinica per l'Ammissione a Trattamenti Intensivi e per la loro Sospensione, in Condizioni Eccezionali di Squilibrio tra Necessità e Risorse Disponibili*. Available at www.siaarti.it/SiteAssets/News/

COVID19-documenti SIAARTI/SIAARTI-Covid19-Raccomandazioni di etica clinica.pdf.

Wang, H. (2017). New multilateral development banks: opportunities and challenges for global governance. *Global Policy* **8**(1), 113–118. https://doi.org/10.1111/1758-5899.12396.

Weinraub, B. (1974). Smallpox grows in India; worst over, officials say. *New York Times*, July 16, p. 3. Available at www.nytimes.com/1974/07/16/archives/smallpox-grows-in-india-worst-over-officials-say-about-26000-deaths.html.

Welch, C. (2009). Inaccurate "swine" flu label hurts industry, pork producers say. CNN, April 30. Available at www.cnn.com/2009/HEALTH/04/30/pork.industry.impact/.

Wolfe, N. D., Dunavan, C. P., & Diamond, J. (2007). Origins of major human infectious diseases., *Nature* **447**(7142), 279–283. https://doi.org/10.1038/nature05775.

World Bank (2018). *World Development Indicators*. Washington, DC: World Bank Group. Available at http://databank.worldbank.org/data/reports.aspx?source=world-development-indicators (accessed August 24, 2018).

World Health Organization (WHO) (2003). *Cumulative Number of Reported Probable Cases of SARS*. Available at www.who.int/csr/sars/country/2003_07_11/en/ (accessed February 7, 2019).

World Health Organization (WHO) (2011). *Pandemic Influenza Preparedness Framework: For the Sharing of Influenza Viruses and Access to Vaccines and Other Benefits*. Geneva: WHO Press. Available at http://apps.who.int/iris/bitstream/handle/10665/44796/9789241503082_eng.pdf;jsessionid=2F9149BC5014B336EF5AC6BD3B00FC87?sequence=1.

World Health Organization (WHO) (2013). *Crimean-Congo Haemorrhagic Fever*. Available at www.who.int/news-room/fact-sheets/detail/crimean-congo-haemorrhagic-fever (accessed February 7, 2019).

World Health Organization (WHO) (2015). *Report of the Ebola Interim Assessment Panel*. Geneva: WHO Press.

World Health Organization (WHO) (2016). *An R&D Blueprint for Action to Prevent Epidemics: Plan of Action*. Geneva: WHO Press. Available at www.who.int/blueprint/about/r_d_blueprint_plan_of_action.pdf.

World Health Organization (WHO) (2017a). *Lassa Fever*. Available at www.who.int/en/news-room/fact-sheets/detail/lassa-fever (accessed February 7, 2019).

World Health Organization (WHO) (2017b). *Marburg Virus Disease*. Available at www.who.int/mediacentre/factsheets/fs_marburg/en/ (accessed February 7, 2019).

World Health Organization (WHO) (2017c). *Methodology for Prioritizing Severe Emerging Diseases for Research and Development*. Available at www.who.int/blue

print/priority-diseases/RDBlueprint-PrioritizationTool.pdf ?ua=1.

World Health Organization (WHO) (2017d). *Multi-Drug Resistant Tuberculosis (MDR-TB): 2017 Update.* Available at www.who.int/tb/challenges/mdr/MDR-RR_TB_factsheet_2017.pdf.

World Health Organization (WHO) (2017e). Plague outbreak Madagascar (External Situation Report 14). Available at https://apps.who.int/iris/bitstream/handle/10665/259556/Ex-PlagueMadagascar04122017.pdf?sequence=1.

World Health Organization (WHO) (2018a). *Ebola Vaccine Frequently Asked Questions.* Available at www.who.int/emergencies/diseases/ebola/frequently-asked-questions/ebola-vaccine.

World Health Organization (WHO) (2018b). *Ebola Virus Disease.* Available at www.who.int/news-room/fact-sheets/detail/ebola-virus-disease (accessed February 7, 2019).

World Health Organization (WHO) (2018c). *List of Blueprint Priority Diseases.* Available at www.who.int/blueprint/priority-diseases/en/ (accessed February 7, 2019).

World Health Organization (WHO) (2018d). *Nipah Virus.* Available at www.who.int/news-room/fact-sheets/detail/nipah-virus (accessed February 7, 2019).

World Health Organization (WHO) (2018e). *Rift Valley Fever.* Available at www.who.int/news-room/fact-sheets/detail/rift-valley-fever (accessed February 7, 2019).

World Health Organization (WHO) (2018f). *Zika Virus.* Available at www.who.int/news-room/fact-sheets/detail/zika-virus (accessed February 7, 2019).

World Health Organization (WHO) (2018g). WHO and World Bank group join forces to strengthen global health security. Available at www.who.int/news-room/detail/24–05-2018-who-and-world-bank-group-join-forces-to-strengthen-global-health-security (accessed December 4, 2018).

World Health Organization (WHO) (2019a). *Cholera.* Available at www.who.int/news-room/fact-sheets/detail/cholera.

World Health Organization (WHO) (2019b). *Ebola in the Democratic Republic of the Congo: Health Emergency Update.* Available at www.who.int/emergencies/diseases/ebola/drc–2019.

World Health Organization (WHO) (2019c). *Global*

Health Observatory (GHO) Data: HIV/AIDS. Available at www.who.int/gho/hiv/en/ (accessed February 12, 2019).

World Health Organization (WHO) (2019d). *Global Outbreak Alert and Response Network (GOARN).* Available at www.who.int/ihr/alert_and_response/outbreak-network/en/.

World Health Organization (WHO) (2019e). *Middle East Respiratory Syndrome Coronavirus (MERS-CoV).* Available at www.who.int/news-room/fact-sheets/detail/middle-east-respiratory-syndrome-coronavirus-(mers-cov) (accessed February 7, 2019).

World Health Organization (WHO) (2019f). *SARS (Severe Acute Respiratory Syndrome).* Available at www.who.int/ith/diseases/sars/en/ (sccessed February 7, 2019).

World Health Organization Initiative for Vaccine Research (2019). *WHO Guide for Standardization of Economic Evaluations of Immunization Programmes.* Geneva: WHO Press.

World Health Organization (WHO) (2020a). *Coronavirus Disease (COVID-19) Training: Simulation Exercise.* Available at www.who.int/emergencies/diseases/novel-coronavirus-2019/training/simulation-exercise (accessed May 11, 2020).

World Health Organization (WHO) (2020b). Prioritizing diseases for research and development in emergency contexts. Available at www.who.int/activities/prioritizing-diseases-for-research-and-development-in-emergency-contexts.

World Health Organization (WHO) in South-East Asia (2020). GOARN Training. Available at origin.searo.who.int/about/administration_structure/hse/GOARN_advocacy/en/.

Yamey, G., Schäferhoff, M., Hatchett, R. et al. (2020). Ensuring global access to COVID-19 vaccines. *Lancet* **395** (10234), 1405–1406. https://doi.org/10.1016/S0140-6736(20)30763-7.

Yang, D. L. (2020). Wuhan officials tried to cover up COVID-19 – and sent it careening outward. *Washington Post*, March 10. Available at www.washingtonpost.com/politics/2020/03/10/wuhan-officials-tried-cover-up-covid-19-sent-it-careening-outward/.

Zhu, T., Korber, B. T., Nahmias, A. J. et al. (1998). An African HIV-1 sequence from 1959 and implications for the origin of the epidemic. *Nature* **391**(6667), 594. https://doi.org/10.1038/35400.

Gender Equality in Science, Medicine, and Global Health
Where Are We At and Why Does It Matter?

Geordan Shannon, Melanie Jansen, Kate Williams, Carlos Caceres,
Angelica Motta, Aloyce Odhiambo, Alie Eleveld, and Jenevieve Mannell

Introduction

We are in the midst of a gender reckoning in the fields of science, medicine, and global health (Clark et al., 2017). Four contemporary social movements have helped shape the global gender and health landscape: online movements against violence, including #MeToo and #NiUnaMenos; intersectional feminism; the evolving recognition of men and masculinities; and the global trans rights movement. These movements are transforming the health sciences, forcing us to grapple with "questions of agency, vulnerability, and the dynamic and changing realities of gendered power relations" (Hilhorst et al., 2018: online). We are living through transformative and challenging times.

It is in this context that we review the evidence for why gender equality matters in science, medicine, and global health. The purpose of this chapter is to provide a high-level synthesis of global gender data; summarize progress toward gender equality in science, medicine, and global health; and review the evidence for why gender equality matters in terms of health and social outcomes. We situate our work in the context of global movements transforming our field, drawing inspiration from trans, feminist, and intersectional scholarship.

BOX 4.1 Key Terms and Definitions

Gender refers to the "socially constructed norms that impose and determine roles, relationships and positional power for all people across their lifetime. Gender interacts with sex, the biological and physical characteristics that define women, men and those with intersex identities" (Global Health 5050, 2018: online).[a]

Gender data are data disaggregated by sex or reporting gendered phenomena.[b]

Gender equality means "equal rights, responsibilities and opportunities of women and men and girls and boys, when the interests, needs and priorities of both women and men are taken into consideration, recognizing the diversity of different groups of women and men" (UN Women, 2011: online).

Trans is "an umbrella term that is used to describe people whose gender is not the same as, or does not sit comfortably with, the sex they were assigned at birth" (Stonewall UK, n.d.).

[a] We have used the Global Health 5050 definition because the definition put forward by the World Health Organization (WHO) does not explicitly recognize trans or non-gender-binary identities.
[b] Some agencies define gender data as data disaggregated by sex or data that affect women exclusively.

Gender, Health, and Society

Restrictive gender norms affect everybody. As a *shared determinant* of health (Hawkes, 2018) for men, women, boys, girls, and gender diverse people, gender inequalities drive large-scale excesses in mortality and morbidity globally (Anderson & Ray, 2000; Sen & Östlin, 2007). Gender inequality is transformed into health risk through discriminatory values, norms, beliefs, and practices; differential exposures and vulnerabilities to disease, disability, and injuries; biases in health systems; and biases in health research (Sen & Östlin, 2007). Gender discrimination at any of these levels detrimentally impacts health and social outcomes (Anderson & Ray, 2000; Sen & Östlin, 2007). For example, interpersonal violence, including violence against women, is influenced by harmful gender norms and broader systems of oppression (Caceres et al., 2002; Shannon et al., 2017); confronting these gendered structures is relevant to all people. More insidiously, gender inequalities contribute to increased levels of stress and anxiety: among women through their socially prescribed role as caregivers (Penning & Wu, 2015), among men through their socially prescribed role as breadwinners (Barker et al., 2011), and among trans people where nonconformity to gender norms is often socially penalized (Health Policy Project, 2015; Winter, 2012).

Gender equality is a human right (Global Health 5050, 2018; United Nations General Assembly, 2018). It is essential "to achieve peaceful societies, with full human potential and sustainable development" (United Nations, 2018: online). After more than a century of feminist advocacy (de Beauvoir, 1949; Gilman, 1971; United Nations, 2018), 40 years of international discourses on gender in development (Beneria et al., 2003; Hillorst & Porter, 2018), and a mounting body of evidence (Clark et al., 2017; Hawkes & Buse, 2013), gender equality is recognized as one of the most significant determinants of health and economic development (Global Health 5050, 2018; Hawkes, 2018; Malhotra et al, 2002). Despite this recognition, gender equality remains a complex issue in health and development. For one, the term *gender* is a "widely used and often misunderstood term. It is sometimes conflated with sex or used to refer only to women" (Momsen, 2010: 2), and it also categorically excludes trans and non-gender-binary people (Hawkes & Buse, 2013). In this chapter, we use the Global Health 5050 definition of gender (Global Health 5050, 2018) and the United Nations (UN) definition of gender equality (UN Women, 2011). Whereas gender equality has been positioned as key to achieving the Sustainable Development Goals (Manandhar et al., 2018; United Nations, 2014), there is "a distinct lack of clarity about how such a goal should be defined or about how it might be achieved" (Doyal, 2000: 931). Gender is an inherently political issue that "is missing from, misunderstood in, and only sometimes mainstreamed into global health policies and programmes" (Hawkes & Buse, 2013: 1783). There has been sluggish progress toward international gender equality targets (Global Health 5050, 2018; Hawkes & Buse, 2013; United Nations, 2014), and conservative campaigns against "gender ideology" threaten to undermine progress (Correa, 2018; Segato, 2016).

The Global State of Gender Equality Data

Gender data matter for women in science, medicine, and global health to both monitor progress and reflect critically on research processes and outputs. A range of gender data has emerged in the last two decades (Barden & Klassen, 1999; Charmes & Wieringa, 2003; Kabeer, 2001). The Organisation for Economic Co-Operation and Development (OECD) reports aggregate gender data on employment, education, entrepreneurship, health development, and governance (OECD, 2019). The World Bank's Gender Data Portal contains over 500 indicators on agency, socioeconomic context, economic opportunities, education, health, public life, and decision making (World Bank, 2019). The UN Statistics Division's Minimum Set of Gender Indicators contains 52 quantitative and 11 qualitative indicators over the domains of economic structures and access to resources, education, health, public life and decision making, and human rights (United Nations Statistics Division, 2018). In addition, there are numerous international gender indexes reflecting composite data over various aspects of gender, health, and development (Dijkstra & Hanmer, 2000; Hawken & Munck, 2013; Klasen, 2007).

Despite the proliferation of indicators, methodological and conceptual shortfalls significantly limit the use of gender data (Charmes & Wieringa, 2003; Cueva Beteta, 2006; Dijkstra & Hanmer, 2000; Hawken & Munck, 2013). Methodological limitations include unequal country coverage, lack of international standards for comparability, insufficient complexity of indicators across gender domains, and insufficient granularity for disaggregation (UN Development Programme [UNDP], 2010; Data2X, 2017; Equal Measures 2030, 2019). Conceptual shortfalls include assumptions of heteronormativity, exclusion of non-gender-binary persons and men, lack of meaningful information about within-household gender dynamics, and inadequate quantification of unpaid and domestic labor (Chant, 2006; Hawkes & Buse, 2013; Hillenbrand et al., 2015; Wood, 2019). Initiatives such as Data2X and Equal Measures 2030 aim to fill these gaps and transform gender data-collection systems through conceptualizing and collecting new data and reorganizing existing data so that they are more actionable by policymakers (Data2X, 2017; Equal Measures 2030, 2019). The Gender Equitable Men Scale (GEMS) offers survey tools that explore attitudes toward gender norms, violence, masculinity, and sexual health (Levtov et al., 2014). With massive national epidemiologic and demographic transitions – combined with the growing recognition of subnational and intraurban heterogeneity and the need for intersectional approaches to the quantification of relative advantage or disadvantage (Chant & McIlwaine, 2016) – gender metrics are moving toward individual-level approaches (Alkire et al., 2013; Ewerling et al., 2017).

Notwithstanding the changing landscape of global gender data, the overall pattern of gender equality for women in science, medicine, and global health is one of mixed gains and persistent challenges.

Gender Equality in Science, Medicine, and Global Health

Progress

In science, the "knowledge gender divide continues to exist in all countries, even those which have a highly-developed knowledge society" (Women in Global Science and Technology, 2012: 1). The United Nations Educational, Scientific, and Cultural Organization (UNESCO) Women in Science data demonstrate that less than 30% of the world's researchers are women, comprising only 19% in South and West Asia, 23% in East Asia and the Pacific, 30% in Sub-Saharan Africa, 32% in North America and Western Europe, and 45% in Latin America (UNESCO, 2018). The proportion of women researchers is increasing worldwide, although they publish fewer research papers on average than men and are less likely to collaborate internationally (Elsevier, 2017). In Europe and North America, men are still more likely to graduate from the natural sciences, mathematics, and information and communication technologies and to translate higher degrees into employment (Catalyst, 2019). Women are often "squeezed out" of science careers by structural barriers: the Science in Australia Gender Equity (SAGE, 2018), the American Association of University Women (AAUW, 2019), and the European Commission (EC, 2015) report that gender inequality is a function of systemic factors unrelated to ability, including bias, organizational constraints, organizational culture, and differential effects of work and family demands. Analysis of Programme for International Student Assessment (PISA) data found, paradoxically, that countries with high levels of gender equality have some of the largest science, technology, engineering, and mathematics (STEM) gaps in secondary and tertiary education (Stoet & Geary, 2018).

In health, issues of occupational segregation, wage and working conditions, and leadership disparities remain pronounced. The health workforce is feminizing, and women's participation is consistently higher than in science or the general workforce, but this is occurring unequally: approximately 75% of the global health workforce is female, yet women disproportionately represent lower cadres of health workers (George, 2007; Shannon et al., 2019; WHO, 2019). In medicine, there are persistent imbalances in specialist training participation, with women remaining the minority in surgical specialties (Australian Institute for Health and Welfare, 2015), and gender pay gaps across all specialties, which are not wholly explained by seniority, career breaks, and part-time work (Connoley & Holdcroft, 2015). Further, wage conditions may deteriorate as more women join the ranks of health professions (Shannon et al., 2019). The High-Level Commission on Health Employment and Economic Growth recognized that working conditions of health workers were affected by poor wages and benefits, the absence of social protection, and unsafe working conditions (High-Level Commission on Health Employment and Economic Growth, 2016). Although women comprise the majority of the health workforce around the world, they hold a small fraction of leadership positions (Schwalbe, 2017). The WHO Global Health Workforce Network Gender Equity Hub recognizes that across the health and social care workforce, women are significantly under-represented in management, leadership, and governance (WHO Gender Equity Hub, 2019).

Global health is defined as "collaborative transnational research and action for promoting health for all" (Beaglehole & Bonita, 2010: 1) and encompasses international governance, research, and health financing. Despite this inclusive definition, global health as a field remains gender unequal or "gender blind." For example, among 140 global health organizations, only 40% mention gender in their governance documents (Global Health 5050, 2018). Only 20% of global health organizations had gender parity on their governing boards (Global Health 5050, 2018), and only two UN agencies related to health have women heads (Schwalbe, 2017). Despite recent commitment by the WHO's director general to gender equality, only a quarter of member state chief delegates to the World Health Assembly or ministers of health are women (Dhatt et al., 2017). Gender has only recently been explicitly recognized by philanthropic bodies and research funders with organizational commitments to gender equality from a range of large international donors (Global Health 5050, 2018). In health financing, gender is insufficiently addressed despite the purported emphasis placed on equity by proponents of universal health coverage (Whitter et al., 2017).

> **BOX 4.2 Search Strategy and Selection Criteria**
>
> We identified published and "gray" literature on gender equality and women in science, medicine, and global health using Medline, Embase, GoogleScholar, Greenfile, and Scopus search engines. Search terms included *gender, gender equ*, gender inequ*, gender disparit*, male, female, gender diversity*, combined with *patient outcomes, research outcomes, morbidity and mortality*, and *differences in practice*. Reference lists of relevant papers were then also searched to identify further relevant papers. The first 30 hits were looked at on Google and Google Scholar searches.

Limits

Gender biases in the health sector "undermine inclusive economic growth, full employment, decent work and the achievement of gender equality. They also create inefficiencies in health systems by limiting the productivity, distribution, motivation and retention of female workers, who constitute the majority of the health workforce" (High-Level Commission on Health Employment and Economic Growth, 2016: 33). Gender discrimination is linked to low morale, low self-esteem, and lower productivity (Newman, 2014; WHO, 2019). In many countries, women lack access to productive resources – including land, finance, technology, and education – necessary to support engagement in science (Women in Global Science and Technology, 2012). Research from East Africa suggests that women scientists face higher burdens of unpaid work and gender violence, with serious sequelae for mental and physical health (Channar et al., 2011; GenderINSITE, 2018; Hafkin, 2019; Women in Global Science and Technology, 2012). Systematic gender inequality leads to health workforce maldistribution and inefficiencies in or barriers to healthcare for those who need it most (Commission on Social Determinants of Health, 2008; Newman, 2014). Unless gender – and its intersections with other social stratifiers – is explicitly recognized, progress toward universal health coverage (UHC) may fail to address or even exacerbate gender inequality (Whitter et al., 2017).

Although men face fewer barriers to career progression in science, medicine, and global health, they also lack systematic support for transforming existing workplace gender structures. Resources such as Men Advocating Real Change (MARC, by Catalyst) exist to support gender equality initiatives, although there are few targeted policies supporting men as carers or other policies supporting men in transforming workplace gender cultures (Cataylst, 2019). A European Union (EU) report found that despite positive effects of paternity leave on economic, social, and demographic outcomes, uptake of leave remained low because of poor compensation, lack of affordable childcare, inflexibility of leave arrangements, gender norms, and cultural expectations (van Belle, 2016).

There is a paucity of information available about trans persons in the science, medicine, and global health workforce. However, a recent study of employment outcomes using the American National Transgender Discrimination Survey found that trans persons experience greater discrimination in hiring and differential treatment once employed (Davidson & Halsall, 2016). Research on the health burden and needs of gender minorities is increasingly available, but trans issues remain marginalized; for example, much data remain blind to trans identities because of the absence of survey items with which to identify as non–gender binary (Reisner et al., 2016).

Why Gender Matters: Opportunities in Science, Medicine, and Global Health

Gender equality in science, medicine, and global health has the potential to lead to significant health, social, and economic gains. There is widespread consensus that gender equality in the community promotes economic growth, lowers fertility, reduces child mortality, and improves nutrition (Abu-Ghaida & Klasen, 2004; Commission on Social Determinants of Health, 2008; McDonald, 2000). There is also evidence, primarily from business and management sectors, that gender-diverse workplaces have improved productivity, innovation, decision making, and employee retention and satisfaction (Chartered Institute of Personnel and Development [CIPD], 2019; Morgan Stanley, 2017). Gender-diverse institutions are more likely to outperform those that are not gender diverse (Dawson et al., 2014; Hunt et al., 2015). If productivity and innovation can be improved by increasing gender diversity, then there is an ethical imperative to do so. Any organization that is not gender diverse is failing to access and leverage talent.

A benefit of diversity in corporate settings is that a workforce that better understands the diverse consumer population can therefore create products and services tailored to clients, leading to increased returns (Tomas, 2004). The same may be true in science, medicine, and global health: a more diverse research team may develop more nuanced and relevant research questions, resulting in research that is applicable (and beneficial) to a broader population. In science research, ethnic diversity of authors is associated with increased impact and citations (Freeman & Huang, 2014). A review article exploring the culture in medicine toward sexual and gender minorities notes that increasing visibility of lesbian, gay, bisexual, and transgender (LGBT) and gender-diverse healthcare providers may promote a welcoming environment for staff and patients (Mansh et al., 2015). In these ways, gender transformation in health and science sectors has the potential to contribute significantly to gains in gender equality in the wider community (Magar et al., in High-Level Commission on Health Employment and Economic Growth, 2016; US Department of Health and Human Services, 2006; Women in Global Science and Technology, 2012).

A gender-diverse medical workforce may also translate into improved patient outcomes. There is evidence that different patients prefer to be treated by a certain-gendered doctor (Alyahya et al., 2019; Cooper-Patrick et al., 1999), which is important for equity of access to care. A study investigating mortality of women patients with acute myocardial infarction found higher mortality rates in women treated by male doctors (Greenwood et al., 2018). Interestingly, the effect was attenuated if male doctors had higher exposure to female patients and physician colleagues (Greenwood et al., 2018). There is also emerging evidence of beneficial differences in the way women doctors practice, leading to lower patient morbidity and mortality (Tsugawa et al., 2017; Wallis, 2017). For example, in a matched cohort study performed in Canada, patients treated by female surgeons had a modest but statistically significant decrease in a composite outcome of 30-day mortality, complications, and readmission (Wallis, 2017). Similarly, Tsugawa et al. (2017) found that hospitalized patients treated by women internists had lower mortality and readmissions compared with those cared for by male doctors. A Canadian study found that patients of women primary care physicians had more consistently received recommended health screening and had fewer emergency department visits than those treated by male primary care physicians (Dahrouge

et al., 2016). The authors of the papers conclude that gender is a marker of other behaviors that lead to better outcomes, pointing to evidence that women doctors tend to follow guidelines more closely, spend more time with patients, and may have more effective communication skills (Dahrouge et al., 2016). In one meta-analysis of the gender effect in medical communication, women primary care physicians had a more patient-centered communication style, but there was no gender difference in the quality of information conveyed to patients, and male obstetrics and gynecology specialists scored higher for emotionally focused talk (Roter et al., 2002). Other gender differences in the medical workforce have been described, from simulated surgical skills tasks to mentorship (Ali et al., 2015). Although gender differences are apparent, it is important not to assume that these are inherent and unchangeable. Instead, we should investigate the drivers of these observed differences to elucidate the positive behaviors that lead to improved outcomes in order to optimize training and development for the entire science and health workforce.

Promoting Gender Equality in Science, Medicine, and Global Health

Specific strategies exist to promote women and girls in health and science. The WHO has catalogued a range of tools to assist with gender analysis in health (WHO, 2002), and outlines gender transformative strategies for programs and policies (WHO, 2011). The Commission on the Status of Women 55th Session (United Nations Population Fund [NFPA], 2011) adopted a report that recognized education and training in STEM, and in 2013, the United Nations General Assembly (UN, 2018) adopted a resolution on science, technology, and innovation for development, recognizing the need for full and equal access by women and girls. The African Union's Science, Technology and Innovation Strategy for Africa 2024 (African Union, 2014) recognizes inclusion of women and youth in the industry (Muthumbi & Sommerfeld, 2015); the East African Community adopted a framework to promote gender in science, technology, and innovation; and the Southern Africa Development Community's (SADC) Gender Policy supports equal access to science education (Muthumbi & Sommerfeld, 2015). Policies such as these are supported by international advocacy networks such as Gender in Science, Innovation, Technology and Engineering (GenderINSITE, 2018) and the Organisation for Women in Science for the Developing World (2019).

However, these policies have not been sufficient to bring about the widespread social changes needed to ensure gender equality in science, medicine, and global health. Social movements, such as the global trans rights movement and online movements against violence, contain important lessons for current efforts for women within science, medicine, and global health. Social movements work by politicizing issues, calling for the rights of marginalized or less powerful groups in ways that transform power relations and create enabling environments for demands to be heard (Campbell et al., 2010). At the turn of the twentieth century, women physicians were very much part of the women's health movement, which led to a groundswell of changes in the exclusionary practices of medical schools (Riska, 2001). However, as women became more integrated into medicine, the focus on feminist principles faded despite the continuation of widespread inequalities in specialization, pay, and career advancement (Riska, 2001). Social movements played a critical role in drawing attention to the voices of women and marginalized groups in global health, particularly in human immune-deficiency virus (HIV) infection and acquired immunodeficiency syndrome (AIDS) populations (Seckinelgin, 2009). For instance, the Treatment Action Campaign mobilized thousands of unemployed black women, medical professionals, students, and academics, reaching across boundaries of race, education, and class, to successfully transform South Africa's HIV/AIDS policy. In science, social collectives and networks play an important role in encouraging women to enter and remain in their careers (Davis, 2001) and may be more important than more individual approaches such as mentorship or "girl-friendly" curricula (Gilbert & Calvert, 2003). Taken as a whole, this literature highlights the critical importance of collective networks in bringing about fundamental changes in gender inequalities and the urgent need for feminist action to transform the position of women in science, medicine, and global health.

Conclusion

Our review has highlighted the evidence for why gender equality matters in terms of health and health-related outcomes, positioning this chapter within a discussion of progress toward gender equality worldwide. We found that better gender data are available, women are making progress but remain considerably disadvantaged, men's roles are expanding but are limited by restrictive gender norms, and information on the trans community is limited. Despite this progress, conceptual and methodological shortfalls in research – including outdated conceptualizations of gender and gender inequalities – persist, meaning that we only understand part of a much more complex whole.

Gender equality matters for health. It is one of the most significant drivers of health and health inequalities of our time. The current gender reckoning in science, medicine, and global health highlights both missed and future opportunities and the need to situate gender analyses in the context of political influences and structural inequalities and draw on contemporary social movements to advance the field. Beyond quantitative gender equality, we must strive for a cultural transformation that allows for the inclusion of values of transparency, honesty, fairness, and justice. With the evolving landscape, we are in the position to demand more from the evidence, to innovate beyond current discourses, and to realize true gender equality for everyone, everywhere. Achieving gender equality is not simply instrumental for health and development; its impact has wide-ranging benefits and is a matter of fairness and social justice for everyone.

Author Contributions

All authors contributed equally to the conceptualization of this study. GS, KW, MJ, and JM performed the literature search. CC and AM contributed to insights on masculinities and transgender communities, whereas AE and AO contributed country-specific insights and supporting case studies. GS drafted the article and collated the figures, with inputs from JM, KW, MJ, CC, AM, AE, and AO.

Declaration of Interests

We declare no competing interests. No funding sources to disclose.

Acknowledgement

This chapter was originally published by the same authors as 'Gender equality in science, medicine, and global health: where are we at and why does it matter? in The Lancet, 2019 Feb 9; 393(10171):560–569., doi: 10.1016/S0140-6736(18)33135-0. Copyright Elsevier. It is reproduced here with the permission of Elsevier with non-exclusive world rights in all languages, and for use in any future editions.

References

Abu-Ghaida, D., & Klassen, S. (2004). The costs of missing the Millennium Development Goal on gender equity. *World Development*, **32**(7), 1075–1107.

African Union (2014). *Science, Technology and Innovation Strategy for Africa 2024*. Addis Ababa: African Union.

Ali, A., Subhi, Y., Ringsted, C., & Konge, L. (2015). Gender differences in the acquisition of surgical skills: a systematic review. *Surgical Endoscopy*, **29**, 3065–3073.

Alkire, S., Meinzen-Dick, R., Peterman, A., et al. (2013). *The Women's Empowerment in Agriculture Index*. Oxford, UK; Oxford Poverty and Human Development Initiative (OPHI).

Alyahya, G., Almohanna, H., Alyahya, A., et al. (2019). Does physicians' gender have any influence on patients' choice of their treating physicians? *Journal of the Nature and Science of Medicine*, **2**(1), 29–34.

American Association of University Women (AAUW) (2019). *Solving the Equation: The Variables for Women's Success in Engineering and Computing* (online). Washington, DC: AAUW. Available at www.aauw.org/research/solving-the-equation/ (accessed November 13, 2019).

Anderson, S., & Ray, D. (2000). Missing women: age and disease. *Review of Economic Studies*, **77**(4), 1262–1300.

Australian Institute of Health and Welfare (AIHW) (2015). *Medical Practitioners Workforce*. Canberra: AIHW.

Barden, K., & Klasen, S. (1999). UNDP's gender-related indices: a critical review. *World Development*, **27**(6), 985–1010.

Barker, G., Contreras, J. M., Heilman, B., et al. (2011). *Evolving Men: Initial Results from the International Men and Gender Equality Survey (IMAGES)*. Washington, DC: International Center for Research on Women (ICRW) and Instituto Promundo.

Beaglehole, R., & Bonita, R. (2010). What is global health? *Global Health Action*, **3**, 5142. DOI:10.3402/gha.v3i0.5142.

Beneria, L., Berik, G., & Floro, M. (2003). *Gender, Development and Globalization: Economics as If All People Mattered*. New York: Routledge.

Caceres, C., Salazar, X., Rosasco, A., & Davila, P. (2002). To be a man in Peru: infidelity, violence and homophobia in the male experience, in Caceres, C. (ed.), *Ser hombre en el Perú de hoy: Una mirada a la salud sexual desde la infidelidad, la violencia y la homofobia*. Lima: REDESS Jóvenes.

Campbell, C., Cornish, F., Gibbs, A., & Scott, K. (2010). Heeding the push from below. *Journal of Health Psychology*, **15**, 962–971.

Catalyst (2019). *Women in Science, Technology, Engineering, and Mathematics (STEM): Quick Take* (online). Available at www.catalyst.org/knowledge/women-science-technology-engineering-and-mathematics-stem (accessed November 2019).

Channar, Z., Abbassi, Z., & Ujan, I. (2011). Gender discrimination in workforce and its impact on the employees. *Pakistan Journal of Commerce and Social Sciences*, **5**(1), 177–191.

Chant, S. (2006). Re-thinking the "feminization of poverty" in relation to aggregate gender indices. *Journal of Human Development*, **7**(2), 201–220.

Chant, S., & McIlwaine, C. (2016). *Cities, Slums and Gender in the Global South: Towards a Feminised Urban Future*, 1st ed. Oxon, UK: Routlidge.

Charmes, J., & Wieringa, S. (2003). Measuring women's empowerment: an assessment of the gender-related development index and the gender empowerment measure. *Journal of Human Development*, **4**(3), 419–435.

Chartered Institute of Personnel and Development (CIPD). (2019). Building inclusive workplaces: assessing the evidence (research report). London: CIPD.

Clark, J., Zuccula, L., & Horton, R. (2017). Women in science, medicine, and global health: call for papers. *Lancet*, **390**(10111), 2423–2424.

Commission on Social Determinants of Health (2008). *Closing the Gap in a Generation: Health Equity Through Action on the Social Determinants of Health* (Final Report of the Commission on Social Determinants of Health). Geneva: Commission on Social Determinants of Health.

Connolly, S., & Holdcroft, A. (2015). *The Pay Gap for Women in Medicine and Academic Medicine*. London: British Medical Association.

Cooper-Patrick, L., Gallo, J. J., Gonzales, J. J., et al. (1999). Race, gender, and partnership in the patient-physician relationship. *Journal of the American Medical Association*, **282**(6), 583–589.

Correa, S. (2018). *Ideología de género: rastreando sus orígenes y significados en la política de género actual*. Rio de Janeiro: Sexuality Policy Watch.

Cueva Beteta, H. (2006). What is missing in measures of women's empowerment? *Journal of Human Development*, **7**(2), 221–241.

Dahrouge, S., Seale, E., Hogg, W., et al. (2016). A comprehensive assessment of family physician gender and quality of care: a cross sectional analysis in Ontario, Canada. *Cancer Medical Care*, **54**(3), 277–286

Data2X (2017). *Ready to Measure: Phase II Indicators Available to Monitor SDG Gender Targets*. New York: Data2X.

Davidson, S., & Halsall, J. (Rev. Eds.) (2016). Gender inequality: nonbinary transgender people in the workplace. *Cogent Social Sciences*, **2**(1), 1236511. DOI:10.1080/23311886.2016.1236511.

Davis, K. S. (2001). Peripheral and subversive: women making connections and challenging the boundaries of the science community. *Science Education*, **85**, 368–409.

Dawson, J., Kersley, R., & Natella, S. (2014). *The CS Gender 3000: The Reward for Change*. Zurich: Credit Suisse Research Institute.

de Beauvoir, S. (1949). *Le deuxième sexe*. Paris: Gallimard.

Dhatt, R., Kickbusch, I., & Thompson, K. (2017). Act now: a call to action for gender equality in global health. *Lancet*, **389**(10069), 602.

Dijkstra, A., & Hanmer, L. (2000). Measuring socio-economic gender inequality: toward an alternative to the UNDP Gender-Related Development Index. *Feminist Economics*, **6**(2), 41–75.

Doyal, L. (2000). Gender equity in health: debates and dilemmas. *Social Science and Medicine*, **51**, 931–939.

Elsevier (2017). *Gender in the Global Research Landscape*. Amsterdam: Elsevier.

Equal Measures 2030 (2019). *Equal Measures 2030* (online). Available at www.equalmeasures2030.org (accessed November 2019).

European Commission (2015). *She Figures*. Brussels: European Commission.

Ewerling, F., Lynch, J., Victora, C., et al. (2017). The SWPER index for women's empowerment in Africa: development and validation of an index based on survey data. *Lancet Global Health*, **5**, e916–e923.

Freeman, R., & Huang, W. (2014). Collaboration: strength in diversity. *Nature*, **513**(18), 305.

George, A. (2007) *Human Resources for Health: A Gender Analysis*. Geneva: WHO.

Gilbert, J., & Calvert, S. (2003). Challenging accepted wisdom: looking at the gender and science education question through a different lens. *International Journal of Science Education*, **25**, 861–878.

Gilman, C. (1971). *The Man-Made World: Or, Our Androcentric Culture*. New York: Johnson.

Global Health 5050 (2018). *Global Health 5050 Report*. London: Global Health 5050.

Greenwood, N., Carnahan, S., & Huang, L. (2018). Patient-physician gender concordance and increased mortality among female heart attack patients. *Proceedings of the National Academy of Sciences USA*, **115**(34), 8569–8574.

Hafkin, N. (2019). *National Assessments on Gender and Science, Technology and Innovation* (online). Available at https://owsd.net/sites/default/files/NH4EastAfricaGEKS.pdf (accessed November 2019).

Hawken, A., & Munck, G. (2013). Cross-national indices with gender-differentiated data: what do they measure? How valid are they? *Social Indicators Research*, **111**, 801–838.

Hawkes, S. Concurrence and Controversy about "gender" and "women and health," in *Women Leaders in Global Health 2018*. London: Women Leaders in Global Health.

Hawkes, S., & Buse, K. (2013). Gender and global health: evidence, policy, and inconvenient truths. *Lancet*, **381**, 1783–87.

Health Policy Project, Asia Pacific Transgender Network, United Nations Development Programme (2015). *Blueprint for the Provision of Comprehensive Care for Trans People and Trans Communities*. Washington, DC: Futures Group, Health Policy Project.

High-Level Commission on Health Employment and Economic Growth (2016). *Working for Health and Growth: Investing in the Health Workforce*. Geneva: WHO.

Hilhorst, D., Porter, H., & Gordon, R. (2018). Challenging humanitarianism beyond gender as women and women as victims #PressforProgress. Africa at LSE blog (online). Available at http://blogs.lse.ac.uk/africaatlse/2018/03/07/challenging-humanitarianism-beyond-gender-as-women-and-women-as-victims-pressforprogress/ (accessed November 2019).

Hillenbrand, E., Karim, N., Mohanraj, P., & Wu, D. (2015). Measuring Gender-Transformative Change: A Review of Literature and Promising Practices. Merrifield, VA: CARE USA.

Hunt, V., Layton, D., & Prince, S. (2015). Why diversity matters. McKinsey (online). Available at www.mckinsey.com/business-functions/organization/our-insights/why-diversity-matters.

Kabeer, N. (2001). Reflections on the measurement of women's empowerment, in Studies, S. (ed.), *Discussing Women's Empowerment: Theory and Practice*. Stockholm: Novum Grafiska AB.

Klasen, S. (2007). Gender-related indicators of well-being, in McGillivray, M. (ed.), *Human Well-Being. Studies in Development Economics and Policy*. London: Palgrave Macmillan.

Levtov, R., Barker, G., Contreras-Urbina, M., Heilman, B., & Verma, R. (2014). Pathways to gender-equitable men: findings from the International Men and Gender Equality Survey in eight countries. *Men and Masculinities*, **17**(5), 1–35.

Malhotra, A., Schuler, S., & Boender, C. (2002). Measuring women's empowerment as a variable in international development. Background paper prepared for the World Bank Workshop on Poverty and Gender: New Perspectives, Geneva.

Mandahar, M., Hawkes, S., Buse, K., Nosrati, E., & Magar, V. (2018). Gender, health and the 2030 agenda for sustainable development. *Bulletin of the WHO*, **96**(9), 644–653.

Mansh, M., Garcia, G., & Lunn, M. R. (2015). From patients to providers: changing the culture in medicine toward sexual and gender minorities. *Academic Medicine: Journal of the Association of American Medical Colleges*, **90**(5), 574–580.

McDonald, P. (2000). Gender equity in theories of fertility transition. *Population and Development Review*, **26**(3), 427–439.

Momsen, J. (2010). *Gender and Development*, 2nd ed. Milton Park, UK: Routledge.

Morgan Stanley (2017). *An Investor's Guide to Gender Diversity* (online). Available at www.morganstanley.com/ideas/gender-diversity-investor-guide (accessed November 2019).

Muthumbi, J., & Sommerfeld, J. (2015). *Africa's Women in Science*. Geneva: WHO.

Newman, C. (2014). Time to address gender discrimination and inequality in the health workforce. *Human Resources for Health*, **12**(25). DOI:10.1186/1478-4491-12-25.

Organisation for Economic Co-operation and Development (OECD) (2019). *Gender Data* (online). Available at www.oecd.org/gender/data/ (accessed November 13, 2019).

Organisation for Women in Science for the Developing World(OWSD) (2019). *Welcome to OWSD* (online). Available at https://owsd.net (accessed November 13, 2019).

Penning, M. J., & Wu, Z. (2015). Caregiver stress and mental health: impact of caregiving relationship and gender. *The Gerontologist*, **56**(6), 1102–1113.

Reisner, S., Poteat, T., Keatley, J., et al. (2016). Global health burden and needs of transgender populations: a review. *Lancet*, **388**, 412–436.

Riska, E. (2001). *Medical Careers and Feminist Agendas: American, Scandinavian, and Russian Women Physicians*. New York: Transaction Publishers.

Roter, D. L., Hall, J. A., & Aoki, Y. (2002). Physician gender effects in medical communication: a meta-analytic review. *Journal of the American Medical Association*, **288**(6), 756–764.

Schüler, D. (2006). The uses and misuses of the gender-related development index and gender empowerment measure: a review of the literature. *Journal of Human Development*, **7**(2), 161–181.

Schwalbe, N. (2017). Global health: generation men. *Lancet*, **390**(10096), 733.

Science in Australia Gender Equity (SAGE) (2019). *Gender Equity in STEMM* (online). Available at www.sciencegenderequity.org.au/gender-equity-in-stem/ (accessed November 13, 2019).

Seckinelgin, H. (2009). Global activism and sexualities in the time of HIV/AIDS. *Contemporary Politics*, **15**, 103–118.

Segato, R. (2016). *La guerra contra las mujeres*. Madrid: Traficantes de sueños.

Sen, G., & Östlin, P. (2007). *Unequal, Unfair, Ineffective and Inefficient Gender Inequity in Health: Why It Exists and How We Can Change It*. Geneva: WHO.

Shannon, G., Motta, A., Cáceres, C., et al. (2017). ¿Somos iguales? Using a structural violence framework to understand gender and health inequities from an intersectional perspective in the Peruvian Amazon. *Global Health Action* **10**(Suppl. 2), 1330458.

Shannon, G., Minckas, N., Tan, D., et al. (2019). Feminization of the health workforce and wage conditions of health professions: an exploratory analysis. *Human Resources for Health*, **17**(72). DOI:10.1186/s12960-019-0406-0.

Stoet, G., & Geary, D. (2018). The gender-equality paradox in science, technology, engineering, and mathematics education. *Psychological Science*, **29**(4), 581–593.

Stonewall UK (n.d.). What does trans mean? Stonewall UK website. Available at www.stonewall.org.uk/what-does-trans-mean (accessed July 2020).

Tomas, D. (2004). Diversity as strategy. *Harvard Business Review* (online). Available at https://hbr.org/2004/09/diversity-as-strategy.

Tsugawa, Y., Jena, A. B., Figueroa, J. F., et al. (2017). Comparison of hospital mortality and readmission rates for medicare patients treated by male vs. female physicians. *JAMA Internal Medicine*, **177**(2), 206–213.

United Nations (2018). *International Day of Women and Girls in Science* (online). Available at www.un.org/en/events/women-and-girls-in-science-day/background.shtml (accessed November 13, 2019).

United Nations (2014). *Sustainable Development Knowledge Platform* (online) Available at http://sustainabledevelopment.un.org (accessed November 13, 2019).

United Nations (2019). *Gender Equality* (online). Available at www.un.org/en/sections/issues-depth/gender-equality/index.html (accessed November 13, 2019).

United Nations Development Programmer (UNDP) (2010). *Human Development Report*. New York: United Nations.

United Nations Educational, Scientific and Cultural Organization (UNESCO) (2018). *Women in Science* (online). Available at http://uis.unesco.org/en/topic/women-science (accessed November 13, 2019).

United Nations General Assembly (1996). *Convention on the Elimination of All Forms of Discrimination against Women*. New York: United Nations.

United Nations Population Fund (UNFPA) (2011). *Commission on the Status of Women, 55th Session* (online). Available at www.unfpa.org/events/commission-status-women-55th-session (accessed November 13, 2019).

United Nations Statistics Division (2019). *Gender Stats* (online). Available at https://genderstats.un.org/#/home (accessed November 2019).

UN Women (2011). *Gender Equality Glossary* (online). Available at https://trainingcentre.unwomen.org/mod/glossary/view (accessed November 2019).

US Department of Health and Human Services Health Resources and Services Administration Bureau of Health Professions (2006). *The Rationale for Diversity in the Health Professions: A Review of the Evidence*. Rockville, MD: USDHHS.

van Belle, J. (2016). *Paternity and Parental Leave Policies across the European Union*. Brussels: RAND Europe.

Wallis, C., Bheeshma, R., Natalie, C., et al. (2017). Comparison of postoperative outcomes among patients treated by male and female surgeons: a population based matched cohort study. *British Medical Journal*, **359**, 4366.

WHO Gender Equity Hub (2019). *Delivered by Women, Led by Men: A Gender and Equity Analysis of the Global Health and Social Workforce* Human Resources for Health Observer Series No. 24). Geneva: WHO.

Witter, S., Govender, V., Ravindran, S., & Yates, R. (2017). Minding the gaps: health financing, universal health coverage and gender. *Health Policy and Planning*, **32**, 4–12.

Winter, S. (2012). *Lost in Transition: Transgender People, Rights and Vulnerability in the Asia-Pacific Region*. Bangkok: UNDP Asia-Pacific Regional Centre.

Women in Global Science and Technology (2012). *National Assessments on Gender and STI*. Toronto: Women in Global Science and Technology.

Wood, S. (2019). *Heteronormativity*. Eldis (online). Available at www.eldis.org/keyissues/heteronormativity#chapter-1084 (accessed November 13, 2019).

World Bank (2019). *Gender Data Portal* (online). Available at http://datatopics.worldbank.org/gender/indicators (accessed November 13, 2019).

World Health Organization (WHO) (2002). *Gender Analysis in Health: A Review of Selected Tools*. Geneva: WHO.

World Health Organization (WHO)(2011). WHO Gender Responsive Assessment Scale: criteria for assessing programmes and policies, in *WHO Gender Mainstreaming Manual for Health Managers: A Practical Approach*. Geneva: WHO.

World Health Organization (WHO) (2019). *Delivered by Women, Led by Men: A Gender and Equity Analysis of the Global Health and Social Workforce* (Human Resources for Health Observer Series No. 24). Geneva: WHO.

Health Systems and Health and Healthcare Reform

Martin McKee

What Are Health Systems For?

It is easy to forget that one of the primary purposes of a health system should be to improve health (McKee et al., 2009). For decades, debates on health systems have been dominated by discussions of how much they cost to run (typically questioning whether they are affordable, as if there were an alternative in a civilized society) or how many resources they require (typically expressed in an arbitrary fashion as people, usually doctors and nurses, but not managers or physiotherapists, or facilities and items of furniture, usually hospitals, but not primary care clinics or beds and not examination couches). The nature of this discourse has meant that health systems have tended to be regarded as a cost to society from which there is little return instead of as an investment whereby appropriately directed expenditure leads to better health.

This chapter is based on a very different vision. It recognizes that although there has long been a debate about the philosophical basis of the right to health, the political reality is that the governments of the world have accepted that this right exists. Thus, in 1946, the constitution of the World Health Organization (WHO) identified "the highest attainable standard of health as a fundamental right of every human being" (Grad, 2002: 981). Subsequently, the right to health has been given force in some national constitutions (Choi et al., 2018; Matsuura, 2013) and in the International Covenant on Economic, Social and Cultural Rights (Forman et al., 2016). Most recently, it has been enshrined in the Sustainable Development Goals (SDGs), specifically Goal 3, in which the world's governments have committed to "[e]nsure healthy lives and promote well-being for all at all ages" (World Health Organization, 2016: 7).

The inclusion of health in the SDGs signifies how it is now viewed as a major contributor to, and indeed marker of, the progress of nations. Yet the SDGs go further than this. By including within SDG3 a target of achieving universal health coverage, they accept the view that health systems make a major contribution to improving health. Of course, commitments must be translated into reality, and in many countries, aspirations are just that. Globally, many millions of people lack access to basic healthcare, and improved access to healthcare remains low on governments' lists of priorities. In some countries, most notably the United States under President Trump, the policy of his predecessors that reduced the numbers of uninsured Americans substantially was threatened with repeal. Those opposed to expanding coverage frequently invoke arguments about costs, arguing that it will be too expensive and cannot be afforded. Yet, as the remainder of this chapter argues, this is based on a false premise. Instead, the question should be whether a country seeking to achieve economic growth and social progress can afford not to.

A ministerial conference organized by the European Region of the WHO in Tallinn, Estonia, in 2008 set out three mutually reinforcing sets of relationships, with better health, stronger health systems, and greater economic growth all contributing to each other (WHO, 2008). The three sets of mutual interrelationships are shown in Figure 5.1, and the evidence supporting each of these relationships can be summarized as follows. First, healthcare delivered appropriately and equitably has achieved substantial gains in population health, and the promotion of better health reduces future demands for healthcare. Second, whereas, in general, wealthy countries have better health than poor ones, better population health leads to faster economic growth because it enables individuals to make a greater contribution to the labor market and to be more productive. Finally, although economic growth makes more resources available for healthcare, the healthcare system can, if harnessed in support of regional development and innovation, contribute to economic growth. These

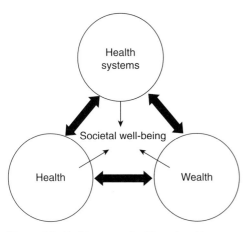

Figure 5.1. Health systems, health, and wealth.
Source: WHO, 2008 (adapted with permission).

mutually beneficial relationships will not, however, emerge spontaneously. Rather, they require collective action by governments and others to create health systems that address the health needs of their populations and respond to them with equitable and effective policies and practices.

The Contribution of Health Systems to Health

In advancing the arguments developed in Tallinn in 2008, it is necessary to recognize that many of those who need to be convinced retain a degree of skepticism. Does healthcare really improve population health? Remarkably, some question this.

Although by the 1970s some writers were making impressive claims for the achievements of modern healthcare, some demographers subscribed to a contrary view. These were exemplified by the work of Thomas McKeown, a British professor of public health who argued that, over the preceding century and a half, therapeutic interventions had added little, if anything, to gains in life expectancy, which instead were driven by improvements in living standards and, especially, nutrition (McKeown, 1976). At the same time, Ivan Illich, in his book *Medical Nemesis,* argued that modern healthcare was actually harmful (Illich, 1976). Coining the term *iatrogenesis,* or doctor created, he described its clinical form in which the growth of diagnostic technology was being used to label variants on normality as illness, leading, in turn, to unnecessary treatment and adverse side effects. He

also described a social and cultural form whereby the increasing medicalization of life encouraged a growing number of essentially normal people to feel that they had something wrong and thus become dependent on doctors. This created a vicious circle whereby the health system expanded, yet the population felt worse.

A consequence was that medicine increasingly took on a role of social control, defining who was normal and who was not. Similar views were being expressed by others working in the field of mental health, where the role of medicine as a form of social control was especially apparent. Laing (2010), for example, saw what was labeled as mental illness as a rational reaction to an abnormal society. Szasz (1974) argued that to qualify as an illness, an entity must be capable of being assessed or measured in a scientific way and be demonstrable at the cellular or molecular level. Many so-called mental illnesses were, in his view, false illnesses, representing a judgment by society about what is or is not acceptable. Hence, "If you talk to God, you are praying; If God talks to you, you have schizophrenia. If the dead talk to you, you are a spiritualist; If you talk to the dead, you are a schizophrenic" (Szasz, 1974: 85). From this perspective, psychiatry is a means of controlling those seen to be deviant, with those deemed to be mentally ill assuming the role previously occupied by witches and certain religious minorities.

All these arguments have some truth. Although McKeown's attribution of much of the improvement in life expectancy in nineteenth-century England to nutrition has been challenged by subsequent, more detailed analyses (Colgrove, 2002), at least until the 1950s, healthcare could do little to address the common causes of premature death. And while Illich may have overestimated the harmful effects of healthcare, his term *iatrogenesis* has become established within mainstream medicine. He was writing at a time when the thalidomide scandal was unfolding, in which a sedative given to pregnant women was found, despite initial denials by its manufacturers, to cause serious birth defects (Rosen, 1979). However, in 2000, a report by the US Institute of Medicine estimated that as many as 44,000 deaths each year could be attributed to medical errors (Institute of Medicine, 2000), findings since replicated elsewhere (Thomson, 2007).

These findings have influenced the development of what is now a global alliance of health professionals seeking to improve patient safety. Similarly, the once firmly opposed camps represented by psychiatry and antipsychiatry have moved closer together, at least in the developed world, as the treatment of people with mental illness is increasingly underpinned by commitments to patients' rights. Yet what healthcare could deliver in the 1960s and 1970s, when McKeown and Illich were writing, has changed almost beyond recognition, as will be described in the following sections.

The Changing Nature of Healthcare

The Antibiotic Era

Perhaps the most spectacular example of how healthcare has changed is the discovery of antibiotics. The early sulfonamides, such as Salvarsan, developed by Domagk, for which he won the 1939 Nobel Prize in Medicine, did work against some common bacteria, but they were of limited effectiveness in severe cases, and they had important side effects. Penicillin, discovered by Fleming and subsequently mass produced following work by Florey and Chain, achievements for which all three shared the 1945 Nobel Prize in Medicine, was much safer and more effective. It now became possible to cure many common but previously often fatal bacterial infections. In time, these compounds were supplemented by new classes of drugs, each with its own mode of action, range of activity against different organisms, and side effects. Thus the advent of aminoglycosides made it possible to treat serious infections with gram-negative bacilli that often followed major abdominal surgery, albeit at a risk of side effects from some of the more effective drugs in this class, such as deafness or kidney damage. The results were especially dramatic with tuberculosis, until then a not-uncommon cause of death in young people.

McKeown's work illustrated the marked influence of the social conditions of life on mortality rates from tuberculosis, showing how the death rate had already fallen substantially even before Koch had identified the tubercle bacillus as the cause of the disease and longer before either immunization with the bacillus Calmette-Guérin (BCG) vaccine or treatment with drugs became available. This was widely cited as evidence that healthcare made little contribution to population health, but an examination of age-specific death rates in England and Wales shows

a further striking year-on-year decline in mortality in young people between 1947, when streptomycin began to be available, and 1954, when it was in widespread use (Nolte & McKee, 2004). This remarkable medical achievement was repeated 40 years later when the introduction of antiretrovirals transformed infection with HIV (another disease with deep links to social conditions of life) from an inevitably fatal illness into one that its victims were as likely to die with as from (Atun et al., 2009).

Unlike some of the other successes of medicine, however, the development of antibiotics has not been without its setbacks. Within a decade of the widespread introduction of antibiotics, it was already becoming clear that humans and microorganisms were engaged in a massive evolutionary struggle because the process of natural selection allowed those few bacteria in which a mutation had conferred resistance to an antibiotic to survive and multiply, a process facilitated in some cases by the transfer of tiny fragments of DNA called *plasmids*. The emergence of resistance was detected early in cases of tuberculosis, leading physicians to employ multiple therapy regimes on the basis that it was extremely unlikely that sufficient organisms would develop resistance against three or more drugs acting on different mechanisms. However, tuberculosis was seen as a special case because of the long duration of treatment, at that time often two years or more, which offered many opportunities for resistance to develop.

Multiple therapy regimes were not seen as an option for more easily cured infections. However, within a few decades, humans had created the conditions that allowed resistance to many common antibiotics to flourish. One factor was the almost ubiquitous use of antibiotics as a growth promoter in the rapidly expanding industrial animal farms, in which tens of thousands of chickens and pigs were kept in appalling conditions where they were at constant risk of growth-retarding infections (Bloomer & McKee, 2018). Another was the inappropriate use of antibiotics for often self-limiting infections, a practice encouraged by widespread over-the-counter sales in many countries. This is exemplified by treatment of respiratory tract infections (many of which are caused by viruses). Another example is *Staphylococcus aureus*, a common bacterium often found on the skin and in the nose that was initially killed rapidly by penicillin. For many years it was possible to keep one step ahead by the development of new antibiotics until finally a strain resistant to methicillin emerged. This is now widespread in hospitals in some countries and is extremely difficult to eradicate.

Problems also arose in treating tuberculosis once antituberculous drugs became widely available in countries with fragile health systems that had weak systems of governance and completion of the full course of treatment could not be assured. These were initially in Latin America and the countries emerging from the Soviet Union but now include many parts of the developing world. The absence of an effective laboratory infrastructure means that patients are treated without knowledge of the drugs to which their infections are sensitive. Patients whose infections are already resistant to two of the usual combination of three drugs are at great risk of developing resistance to the third drug, a risk that could be countered by giving them one or more second-line drugs to which their infections are still sensitive. The resulting multidrug-resistant tuberculosis (MDR-TB) and, initially in South Africa, extensively resistant tuberculosis (XDR-TB) were the inevitable consequences. The emergence of antibiotic-resistant organisms is a major threat to health problem, and the challenges related to both ethics and practicalities arising in the prevention and treatment of infectious diseases remain (Viens & Littmann, 2015).

Advances in the Treatment of Chronic Diseases

The situation is rather more encouraging with regard to drugs for chronic diseases. The discovery of insulin in the early 1920s by Banting and Best transformed the management of type 1 diabetes. Children who, until then, had been dying slowly over a period of about 18 months after diagnosis could be treated, enabling them to achieve an almost normal life expectancy (at least after subsequent developments allowed prevention or treatment of many of the long-term complications of this disease). This was the first time ever that a disease was treated by a drug that the patient would remain on for the rest of his or her life. Sadly, the ascent of the profit motive has taken the cost of insulin to ridiculous heights in some countries, making it almost inaccessible to many even in wealthy countries (Reuters, 2019). The introduction of progressively purified thyroid hormones in the 1930s followed for patients with myxedema, but in both cases, the numbers of people in the population affected by these disorders were relatively small. By the 1950s, however, the first drugs that were both effective and well tolerated in treating hypertension were becoming available. The subsequent discovery of safe and effective bronchodilators for people with asthma and chronic obstructive airways disease, major tranquillizers for those with mental disorders, and anti-inflammatory drugs for those with arthritis led to a situation whereby a substantial share of the middle-aged population would be started on medications they would take for the rest of their lives. Progress was gradual. For example, treatment of hypertension was initially prescribed only for those whose blood pressure was extremely high and who were clearly suffering adverse consequences, manifest as cerebrovascular, ocular, and renal dysfunction. In the early 1960s, research showed how the treatment of asymptomatic hypertension could reduce the subsequent incidence of stroke (Hamilton et al., 1964). The new thiazide diuretics and later beta blockers were initially prescribed predominantly for younger men with substantially elevated blood pressure, reflecting both the widespread tendency to undertreat cardiovascular disease in women and an erroneous view that the observed increase in blood pressure with age was both natural and of little danger. In time, the population offered treatment expanded, and the threshold for treatment fell, accompanied by a steady decline in mortality from stroke in developed countries that continues to this day (GBD 2016 Stroke Collaborators, 2019).

Advances in Surgery

Progress was also seen in the outcome of surgery. The development of anesthesia and asepsis in the nineteenth century made it possible to operate inside the abdominal and thoracic cavities. Over the subsequent century, surgical, anesthetic, and postoperative techniques progressively developed. Over the past three to four decades, rates of perioperative mortality associated with many procedures have fallen markedly. A major factor has been the ability to recognize and treat complications, as is apparent from studies using a measure of *failure to rescue*, which assesses mortality in those suffering complications (Silber et al., 2007). At the same time, advances in surgical technique have reduced the trauma associated with surgery, in particular through the use of minimally invasive techniques. Although there is little evidence that these methods are, overall, safer than open procedures, they reduce suffering from more invasive surgery and increase the number of otherwise unfit patients who can benefit from surgery. A related development is the introduction of medical alternatives to surgery, most notably the introduction of H_2 blockers and proton pump inhibitors for peptic ulcers, followed later by the use of drugs to eradicate *Helicobacter* infection, now known to be the cause of most ulcers.

Cancer Therapy

Although less successful overall, there have also been achievements in the struggle against cancer. Within a decade of the discovery of x-rays by Röntgen in 1895, electromagnetic radiation was being used to treat cancers. However, its use was limited to tumors that were radiosensitive, such as lymphomas and germ cell tumors, rather than those developing from epithelial cells, and to those that were localized to one part of the body. By the 1940s, a number of chemotherapeutic agents were being used, initially derived from chemical weapons such as mustard gas. The combination of chemotherapy and radiotherapy transformed the management of some cancers, such as Hodgkin's disease and testicular cancer, but for many others the only option was surgical removal. This was only successful where resection was complete and before metastases had developed. From the 1980s, advances in understanding of cell biology and, in particular, the role of hormones and the complex relationship between tumors and their blood supply have progressively extended the pharmacologic armamentarium, with drugs such as tamoxifen transforming the survival of patients with the form of breast cancer that is estrogen receptor positive. The development of new *biologicals* has had a striking effect on fatality from several malignancies (National Cancer Institute, 2018). Deaths from some cancers have also been reduced by the development of screening programs that have enabled tumors or premalignant lesions to be detected and treated at an early stage, exemplified by population-based breast and cervical cancer screening, although many health systems still struggle to implement the well-organized programs required for optimal results (Priaulx et al., 2018).

Technological Advances in Diagnosis and Treatment

There have also been a number of technological developments that have impacted substantially on the ability to improve health or prevent premature death more generally. These include a wide range of diagnostic methods, such as improved imaging that facilitates the targeting of radiotherapy. In other cases, the benefits have been unexpected. For example, the widespread use of new forms of abdominal imaging may have detected many early cancers of the kidney that would have been missed using barium enemas. In other cases, technology has provided a new form of treatment, with dialysis enabling those with renal failure to remain alive, ideally until they can receive a transplant.

The Influence of Evidence on Medical Practice

Finally, it is necessary to consider the massive expansion of evidence-based medicine. The expansion of randomized, controlled trials into areas such as surgery and organizational interventions (such as the evaluation of stroke units) has generated a vastly increased body of knowledge on the effectiveness of healthcare. This, in turn, has been taken advantage of by those engaged in the synthesis of evidence, most notably by the Cochrane Collaboration. Its use of meta-analysis to combine the results of multiple studies has made it possible to identify effective treatments where single trials have been inconclusive and to reject treatments previously thought to be effective, while also delineating areas where more primary research is required. These activities are not, however, limited to synthesizing knowledge. There is increasing emphasis on the translation of evidence into practice, encouraged in some countries by the creation of specialized agencies such as the English National Institute for Health and Clinical Evidence (NICE) and the German Institut für Qualität und Wirtschaflichkeit im Gesundheitswesen (IQWiG), both generating guidelines tailored to the needs of practicing clinicians. This is supported by a growing body of research on how to influence clinical practice. The consequences can be seen in a study of the outcomes of major trauma in British hospitals, where steadily improving outcomes could not be attributed to a single intervention but rather to the increased seniority and skills of the doctors involved, coupled with greater use of evidence-based guidelines (Lecky et al., 2000). Together these advances illustrate the importance of strong institutions committed to the generation, synthesis, and transmission of evidence in modern health systems (Moon et al., 2010).

Measuring the Health Impact of Health Systems

The advances in healthcare described in the preceding section are impressive, but what impact have they had on population health? The concept of mortality amenable to healthcare was developed by Rutstein et al. (1976) in the mid-1970s. They identified a number of conditions from which premature death should not occur in the presence of timely and effective care. Such deaths were termed *avoidable*. The initial list included many infectious diseases; common surgical conditions, such as acute appendicitis and cholecystitis; and some chronic conditions for which life-sustaining medication was available, such as diabetes or hypertension. They were writing at a time when the scope of medical practice had changed beyond all recognition. This concept has been refined and updated, taking account of factors such as the increase in life expectancy (Rutstein considered only those deaths before 65 years of age as avoidable, whereas life expectancy at birth now exceeds 80 years in many industrialized countries) and the greater scope of medicine to prevent premature death, as discussed earlier (Nolte & McKee, 2004).

The concept of amenable mortality has since been developed even further, following its adoption by the Global Burden of Disease (GBD) initiative. The Healthcare Access and Quality Index (HAQI) is a composite measure of deaths from conditions amenable to healthcare (GBD 2015 Healthcare Access and Quality Collaborators, 2017). By using the vast amount of data gathered by the GBD program, the HAQI has achieved global coverage, albeit with caveats given the continued variability in quality and coverage of information from some countries. It also includes important refinements, such as adjusting performance for the prevalence of risk factors, recognizing that it is easier for a health system to reduce such deaths where the underlying risks are lower, and establishing a measure (frontier) of what each country can realistically be expected to achieve with its health system, given its underlying level of economic and social development.

The data from the GBD initiative show quite remarkable improvements worldwide, continuing to the present. For example, between 2006 and 2016, age-standardized death rates from tuberculosis and diarrheal diseases each fell by 36% (GBD 2016 Causes of Death Collaborators, 2017). Deaths from measles fell by 74%, from appendicitis by 20%, and from epilepsy by 14%.

The analysis using the HAQI reveal that almost all countries have achieved substantial reductions in death rates from conditions amenable to healthcare, with 167 of the 195 countries and territories studied showing statistically significant improvements. Given the differences in levels of development, the results were grouped into broad categories based on the Social Development Index (SDI), a composite measure including education, fertility, and income. The countries achieving the greatest progress were South Korea (high SDI), Turkey and Peru (high-middle SDI), China and the Maldives (middle SDI), and Laos and Ethiopia (low-middle and low SDI).

As understanding has grown as to how health systems vary in their ability to improve health, attention has focused on those that are performing particularly well. Over 30 years ago, the Rockefeller Foundation led a study into what it termed "Good Health at Low Cost," seeking to understand why some countries, such as Costa Rica and Sri Lanka, achieved much better outcomes than others at similar levels of development. Twenty-five years later, the study was repeated with a different set of countries (Balabanova et al., 2013). Success was associated with a strong political commitment to health, investment in capacity to develop and implement health policy, and an ability to innovate and take advantage of changing circumstances. The potential to learn from these successes has led to a number of new initiatives to identify countries that are "punching above their weight" and to understand how they have done it (Baum et al., 2018: 117). However, what is clear is that there is now extensive evidence that health systems can, when working well, make a substantial contribution to population health.

The Contribution of Health to Health Systems

So far this chapter has focused on the evidence that healthcare can contribute to population health. However, there is a potential reciprocal relationship, whereby the level of health has an impact on health systems. This is intuitively important; if everyone were to live to 100 years without significant illness and then die suddenly, there would be no need for organized healthcare. However, the implication of the possibility that efforts to improve the health of a population may save future costs of healthcare has attracted surprisingly little attention. In fact, some have argued quite the contrary. In a now notorious example, consultants acting on behalf of a major tobacco company sought to persuade the Czech government not to implement antismoking measures on the grounds that the resulting increase in people surviving into old age would increase the cost to the taxpayer.

The Wanless Report, prepared for the UK Treasury, was a seminal document in this respect (Wanless, 2001). Asked to assess future options for funding the National Health Service, Wanless, a banking executive, developed a series of scenarios of future expenditure on healthcare varying according to the nature and extent of adoption of policies to promote health and ensure timely and effective care. He concluded that the difference in expenditure between slow progress on these policies compared with what was described as "full engagement" would be £30 billion by 2022–2033, representing approximately 40% of the total National Health Service budget in 2002. This evidence was seen as compelling by the Treasury, contributing to a substantial increase in healthcare funding in the United Kingdom, a necessary measure given the need to make up for the long-term effects of underspending over several decades.

There are others who are more pessimistic, arguing that an aging population will inevitably render healthcare unaffordable. This argument is based, in large part, on the evidence that older people incur greater healthcare costs. However, initial research on the costs of aging was cross-sectional. Longitudinal studies have since confirmed that it is proximity to death that drives costs, with those dying at older ages actually being less expensive because they are treated less intensively (McGrail et al., 2000). Furthermore, there is much that can be done to encourage healthy aging and thus mitigate the economic consequences (Doyle et al., 2009). This suggests that it may be possible to create a mutually beneficial situation whereby investments in health reduce future costs of healthcare, while effective healthcare, especially where it prevents the onset or progression of disease and avoids the emergence of complications, may be mutually reinforcing.

Bring the Economy into the Equation: Health Systems and Wealth

This concept, whereby health and health systems are mutually beneficial, has recently been extended to links with the wider economy. Self-evidently, there is a relationship between economic development and the ability to provide healthcare, although this is complicated by the fact that some inputs to healthcare have local prices, such as salaries (although even here there is to some degree a global market, depending on the ease with which health workers can migrate), whereas other inputs, such as technology and pharmaceuticals, have international prices. A key question is how much to spend. This cannot be answered easily, and to some extent, the answer will depend on the political priorities of each government, especially because healthcare spending is fundamentally redistributive not only from healthy to ill but also, because the latter are typically concentrated among the most deprived, from rich to poor.

Once again, there is a reciprocal relationship. Paying for healthcare, especially when serious illness strikes, is a major burden in many developing countries. Consequently, health systems are increasingly seen as playing a role in macroeconomic policy by lifting the fear of catastrophic expenditure (Anand & Ravallion, 1993). Provision of funds for healthcare not only will benefit the poor directly but also will give them the security to invest their meager resources in wealth creation rather than hoarding it to protect their families from possible disaster. This is also becoming a concern in the United States, the only industrialized country unwilling to pay for healthcare for all its citizens, where medical expenses are the leading cause of personal insolvency. The provision of health infrastructure is also being recognized increasingly as one component of a comprehensive approach to regional development, especially where procurement systems are established that provide a level playing field for local suppliers, for example, by breaking up large tenders into smaller packages that enable small and medium-sized enterprises to bid. Health infrastructure can also support regional development through tie-ups with the health industry, for example, through academic medical centers linked to biotechnology start-ups.

Health and Wealth

There is a considerable body of evidence, reviewed in the report of the Commission on Social Determinants of Health, that greater wealth is, all else being equal, associated with better health (Commission on

Macroeconomics and Health, 2001). There is also evidence that relative wealth has significant impacts on health and other indicators of social stability (Wilkinson & Pickett, 2010). Those with greater command over resources are better able to make healthy choices, enabling them to live healthier lifestyles and access timely and effective healthcare.

The key question is, however, whether better health leads to greater wealth. This has already been answered in developing countries by the Commission on Macroeconomics and Health (2001), which assembled an impressive body of evidence that poor health is an important constraint on economic growth. It also showed that the return on investment from many basic health interventions is considerable. However, it was by no means clear that the Commission's conclusions could be applied to high-income settings. One reason is that the nature of work differs. In poor countries, much work involves physical activity, in agriculture, extractive industries, and nonmechanized manufacturing, whereas in rich countries, much work is sedentary. Another reason is that in poor countries substantial health gains can be achieved by scaling up basic interventions, such as immunization and treated bed nets, whereas in rich countries the burden of disease is dominated by chronic disorders so that the interventions needed are complex, multifaceted, and often expensive.

Subsequent work, however, has examined the situation in both high-income and transition countries in Europe (Suhrcke et al., 2005, 2007). This work explores several pathways by which better health can increase economic growth. First, healthy people are more likely to be employed and are less likely to take sickness absence or retire early. Second, they are more productive at work. It has been suggested that as people realize that they are likely to live longer, they invest more time and money in their education, itself a driver of economic growth, and although the available evidence is limited, what does exist supports this pathway. Finally, in poor countries, people expecting to live longer are likely to save more for retirement, providing greater resources for capital investment. Here the evidence from rich countries remains inconclusive. Contemporary research is consistent with historical studies that have shown that how a substantial share of the economic wealth in rich countries today can be linked to gains in health and nutrition in the past two

centuries (Arora, 2001; Fogel, 1994), with several cross-country growth studies documenting a significant effect of better health on economic growth (Sala-I-Martin et al., 2004).

This work has been complemented by research on the economic losses attributable to health inequalities in Europe in terms of both the additional cost of health care and the wider impact on productivity (Mackenbach et al., 2007). It is estimated that if European Union (EU) governments could raise levels of good health among the least well educated to those of the best educated, they could achieve a 22% reduction in hospitalizations and gain €141 billion in productivity (equivalent to 1.4% of gross domestic product) each year.

Health Systems for Prosperity and Solidarity

The spirit of optimism that was encapsulated in the 2008 Tallinn Charter was soon dispelled as the global financial crisis erupted. Some countries in Europe developed a collective amnesia about the commitments they had just made, instead imposing deep austerity, cutting budgets for healthcare and public health. This provided empirical support for the arguments set out in Tallinn. Rather than achieving a virtuous circle of improved health and economic growth, they entered a downward spiral, with those making the deepest cuts suffering the largest declines in economic performance (Reeves et al., 2014).

When, in 2018, the WHO reconvened European governments in Tallinn for a high-level meeting, the financial crisis had largely abated, although the legacy of underinvestment remained in many countries. However, the discourse about health had moved on. Increasingly, governments were seeing the health sector as an important contributor to the economy, featuring prominently in their industrial strategies (Rawlins, 2018). The argument that better health reduces the demand and thus the cost of healthcare has been accepted by many governments, leading some to adopt measures such as sugar taxes that would once have been unimaginable (Burki, 2016). But health was also being seen as a means to promote social cohesion. The finding that worsening health in the United States, and especially the growth of the "diseases of despair," was closely correlated with a shift in support for Donald Trump sounded an alarm among European politicians concerned about the increasing support for populist politicians promoting divisive policies (Bor, 2017).

The subject of the 2018 Tallinn meeting was "Health Systems for Prosperity and Solidarity: Leaving No-One Behind." It reiterated messages from 2008 but with a renewed emphasis on inclusiveness, recognizing that not everyone in an increasingly diverse Europe had benefited to the same extent from the progress that had been made. Life expectancy in the European region as a whole had increased by two years in the intervening period, but some countries, such as the United Kingdom, have experienced stagnation since 2010, with some groups, such as the very old, even experiencing increasing mortality (Hiam et al., 2018a). Even though European countries are often considered to have achieved universal coverage, some groups remain excluded, in particular undocumented migrants, who are facing an increasingly "hostile environment" (Hiam et al., 2018b). While the European countries provide a high level of financial protection, many people are still left behind, with some of the poorest facing large out-of-pocket payments and even catastrophic expenditures (WHO, 2018). As those present at the meeting noted, "some of the attributes we assign to European health systems – solidarity, equity, and universalism – are now at risk."

The response, as set out by those present, involved three imperatives: include, invest, and innovate. Inclusion requires that governments measure and reduce inequalities in financial protection and unmet needs, a goal now endorsed by the EU, which is developing measures that can be incorporated into health system performance assessment (Expert Panel on Effective Ways of Investing in Health, 2018). This imperative to reduce unmet needs is gaining traction, with some countries reversing reductions in entitlement introduced during the financial crisis (Legido-Quigley et al., 2018).

Investment is necessary to ensure that there are adequate funds to provide inclusive services that can protect the poorest in society. It is important to consider not just how much money is raised but also how it is raised. Financing health systems inevitably involves redistribution because many of those most in need of healthcare are least able to pay for it. Health systems funded by user charges or regressive indirect taxes achieve poorer health outcomes than those funded by progressive taxation (Reeves et al., 2015). It is also important to look to the future to ensure that services can be provided in the future. Cuts to training of health professionals and procurement and maintenance of facilities and equipment and a failure to invest in the knowledge needed to provide a modern health system are false economies.

The final imperative is innovation. The demands on health systems are constantly changing, with aging populations and the growth of multimorbidity. This means that countries must establish mechanisms to generate and implement new knowledge, medicines, technologies, and models of care. Governments must also step in where there are market failures. A contemporary example is the failure of the existing model of drug discovery and development to produce truly innovative medicines and especially antibiotics (Mazzucato, 2015). Innovation also demands ways of scaling up beneficial innovations rapidly while ensuring that technological advances narrow rather than widen the health divide.

Summary

Too often health systems have been seen as a safety net, dealing with the immediate effects of illness but not actually enhancing health or contributing to economic growth. This chapter sets out a vision in which health, health systems, and economic growth can exist together in a mutually supportive virtuous circle.

The importance of well-functioning health systems has been accepted by the global community of nations when they agreed to the Sustainable Development Goals. It has also been accepted by governments of the EU when they decided to invest in the health of their citizens as a key element of their Lisbon Strategy that seeks to make Europe the most competitive economy in the world (European Commission, 2008), by the World Bank's approach to investing in health-in-transition countries (World Bank, 2005), and by the governments of the WHO's European region, meeting in Tallinn in 2008 and 2018 (McKee & Kluge, 2018; McKee et al., 2009). Increasingly, health systems are being seen as a driver of economic growth and a means to promote social cohesion.

This chapter has described the enormous strides that have been made over recent decades by medical science. Yet these advances can only be dreamt of by the majority of the world's populations, and even in the United States, one of the richest countries in the world, those striving to provide universal health coverage face an enormous struggle against powerful vested interests. Governments and international agencies now need to deliver on the commitments that have been made, developing coordinated policies to structure effective health systems that meet the needs of their populations while establishing systems to monitor whether they are achieving what they promise.

References

Anand, S., & Ravallion, M. (1993). Human development in poor countries: on the role of private incomes and public services. *Journal of Economic Perspectives* 7, 133–150.

Arora, S. (2001). Health, human productivity, and long-term economic growth. *Journal of Economic History* **61**, 699–749.

Atun, R. A., Gurol-Urganci, I., & McKee, M. (2009). Health systems and increased longevity in people with HIV and AIDS. *British Medical Journal*, **338**:b2165.

Balabanova, D., Mills, A., Conteh, L., et al. (2013). Good health at low cost 25 years on: lessons for the future of health systems strengthening. *Lancet* **381**, 2118–2133.

Baum, F., Popay, J., Delany-Crowe, T., et al. (2018). Punching above their weight: a network to understand broader determinants of increasing life expectancy. *International Journal of Equity Health* **17**, 117.

Bloomer, E., & McKee, M. (2018). Policy options for reducing antibiotics and antibiotic-resistant genes in the environment. *Journal of Public Health Policy* **39**, 389–406.

Bor, J. (2017). Diverging life expectancies and voting patterns in the 2016 US presidential election. *American Journal of Public Health* **107**, 1560–1562.

Burki, T. K. (2016). Sugar tax in the UK. *Lancet Oncology* **17**, e182.

Choi, S., Park, S., & Kim, S. Y. (2018). A comparative study on the constitutional right to health in the western Pacific region countries. *Asia Pacific Journal of Public Health* **30**, 458–469.

Colgrove, J. (2002). The McKeown thesis: a historical controversy and its enduring influence. *American Journal of Public Health* **92**, 725–729.

Commission on Macroeconomics and Health (2001). *Macroeconomics and Health: Investing in Health for Economic Development: Report of the Commission on Macroeconomics and Health*. Geneva: WHO.

Doyle, Y., McKee, M., Rechel, B., & Grundy, E. (2009). Meeting the challenge of population ageing. *British Medical Journal* 339, b3926.

European Commission (2008). *Lisbon Strategy*. Brussels: European Commission.

Expert Panel on Effective Ways of Investing in Health (2018). *Benchmarking Access to Healthcare in the EU*, Brussels: European Commission.

Fogel, R. W. (1994). Economic growth, population theory, and physiology: the bearing of long-term processes on the making of economic policy (NBER Working Paper No. 4638), National Bureau of Economic Research, Cambridge, MA.

Forman, L., Beiersmann, C., Brolan, C. E., et al. (2016). What do core obligations under the right to health bring to universal health coverage? *Health and Human Rights* **18**, 23–34.

GBD 2015 Healthcare Access and Quality Collaborators (2017). Healthcare Access and Quality Index based on mortality from causes amenable to personal health care in 195 countries and territories, 1990–2015: a novel analysis from the Global Burden of Disease Study 2015. *Lancet* **390**, 231–266.

GBD 2016 Causes of Death Collaborators (2017). Global, regional, and national age-sex specific mortality for 264 causes of death, 1980–2016: a systematic analysis for the Global Burden of Disease Study 2016. *Lancet* **390**, 1151–1210.

GBD 2016 Stroke Collaborators (2019). Global, regional, and national burden of stroke, 1990–2016: a systematic analysis for the Global Burden of Disease Study 2016. *Lancet Neurology* **18**, 439–458

Grad, F. P. (2002). The preamble of the constitution of the World Health Organization. *Bulletin of the WHO* **80**, 981–981.

Hamilton, M., Thompson, E., & Wisniewski, T. (1964). The role of blood-pressure control in preventing complications of hypertension. *Lancet* **283**, 235–238.

Hiam, L., Harrison, D., McKee, M., & Dorling, D. (2018a). Why is life expectancy in England and Wales "stalling"? *Journal of Epidemiology and Community Health* **72**, 404–408.

Hiam, L., Steele, S., & McKee, M. (2018b). Creating a "hostile environment for migrants": the British government's use of health service data to restrict immigration is a very bad idea. *Health Economics, Policy and Law* **13**, 107–117.

Illich, I. (1976). *Medical Nemesis: The Expropriation of Health*. New York: Pantheon Books.

Institute of Medicine (2000). *To Err Is Human: Building a Safer Health System*. Washington, DC: National Academy Press.

Laing, R. (2010). *The Divided Self: An Existential Study in Sanity and Madness*. London: Penguin Books.

Lecky, F., Woodford, M., & Yates, D. (2000). Trends in trauma care in England and Wales 1989–97. *Lancet* **355**, 1771–1775.

Legido-Quigley, H., Pajin, L., Fanjul, G., Urdaneta, E., & McKee, M. (2018). Spain shows that a humane response to migrant health is possible in Europe. *Lancet Public Health* **3**, e358

Mackenbach, J., Meerding, W. J., & Kunst, A. (2007). *Economic Implications of Socio-economic Inequalities in Health in the European Union*. Brussels: European Commission.

Matsuura, H. (2013). *The Effect of a Constitutional Right to Health on Population Health in 157 Countries, 1970–2007: The Role of Democratic Governance.* Cambridge, MA: Program on the Global Demography of Aging.

Mazzucato, M. (2015). *The Entrepreneurial State: Debunking Public vs. Private Sector Myths*. London: Anthem Press.

McGrail, K., Green, B., Barer, M. L., et al. (2000). Age, costs of acute and long-term care and proximity to death: evidence for 1987–88 and 1994–95 in British Columbia. *Age and Ageing* **29**, 249–253.

McKee, M., & Kluge, H. (2018). Include, invest, innovate: health systems for prosperity and solidarity. *Journal of Health Services Research & Policy* **23**, 209–211.

McKee, M., Suhrcke, M., Nolte, E., et al. (2009). Health systems, health, and wealth: a European perspective. *Lancet* **373**, 349–351.

McKeown, T. (1976). *The Role of Medicine: Dream, Mirage, or Nemesis?* Princeton, NJ: Princeton University Press.

Moon, S., Szlezák, N. A., Michaud, C. M., et al. (2010). The global health system: lessons for a stronger institutional framework. *PLoS Medicine* **7**, e1000193.

National Cancer Institute (2018). *Biological Therapies for Cancer* (online). Available at www.cancer.gov/about-cancer /treatment/types/immunotherapy/bio-therapies-fact-sheet (accessed April 4, 2019).

Nolte, E., & McKee, M. (2004). *Does Health Care Save Lives? Avoidable Mortality Revisited*. London: Nuffield Trust.

Priaulx, J., de Koning, H. J., de Kok, I., Szeles, G., & McKee, M. (2018). Identifying the barriers to effective breast, cervical and colorectal cancer screening in thirty-one European countries using the Barriers to Effective Screening Tool (BEST). *Health Policy* **122**, 1190–1197.

Rawlins, M. D. (2018). The UK's life sciences strategy: opportunities for clinical pharmacology. *British Journal of Clinical Pharmacology* **84**(10), 2175–2177.

Reeves, A., Gourtsoyannis, Y., Basu, S., et al. (2015). Financing universal health coverage – effects of alternative tax structures on public health systems: cross-national modelling in 89 low-income and middle-income countries. *Lancet* **386**, 274–280.

Reeves, A., McKee, M., Basu, S., & Stuckler, D. (2014). The political economy of austerity and healthcare: cross-national analysis of expenditure changes in 27 European nations 1995–2011. *Health Policy* **115**, 1–8.

Reuters (2019). U.S. insulin costs per patient nearly doubled from 2012 to 2016, study finds (online). NBC News. Available at www.nbcnews.com/health/diabetes/u-s-insu lin-costs-patient-nearly-doubled-2012–2016-study-n961296 (accessed April 4, 2019).

Rosen, M. (1979). *The Sunday Times Thalidomide Case: Contempt of Court and the Freedom of the Press*. London: Writers and Scholars Educational Trust in association with the British Institute of Human Rights.

Rutstein, D. D., Berenberg, W., Chalmers, T. C., et al. (1976). Measuring the quality of medical care: a clinical method. *New England Journal of Medicine* **294**, 582–588.

Sala-I-Martin, X., Doppelhofer, G., & Miller, R. I. (2004). Determinants of long-term growth: a Bayesian averaging of classical estimates (BACE) approach. *American Economic Review* **94**, 813–835.

Silber, J. H., Romano, P. S., Rosen, A. K., et al. (2007). Failure-to-rescue: comparing definitions to measure quality of care. *Medical Care* **45**, 918–925.

Suhrcke, M., McKee, M., Sauto Arce, R., et al. (2005). *The Contribution of Health to the Economy in the European Union*. Brussels: European Commission.

Suhrcke, M., Rocco, L., & McKee, M. (2007). *Health: A Vital Investment for Economic Development in Eastern Europe and Central Asia*, Copenhagen: WHO Regional Office for Europe on behalf of the European Observatory on Health Systems and Policies.

Szasz, T. S. (1974). *The Second Sin*. London: Routledge & Kegan Paul.

Thomson, R. P. (2007). *Safer Care for the Acutely Ill Patient: Learning from Serious Incidents*. London: National Patient Safety Agency.

Viens, A. M., & Littmann, J. (2015). Is antimicrobial resistance a slowly emerging disaster? *Public Health Ethics* **8**, 255–265.

Wanless, D. (2001). *Securing Our Future Health: Taking a Long-Term View (Interim Report)*. London, Her Majesty's Treasury.

Wilkinson, R., & Pickett, K. (2010). *The Spirit Level: Why Equality Is Better for Everyone*. London: Penguin Books.

World Bank (2005). *Dying Too Young*. Washington DC, World Bank.

World Health Organization (WHO) (2008). *The Tallinn Charter: Health Systems for Health and Wealth.* Copenhagen: WHO Regional Office for Europe.

World Health Organization (WHO) (2016). *World Health Statistics 2016: Monitoring Health for the Sustainable Development Goals.* Geneva: WHO.

World Health Organization (WHO) (2018). *Financial Protection Country Reviews* (online). Available at www.euro.who.int/en/media-centre/events/events/2018/ 06/health-systems-for-prosperity-and-solidarity-leaving-no-one-behind/documents/background-resources/ financial-protection-country-reviews (accessed June 27, 2018).

Is There a Need for Global Health Ethics?
For and Against

David Hunter and Angus J. Dawson

Introduction

To provide an answer to the question of whether we need global health ethics, we set ourselves three goals in this chapter. First, we explore a number of different ways that we might understand the term *global health ethics*. Second, we consider the arguments that could be used either to support or dismiss what we call *substantive accounts* of global health ethics. Finally, we make some suggestions in relation to what (if any) *global* obligations may bind us. Our discussions will use public health as an example throughout to illustrate our points. The reason for this focus is that, in our view, we ought to think of public health as providing systematic structural support for population health, with the key aim of fulfilling the basic requirements to protect health and prevent illness. This is not to suggest that other forms of healthcare are unimportant, just that public health will fulfill a primary role in any attempt to address questions of global justice in relation to existing health inequalities.

Global health ethics is an important topic. We do not need to accept the view that health is of special consideration in a range of possible aims or outcomes to accept that it is, nevertheless, a key constitutive part of how well our lives go (Daniels, 1985, 2007; Segall, 2007; Wilson, 2009). Health may not be the only or the primary good to be promoted, but it is important for both prudential and ethical reasons. One reason to explore global health ethics is that it is a striking feature of many healthcare issues, particularly in the field of public health, that they fail to respect national boundaries. For example, if we look at the ethical issues in infectious disease control, given that epidemics often spread between countries, policies adopted in one country have cross-border effects. Likewise, issues in resource allocation for individual countries can exacerbate or ameliorate health outcomes depending on what their neighbors do. Similarly, issues about the control and regulation of new medical technologies can be affected by cross-border

considerations (Hunter & Oultram, 2008). Global and cross-border considerations therefore have clear implications for individual and population health. If we assume that this is true, what does this mean for thinking about the ethics of health and healthcare? The place to start is with trying to become clearer about what we mean by *global health ethics*.

What Is Global Health Ethics?

The term *global health ethics* has been used and conceptualized in different ways in the literature (Robson et al., 2019). In this section, we will consider three possible ways of interpreting the phrase *global health ethics*, first as a purely geographic account, second as an account focused on content, and finally, as a normative account.

A Geographic Account

When thinking about how we might define global health ethics, we might focus on the *global* aspects of the phrase to give a purely descriptive definition. On this view, global health ethics is defined spatially. It is about ethical issues related to health at the global level. This, in turn, may be filled out by specifying that such issues might be global in two senses: issues that spatially *affect* the world (e.g., climate change, global pandemics, etc.) or issues that can perhaps only be *solved* by worldwide activity and collaboration (e.g., infectious disease control, global tobacco control, etc.).

On this view, then, global health ethics would be an area of study within the broader field of healthcare ethics – one with a particular focus on ethical issues that span or sit outside of national boundaries or require global solutions. The main strength of this approach is that it is relatively uncontroversial. It requires people discussing global health ethics to make few normative assumptions or commitments and relies on a clear and generally accepted definition of *global*. It might, arguably, also help to refocus attention on issues that are neglected in mainstream medical ethics, where there is often a tendency to focus on micro-level interactions between patients and healthcare practitioners with minimal concern for more macro-level considerations (Dawson, 2010; Hunter, 2007).

However, this definition applies, uncontroversially, only to a limited set of issues. This may leave the field of global health ethics as relatively small and unimportant, possibly reinforcing its neglect. Furthermore, there is a risk here of creating a silo of thought that is then difficult to integrate into our thinking about healthcare ethics in other contexts. Given that there will be issues that impact both on the global and the local scale, we must ensure that we have an integrated approach.

Finally, it is difficult to see how one could be either for or against global health ethics on this definition because it is largely descriptive and assumes that we can agree that such global problems and solutions exist. It may seem trivially true to state that they are important and need to be addressed.

A Content Account

Rather than defining global health ethics in terms of geography, we might instead define it in terms of the issues it addresses. In other words, we could consider global health ethics to be specified by discussion of a set of important issues that might include global justice, health inequalities, infectious diseases, resource allocation, international research, and so on. On this view, global health ethics would be a field of study or area of activity with a range of different topics and focal areas within it. The relevant content would be specified by convention, in the sense that whichever topics were the focus of those involved in the discussions would count as *being* global health ethics. This would mean that such issues might well change over time. For example, smallpox may once have counted as a relevant issue, but since its elimination, it does no longer.

This content approach contrasts with the descriptive focus of the geographic account we gave previously and provides for an arguably richer approach that allows for greater normativity to be built in, because including something in the range of topics immediately calls attention to it.

This view has the advantage of focusing on specific issues and allows for considerable flexibility in the approaches taken to each issue. In principle, because its concerns are not just limited to the global sphere but also address issues that cut across the global sphere and into the realms of individual countries, it is less likely to encourage silos of thought than the previous approach.

However, this focus on specific issues could be accused of being vague and lacking both coherence and unity in its approach. This objection is seen most clearly when we consider which issues might be held to be the core issues of global health ethics. Without a coherent account of why something would count as a global health ethics issue, it seems difficult to appropriately limit the scope of the field. Indeed, on this view, global health ethics might be seen not as a part of medical ethics/bioethics but instead as a competitor – an entirely new field of study that encompasses the concerns of conventional healthcare ethics as well as other concerns, topics, and issues.

As with the first account, the conventional nature of the account seems to make nonsense of the question of whether global health ethics is something we ought to be either for or against. As a field of study, as long as we agree that the topics within it are worthy of consideration, there seems little to say in regard to whether we ought to be for it or against it. All interesting debate switches to arguments about which items ought to be on the list and what we ought to do in relation to each particular topic.

A Normative Account

The third alternative way to approach the definition is to see global health ethics as being, explicitly, a normative project. On this view, to be working on global health ethics is to be committed to and engaged in identifying global wrongs related to health and seeking to have them redressed. For example, we might take global health ethics to be an approach requiring us to address global injustice in regard to health, motivated by existing and historical wrongs characteristic of global trade, structural global inequalities, inequalities in global power, and so on.

This approach has the strong advantage of being a clearly defined project, with key aims, rather than merely being a field of study. However, this strength comes with a parallel weakness in that this account of global health ethics requires substantive normative commitments, and these commitments are not merely conclusions to arguments but serve as premises, often taking it as given, for example, that global injustice has occurred and that such a fact provides us with good (even overriding) reasons to act. There is a significant danger here of an unjustified drift into mere ideology, where writers in the field of global health ethics move from addressing arguments and evidence into prioritizing their role as activists.

Nonetheless, in terms of an account of global health ethics, here is something one could be either for or against. This account seems to be the most plausible candidate for being a distinctive account of global health ethics, but it is also the most contentious. If this is what global health ethics is (and ought to be), then we need some strong arguments in favor of such views. Let us call such a view *substantive global health ethics*.

Arguments in Favor of Substantive Global Health Ethics

To be successful, an argument for substantive global health ethics needs to provide compelling normative reasons for being concerned about global inequalities in health outcomes. The starting point for such a view may be establishing plausible empirical claims about the existence of inequalities in global health outcomes. Fortunately (at least for the argument), there is considerable evidence of significant disparities in global health outcomes.

For example, children have dramatically different life expectancies depending on where they are born. In Japan and Sweden, they can expect to live more than 80 years; in India, 63 years; and in several African countries, fewer than 50 years (Commission on Social Determinants of Health [CSDH], 2008). The infant mortality rate is just 2 in every 1,000 babies born in Iceland, but it is over 120 in every 1,000 babies born in Mozambique. And it is no better for mothers in developing nations. The lifetime risk of maternal death is 1 in 8 in Afghanistan, and it is 1 in 17,400 in Sweden (WHO et al., 2007).

If we switch from children to adults, we see that low- and middle-income nations fare no better here. It was estimated that 17.5 million people died from cardiovascular diseases in 2005, representing 30% of all global deaths. Over 80% of these deaths occurred in developing countries (WHO, 2010a). Of people with diabetes, a disease that is making a rapidly increasing contribution to the global disease burden and mortality rate, 80% live in developing countries (WHO, 2010b). These are only a few examples of the evidence available outlining the significant inequalities in the global disease burden, but it serves to illustrate the key point in relation to the reality of the inequalities that currently exist.

Merely demonstrating the existence of global inequalities in health outcomes does not provide us with the normative grounding necessary for the substantive claim we are interested in. It would need to be shown that there was something ethically problematic about such inequalities, either in and of themselves or because of the nature of their causes. There are several arguments that can be made to show that we ought to take the existence of global inequalities in health outcomes as being ethically troubling, and we will canvass some of the more compelling arguments here to assess whether they show that we ought to be committed to substantive global health ethics. We will consider beneficence, harm, and certain accounts of justice as plausible a priori grounds for such a substantive view.

Beneficence

There are a number of ethical positions that consider global inequalities in health outcomes as morally objectionable in and of themselves because they hold that differences in outcomes need to be morally justified and that there does not seem to be a justification in this case (Unger, 1996). These views might focus on our claims relating to common humanity, needs, capabilities, or disadvantages. However, we focus here on a beneficence claim deriving from a particular form of consequentialism as an example of this kind of approach to ethics. We discuss Peter Singer's account of the obligation of the developed world to those in dramatic need in the developing world. Singer argues in an influential paper titled "Famine, Affluence and Morality" that those in the developed world have direct responsibilities to aid those in the developing world (Singer, 1972). While Singer was not directly discussing healthcare needs, his account straightforwardly applies to these as well as other forms of aid. What makes such accounts relevant for supporting substantive global health ethics is their impartiality toward individuals. On this view, given that the possession of a given property entails moral relevance or value, we are provided with a reason to support an account of our obligations that responds to cross-border and global issues where global health inequalities exist.

Singer's argument is relatively simple yet compelling. He suggests that we ought to accept one of two versions of a principle of comparable moral importance. The weaker version of this principle, which Singer argues should be broadly acceptable to someone from any moral perspective, holds that

> If it is in our power to do or prevent something bad from happening, without thereby sacrificing anything of moral importance, we ought, morally, to do it.
>
> *(Singer, 1972: 235)*

Singer himself holds a stronger version of this principle:

> If it is in our power to do or prevent something bad from happening, without thereby sacrificing anything of comparable moral importance, we ought, morally, to do it. *(Singer, 1972: 231)*

It is this stronger version that is most discussed in the literature, and we will focus on this version here.

From here, the argument for redistributing from those in the developed world toward those in the developing world is relatively simple:

1. Suffering and death from lack of food, shelter, and medical care are bad.
2. "If it is in our power to do or prevent something bad from happening, without thereby sacrificing anything of comparable moral importance, we ought, morally, to do it" (Singer, 1972: 231).
3. It is within our power to prevent such suffering.

Conclusion: Therefore, we ought to prevent such suffering.

The first premise seems, in light of the evidence we have already given, uncontroversial. Such suffering and death clearly do occur and can only be counted as bad. Likewise, the third premise is empirical in nature, and although we do not want to address it in detail here, it seems plausible. Even if it is the case that a significant amount of suffering cannot be prevented, nonetheless, a significant amount could be. For these reasons, discussion of Singer's argument usually focuses on the second premise, either by debating whether it holds true or, alternatively, whether Singer is right to claim that nothing of comparable moral worth would be sacrificed in this case.

To justify this premise, Singer offered a thought experiment to help guide our intuitions:

> If I am walking past a shallow pond and see a child drowning in it, I ought to wade in and pull the child out. This will mean getting my clothes muddy, but this is insignificant, while the death of the child would presumably be a very bad thing. *(Singer, 1972: 231)*

He notes that saving the child in this case would be supported and explained by the principle of comparable moral importance. We will not focus on criticisms of Singer's view here, although we will address some of these later in this chapter. Instead, we will simply conclude that Singer's beneficence-based argument is likely to give us a prima facie reason to accept substantive global health ethics.

Justice and Harm

Thomas Pogge agrees with Singer that we have demanding obligations to respond to those in need in the developing world. However, contrary to Singer, he argues that our duties to aid do not derive from our positive obligations to *benefit* others but rather from claims of justice and our negative duties to both not harm others and to provide restitution when we have harmed them (Pogge, 2008). This is potentially a very powerful argument because some theorists argue (as we will see in the following section) that negative duties (e.g., do not harm) bind strictly (they must always be followed), whereas while individuals are bound by positive duties (e.g., give to charity), they have latitude to decide when they ought to act from them.

There are two primary strands to Pogge's argument, an appeal to historical injustices and an appeal to present injustices, although these two strands are conceptually linked. It seems unarguable that the present global world order rests in part on the back of significant and systemic historical injustices stemming from a shared global history. Many developing nations were colonized by developed nations, and their resources and people were exploited for economic gain by the developed nations. Pogge argues that this creates obligations that bind those countries that were involved in exploitation to aid those which were historically exploited. However, in response, it can be argued that there are significant epistemic difficulties both with tracing the causal pathway of past harms and in assigning the degree of responsibility of restoration given that the present members of the "relevant" group are distinct from the past members of that "same" group.

However, if we choose to focus on the impact of past injustice in the present, we can sidestep these epistemic concerns to some degree. First, it is clear that whoever is present in a developed nation is likely to have benefited from the effects of historical injustice. This fact, in turn, generates some obligations to aid those who are likely to have been harmed by such injustice. Furthermore, as Jeremy Waldron argues, unjust transactions are particularly pernicious because they have an impact on all the other transactions in a market (Waldron, 1992). To see this point, consider the market for car stereos. Given that a significant number of probably stolen car stereos are available secondhand through such outlets as eBay, someone who wants to sell a legitimate second-hand car stereo will have to price their stereo at a lower price point to be able to compete with the stolen car stereos on the market. Hence, the availability of some unjust transactions in a market has an effect on all prices in a market.

Second, the relative power relationships that have developed (based on economies bolstered by historical unjust acts) have allowed the negotiation of a world order that heavily favors the powerful, and disadvantages the weak. Pogge argues that this is a systemic problem and notes, for example, that the way we have decided to recognize people as having the right to alienate the resources of a country if they have effective military control creates strong incentives for dictators to seize control of developing countries, financing their revolution on the basis of future profits from selling off the country's resources to the highest bidder.

As Pogge puts it:

> It is hardly obvious that the basic institutions we participate in are just or nearly just. In any case, a somewhat unobvious but massive threat to the moral quality of our lives is the danger that we will have lived as advantaged participants in unjust institutions, collaborating in their perpetuation and benefiting from their injustice. *(Pogge, 1989: 36)*

To give an example of this in the context of healthcare, Pogge, in his paper "Human Rights and Global Health: A Research Program," argues that the present medical patenting system formed by the trade-related aspects of intellectual property rights (TRIPs) agreement is patently unjust because of the avoidable mortality and morbidity it produces (Pogge, 2005). At present, medical research is overwhelmingly focused on the needs of those in relatively affluent nations because there is little incentive for innovation if there is no market that can afford to purchase that innovation. For example, statistics from the Global Forum for Health Reform show that only 0.31% of all public and private funds devoted to health research is spent on research into medication for malaria, pneumonia, diarrhea, and tuberculosis, which together account for 21% of the global burden of disease (Global Forum for Health Research [GFHR], 2004). But this means that much of new medical research makes little impact on the global disease burden because this burden is disproportionately borne by those in relatively poor nations (Pogge, 2008). This has led to what is often referred to as the 90/10 gap: 90% of medical research funding is spent on conditions affecting only the top 10% of people in terms of wealth. As Pogge notes in his paper, the TRIPs agreement developed out of the Western pharmaceutical industry's concerns that companies in the developing world failed to respect patents and produced considerably cheaper versions of their drugs for local markets.

Whereas Pogge, like Singer, has critics, some of whom we will discuss later in this chapter, it nonetheless appears that considering harms and justice, likewise, can provide a prima facie reason for accepting a substantive global health ethics.

Cosmopolitan Justice

Cosmopolitanism is a term that applies to a broad range of views perhaps best summed up by the quote from the fourth-century BC cynic Diogenes, who, when asked where he came from, replied, "I am a citizen of the world" (Kleingeld & Brown, 2009: online). The essence of cosmopolitanism can be found in either the denial or reduction of the importance of nations and nationality (Scheffler, 1999). For our purposes, this range of views can be divided into moral cosmopolitanism and political cosmopolitanism.

Moral cosmopolitanism focuses on moral judgments and obligations as being universal and impartial in nature. Singer's account of our obligations counts as a version of moral cosmopolitanism, so we will not discuss moral cosmopolitanism further here.

Political cosmopolitanism, by contrast, generally focuses on institutions and argues for no or a weakened role for the state in politics (although not all political cosmopolitans argue for this; see Brock [2009] for example). This is then replaced either with a world government or global institutions such as the United Nations or the International Court of Justice. Such global institutions mitigate and limit the power of individual nation-states (in terms of interfering with their neighboring states and also in regard to states acting on their own citizens). Because political cosmopolitanism downplays the importance of individual nation-states and focuses instead on fair world governance, it might, indirectly, provide a possible grounding for a substantive global health ethics. This is because injustices in health outcomes that may exist across the globe are to be assessed in terms of comparisons across the world and are therefore a concern for all.

A number of different arguments can be offered for political cosmopolitanism. In his book *Realizing Rawls*, Thomas Pogge (1989) develops a strong case for political cosmopolitanism, arguing, ironically, that Rawls himself is mistaken about the implications of his views in the international context. Pogge suggests that precisely the same arguments that Rawls makes for the (potentially radical) reformation of the nation-state likewise apply in the global context. The argument can be established through an intuitive appeal to a revised version of the "veil of ignorance" example, wherein the participants do not know which society they will end up in (Rawls, 1971). This results in the establishment of principles of international governance similar to the principles that Rawls derives for the internal governance of nation-states. Or it can be established on the basis of the moral argument offered by Rawls (1971) in *A Theory of Justice* for a certain model of a just state, abstracted to the worldwide level. In either case, this would lead to a global system that protected basic liberties and, critically in terms of supporting substantive global health ethics, would call for a redistribution of global resources on the basis of the difference principle: namely that the distribution of resources ought to be such that the person in the worst-off position is as well off as possible.

Another possible ground for the establishment of political cosmopolitanism is *luck egalitarianism* (Caney, 2005). Luck egalitarianism is (broadly) the view that the distribution of resources ought to be such that it is insensitive to matters of brute luck (Dworkin, 2000). As Ronald Dworkin puts it, the distribution of resources ought to be ambition sensitive but insensitive to natural endowments (Dworkin, 2000). When this view is applied to questions of global justice, it appears to straightforwardly lead to cosmopolitan conclusions (at least in relation to the, presumably, quite extensive elements of global health injustice related to brute luck).

As Simon Caney puts it:

Underpinning our commitment to equality of opportunity is the deep conviction that it is unfair if someone enjoys worse chances in life because of class or social status or ethnicity. This deep conviction implies, however, that we should also object if some people have worse opportunities because of their nationality or civic identity. The core intuition, then, maintains that persons should not face worse opportunities because of the community or communities they come from. This point can be expressed negatively: people should not be penalized because of the vagaries of happenstance, and their fortunes should not be set by factors like nationality or citizenship. Or it can be expressed positively: People are entitled to the same opportunities as others. If, then, we object to an aristocratic or medieval scheme that distributes unequal opportunities according to one's social standing, or to a racist scheme that distributes unequal opportunities according to one's race, we should, I am arguing, also object to an international order that distributes unequal opportunities according to one's nationality. In short, then, the rationale for accepting equality of opportunity within the state entails that we should accept global equality of opportunity. *(Caney, 2001: 115–116)*

Alternatively, a republican justification could be offered for political cosmopolitanism. This view is centered on the claim that the common understanding of political freedom as a claim about noninterference is a mistake (Pettit, 1997). Instead, we should consider true political freedom to be what Phillip Pettit (1997: 4) dubs "freedom as nondomination." Pettit argues that the usual characterization of liberty as either positive or negative leaves out an important alternative, namely freedom from the ability of others being able to arbitrarily interfere with us – freedom from domination. Because the state is an important potential source of domination, republicans argue that we need to have a state that has a significant division of powers to ensure that checks and balances are in place. In the international arena, strong global institutions provide a reassuring limitation on governments for republicans, and because those who are unhealthy are often vulnerable to domination, this provides a ground for a concern about global health inequalities.

Whichever of these grounds we accept for political cosmopolitanism may provide, once again, a prima facie ground for substantive global health ethics. Thus, in this section, we have shown that there are several arguments that might be offered for a substantive global health ethics. However, there are also several arguments that are often offered against any substantive view of global health ethics. These either aim to show that the arguments we have thus far given are mistaken or that there is some independent reason for denying the legitimacy of the obligations that supposedly derive from substantive global health ethics.

Arguments Against Substantive Global Health Ethics

Obligations of Charity Are Imperfect Duties

One argument that might be offered against substantive global health ethics is that, as has already been mentioned, on some views of morality, a positive duty to assist others is of a different nature to a negative duty not to cause harm. One way of putting this position forward is in regards to Kant's distinction between what he calls perfect and imperfect duties. A *perfect* duty is one that you can fulfill all the time, simply by refraining from doing something. Not lying is a good example of such a duty. By contrast, an *imperfect* duty is one that you have latitude over when you can choose to fulfill it. Benefiting others through charitable activity might be a good example of such an imperfect duty. Such a duty is binding on you, but you cannot be expected to always be acting charitably.

Given the imperfect nature of the obligation of charity, some have argued that it is a matter of choice how and where we ought to carry it out. Although we may choose to give charity to developing nations, there would be nothing wrong in choosing to fulfill our obligation of charity in other ways, such as donating money to allow a local child to travel overseas to receive potentially lifesaving, but expensive, treatment.

If this truly is the nature of our obligation to give, then it undermines arguments such as that offered by Singer. Even if he is able to establish that we have a duty to give to those in need, it might be argued that the obligation is not of the nature he suggests, and so we are not necessarily obliged to give to anything like the extent he suggests. However, in the face of massive global inequalities in health outcomes, it is worth considering how compelling this argument might be. Is it really the case that what matters is the mere fact *that* we act charitably rather than *how* and *when* we

act charitably? For this objection to be entirely telling, it would have to be the case that it did not matter what the subject of our charity was, only that we engaged in some charitable act or other. However, even if it is the case that our duty to give charitably is weaker than that which Singer defends, it is surely the case that the nature of our charitable actions will still matter morally. Is it really the case that we ought to just give to someone on some occasion rather than focusing on potentially life-threatening health inequalities? Perhaps what has convinced some people of this argument is a misunderstanding about the differences between praiseworthy actions and right actions. It seems that while the giving of large but inefficient donations to individuals may be praiseworthy, we may not see it as being the right action, given what else that money could do. Even if we think the positive/negative duties distinction is morally relevant, we have a choice about priorities when it comes to our actions, and it is hard to imagine a more pressing priority than at least some of the inequalities in relation to global healthcare.

Furthermore, this objection is not telling against all the arguments for substantive global health ethics because some, such as Pogge's position, focus on negative rather than positive duties. Nonetheless, this objection may cause some doubt about an argument for a substantive global health ethics. At the very least, we are pushed into the necessity of grappling with deep and contested normative theory, and it certainly looks as though there is no easy intuitive support for the radical conclusions that some supporters of global health ethics wish for.

We Have No Obligations to the Distant Needy

Some theorists have argued, contra Peter Singer, that the distance we are from those in need does make a moral difference. Our duties to aid decrease as the needy become further away from us (Kamm, 2000).

This might be based on the ease of aiding those who are closer or in determining their need. Kamm puts forward an argument to claim that distance does make a moral difference in her paper "Does Distance Matter Morally to the Duty to Rescue?" (Kamm, 2000), where she criticizes Singer for relying on single cases to try to show that distance does not matter (because single cases only show that distance does not matter in that case, not all cases). Kamm suggests that we have to carefully construct cases to test our intuitions and that the following example is a better test of our intuitions in regard to the role of distance:

> Near Alone Case: I am walking past a pond in a foreign country that I am visiting. I alone see many children drowning in it and I alone can save one of them. To save the one, I must put the $500 I have in my pocket into a machine that then triggers (via electric current) rescue machinery that will certainly scoop him out.
>
> Far Alone Case: I alone know that in a distant part of a foreign country that I am visiting, many children are drowning, and I alone can save one of them. To save the one, all I must do is put the $500 I carry in my pocket into a machine that then triggers (via electric current) rescue machinery that will certainly scoop him out. *(Kamm, 2000: 657)*

Kamm concludes that it is intuitive to recognize a difference in our moral obligations between these two cases. Singer, however, defends the idea that distance is irrelevant. This underlies his argument that we outlined earlier. He insists that if you accept "any principle of impartiality, universalizability, equality, or whatever," then you ought to hold distance as morally irrelevant (Singer, 1972: 232). He suggests that to hold otherwise is to be guilty of a form of discrimination. He allows that *psychologically* it might make a difference whether an individual is starving to death in front of your eyes or in a far-away country but that it makes no *moral* difference.

As with the previous objection, at best, this argument undermines only some of the arguments for substantive global health ethics – namely those founded on beneficence and other such positive obligations.

Property Rights as Trumps

Perhaps a more powerful argument against substantive global health ethics is a libertarian argument based around the ideal of freedom and the notion of the ownership of property. On this view, we only can have positive duties if we ourselves have caused harm. Although the suffering of others is unfortunate, it is not unfair. On this view, it would be good of us to intervene, but it is not, and cannot be, compulsory to give, for that would violate our property ownership rights. If this position can be defended, then this is a problem for champions of substantive global health ethics because it would block the significant redistribution that substantive global health ethics requires.

Typically, such a response is based on Nozick's account of Lockean property rights (Locke, 1690 [1960]; Nozick, 1974). Such a view starts from an account of the fair initial acquisition of property and then holds that as long as procedurally fair transactions led us from that initial distribution of resources to the current distribution of resources, then the current distribution is just and fair, and interference with it would be illegitimate. The account of initial acquisition relies on the idea that prior to anyone owning anything, it is reasonable to believe that we all have a right to everything. In other words, everything is owned in common. This generates a puzzle, though, because to be able to use something, we usually need to alienate it: to make it ours and ours alone. While in a small group, we could simply ask if anyone minded, but when everything is owned in common, we would need to ask everyone. Locke thought that no one could object to the alienation of some bit of property provided that two conditions were met: first, that you left enough for others and that what was left was as good for them and, second, that you didn't just waste the common stock.

Similar to the last objection, if this argument holds, then this would seem to undermine some of the arguments put forward for substantive global health ethics. However, there seem to be three main objections that could be raised to it.

The first objection is to point out, as Pogge does, that there is *in fact* a systemic history of the violent and unjust acquisition of resources (Pogge, 2008). In the face of this undeniable fact, it seems difficult to justify resisting redistribution.

The second objection challenges the first condition of initial acquisition – that enough and as good has been left. Given that all or most resources have been acquired, is it really possible to leave enough and as good? The typical libertarian response to this is to point to the benefits for all of economic development that depends on the alienation of the means of production and the notion that people who have worked hard deserve a reward for their work. However, this seems based on the notion of first come, first served, and it is hard to see why latecomers would automatically accept that this is a fair way to determine who owns resources, especially if there are no limits on the control of those resources.

The final objection is that the appeal to desert leaves libertarians open to a desert-based challenge. This challenge is commonly made by egalitarians, who point out that some of the income we earn does not seem to be deserved because it is just a matter of luck. This is the part of our income that is derived from the exercise of our natural talents. Which talents we have, and which talents are valued, is a matter of brute luck, and if a distribution should reflect deservingness, then natural talents and differences ought not make a difference to who gets what. Thus, while we might not be in a position to tax people and remove all their income, we might still be able to justly redistribute (at least) some of it.

As with the last argument, at best, this is only telling against some of the positive arguments for substantive global health ethics. Nonetheless, in so far as it is compelling, it does provide reasons to question the acceptance of a substantive global health ethics.

We Have a Duty to Prioritize Our Compatriots

There seem to be two main versions of this objection, the first of which argues that we have more significant duties to our compatriots than to others. The second version argues that we have duties not to interfere directly in the governance of other societies. This is a different sort of objection to the first three because if it works, it is a global objection to substantive global health ethics.

Broadly, the first version of the objection might be called *nationalism* and might seem to run directly counter to the claims made by cosmopolitans that we discussed earlier. On this view, there is something central and important about the nation-state. To maintain and develop our nations, we are required to prioritize the needs of our citizens first, even if others are in greater need (Miller, 1995).

A number of arguments might be offered for this claim; for example, we might claim that there is something important about the shared cultural and moral understandings that flourish in a common culture. Alternatively, we might argue that to properly flourish, individuals need a cultural context within which they are comfortable and that the nation-state is an essential part of this. Or we might simply claim that nationality is an important constitutive part of our personal identity, and if we allow our nation to be undermined, then, in a sense, we are undermining our own identity. On each of these claims there is the underlying notion that the nation is important psychologically to underwrite our behavior, moral or otherwise. Although this position does seem to weaken the strength of substantive global health ethics, it does not seem to negate it entirely. Even if we must prioritize our compatriots, given, as we pointed out earlier, the scale of health inequalities between nations, even a nationalist might admit that there are significant opportunities to aid others without undermining our own nation.

The second version of these arguments, if compelling, would be more telling against substantive global health ethics because it would establish that there is no obligation to aid those individuals outside our nation or even a positive obligation to not interfere in others' ways of life. These arguments tend to be based on social contract theory that sees both political and moral obligations as based on an unspoken agreement as the basis for society. Hobbes, one of the early social contract theorists, held that moral obligations were only possible within the context of a society, but modern social contract theorists often see our obligations to our compatriots as being far stronger than our obligations to those in other countries (Hobbes, 1651 [1992]). We focus on John Rawls as the exemplar of this sort of position.

Rawls has been a very influential writer on justice within liberal societies, and his position on justice inside liberal societies, as we outlined earlier, had been applied to the global context. However, Rawls felt that these approaches misconstrued an appropriate approach to global considerations because they applied his theory, which was targeted at individuals within a particular context, in a parallel way to countries within the global context.

As Rawls says:

Two main ideas motivate the Law of Peoples. One is that the great evils of human history – unjust war and oppression, religious persecution and the denial of liberty of conscience, starvation and poverty, not to mention genocide and mass murder – follow from political injustice, with its own cruelties and callousness . . . . The other main idea, obviously connected with the first, is that, once the gravest forms of political injustice are eliminated by following just (or at least decent) social policies and establishing just (or at least decent) basic institutions, these great evils will eventually disappear. *(Rawls, 1999: 6–7)*

On the basis of this, Rawls put forward eight principles for ordering the international basic structure:

1. Peoples are free and independent, and their freedom and independence are to be respected by other peoples.
2. Peoples are to observe treaties and undertakings.
3. Peoples are equal and are parties to the agreements that bind them.
4. Peoples are to observe the duty of nonintervention (except to address grave violations of human rights).
5. Peoples have a right of self-defense, but no right to instigate war for reasons other than self-defense.
6. Peoples are to honor human rights.
7. Peoples are to observe certain specified restrictions in the conduct of war.
8. Peoples have a duty to assist other peoples living under unfavorable conditions that prevent their having a just or decent political and social regime.

(Rawls, 1999)

Many theorists, who held that the difference principle ought to be applied globally, were surprised by Rawls' rejection of this idea and his insistence instead on a much more limited set of obligations. The aim of aid was not to achieve global equality but to ensure instead that nations could achieve and maintain liberal or decent political institutions.

As we mentioned earlier, Rawls' views have been criticized by Pogge, pointing out that while starvation and poverty are related to internal political injustice, they are not solely derived from this – unjust international institutions and a lack of natural resources also have an impact. And it seems that the points that Simon Caney made in favor of global equality of opportunity earlier still hold. It seems unfair that an arbitrary factor such as where one is born ought to have a significant role to play in determining how well one's life goes. Nonetheless, although Rawls' position might weaken support for a substantive global health ethics, it need not remove it because Rawls does recognize that there is a duty to assist those who are living in conditions that prevent them living in a just or decent political and social regime, which, arguably, is the case in countries with the severest needs.

Practical: What Obligations Bind Us Here?

So what can we now say about substantive global health ethics? At best, the arguments for substantive

global health ethics could not be described as uncontroversial, and although we have expressed doubt about whether the arguments against are decisive, the case for, likewise, does not seem entirely compelling. Given this, it seems inappropriate, at the very least, to take substantive and controversial normative conclusions as our starting point and to approach issues in global health ethics from there.

However, it might be asked, do we have to accept substantive global health ethics to achieve many of the goods it aims to achieve? It seems to us that the answer to this question is clearly no.

As we saw in our discussion of the arguments for substantive global health ethics, there are powerful ethical arguments for being concerned with global issues. Even if these do not carry us as far as someone committed to substantive global health ethics would like us to go, nonetheless, any reasonable theory/view is going to accept that global ethical and political concerns need to be addressed, if only because when they are not, there is a tendency for this to end up in our own backyard, as can happen, for example, in regard to infectious diseases and other public health issues. Drug-resistant tuberculosis or increasingly ineffective antibiotics ought to be a concern to us all. Given that healthcare issues rarely respect borders, even the staunchest nationalist will have to sometimes consider taking action on healthcare issues while they are still "someone else's problem."

Indeed, taking a purely prudential approach might lead even the purely self-interested to address significant global ethical and political concerns. It has been argued that this might arise out of consideration of global public goods.

Public goods are classically defined as being

1. *Nonrival* (my enjoyment of clean air has no consequences for your enjoyment of the same thing), and
2. *Nonexcludable* (it is not possible to exclude others from enjoying the benefits of clean air).

Global public goods are public goods that benefit a substantial region of the world or the whole world. Suggested candidates include climatic and environmental stability, financial stability, infectious disease control, and human rights. If we accept these as global public goods, then it is in *each individual state's interests* to create and maintain such goods. Whatever the merits of such an approach, discussion of global public goods is one way to motivate self-interested nation-states to act to improve (at least some) global health inequalities.

Thus, we conclude that it seems that there is something to be said for the aims of substantive global health ethics. However, even if we choose to interpret the phrase *global health ethics* in either the geographic or content sense, we might end up with significant overlap with a more substantive account when it comes to justifying many actions.

It is also worth noting how a focus on the wider issue of global inequalities can, helpfully, stress the problems for more narrow approaches, such as the autonomy-obsessed state of present medical ethics. Hence, even if we adopt one of the less substantive approaches to global health ethics that we have outlined, there are still things to be said in favor of giving a higher priority to justice in relation to health outcomes. Such an approach focused on considering issues broadly within the field of global health ethics might give us new ideas and approaches that can then be used to critique and develop traditional medical ethics (Dawson, 2010).

This chapter has focused on the moral/political case for being concerned about inequalities and justice in health across the world (particularly in relation to public health). We can call this global health ethics if we wish, but it is the issues that require action. Labels are far less important. We have argued that we are obligated to respond to global inequalities (whatever you think of the idea of global health ethics).

References

Brock, G. (2009). *Global Justice: A Cosmopolitan Account.* Oxford, UK: Oxford University Press.

Caney, S. (2001). Cosmopolitan justice and equalizing opportunities. *Metaphilosophy* 32, 113–134.

Caney, S. (2005). *Justice Beyond Borders: A Global Political Theory.* Oxford, UK: Oxford University Press.

Commission on Social Determinants of Health (CSDH) (2008). *Closing the Gap in a Generation: Health Equity through Action on the Social Determinants of Health. Final Report of the Commission on Social Determinants of Health.* Geneva: WHO.

Daniels, N. (1985). *Just Health Care.* Cambridge, UK: Cambridge University Press.

Daniels, N. (2007). *Just Health: Meeting Health Needs Fairly.* New York: Cambridge University Press.

Dawson, A. (2010). The future of bioethics: three dogmas and a cup of hemlock. *Bioethics* 24, 218–225.

Dworkin, R. (2000). *Sovereign Virtue.* Cambridge, MA: Harvard University Press.

Global Forum for Health Research (GFHR) (2004) *The 10/90 Report on Health Research 2003– 2004.* Available at www.globalforumhealth.org/filesupld/1090_report_03_04/1090 04_chap_5.pdf (accessed March 11, 2010).

Hobbes, T. (1651). *Leviathan*, trans. E. Curley (1992). London: Hackett.

Hunter, D. (2007). Am I my brother's gatekeeper? Professional ethics and the prioritisation of healthcare. *Journal of Medical Ethics* 33, 522–526.

Hunter, D., & Oultram, S. (2008). The challenge of "sperm ships": the need for the global regulation of medical technology. *Journal of Medical Ethics* 34, 552–556.

Inge, K., Conceicao, P., Le Goulven, K., & Mendoza, R. (2003). *Providing Global Public Goods: Managing Globalization.* New York: Oxford University Press.

Kamm, F. M. (2000). Does distance matter morally to the duty to rescue? *Law and Philosophy* 19, 655–681.

Kleingeld, P., & Brown, E. (2009). Cosmopolitanism, in Zalta, E. N. (ed.), *The Stanford Encyclopedia of Philosophy*, Summer 2009 ed. http://plato.stanford.edu/archives/su m2009/entries/cosmopolitanism/ (accessed March 11, 2010).

Locke, J. (1690 [1960]). *Two Treatises of Government*, P. Laslett (ed.). New York: Cambridge University Press.

Miller, D. (1995). *On Nationality.* Oxford, UK: Oxford University Press.

Nozick, R. (1974). *Anarchy, State, and Utopia.* New York: Basic Books.

Pettit, P. (1997). *Republicanism: A Theory of Freedom and Government.* Oxford, UK: Clarendon Press.

Pogge, T. (1989). *Realizing Rawls.* Ithaca, NY: Cornell University Press.

Pogge, T. (2005). Human rights and global health: a research program. *Metaphilosophy* 36, 182–209.

Pogge, T. (2008). *World Poverty and Human Rights: Cosmopolitan Responsibilities and Reforms*, 2nd ed. Cambridge, UK: Polity Press.

Rawls, J. (1971). *A Theory of Justice.* Cambridge, MA: Harvard University Press.

Rawls, J. (1999). *The Law of Peoples.* Cambridge, MA: Harvard University Press.

Robson, G., Gibson, N., Thompson, A., et al (2019). Global health ethics: critical reflections on the contours of an emerging field, 1977–2017. *BMC Medical Ethics*, 20, 1–10.

Scheffler, S. (1999). Conceptions of cosmopolitanism. *Utilitas* 11, 255–276.

Segall, S. (2007). Is health care (still) special? *Journal of Political Philosophy* 15, 342–361.

Singer, P. (1972). Famine, affluence, and morality. *Philosophy and Public Affairs* 1, 229–243.

Unger, P. (1996). *Living High and Letting Die*. Oxford, UK: Oxford University Press.

Waldron, J. (1992). Superseding historic injustice. *Ethics* **103**, 4–28.

Wilson, J. (2009). Not so special after all? Daniels and the social determinants of health. *Journal of Medical Ethics* **35**, 3–6.

World Health Organization (WHO) et al. (2007). *Maternal Mortality in 2005: Estimates Developed by WHO, UNICEF, UNFPA and the World Bank*. Geneva: WHO. Available at www.who/reproductive-health/publications/maternalmortality2005/mme2005.pdf (accessed March 11, 2010).

World Health Organization (WHO) (2010a). *Cardiovascular Diseases: What Are Cardiovascular Diseases?* Geneva: WHO. Available at www.who.int/mediacentre/factsheets/fs317/en/index.html (accessed March 11, 2010).

World Health Organization (WHO) (2010b). *Quick Diabetes Facts*. Geneva: WHO. Available at www.who.int/diabetes/en/ (accessed March 11, 2010).

The Human Right to Health

Jonathan Wolff

Introduction: The Global Health Duty

It is hardly news that the health and life expectancy of many of the peoples of the developing world fall well below what we might think should be a reasonable standard. Health inequalities remain stark. For example, according to one source, in 2018 life expectancy at birth was 85.5 years for those born in Japan but a depressingly low 52 years for those born in Afghanistan (Central Intelligence Agency [CIA], 2019). This gap is highly significant, although it represents a great improvement for those at the bottom compared with the situation merely 10 years ago, where a life expectancy of 32 years was reported for Eswatini (then known as Swaziland; CIA, 2009). If this figure is to be believed, then it may well be that adult male life expectancy in Swaziland was the lowest it had ever been in history, or at least not far above.[1] The progress since then has been remarkable, primarily because of the rapid improvements in treatment for HIV, although much needs to be done.

At its worst, the depth of the crisis in health in the developing world was staggering, and it remains an issue of deep concern. It is no surprise, therefore, that it has been an increasing topic of concern at all levels. In the case of academic political philosophy, the global health crisis intersects with the topic of global justice, which has seen a huge surge in interest and attention in recent years (see, e.g., Brock, 2009a; Caney, 2005; Nussbaum, 2006; Pogge, 2002; Rawls, 1999; Valentini, 2011; Ypi, 2012). The health agenda is beginning to receive the attention it deserves in this context, broadening from a concern about financial redistribution (Sreenivasan, 2002), the health brain drain (Brock, 2009b), access to medicine, and drug discovery (Hassoun, 2012; Pogge, 2005) to issues of health capability (Venkatapuram, 2011) and, the topic of this chapter, the human right to heath (Wolff, 2012a).

Philosophical debates need to absorb a wave of critical examination of existing policies both from development commentators (Collier, 2007; Easterley, 2006; Moyo, 2009) and from the health activist literature (Global Health Watch, 2008), which suggests that traditional forms of assistance are far less effective than their proponents hope or believe. For example, it is said that the research effort has been driven by the agenda of the funders and researchers looking for glamorous, headline-grabbing, potentially prize-winning outcomes and concentrating on a "technological fix" when community and health system strengthening may be more effective.

These criticisms of development aid should not stop philosophers arguing that there is a duty for wealthy nations and their citizens to take steps to attempt to remedy the global health crisis. Moreover, we should acknowledge that while finding solutions will be complex, these solutions should not exclude seeking imaginative ways of improving financial flows, changing drug discovery and migration incentives, and funding health interventions. Nevertheless, work connecting political philosophy and global health remains at a relatively early stage.

Possible Foundations of the Global Health Duty

Yet, before deciding which global health programs to support, there is a prior question. Why should peoples of the developed world take an interest in the health of those in the developing world? What, to put the point bluntly, business is it of ours? Possible answers can be divided into three types (which, we should note, are not exclusive of each other; Wolff, 2012b). First, taking on this duty may be in our own interests, either as nations or as particular individuals. For example, perhaps the best protection against global pandemics

---

[1] I have used the example of an adult male to abstract from the benefits of improved infant and maternal survival.

is to strengthen public health in the developing world. Or, for an individual, it may be that attending to the health needs of others is highly fulfilling.

This individualized self-interest argument shades into another – that there is a humanitarian duty of assistance to help people in the developing world. Such a moral duty could be grounded in arguments such as Peter Singer's claim that if we can save a life without sacrificing anything of significant moral importance, we have a duty to do so (Singer, 1972). Many international charities implicitly appeal to such considerations, especially in times of emergencies. Third, there are arguments from justice that go beyond humanitarian claims by positing not only a duty to act but also a right of those in the developing world to receive assistance.

Three forms of justice arguments seem particularly salient. First, "cosmopolitans" argue that there is no moral significance to distinctions between countries and that each person has duties of justice to all others regardless of where they live (Steiner, 2005). Second, it is argued that many of the problems of the developing world are either the legacy of shamefully brutal colonization or the consequence of unfair contemporary international trade policies, for which justice requires reparation (Benatar, 2003; Pogge, 2002). Finally, it is also increasingly argued that each person on Earth has a set of human rights and that these rights include the human right to health. It is the responsibility of the global community to advance and protect the human rights of all. Therefore, we each have a justice-based responsibility to act in accordance with the human right to health (Clapham & Robinson, 2009; Wolff, 2012a). The claim that there is a human right to health will be the focus of the remaining discussion here.

Why Do Foundations Matter?

Each of the arguments set out in the preceding section appeals to a plausible consideration. However, given the convergence on the result that there is a global health duty, it may be reasonably asked why it is worth pursuing the philosophical debate. How can it matter? It seems indulgent to spend time and energy on obtuse philosophical questions when our duties are so clear and so pressing.

I have a great deal of sympathy for this objection (Wolff & de-Shalit, 2007). Indeed, I will make a version of this argument later in this chapter. However, in the present case, in the words of health

activist James Orbinski, "language matters" (Orbinski, 2008: 341). It matters not only because it can be important, for its own sake, to get the philosophical details right but also because different ways of understanding the basis of the duty can lead to different outcomes.

Consider the question of agency. Who has a duty to act? Cosmopolitan justice arguments put the duty on everyone, whereas reparative justice arguments put the duty on those who have caused or have benefited from previous injustice, while humanitarian arguments place the duty on those who are best able to help. (Human rights arguments raise more complex issues of agency, to which we will return later.) Another issue is one of enforcement. Human rights and, in some cases, reparative justice arguments have international institutions associated with them, so they offer some hope of judicial remedy, whereas none of the others do (Wolff, 2012b). Indeed, the pragmatic advantages of using the idea of a human right to health are clear: human rights are an international respected currency, backed by 60 years of institution building, an enforcement mechanism, and ever-growing in influence (Wolff, 2012c).

Human Rights Conventions

Various declarations and conventions have attempted to establish the human right to health (Tobin, 2012; Yamin, 2017). Perhaps the boldest statement is to be found, not surprisingly, in the constitution of the World Health Organization (WHO):

> The enjoyment of the highest attainable standard of health is one of the fundamental rights of every human being without distinction of race, religion, political belief, economic or social condition.
> *(WHO, 1946 [2006])*

The same year that the WHO constitution came into effect, 1948, also saw the Universal Declaration of Human Rights, article 25(1) of which reads

> Everyone has the right to a standard of living adequate for the health and well-being of himself and of his family, including food, clothing, housing and medical care and necessary social services, and the right to security in the event of unemployment, sickness, disability, widowhood, old age or other lack of livelihood in circumstances beyond his control.
> *(United Nations, 1948)*

The Universal Declaration, therefore, while recognizing the right to medical care as a determinant of well-being, falls short of the expansive right to health set out by the WHO.

However, in 1966, the International Covenant on Economic, Social, and Cultural Rights was adopted, coming into force only in 1976 when ratified by the required 30 countries. Here, in article 12, we see the most elaborate statement of the human right to health:

1. The States Parties to the present Covenant recognize the right of everyone to the enjoyment of the highest attainable standard of physical and mental health.
2. The steps to be taken by the States Parties to the present Covenant to achieve the full realization of this right shall include those necessary for:

    (a) The provision for the reduction of the stillbirth-rate and of infant mortality and for the healthy development of the child;
    (b) The improvement of all aspects of environmental and industrial hygiene;
    (c) The prevention, treatment and control of epidemic, endemic, occupational and other diseases;
    (d) The creation of conditions which would assure to all medical service and medical attention in the event of sickness. *(United Nations, 1966)*

Furthermore, at least for children, the WHO right was recognized in the United Nations (UN) Convention on the Rights of the Child, which came into force in 1990. Article 24(1) reads

> States Parties recognize the right of the child to the enjoyment of the highest attainable standard of health and to facilities for the treatment of illness and rehabilitation of health. States Parties shall strive to ensure that no child is deprived of his or her right of access to such health care services
> *(United Nations Treaty Collection n.d.)*

Although the International Covenant on Economic, Social and Cultural Rights (ICESCR) has not been universally adopted, the position is rather more encouraging for the Convention on the Rights of the Child. According to the United Nations, now that the Convention on the Rights of the Child has been ratified by Somalia and South Sudan, the only country in the world that has not ratified it is the United States of America (United Nations Treaty Collection, n.d.). In consequence, virtually all countries in the world have accepted the right to the highest attainable standard of health for children, and many have accepted it for all

their citizens as part of ratification of international human rights treaties.

Yet, looking at the terms in which these treatises are stated, one may be filled with a sense of hopelessness. What could it mean to guarantee to all the people of the world "the right to the highest attainable standard of health"? Does everyone in the world have the right to the health and life expectancy of the Japanese? How could that be achieved? Without a huge increase in budgets, which is not in prospect, attempting to provide everyone with the right to health would drain all resources from other areas, such as education and housing. Many will view such conventions as collections of fine words and sentiments that will have to be ignored in practice.

In response, the ICESCR explicitly adopts the notion of "progressive realization" rather than "full immediate realization" of the rights (article 2(1); United Nations, 1966; see also Hessler & Buchanan, 2002). In 2000, this was further clarified when the Committee on Economic, Social and Cultural Rights issued General Comment 14 to explain how the human right to health can be approached in practice. The committee producing the comment understood the difficulties of the task, writing, in article 5,

> [t]he Committee is aware that, for millions of people throughout the world, the full enjoyment of the right to health still remains a distant goal. Moreover, in many cases, especially for those living in poverty, this goal is becoming increasingly remote. The Committee recognizes the formidable structural and other obstacles resulting from international and other factors beyond the control of States that impede the full realization of article 12 [of the ICESCR] in many States parties. *(United Nations, 2000)*

Accordingly, General Comment 14 clarifies that the right to health is not the right to be healthy (article 8). Nevertheless, the right to health is not merely the right to access to medical care, for medical care is only one of the many determinants of health. Healthy living and working conditions, for example, are just as vital (article 11).

Resource constraints can be a legitimate reason why a particular state may not be able to do as much as another to realize the right to health for its people. Nevertheless, General Comment 14 insists that

> 30. ... States parties have immediate obligations in relation to the right to health, such as the guarantee that the right will be exercised without discrimination

of any kind (art. 2.2) and the obligation to take steps (art. 2.1) towards the full realization of article 12 [of the ICESCR]. Such steps must be deliberate, concrete and targeted towards the full realization of the right to health. *(United Nations, 2000)*

This is known as *progressive realization*, but in the earlier General Comment 3, the notion of a state's "minimum core obligations" is clarified, which requires states to use whatever resources they have to supply essential primary healthcare (United Nations, 1990). To help promote, protect, and advocate for the human right to health, in 2002, a Special Rapporteur on the right to health was appointed, with the obligation to undertake country-based missions and produce reports.

Skepticism About the Human Right to Health

The covenants are full of fine words. General Comment 14 attempts to translate those words into action, and we saw in the "Introduction" that the health situation of the most disadvantaged people in the world is, on aggregate, now improving. Perhaps the human right to health has already helped, despite earlier skepticism (Benatar, 2002). Nevertheless, a range of criticisms has been made, and it has even been alleged that philosophers do themselves no credit by associating themselves with the human right to health (Baumrin, 2002). In response, it is commonly argued that although there is room for improvement, the human right to health is perhaps the most promising route available to address global health problems.

Many arguments against the human right to health are parasitic on a more general argument against human rights in general – that they are in some way confused, empty, useless, or damaging. Some of these arguments go back several centuries. (Bentham, 1796 [1987]; Marx, 1843 [1975]) though here we will concentrate on more recent arguments, such as that once we accept a wide range of human rights, and also that states do not have an obligation to realize them all fully, then we have devalued the currency of human rights. This is the criticism of *rights inflation*, that once rights such as the right to health are accepted, then rights against arbitrary arrest, even rights against torture, will be taken less seriously and abused (for discussion, see Nickel, 2017). To guard against this, it is said, human rights must be limited to a relatively small set of absolutely indispensable rights that should always be fully, rather than progressively, realized.

It is unclear whether there is evidence that rights inflation has devalued the currency, but to guard against it, rights-based claims and actions must be made sparingly. And still it is not obvious that a minor weakening of civil and political rights is too high a price to pay for the establishment of the right to health and other social and economic rights. This is controversial, but there are costs and benefits on both sides. However, it is important to use rights claims sparingly for a different reason: that a quick recourse to rights will encourage an unattractive and unproductive legalistic culture in which people encounter each other as opponents rather than as fellow citizens who jointly need to negotiate their way out of a collective difficulty (O'Neill, 2005). Human rights are something close to a last resort, for when all else has failed, rather than the first moral weapon to hand. It would be a better world if we never had to mention human rights. But, unfortunately, this is not the world we are in.

Proliferation of rights makes conflicts more probable (Freeman 2002: 5). So, for example, the right for people to choose to spend their resources their own way may lead to wealthy people looking to the private sector for healthcare, leaving the public sector in a state of political and economic neglect. Hence, one right may undermine another. Once more, we must accept that this may happen. But it is not clear that the solution is to restrict the list of human rights in advance, for even if that does have the virtue of ruling out conflict by privileging one set of values, avoidance of conflict is not the highest good if it comes at a high price.

It has also been argued that it is incoherent to claim that a person has a right unless it is possible to identify a duty holder in respect of that right, and in the case of the claimed human right to health, it is not obvious who the duty holder will be (this returns us to the vexing question of *agency* raised earlier; Baumrin, 2002; O'Neill, 2005; see also Benatar, 2002). However, it is possible to deny that it is always necessary to identify a particular duty holder. Or, more concessively, it could be said that the duty holder is the government of the state in which the person resides. Now this can be problematic. Some people are stateless or are refugees across borders, and this is where some of the greatest human rights challenges are to be found. Furthermore, some states are unwilling or unable to act, whereas others that may be willing to act are restricted by international organizations that constrain how they can spend their budgets. Nevertheless, we can still say that in the first instance the duty falls on the state of which the person is a citizen – if that is problematic, then the country of residence and, as a last resort, the international community.

Other critics have focused on the individualism of human rights discourse, suggesting, instead, that it can be a grave obstacle to achievement of global health (Benatar et al., 2003). First, a focus on individual rights inevitably tends to bring issues of access to healthcare into sharper focus than public health, which, from the point of view of global health, is far more important. Second, access to human rights courts is likely to be the exclusive recourse of those who are wealthy or have powerful connections. Hence, it appears, a human right to health agenda threatens to reduce health to healthcare and to reinforce health inequalities. These are serious problems. The question is whether they are intrinsic to the human rights approach. It may be possible to refocus the human rights agenda to include the rights of groups of individuals, and to some degree, this is already in process, as we will see later. Furthermore, although court action is the ultimate sanction for human rights abuse, how common it is varies considerably from country to country, whereas policies of "naming and shaming" can be more effective (Birn, 2008) and may be pursued with respect to the poor and vulnerable. Consider, for example, the study of "excess deaths" in the aftermath of the invasion of Iraq, which, although it was not explicitly part of a human rights agenda, is highly appropriate for that purpose (Burnham et al., 2006).

Naturally following on from this observation, however, is a quite different argument based on the political sociology of human rights and, in particular, rights advocacy and empowerment. Human rights organizations such as Amnesty International and Human Rights Watch campaign, lobby, and take action on behalf of those whose rights have been violated. This, it is said, while often highly beneficial and effective, nevertheless has the effect of continuing to marginalize disadvantaged people. Human rights activists will tend to be relatively privileged people from the developed world acting on behalf of others, who are passive beneficiaries of their activities. Once more we must

admit that this is a danger. For this reason, some of the most encouraging developments in human rights activism are those facilitating disadvantaged people's self-advocacy. The role for nongovernmental organizations (NGOs) is to provide training and support and to help form a radicalized and empowered community, able to fight its own battles. It is important for NGOs to focus not only on the goals of their campaigns but also on the means by which those goals are obtained. Every NGO should consider whether making itself redundant should be part of its mission statement.

However, it has been argued that advocacy for the human right to health has done more harm than good by distorting health priority setting, diverting resources, effectively, to those who shout the loudest and are most effective in their advocacy, to the detriment of general health promotion (Easterley, 2009). Easterley (2009) claims that societies – developed and developing – would be better off with cost-effective health-maximizing strategies.

Single-issue advocacy can be damaging to health systems. For example, in some areas of Sub-Saharan Africa, as ever more money is spent on HIV/AIDS programs, the proportion of attended births has gone down (Haacker, 2010; see also WHO, 2009). Health workers are drawn to the well-funded campaign areas, away from general practice, which is left depleted. This is a very serious problem. It is unclear, though, that it is somehow intimately connected with the right to health. Human right to health advocacy is as likely to be addressed to health system strengthening as to single-issue projects. We will consider later the degree to which human right to health litigation has distorted spending priorities. But the lesson from Easterley's challenge is important. We should never complacently assume that attempts to do good can do no harm. This is as true for rights advocacy as it is for anything else.

Philosophical Foundations of Human Rights

Skepticism about human rights, we saw, takes many forms. Philosophers, whose training instructs them to take nothing for granted, have often led the skeptical charge. Yet this is puzzling, for it is possible to see the Universal Declaration of Human Rights (UDHR) as a philosophical triumph. After two and a half thousand years of dispute about the fundamental terms on which human beings should live together, a series of international discussions, meetings, and debates arrived at a detailed consensus statement of the fundamental rights of human beings.

Yet, until very recently, philosophers have tended to treat the UDHR as if it had very little to do with philosophy. If one looks at some of the most important works of twentieth-century political philosophy, such as John Rawls' *A Theory of Justice* (Rawls, 1971) and Robert Nozick's *Anarchy, State, and Utopia* (Nozick, 1974), almost nothing is said about human rights. The general attitude among philosophers seems to have been that there is something problematic either about the idea of human rights or in the catalog of rights included. This can be seen, for example, even in the title of James Griffin's paper "Discrepancies Between the Best Philosophical Account of Human Rights and the International Law of Human Rights" (Griffin, 2001).

Griffin argues that when one properly understands the foundations of human rights, not all of the rights in the standard list can be justified. Griffin believes that human rights must be seen as "protections of our normative agency" (Griffin, 2008: 2) and, for example, pours scorn on the "human right" to "periodic holidays with pay," as stated in article 24. But much more important, Griffin acutely observes that the convention documents provide the *names* of rights but typically say very little about their *content*, and so, it appears, philosophical and ethical reflection is needed to complete the account of human rights, as well as to refine it (Griffin, 2008: 5). In the case of the right to health, Griffin argues, its contours must be determined by what is necessary to preserve agency: a decent life span and protection of the capacities that promote agency. This will have consequences, for example, for the right to healthcare at the end of life, when agency cannot be restored in any meaningful way (Griffin, 2008: 98–99). This is important, for if it were thought that the correct ethical foundation for the human right to health was that of need, then there is no special reason to give priority to interventions that would protect or promote individual agency.

It may seem, therefore, that strengthening the philosophical foundations of the rights is necessary to provide a concrete account of the rights. Yet the matter is problematic. There is no ultimate agreement on the foundation of human rights. Is it normative agency? Human dignity? Vital human interests? Each of these may provide subtly different accounts of the precise contours of human rights, and how are such disputes to be settled?

However, this repeats a debate that took place in the context of drafting the UDHR, for what is as true now as 70 years ago is that there is much greater agreement on the list of human rights than on their moral foundations. Of course, there are disagreements about content, but the convergence on doctrine is remarkable, given the divergence on foundations.

Jacques Maritain, who helped provide background material for the convention at which the UDHR was drafted, commented:

> During one of the meetings of the French National Commission of UNESCO at which the Rights of Man were being discussed, someone was astonished that certain proponents of violently opposed ideologies had agreed on the draft of a list of rights. Yes, they replied, we agree on these rights, *provided we are not asked why.* (Maritain, 1951: 77, emphasis in original)

Indeed, Maritain names the section heading in which this discussion is contained "Men Mutually Opposed in Their Theoretical Conceptions Can Come to a Merely Practical Agreement Regarding a List of Human Rights" (Maritain, 1951: 76). Unfortunately, the point is rather spoiled by the inclusion of the words "merely practical." To use Rawlsian terminology, we might argue that the UDHR is a superb example of an overlapping consensus, in which each person can endorse a political doctrine for his or her own moral reasons (Rawls 1993 [1996]: 135–172). Although they share the political doctrine and can justify it on the basis of their own moral reasons, none of the moral perspectives has a privileged place as providing the core foundation for the doctrine. Different people will find their own justifications. In sum, then, on this view, human rights have moral foundations, but no particular moral foundation. This, perhaps, explains the appeal of human rights doctrine within a broadly liberal framework.

But what do we do about residual differences in interpretation? Arguably, however, the right response at this point is simply to acknowledge the limits of philosophical argument and allow the resulting disputes to be resolved through the development of democratic politics and legal doctrine (Hessler & Buchanan, 2002). Such a proposal fits well with the account of human rights provided by Joseph Raz (2010; see also Beitz, 2009). In summary, Raz believes that human rights should now be seen as a branch of international law and, luckily, a branch of law in reasonably good order. This is essential, Raz argues, if the discussions of philosophers are to engage with the concerns of human rights practice. Seeing matters this way allows us to draw an analogy with other branches of law, such as family law or property law. In such cases, the broad contours of the law can be seen as having a philosophical foundation, setting limits to what can reasonably be part of the law. Thus, for example, no doubt any reasonable view would wish to give parents duties of care toward their children. Yet it would be unrealistic to think that precise details of maintenance payments for children in case of divorce can be given a philosophical foundation. Such issues will be worked out in the practical context of politics and legal casework. The same is possible for the details of human rights. Whereas the overall framework can be justified from a range of philosophical positions, it is not necessary to think that each particular human right needs a single philosophical justification or even that the details of its determinate content need to be acceptable from all points of view.

Of course, this does not settle all disputes. For example, the United States has complained that General Comment 14 has expanded the human right to health beyond its initial basis in an arbitrary and unaccountable fashion (United States Government, n.d.).[2] But it is unrealistic to think that all disputes about doctrine can be settled. Sometimes we have to accept that doctrine is living – contested and permanently developing rather than entirely static and stable.

Still, this understanding of the doctrine of human rights raises the question of what human rights are for: why, exactly, do we have this branch of international law? Raz takes his cue, initially, from John Rawls' account (Rawls, 1999: 80–81) that the point of human rights law is to legitimate one state's interest, and possible interventions, in the affairs of another. Such interventions can, of course, take a variety of forms, from sending a note expressing concern to the ambassador, through public criticism and sanctions, to full-scale invasion (Raz, 2010). Beitz points out the importance of mechanisms such as reporting requirements and trade incentives (Beitz, 2009: 31–47). Naturally, many aspects of a state's internal arrangements are simply not the business of other states. For example, the particular pension regime one country has may seem unacceptable from the point of view of another country, but still, attempts to influence it may

seem an illegitimate interference with a sovereign state's internal affairs. No such defense may be available if a country tortures prisoners or, arguably, fails to take steps progressively to realize universal access to healthcare.

The international law understanding of human rights allows both outsiders and insiders to criticize a regime for failing to meet the human rights of its citizens and to exert pressure. On this understanding, a human right is claimed against a particular government, which has the duty to meet the right. The international community is not directly expected to meet the claim itself but has the second-order duty to help enforce the duty of the national government and come to assistance if the relevant national government cannot fulfill the right. It is this second-order character, placing duties of enforcement on the international community, that arguably marks the distinction between a *human right* to heath and a *right* to health.

Case Law

The human right to health has been seen from two perspectives. From a philosophical point of view, it is a right that, in outline, can be justified from a variety of perspectives as an overlapping consensus. However, in trying to go further to specify the right, and to connect it with human rights practice, philosophy runs out, and the second perspective needs to be engaged, that of the development of legal doctrine. Accordingly, to explore the detailed contours of the human right to health, it is necessary to look at case law, in addition to the conventions, declarations, and general comments outlined earlier.

Some instructive cases come from South Africa, where the right to health is included in article 27 of the South African Constitution, which took effect in 1997 and includes "the right to have access to health care services, including reproductive health care" and the right to "emergency medical treatment" (Republic of South Africa, 1996).

One critically important case, *Soobramoney v. Minister of Health*, was brought very soon after the adoption of the new constitution in 1997 [(KwaZulu Natal) CCT32/97 (1997) ZACC 17: 1998 (1) SA 765 (CC)]. The claimant, Thiagraj Soobramoney, who was just 41, was unemployed and suffering from many health problems. In 1996, his kidneys failed, and his life was in danger. He sought access to dialysis treatment, at public expense, in the hospital in Durban, but dialysis machines, which are very expensive, were in

---

[2] I owe this reference to Douglas Reeve

short supply. The hospital had set up tight guidelines for access, but sadly, Soobramoney fell outside the criteria. He had managed to pay for private dialysis to keep him alive but was running out of money. Accordingly, he brought a legal action under article 27 and, in particular, the right not to be denied emergency medical treatment, as well as article 11, which states, bluntly enough, that "[e]veryone has the right to life."

The court emphasized, however, that even the right to life has to be understood in the context of resource constraints and followed other precedents that it simply is not the right authority to make resource-allocation decisions. Consequently, the judges concentrated on the question of whether the rules applied by the hospital for access to scarce dialysis machines could be justified, and here they found no objection. Hence the case did not succeed.

Given the courts' reasonable reluctance to make decisions concerning resource allocation, one might wonder whether there will be anything to be gained by pursuing a human right to health action. However, the position is not entirely bleak. In the *Soobramoney* case, the judges referred to the Indian case of *Paschim Banga Khet Mazdoor Samity and others v. State of West Bengal and another*, where it was argued that the right to medical treatment falls under the constitutionally protected right to life. In this case, a patient with severe head injuries was turned away from a number of state-funded hospitals and had to seek treatment at a private hospital. But at least some of these hospitals did in fact have available facilities and denied him access on arbitrary grounds. Hence the court felt that it could determine the case in the claimant's favor without distorting health resource-allocation decisions.

Another important and well-known case in which the court found in favor of the claimant also comes from South Africa and is part of a series of activities led by the Treatment Action Campaign (TAC), which took up the vital issue of HIV/AIDS in South Africa. It was founded in late 1998 to demand right of access to treatment for HIV/AIDS, believing this to be supported by article 27(a) of the South African Constitution, providing "access to health care services including reproductive health," which was especially important for mothers with HIV infection.

In 1999, TAC pressed for the government to make nevirapine – the leading antiretroviral (ARV) drug – available to HIV-infected pregnant women. The manufacturers had, in fact, offered the drug to the government free of charge for a period, so the resource implications were very limited. The treatment is very simple: the administration of a single dose to the mother and a few drops to the baby. However, even after treatment, there remains a risk of passing on infection through breast-feeding. Therefore, a comprehensive package of treatment involves replacing breast-feeding with bottle feeding, which is not a trivial matter, especially given the strong cultural attachment to breast-feeding, advocacy of breast-feeding by the WHO, the cost of formula milk, and the difficulty of obtaining safe water in some parts of the country. There would also be the need for infrastructural change and staff training. Citing concerns about safety and efficacy, as well as the need to assess management issues, the government allowed only small-scale pilot studies, which it was very slow to implement. The Constitutional Court accepted that there were good public health reasons for having a pilot program but was dismayed that the infants of mothers without access to private healthcare were suffering while the government dragged its feet. The court did not accept the government's contention that providing less than the more comprehensive package would be ineffective or harmful. Accordingly, the court ordered the government to make nevirapine available where it was clinically indicated to prevent transmission to infants (Heywood, 2009).

There are a number of important differences between *Soobramoney* and the *TAC* case. First of all, Soobramoney was an individual with a specific, fatal condition that the health service chose not to treat, even though it could have done. However, to have chosen to treat Soobramoney would have left another person facing the same plight as him, so it was declared appropriate for the health authorities to make these decisions, as long as they did so on defensible and rational grounds. In the *TAC* case, the government's stand is much harder to understand. Although the government appealed to the importance of providing a more comprehensive package of care, which was unaffordable as well as having other difficulties, the court was persuaded by the evidence that drug treatment, alongside testing and counseling, would save the lives of thousands and would have minimal cost implications. Indeed, it was argued, there would eventually be cost savings, compared with the burden on the health system of caring for thousands of HIV-positive infants. Some commentators have attempted to explain the government's position as being linked to Mbeki's "AIDS denialism" or even the African National Congress's hope to be able to provide its own, lucrative therapy for AIDS, although such issues were not discussed in the judgment (Heywood, 2009).

Legally, then, the difference appears to be that in the *Soobramoney* case, the authorities acted reasonably in difficult circumstances, whereas in the *TAC* case, no such defense was available. A further difference is that TAC is, after all, a campaign, building up a groundswell of support among people who themselves were suffering from adverse government policy. TAC was able to ride on the support of a people's movement. There was no equivalent support for Soobramoney, even though no doubt there was great public sympathy.

It should be made clear too that *TAC* is not the only human right to health success story. For example, Brazil extended many lives by manufacturing generic ARV drugs, defending its action in international forums against accusations of patent violation in terms of protecting the human rights of its citizens. Here, too, a constitutional right to health and human rights case law have strengthened human rights campaigns (Galvao, 2005).

Yet, Brazil, Colombia, and other countries in South America provide a disturbing contrast to the orderly way in which the right to health has been dealt with in South African courts. In these countries, individual claims under the right to health are very common and also often succeed to the point where a significant percentage of the health budget is spent meeting the costs of judgments (Ferraz, 2009). Here we see a stark illustration of both Easterley's warnings that the right to health can disrupt orderly health planning (Easterley, 2009) and Benatar's point that it can increase inequality by giving extra health resources to those with the financial resources to fight cases (Benatar, 2002). In response, it can be argued that all this shows is that a constitutional right to health can require more than the human right to health (Wolff, 2015), but in any case, it is very important not to be complacent, to continue to monitor how international case law develops, and to try to rein in the worst abuses (Tobin, 2012; Yamin & Gloppen, 2011).

Realizing the Right to Health

While philosophers may continue to puzzle over the foundation, even the existence, of human rights, and philosophers and lawyers wrangle over their content, activists are most concerned about their realization (Backman et al., 2008; Clapham & Robinson, 2009). Nevertheless, the TAC example is in some respects very encouraging. It was, after all, a successful human rights case, saving many lives. Yet it is also limited. The South African context was very unusual, and the government stance appeared quite unreasonable. In legal terms, the situation appears unlikely to reoccur, and the case will rarely, if ever, be used as a precedent. And elsewhere, as we have seen, individualist claims proliferate.

By contrast, the organization of TAC provides a model for activism in which legal action could be a useful threat, even if it is rarely taken forward. At its foundation, TAC was originally concerned about the high price of HIV/AIDS-related pharmaceuticals. Later it broadened out as it became clear that realizing human rights requires governments to act over a much wider range of areas. In contrast to other NGO campaigns, which often work through elites, academics, professionals, the press, and communications, TAC aimed to set up a situation in which "poor people become their own advocates" (Heywood, 2009:17) and build a political movement for health, with an understanding both of health and governance. A rights approach, backed by a popular movement, can have considerable power and influence. Yet the right to health is still at a relatively early stage – realization is at present a struggle.

Nevertheless, it is worth reminding ourselves of some of the criticisms explored earlier. Used the wrong way, a human right to health approach can prioritize the claims of powerful, vocal, troublesome, and well-organized groups, leaving the most vulnerable unprotected. Health system strengthening, rather than single-issue campaigning, would surely be far more generally beneficial, but there is, no doubt, great difficulty in organizing campaigns and popular movements in such a way.

Conclusion

Whatever philosophical or practical doubts one may have about human rights in general or the human right to health in particular, there can be no doubt that they exist, at least in the sense of being objects of international agreement, with some mechanisms of enforcement. This gives the human rights approach a powerful advantage over other philosophical arguments aimed at improving the health status of the poor and vulnerable. The general point has been made with great force by health activist Gorik Ooms:

[We are] trying to achieve a goal: to describe a bad situation, to explain why it is as bad as it is, and to convince decision-makers to change their decisions. So the very pragmatic question for me is: which are the arguments most likely to convince these decision-makers? One line of arguments could be: "what goes around comes around, if you continue to abandon a huge part of humanity in its present misery, it will come back to you." Another line of arguments could be: "this is really extremely unfair." Or it could be: "the way you (leaders of high-income countries) are organising the global economy, refusing to share your or our wealth, and using your powers in the World Bank and the IMF [International Monetary Fund] to make countries invest less in social expend-iture, is in fact a permanent and deliberate violation of human rights, for which you should be put on trial." Perhaps that would help?

(Ooms, private communication)[3]

Of course, Ooms and other activists would not wish to suggest that human rights abuses are a consequence purely of the negligence or corruption of public officials. Much more important is creating resilient and support-ive national and international health and governance structures and systems. Yet even the reform of struc-tures has to be initiated, in the first instance, through the action of individuals with the power – individually or collectively – to bring about those reforms.

References

Backman, G., Hunt, P., Khosla, R., et al. (2008). Health systems and the right to health: an assessment of 194 countries. *Lancet* **372**, 2047–2085.

Baumrin, B. (2002). Why there is no right to health care, in Rhodes, R., Battin, M. P., & Silvers, A. (eds.), *Medicine and Social Justice: Essays on the Distribution of Health Care*. Oxford, UK: Oxford University Press.

Beitz, C. (2009). *The Idea of Human Rights*. Oxford, UK: Oxford University Press.

Benatar, S. R. (2002). Human rights in the biotechnology era 1. *BMC International Health and Human Rights* **2**, 3.

Benatar, S., Daar, A. & Singer P.A. (2003). Global health: the rationale for mutual caring. *International Affairs* **79**, 107–138.

Bentham, J. (1796 [1987]). "Anarchical Fallacies" and "Supply Without Burden," in Waldron, J. (ed.), *Nonsense Upon Stilts*. London: Methuen.

Birn, A.-E. (2008). Health and human rights: historical perspectives and political challenges. *Journal of Public Health Policy* **29**, 32–41.

Brock, G. (2009a). *Global Justice*. Oxford, UK: Oxford University Press.

Brock, G. (2009b). Health in developing countries and our global responsibilities, in Dawson, A. (ed.), *The Philosophy of Public Health*. Farnham: Ashgate, pp. 73–83.

Burnham, G., Lafta, R., Doocy, S., & Roberts, L. (2006). Mortality after the 2003 invasion of Iraq: a cross-sectional cluster sample survey. *Lancet* **368**, 1421–1428.

Caney, S. (2005). *Justice Beyond Borders*. Oxford, UK: Oxford University Press.

Central Intelligence Agency (CIA) (2009). *The World Factbook: Life Expectancy at Birth*. Available at www.cia.gov/library/publications/the-world-factbook/rankorder/2102rank.html (accessed November 25, 2009).

Central Intelligence Agency (CIA) (2019). *The World Factbook: Life Expectancy at Birth*. Available at www.cia.gov/library/publications/the-world-factbook/fields/355rank.html#WZ (accessed March 30, 2019).

Clapham, A., & Robinson, M. (eds.) (2009). *Realizing the Right to Health*. Zurich: Rüffer & Rub.

Collier, P. (2007). *The Bottom Billion*. Oxford, UK: Oxford University Press.

Easterley, W. (2006). *The White Man's Burden*. Oxford, UK: Oxford University Press.

Easterley, W. (2009). Human rights are the wrong basis for health care. *Financial Times*, October 12, 2009. Available at www.ft.com/content/89bbbda2-b763-11de-9812-00144fea b49a (accessed April 2, 2019).

Ferraz, O. (2009) The right to health in the courts of Brazil: worsening health inequities? *Health and Human Rights* **11**, 33–45.

Freeman, M. (2002). *Human Rights*. Cambridge, UK: Polity.

Galvao, J. (2005). Brazil and access to HIV/AIDS drugs: a question of human rights and public health. *American Journal of Public Health* **95**, 1110–1116.

Garrett, L. (1995). *The Coming Plague*. London: Virago.

Global Health Watch (2008). *Alternative World Health Report 2*. London: Zed Books.

Griffin, J. (2001). Discrepancies between the best philosophical account of human rights and the International Law of Human Rights. *Proceedings of the Aristotelian Society* **101**, 28.

Griffin, J. (2008). *On Human Rights*. Oxford, UK: Oxford University Press.

---

[3] I am extremely grateful to Gillian Brock, Solly Benatar, Douglas Reeve, and Gorik Ooms for their comments on an earlier draft.

Haacker, M. (2010). The macroeconomics of HIV/AIDS, in Hannam, M., & Wolff, J. (eds.), *Southern Africa: 2020 Vision*. London: e9 Publishing.

Hassoun, N. (2012). Global health impact: a basis for labeling and licensing campaigns? *Developing World Bioethics* **12**, 121–134.

Hessler, K., & Buchanan, A. (2002). Specifying the content of the human right to health care, in Rhodes, R., Battin, M. P., & Silvers, A. (eds.), *Medicine and Social Justice: Essays on the Distribution of Health Care*. Oxford, UK: Oxford University Press.

Heywood, M. (2009). South Africa's Treatment Action Campaign: combining law and social mobilization to realize the right to health. *Journal of Human Rights Practice* **1**, 14–36.

Maritain, J. (1951). *Man and the State*. Chicago: University of Chicago Press.

Marx, K. (1843 [1975]). On the Jewish Question, in Colletti, L. (ed.), *Early Writings*. Harmondsworth, UK: Penguin.

Moyo, D. (2009). *Dead Aid*. London: Allen Lane.

Nickel, J. (2017). Human rights, in Zalta, E. N. (ed.), *The Stanford Encyclopedia of Philosophy*. Available at http://plato.stanford.edu/archives/spr2017/entries/rights-human/.

Nozick, R. (1974). *Anarchy, State, and Utopia*. Oxford, UK: Blackwell.

Nussbaum, M. (2006). *Frontiers of Justice*. Cambridge, MA: Harvard University Press.

O'Neill, O. (2005). The dark side of human rights. *International Affairs* **81**, 427–439.

Orbinski, J. (2008). *An Imperfect Offering*. London: Rider.

Pogge, T. (2002). *World Poverty and Human Rights*. Cambridge, UK: Cambridge University Press.

Pogge, T. (2002). *World Poverty and Human Rights*. (Cambridge, UK: Cambridge University Press).

Pogge, T. (2005). Human rights and global health: a research programme. *Metaphilosophy* **36**, 182–209.

Rawls, J. (1971). *A Theory of Justice*. Oxford, UK: Oxford University Press.

Rawls, J. (1993/1996). *Political Liberalism*. New York: Columbia University Press.

Rawls, J. (1999). *The Law of Peoples*. Cambridge, MA: Harvard University Press.

Raz, J. (2010). Human rights without foundations, in Tasioulas, J., & Besson, S. (eds.), *The Philosophy of International Law*. Oxford, UK: Oxford University Press.

Republic of South Africa (1996). Constitution. Available at www.gov.za/documents/constitution-republic-south-africa-1996 (accessed April 2, 2019).

Singer, P. (1972). Famine, affluence and morality. *Philosophy and Public Affairs* **1**, 229–243.

Sreenivasan, G. (2002). International justice and health: a proposal. *Ethics and International Affairs* **16**, 81–90.

Steiner, H. (2005), Territorial justice and global redistribution, in Brock, G., & Brighouse, H. (eds.), *The Political Philosophy of Cosmopolitanism*. Cambridge, UK: Cambridge University Press, pp. 28–38.

Tobin, J. (2012) *The Right to Health in International Law*. Oxford, UK: Oxford University Press.

United Nations (1948). Universal Declaration of Human Rights. Available at www.un.org/en/universal-declaration-human-rights/index.html (accessed April 2, 2019).

United Nations (1966). International Covenant on Economic, Social and Cultural Rights. Available at www.ohchr.org/en/professionalinterest/pages/cescr.aspx (accessed April 2 2019).

United Nations (1990). General Comment 3. Available at www.unhchr.ch/tbs/doc.nsf/(symbol)/E.C.12.2000.4.En (accessed November 26, 2009).

United Nations (2000). General Comment 14. Available at www.unhchr.ch/tbs/doc.nsf/(symbol)/E.C.12.2000.4.En (accessed November 26, 2009).

United Nations Treaty Collection (n.d.). Convention on the Rights of the Child. Available at https://treaties.un.org/pages/ViewDetails.aspx?src=TREATY&mtdsg_no=IV-11&chapter=4&lang=en (accessed March 30, 2019).

United States Government (n.d.). Response to Request. Available at www.state.gov/documents/organization/138850.pdf (accessed April 2, 2019).

Valentini, L. (2011). *Justice in a Globalized World*. Oxford, UK: Oxford University Press.

Venkatapuram, S. (2011). *Health Justice*. Cambridge, UK: Polity.

Wolff, J. (2012a). *The Human Right to Health*. New York: Norton.

Wolff, J. (2012b). Global justice and health: the basis of the global health duty, in Emanuel, E., & Millum, J. (eds.), *Global Justice and Bioethics*. Oxford, UK: Oxford University Press.

Wolff, J. (2012c). The demands of the human right to health. *Proceedings of the Aristotelian Society: Supplementary Volume* **86**, 217–237.

Wolff, J. (2015). The content of the human right to health, in Cruft, R., Liao, S. M., & Renzo, M. (eds.), *The Philosophical Foundations of Human Rights*. Oxford, UK: Oxford University Press. pp. 491–501.

Wolff, J., & de-Shalit, A. (2007). *Disadvantage*. Oxford, UK: Oxford University Press.

World Health Organization (WHO) (1946 [2006]). Constitution. Available at www.who.int/governance/eb/who_constitution_en.pdf (accessed April 2, 2019).

World Health Organization (WHO) (2009). *Positive Synergies*. Available at www.who.int/healthsystems/GHIsynergies/en/index.html (accessed April 2, 2019).

Yamin, A. (2017). *Power, Suffering and the Struggle for Dignity*. Philadelphia: University of Pennsylvania Press.

Yamin, A., & Gloppen, S. (2011). *Litigating Health Rights*. Cambridge MA.: Harvard University Press.

Ypi, L. (2012). *Global Justice and Avant-Garde Political Agency*. Oxford, UK: Oxford University Press.

8 International Human Rights Law and the Social Determinants of Health[*]

Chapter

Lisa Forman

Introduction

In its proclamation that "social injustice is killing people on a grand scale," the 2008 World Health Organization (WHO) Commission on the Social Determinants of Health (CSDH) squarely locates the achievement of global health equity within the realm of ethics, social justice, and human rights (WHO, 2008: 26). The report is explicit about the human rights aspect of this injustice, continuing that while "[t]he right to the highest attainable standard of health is enshrined in the Constitution of the World Health Organization (WHO) and numerous international treaties ... the degree to which these rights are met from one place to another around the world is glaringly unequal" (WHO, 2008: 26). Links between human rights and the social determinants of health have been reiterated in subsequent global health policies, including the 2011 Rio Declaration on the Social Determinants of Health and the 2015 Sustainable Development Goals (SDGs). These references reinforce that human rights and the social determinants of health are "different yet overlapping measures and languages of human well-being and self-actualization" (Kenyon et al., 2018: 1).

Yet what does it really mean to locate the advancement of the social determinants of health within human rights and the right to health in particular? These are pressing questions given that the right to health has long been critiqued for being overly individualistic and legally unenforceable, state-centric, vague, ineffective, and even damaging to population health outcomes, and given widespread perceptions that international legal treaties inadequately address the meagerness of domestic and global efforts to address poverty and achieve

better health and well-being. These critiques have been joined by contemporary arguments that this body of law has not sufficiently focused on neo-liberal economic policies and their resulting amplification of economic inequality globally, increasingly understood as itself a significant adverse health determinant. These critiques contradict the idea that the right to health offers a potentially powerful corrective to globalization's ills, capable of advancing health equity and more equitable access to affordable and good-quality healthcare. Yet international human rights law offers a range of legal protections relevant to the social determinants of health, and civil society in countries around the world is successfully using the right to health in litigation, advocacy, social mobilization, and participation. How should we understand these experiences in light of critiques of this right? More broadly, what capacity does the right to health hold to respond to changing global conditions, realize health equity on the ground, and respond to rising health inequality?

This chapter explores some of these questions by focusing on how the right to health in international law addresses health and its social determinants and exploring instances in which rights are being used to advance health equity. It first overviews legal protections of the right to health in international and regional treaties, as well as interpretations of this right in international conferences and United Nations (UN) commentary. It then considers critiques of international human rights law and the right to health, particularly in relation to the social determinants of health. It turns to consider various human rights tools for achieving accountability in this domain, including judicial, administrative, political, and social mechanisms. The chapter concludes by returning to key questions about the utility of the right to health in addressing the social determinants of health.

---

[*] This chapter has been adapted from Forman, L. (2013). A rights-based approach to global health policy, in Brown, G., Yamey, G., & Wamala, S. (eds.), *The Handbook of Global Health Policy*. West Sussex, UK: Wiley-Blackwell, pp. 459–482.

International Human Rights Law and the Social Determinants of Health

The WHO CSDH report suggests that achieving the social determinants of health requires improving both "the immediate, visible circumstances of people's lives – their access to health care, schools, and education, their conditions of work and leisure, their homes, communities, towns, or cities" as well the distributions "of power, income, goods, and services, globally and nationally" that affect their chances of leading a flourishing life (WHO, 2008: 1). Contemporary international human rights law offers several protections that aim to improve daily life and the inequitable distributions of power and resources related to them through inalienable human rights guarantees: rights to health, education, housing, social security, and work are extensively codified in international human rights treaties, sometimes as integrated sets of rights. This interdependence between health and a range of other human rights has long been theorized, most influentially by Jonathan Mann, who argued that human rights are in inextricable relationships with health (and vice versa) (Mann et al., 1999).

The right to health is intimately connected to other enumerated international human rights, including rights to life, privacy, an adequate standard of living, and nondiscrimination (Stronks et al., 2016: 28). This integration is partially reflected within legal iterations of the right to health, and the next section considers how this right has been legally entrenched in international and regional human rights law, considering also influential interpretations emerging from international conferences as well as the UN Committee on Economic, Social and Cultural Rights (UNCESCR), which oversees a key treaty that contains the right to health. This exploration of legal text does not suggest its efficacy – it simply seeks to establish the legal framework as it exists within international law.

International Human Rights Treaties and the Right to Health

The first international iteration of the right to health is found in the Constitution of the World Health Organization (WHO Constitution), which makes a range of significant contributions to the elaboration of an international right to health. First, it provided the first international recognition that "the enjoyment of the highest attainable standard of health is a fundamental right of every human being without distinction of race, religion, political belief, economic or social condition" (UN, 1946: preamble) and that governments have a responsibility "for the health of their peoples which can be fulfilled only by the provision of adequate health and social measures" (UN, 1946: preamble). Second, the WHO Constitution adopted an expansive definition of health as "a state of complete physical, mental and social well-being and not merely the absence of disease or infirmity" (UN, 1946: preamble), a definition which clearly understands health as extending beyond the biomedical.

A similarly broad construction of health as a socially determined right is articulated in the Universal Declaration of Human Rights (UDHR), which in article 25.1 recognizes that "everyone has the right to a standard of living adequate for the health and well-being of himself and of his family, including food, clothing, housing and medical care and necessary social services" (UN, 1948). The recognition that health and well-being depend on an adequate standard of living that includes these basic necessities presages a considerably social conception of the determinants of health and well-being. It also illustrates the interdependence of health with a range of other human rights.

The International Covenant on Economic, Social and Cultural Rights (ICESCR) provides the most authoritative formulation of the right to health in international law (UN, 1976a). In contrast to the UDHR, it separates out health from the minimum preconditions of an adequate standard of living (albeit not of well-being, as elaborated in article 11) and (in article 12.1) recognizes "the right of everyone to the enjoyment of the highest attainable standard of physical and mental health." It proceeds to elaborate steps to be taken to fully achieve this right, including in relation to child health, environmental and industrial hygiene, disease control, and ensuring medical service to all (UN, 1976a, article 12.2).

This articulation of the right to health is thus considerably broader than an entitlement to medical care, recognizing that the achievement of the highest attainable standard of health requires considerable attention to disease prevention and environmental "hygiene." Yet these broad duties are undercut by article 2 of the ICESCR, where states agree

> to take steps, individually and through international assistance and cooperation, especially economic and technical, to the maximum of [their] available

resources, to achieve progressively the full realization of Covenant rights by all appropriate means, including particularly legislation.

The notion of progressive realization within available resources places considerable limits on the promise of a right to the highest attainable standard of health and has been critiqued not only as creating a loophole capable of nullifying the covenant's guarantees (Chapman & Russell, 2002: 5) but as effectively disabling enforcement of this treaty from the start (Moyn, 2018: 199–200).

Subsequent human rights treaties entrench health rights for specific groups, including racial minorities, women, children, and people with disabilities, and in so doing incrementally advance the scope and content of the right to health in relation to both healthcare and aspects of the social determinants of health. This dual focus is apparent, for example, in the 1969 International Convention on the Elimination of All Forms of Racial Discrimination (ICERD), which obligates state parties to prohibit racial discrimination and guarantee everyone's right to equality before the law, including their enjoyment of their rights to public health and medical care (UN, 1969: article 5.e.iv). This convention not only identifies medical care as an individual entitlement but also suggests a collective right to public health. The Convention on the Elimination of All Forms of Discrimination Against Women (CEDAW) adopts a narrower conception of a right to healthcare services, requiring that state parties undertake measures to ensure women's equal access to healthcare services, including appropriate services for "pregnancy, confinement and the postnatal period, granting free services where necessary, as well as adequate nutrition during pregnancy and lactation" (UN, 1979: article 12.1–2). Despite the lacuna around recognition of public health or the determinants of health, the CEDAW does advance extant interpretations of the right to health by specifically elaborating women's reproductive rights.

The 1989 Convention on the Rights of the Child (CRC) contains an extensive identification of specific state obligations regarding health and is distinctive in its reach: 196 countries have ratified it (only the United States has not done so), giving it an effectively universal reach. In the CRC, states recognize children's right to the highest attainable standard of health and to facilities for the treatment of illness and rehabilitation of health and commit to strive to ensure that no child is deprived of his or her right to

access such healthcare services (UN, 1989: article 24.1). States undertake to pursue appropriate measures to achieve this goal, which straddle the provision of healthcare and the social determinants of health, including reducing infant and child mortality; ensuring healthcare for all children, especially through primary healthcare; and combating disease and malnutrition within primary healthcare by providing "adequate nutritious foods and clean drinking-water, taking into consideration the dangers and risks of environmental pollution" (UN, 1989: article 24.2). In contrast to the CEDAW, which aims to provide women with additional protection as required, the CRC instead restates the standards of the WHO Constitution and the ICESCR in relation to children (Stronks et al., 2016: 29).

The 2008 Convention on the Rights of Persons with Disabilities (CRPD) aims to protect people with disabilities from a variety of social and political obstacles that may impair their full and equal participation in society (UN, 2008). Its provisions on health, however, are significantly more focused on healthcare than on the social determinants of health, albeit that the convention includes a number of articles that directly or indirectly concern health, including the right of people with disabilities to access health facilities (UN, 2008: article 9) and their "right to the enjoyment of the highest attainable standard of health without discrimination on the basis of disability" (UN, 2008: article 25). Yet, rather than incorporating a social determinants of health perspective in relation to health, as in previous treaties, the CRPD separately articulates a right to an adequate standard of living and social protection that includes food, clothing, housing, and adequate social protection (UN, 2008: article 28).

The Right to Health in Regional Human Rights Treaties

Rights to health are recognized in each of the three regional human rights systems that developed after the creation of the UN, and again these rights combine entitlements to healthcare and the social determinants of health. This dual focus is apparent in the African (Banjul) Charter on Human and Peoples' Rights (1981), which provides for every individual's right to enjoy the "best attainable state of physical and mental health," with states undertaking to take the necessary measures to protect the health of their people and to ensure that they receive medical attention when they are sick (Organization of African Unity [OAU], 1986: article 16). The African Charter on the Rights and Welfare of the Child (1999) protects every child's right to enjoy the best attainable state of physical, mental, and spiritual health and specifies necessary measures to achieve this, which extend to obligations to ensure the provision of adequate nutrition and safe drinking water (OAU, 1999: article 14).

In the European system, health rights are not recognized in the European Convention on Human Rights and Fundamental Freedoms, which contains only civil and political rights, thereby excluding enforcement of these rights by the European Court of Human Rights in Strasbourg (Stronks et al., 2016: 29). Instead, these rights are contained in the 1965 European Social Charter, where states undertake to realize both rights to broadly protect health and to provide healthcare (article 11 and 13).

In the Inter-American system, the Protocol of San Salvador provides that "everyone shall have the right to health, understood to mean the enjoyment of the highest level of physical, mental and social well-being" (Organization of American States [OAS], 1999: article 10.1). Its provisions integrate healthcare and the social determinants of health: state parties recognize "health as a public good" and agree to adopt a range of measures including ensuring primary healthcare; health services for all individuals within a state's jurisdiction; universal immunization against the principal infectious diseases; prevention and treatment of endemic, occupational, and other diseases; health education; and the satisfaction of health needs of the highest-risk groups and those whose poverty makes them the most vulnerable (OAS, 1999: article 10.2).

There is no formal regional human rights system in Asia, but in 1998, more than two hundred nongovernmental organizations (NGOs) drafted a "people's charter" of Asian human rights, which rather than recognizing a free-standing right to health includes health-related provisions within rights to life, rights to development and social justice, and rights of women (Asian Human Rights Commission, 1998: articles 3.2, 7.1, 9.3; Forman, 2014). In the Middle East, the Cairo Declaration on Human Rights in Islam protects an integrated right recognizing that "everyone shall have the right to medical and social care, and to all public amenities provided by society and the State within the limits of their available resources" (Forman, 2014; World Conference on Human Rights, 1993: article 17).

The Right to Health in International Health Conferences

The international legal interpretation of the right to health has been assisted by conceptual advances in international health conferences over the last 40 years. In 1978, the seminal International Conference on Primary Health Care (ICPHC) issued the Declaration of Alma-Ata, which declared primary healthcare the principal vehicle for achieving health for all by the year 2000 (ICPHC, 1978). Alma-Ata recognized health as a fundamental human right that "requires the action of many other social and economic sectors in addition to the health sector" (ICPHC, 1978: paragraph I). It is also distinctive in its recognition that "[t]he existing gross inequality in the health status of the people particularly between developed and developing countries as well as within countries is politically, socially and economically unacceptable and is, therefore, of common concern to all countries" (ICPHC, 1978: paragraph II). The declaration sees economic and social development as basic to achieving health for all and reducing gaps in health status between countries (ICPHC, 1978: paragraph III), and moreover, it also states that "[g]overnments have a responsibility for the health of their people which can be fulfilled only by the provision of adequate health and social measures" (ICPHC, 1978: paragraph V). As the following discussion illustrates, this declaration was highly influential on the UN Committee on Economic, Social and Cultural Rights' interpretation of the right to health, including insofar as it defined core obligations under this right. However, as the following discussion illustrates, Alma-Ata's broader recommendations for addressing health gaps between countries has not been recognized as effectively within the UN committee's interpretation of the right to health.

The 1986 Ottawa Charter for Health Promotion elaborates that the social conditions that influence and determine health include "peace, shelter, education, food, income, a stable eco-system, sustainable resources, social justice, and equity" (First International Conference on Health Promotion, 1986: 1). The charter's recommendations for actions on health include intersectoral policy development, individual and community empowerment, and restructuring health services toward preventative rather than curative services. Subsequent international health conferences reinforced and expanded this emphasis on primary healthcare and the social determinants of health. The 1994 International Conference on Population and Development (ICPD), held in Cairo, saw 179 states agree to health-related goals to be achieved by 2004 and established global indicators for those goals (UN, 1994: chapter VII, objective 8.3). The 1995 Fourth World Conference on Women, held in Beijing, saw 189 states endorse the Beijing Declaration and Platform for Action, which elaborated state commitments to increase women's access to appropriate, affordable, and quality healthcare and services that were later applied to the international human right to health (UN, 1995). Most recently, the 2015 SDGs integrate an explicit health goal in SDG3 and around ten other goals concerned with health, as well as more than fifty indicators to "measure health outcomes, proximal determinants of health or health service provision" (WHO, 2018).

General Comment 14 on the Right to the Highest Attainable Standard of Health

In 2000, the UNCESCR, a group of independent experts tasked with monitoring state implementation of the ICESCR, released a seminal interpretation of the international right to health (UN, 2000). General Comment 14 attempts to answer key questions about the normative scope and content of the right to health and makes important conceptual advances by elaborating on individual entitlements and state duties under the right to health. It is notable that the committee's interpretation draws from several of the international conferences described earlier (including Alma-Ata, ICPD, and Beijing).

From a social determinants of health perspective, General Comment 14 is distinctive for how it almost from the start locates the right to health in a far broader perspective than simply healthcare. First, the committee indicates how closely related the right to health is to other fundamental human rights, including "the rights to food, housing, work, education, human dignity, life, non-discrimination, equality, the prohibition against torture, privacy, access to information, and the freedoms of association, assembly and movement. These and other rights and freedoms address integral components of the right to health" (UN, 2000: paragraph 3). The committee argues, in fact, that the social and economic determination of health is the primary

way to understand why the drafters of article 12 of the ICESCR defined this as a right to the highest attainable standard of health rather than the WHO conception of health as "a state of complete physical, mental and social well-being and not merely the absence of disease or infirmity" (UN, 2000: paragraph 4). This choice, the committee suggests, acknowledges "that the right to health embraces a wide range of socio-economic factors that promote conditions in which people can lead a healthy life, and extends to the underlying determinants of health, such as food and nutrition, housing, access to safe and potable water and adequate sanitation, safe and healthy working conditions, and a healthy environment" (UN, 2000: paragraph 4). In this context, the committee recognized "the formidable structural and other obstacles resulting from international and other factors beyond the control of States that impede the full realization of article 12 in many States parties" (UN, 2000: paragraph 9). As indicated earlier, the committee thus defines the right to health as an inclusive right that extends both to timely and appropriate healthcare and to what it terms the "underlying determinants of health," which include access to safe and potable water and adequate sanitation; an adequate supply of safe food, nutrition, and housing; healthy occupational and environmental conditions; access to health-related education and information, including on sexual and reproductive health; and the participation of the population in health-related decision making at the community, national, and international levels (UN, 2000: paragraph 11).

Thus, in place of the social determinants of health, the UNCESCR incorporates the notion of the "underlying determinants of health," a notion congruent with but not necessarily synonymous with the broader conception of the former (Hunt, 2009; Stronks et al., 2016: 33). These underlying determinants (food, housing, access to water and adequate sanitation, safe working conditions, and a healthy environment) are almost all the subject matter of separate rights entrenched in the ICESCR. Indeed, this narrower interpretation of health determinants may have purposefully avoided reading into the ICESCR obligations not explicitly already agreed to in other provisions within the ICESCR.

What is notable about General Comment 14 is that these determinants are integrated into the committee's interpretation of the right to health, including those areas of the right to health it defines as the most critical and prioritized aspects of this right. For example, the committee recognizes that while the highest attainable standard of health and the health system will vary from country to country depending on national resources, the right "will include, however, the underlying determinants of health, such as safe and potable drinking water and adequate sanitation facilities, hospitals, clinics and other health-related buildings, trained medical and professional personnel receiving domestically competitive salaries, and essential drugs, as defined by the WHO Action Programme on Essential Drugs (UN, 2000: paragraph 12.a). The committee defines these elements as those essential to the right to health, requiring that healthcare facilities, goods, and services and the social determinants of health are available, accessible, acceptable, and of good quality (AAAQ; UN, 2000: paragraph 12). These elements provide important practical guidance to states on what might constitute adequate compliance with this right.

In addition, the committee identifies core obligations that a state party cannot "under any circumstances whatsoever, justify ... non-compliance" with, an interpretation widely viewed as an overreach (UN, 2000: paragraph 47). The intentions of core duties are to safeguard against progressive realization within available resources being cited to deny any level of healthcare, including in particular those necessary to address the essential health needs of the most vulnerable (Forman, 2014). Again, the underlying determinants of health are central to this definition: states' core obligations are to "ensure the satisfaction of, at the very least, minimum essential levels of each of the rights," including

- Nondiscriminatory access to health facilities, goods, and services
- Access to minimum essential food
- Access to basic shelter, housing, and sanitation and an adequate supply of safe and potable water
- Essential drugs as defined by the WHO
- Equitable distribution of all health facilities, goods, and services
- Adopting and implementing a national public health strategy and plan of action addressing the health concerns of the whole population, with particular attention to vulnerable or marginalized groups (UN, 2000: paragraph 43).

These interpretations of essential elements and core obligations of the right to health thus place social determinants of health at the very heart of this right. The committee also identifies state obligations to respect, protect, and fulfill the right to health that apply equally to realizing the underlying determinants of health (UN, 2000: paragraph 33). *Respecting* the right to health requires governments not to interfere with this right, including through policies that are discriminatory or that are likely to cause unnecessary morbidity and preventable mortality (UN, 2000: paragraphs 34, 50). *Protecting* the right to health requires states to take measures to ensure equal access to health services provided by third parties, including controlling the marketing of health goods and services by third parties (UN, 2000: paragraph 35). State obligations to *fulfill* the right to health arise "when individuals or a group are unable, for reasons beyond their control, to realize that right themselves by means at their disposal" (UN, 2000: paragraph 37) and include duties to "ensure provision of health care, including immunization programmes against the major infectious diseases, and ensure equal access for all to the underlying determinants of health, such as nutritiously safe food and potable drinking water, basic sanitation and adequate housing and living conditions" (UN, 2000: paragraph 37).

Contestation and Critiques of Human Rights and Right to Health

Despite the extensive legalization just outlined, the right to health has been subject to considerable contestation and critique: for being overly individualistic and legally unenforceable, state-centric, vague, ineffective, and even damaging to population health outcomes (De Cock et al., 2002; Easterly, 2009; Forman, 2014). These arguments join older criticisms that social rights in particular are inappropriately legal rights within international human rights law (Cranston, 1973). More recently, contemporary critiques suggest that there has not been sufficient focus on either neoliberalism or its resulting widening of economic and health inequalities within and between countries. Certainly some of these critiques of the right to health are poorly supported factually and undercut by emerging interpretations and enforcement (Forman, 2014). Yet other critiques outline credible weaknesses that limit the potential force of these rights when it comes to advancing the social determinants of health (Chapman, 2017; Kapczynski, 2019; Moyn, 2018). This section interrogates the validity of these critiques, particularly insofar as they relate to the social determinants of health.

The critique of rights inflation argues that adding rights such as health to the pantheon of accepted human rights devalues all human rights (Cranston, 1973; Forman, 2014; Griffin, 2010; Orend, 2002;). There is little basis to this argument to the extent that it asserts that the right to health protects human interests less grave than those protected in traditional civil and political rights (such as rights to life, privacy, etc.; Forman, 2014). The right to health addresses essential human needs rooted in fundamental human rights to life, dignity, and nondiscrimination that are clearly appropriately protected *as* human rights. Yet rights inflation arguments also target the legitimacy of the right to health as a social right (Cranston, 1973). Arguments such as these rely on sharp distinctions between civil and social rights that characterize civil rights as negative rights that are relatively cheap and easy to achieve versus social rights, which are viewed as positive rights that are very expensive and require considerable state action to realize (Forman, 2014). This argument holds little merit today given scholarship showing the considerable costs and action required to realize civil rights (Holmes & Sunstein, 2000; Hunt, 1996). Moreover, the extent to which this right is already legally entrenched in international and regional treaties, as well as in domestic constitutions, significantly undermines arguments against its legal recognition.

Other critiques focus on the relative unenforceability of a vague and expansive formulation of a right to the "highest attainable standard of health," with even human rights scholars initially arguing that it made more sense to talk about a right to *healthcare* rather than a right to health (Kass, 1975, in Toebes, 1999: 17; see also Forman, 2014). The challenges of scope are deepened by the requirement of progressive realization within available resources, which unwittingly provides states with ample room to evade their legal obligations. Although General Comment 14 has offered considerably greater clarity on entitlements and duties under this right, it has not necessarily resolved all remaining questions about the scope and legitimate restrictions of this right.

Other criticisms suggest that the legalization of the right to health is ineffective in the context of a global governance displaying a hypocritical attitude toward poverty and a parsimonious definition of what it extends to (Benatar, 2016). Others suggest that the right to health is not just ineffective but also damaging to public health interests in its favoring of individual needs. It is argued that the overly individualistic nature of the right to health undermines both population health outcomes and democratic allocations of limited resources (De Cock et al., 2002; Easterly, 2009; Goodman, 2005). These critiques are buttressed by the mixed evidence of the public health impacts of the rising trend of right to health litigation, especially as exemplified in the Brazilian and Colombian case studies that have seen dramatic rates of litigation that have favored relatively privileged litigants and individual claims irrespective of budgetary or population impacts (Ferraz, 2009; Moestad et al., 2011; Yamin & Gloppen, 2011). These cases have prompted deep interrogations of the equity impacts of right to health litigation and indeed of the imperative to consider more optimal conceptual frameworks for litigation and the realization of the right to health going forward (Forman, 2013; UN General Assembly, 2008).

The most powerful contemporary critiques of economic, social, and cultural rights such as the right to health argue that these rights have failed to adequately respond to rising inequality, to powerful transnational corporations (Garret, 1995) and to the neoliberal economic system itself (Chapman, 2017; Hopgood, 2014; Klein, 2007; Moyn, 2018). Samuel Moyn argues that after the Cold War, economic and social rights such as health dropped ambitions of material equality and instead adopted a "moral focus on a floor of sufficient protection in a globalizing economy … while doing nothing to interfere with the obliteration of any ceiling on distributive inequality" (Moyn, 2018: 176). In this context, "human rights emerged in a neoliberal age as weak tools that aim at sufficient provision alone [and the] political and legal project in their name became a powerless companion of the explosion of inequality" (Moyn, 2018: 176). Stephen Hopgood makes an even stronger critique of human rights, arguing that "we are on the verge of the imminent decay of the Global Human Rights Regime" (Hopgood, 2014: ix). Hopgood suggests that this decline began when human rights became intimately tied to American power and to "the export of neoliberal democracy using American state power" (Hopgood, 2014: xi–xii). Hopgood argues that "Human Rights, handmaiden to neoliberal democracy, are unveiled as ideological, opening a legitimacy that has allowed their opponents to make increasing inroads against them" (Hopgood,

2014: xiii). Naomi Klein goes further, arguing that through the 1970s and 1980s, authoritarian regimes in Latin America deliberately used terror to blunt opposition to their introduction of neoliberal economic policies and that human rights activists effectively enabled this effort by failing to identify this motive and instead treating these actions as human rights abuses (Klein, 2007: 147).

Moyn critiques the right to health in particular as an example of "how norms were elaborated as part of an expansion of humanitarianism after decolonization, in a world in which originally imperial global health enterprises were retained amid profound continuing hierarchy" (Moyn, 2018: 197). He argues that the emergence of the right to health in the 1990s with the AIDS pandemic and Jonathan Mann's work "was a bid to give outrageous need more visibility, but ultimately global health remained the philanthropic and technocratic enterprise it had long been and still is" (Moyn, 2018: 197). He argues that even its most successful campaigns around access to medicines "did little to challenge inequities of power or wealth on a global scale" (Moyn, 2018: 197–198). Amy Kapczynski argues that the right to medicines within the right to health is "imbricated" within the prevailing neoliberal regime and "is plausibly regressive: it places significant strain on healthcare budgets, redistributes upwards, and provides medicines on terms largely dictated by one of the most profitable industries in the world. ... It mandates discrete individual relief, but rarely sees, much less disrupts, the underlying legal logics and structures that help produce radical health inequities" (Kapyczynski, 2019: 81).

These are damning critiques given growing understanding that neoliberalism is causally connected to increased global inequality, with a well-established evidence base now illustrating that the social gradient in health is causally related to status and income differences and that "bigger income differences make status differences more potent" with regard to negative health effects (WHO, 2008; Pickett & Wilkinson, 2009; Marmot, 2015; Wilkinson & Pickett, 2018: 5–6). Indeed, it is arguable that in an age of rampant inequality and deteriorating respect for human rights, the right to health's ability to frontally address these issues poses existential threats to its legitimacy and perhaps even its future.

Realization of the Right to Health

Given these critiques, what utility should we understand the right to health to hold in advancing health and its social determinants? To make this assessment, it is useful to consider a broader continuum of accountability mechanisms than judicial action alone. Stronks et al. (2016: 45) identify five types of national and international accountability mechanisms capable of holding states to account for their failures to realize human rights: judicial (national and international courts), quasi-judicial (national human rights institutions and ombudspersons), administrative (human rights impact assessment), political (parliamentary committees, UN and regional human rights bodies), and social (national and international NGOs, mass media). Several case studies in these domains illustrate the potential utility of the right to health to hold state as well as nonstate actors accountable for action on the social determinants of health.

Judicial Accountability for the Right to Health and the Social Determinants of Health

There are several instances of effective enforcement of the right to health to claim social determinants of health through regional human rights bodies. The earlier African Commission on Human and People's Rights found violations of the African Charter's right to health in the Democratic Republic of the Congo (then Zairean) government's failure to provide safe drinking water, electricity, and medicines (*Free Legal Assistance Group and Others v. Zaire*, 1995) and the Malawian government's failure to provide medical treatment and other adequate living conditions to prisoners (*Malawi African Association and Others v. Mauritania*, 2000; see also Forman, 2014). In 2000, the commission held the Nigerian government in violation of the Ogoni people's right to health for its failure to prevent pollution and ecological degradation and to monitor the national petroleum company's oil activities, which was a majority shareholder in a consortium with Shell Petroleum (*Social and Economic Rights Action Centre and the Centre for Economic and Social Rights v. Nigeria*, 2001). Although the European Court of Human Rights enforces civil and political rights alone, several of its decisions have resulted in governmental law and policy changes in relation to health (Stronks et al., 2016: 50). For example, in *Oneryildiz v. Turkey*, the Court found that a methane explosion that killed almost forty slum dwellers was an instance of inadequate environmental health and housing safety that violated the right to life protected in the European Convention on Human Rights and Fundamental Freedoms (European Court, 2004).

National court decisions are the most strictly binding methods of enforcing the right to health, and the last few decades have seen an exponential growth of litigation based on the right to health in low- and middle-income countries (Hogerzeil et al., 2006; Gauri & Brinks, 2008; Gloppen, 2008; Yamin & Gloppen, 2011). This growth is explained in part by the growing number of states ratifying the ICESCR and entrenching this right domestically (Hogerzeil et al., 2006), as well as by transnational civil society coordination of legal and political strategies. In successful cases of litigation, civil society has effectively claimed access to antiretroviral drugs for people with HIV/AIDS, access to generic drugs, prisoners' rights to healthcare services, reproductive rights, and rights to water, food, and a healthy environment (Forman, 2014; Yamin & Gloppen, 2011: 2). Yet, as indicated earlier, evidence on the equity impacts of this litigation is mixed.

South African litigation offers a key illustration of how domestic litigation can produce larger benefits: In 2002, the Constitutional Court held that constitutional and international protections of rights to health and life required the government to ensure broad access to medicines to prevent mother-to-child transmission (MTCT) of HIV (*Minister of Health and Another v. Treatment Action Campaign and Others*, 2002). Today, a national program provides these medicines in almost 100% of government clinics (South African Department of Health, 2014). This case also led to the establishment of a national AIDS treatment program that by 2016 was treating 61% of people in need with antiretrovirals (UNAIDS, 2017). The South African case attests that individual claims can benefit collective health interests and assist in reducing systematic disparities in health and healthcare (Forman, 2011). In another case, the Latvian Constitutional Court found the state in violation of the right to social security by failing to ensure that employers pay premiums for their employees' social security (Constitutional Court of Latvia, 2000).

Yet domestic litigation has not always had positive outcomes. In Colombia, almost a million health rights claims have been lodged under the *tutela* system (an informal fast-track petition procedure that does not create precedents; Lamprea, 2014). As a result, Colombia has the highest per capita rate of right to health litigation in the world (Moestad et al., 2011: 282; see also Forman, 2014). These cases are critiqued for reinforcing existing inequities by favoring individual claims without consideration of their broader impacts (Lamprea, 2014; Yamin & Gloppin, 2011). However, others argue that the scale of litigation did not create the problems, as opposed to responding to preexisting institutional dysfunctions (Lamprea, 2014; Yamin & Gloppin, 2011).

The Colombian Constitutional Court responded in 2008 by issuing a landmark judgment ordering institutional reform to reduce litigation rates and extensively restructure the health system (Lamprea, 2014; Yamin and Parra-Vera, 2009). The Colombian experience reinforces that litigation favoring individual interests may do so at the expense of population health. The Colombian experience nonetheless underscores that courts can play a key role in ensuring health equity within domestic health policy.

Administrative Accountability Mechanisms

Over the past decade, there has been growing interest in health and human rights impact assessments (HHRIAs) within public health and human rights communities and within the established domain of impact assessment practice (Forman & MacNaughton, 2015; Kemp & Vanclay, 2013). The development of HHRIA methodologies has arisen from the practical imperative to mitigate the health and human rights impacts of policy and trade. They have been used to predict the health and human rights consequences at the level of clinic operations, state and local policy, and foreign direct investment projects (Bakker et al., 2009; Rights and Democracy, 2007).

HHRIAs have extended to enhancing recognition of the social determinants of health, promoting intersectoral responsibility for health, and increasing awareness of the need for transparent and accountable policymaking (Krieger et al., 2003: 659–660). These broader aspirations are reflected in the 2008 CSDH report's endorsement of health equity impact assessment as a key practical strategy to prevent market pressures from impeding action on health equity (WHO, 2008: 46, 135–137, recommendations 12.1, 10.3, 16.7; see also Forman & MacNaughton, 2015).

The Health Rights of Women Assessment Instrument (HeRWAI) is the most widely used of these tools. It was developed from 2002 to 2006 by a group of NGOs located in the Netherlands, Kenya, Malaysia, Nicaragua, and Bangladesh as an advocacy tool to assist organizations to link policies to human rights issues, gather data and assess human rights impacts of policies, and pressure governments to address their concerns (Bakker et al., 2009: 443; Forman & MacNaughton, 2015). Groups in numerous countries have conducted studies using the HeRWAI as the basis for their advocacy efforts, including in Holland, where a prospective change to a healthcare insurance law was analyzed using this tool, finding that it would reduce access to healthcare among undocumented women in particular, resulting in corresponding changes to the proposed law (Stronks et al., 2016: 55). These tools offer particular utility in advocacy efforts to mitigate the health impacts of trade and investment agreements, particularly in relation to their potential impact on pharmaceutical pricing (Forman & MacNaughton, 2015).

Political Accountability Mechanisms

Human rights offer norms, standards, and frameworks that can guide policy even in countries that do not recognize economic, social, and cultural rights such as health. Canada offers several examples in this regard. Although Canada does not entrench rights such as health in its national Charter of Rights and Freedoms, government policy has relied on rights-based framing in relation to the social determinants of health. The lobbying of several UN special rapporteurs (independent experts appointed at the UN to address specific rights and issues) resulted in the government's adoption in 2017 of its first ever National Housing Strategy, which suggests that "the federal government is taking . . . steps to progressively implement the right of every Canadian to access adequate housing" and that their "plan is grounded in the principles of inclusion, accountability, participation and non-discrimination, and will . . . affirm the International Covenant on Economic, Social and Cultural Rights" (Government of Canada, 2018: 8).

Social Accountability Mechanisms

As the preceding litigation examples suggest, civil society actors are key players in enforcing health rights in a variety of forums, and one of the primary longest-standing mechanisms for doing so is via social advocacy and mobilization. One of the most successful instances of social accountability is found in the AIDS treatment movement, where social movements used rights-based approaches to advance access to affordable antiretroviral treatment in low- and middle-income countries. These efforts not only achieved a dramatic global reduction in the price of AIDS drugs but also saw corporations, governments, and international organizations shift toward advocating universal access to antiretroviral treatment (Forman, 2011). As a result, access to these medicines has increased from several thousand people in 1999 to almost 21 million people in 2017 (WHO, 2018). Access to antiretroviral treatment has resulted in declining mortality from AIDS for the first time, with a 48% decline since 2005 (WHO, 2018). The AIDS medicines experience therefore illustrates how rights-based methods can effectively challenge economic and political interests that may sustain gross health inequities and in so doing positively impact population health, albeit with uncertain sustainability (Forman, 2011).

Smaller-scale examples show the utility of integrating human rights and the social determinants of health. In Alaska, civil society and researchers established the Maniilaq Social Medicine Center, which attempts to align healthcare with a rights-based approach acknowledging the social determinants of health (Trout et al., 2018). The center uses an integrated approach that connects governance, social services, primary care, local knowledge, academic research, and policy advocacy around social determinants and human rights in order to both provide healthcare and redress "larger structures of inequity that both produce and are propagated by poor health" (Kenyon et al., 2018; Trout et al., 2018: 26).

These mechanisms reinforce the critical role of social participation and action in governance related to the social determinants of health and their potential to nudge policy initiatives toward equity. The role of social actors in enforcing human rights is particularly important given growing recognition that law alone is a poor causal mechanism for advancing transformative human rights change and that social action is key to such outcomes (Koh, 1997; Risse et al., 1999; Finnemore & Sikkink, 2001). Indeed, social action is increasingly understood to be intimately intertwined with the production of international law (Baxi, 2002; Rajagopal, 2003; Siegel, 2004).

Conclusion

The right to health in international law offers an extensive legal framework relevant to advancing the social determinants of health, as well as practical tools and strategies with some efficacy in advancing the social determinants of health at various levels. These experiences suggest that the right to health and its allied entitlements to healthcare, water, sanitation, food, and access to housing can ensure benefits that assist in advancing toward health equity. The AIDS treatment struggle is perhaps the most successful human rights campaign in this regard, and its trans-formation of the global policy arena in this domain, as well as of treatment access on the ground, has saved millions of lives and, for the first time in multiple decades, halted and reversed the global incidence of HIV infection. These are transformative outcomes by any measure, suggesting the potential for human rights frameworks in conjunction with social move-ment to advance global health equity. Smaller-scale victories in the enforcement and monitoring of rights similarly reinforce their capacity to incrementally advance the social determinants of health and achieve material gains with potentially polycentric social benefits.

Yet these rights are less explicit or effective when it comes to addressing the more distal political and economic determinants of health, including those that enable inequitable distributions of power, money, and resources. It is arguable that the extent to which they are able to influence the latter depends on how effectively civil society can enforce the former and that even in the most successful instances of realizing these rights, the distal structural determin-ants may remain untouched. The AIDS treatment struggle again exemplifies these lacunae: despite its successes, the campaign could do little to alter inter-national trade rules that sustain prohibitive drug pri-cing (Forman, 2019), nor challenge "inequities of power or wealth on a global scale" (Moyn, 2018: 197–198). At the same time, skyrocketing litigation in Latin America illustrates how rights frameworks can negatively impact health equity by favoring indi-vidual litigants and creating unsustainable budgetary burdens. These contrasting experiences reinforce that rights and law of any nature can be wielded either as a regulating force to sustain the status quo or an emancipatory force for social transformation (De Sousa Santos, 2002: 2–3). Moreover, these experiences suggest that without explicit attention to the distal determinants of health, and especially to inequities of power and wealth, the gains promised by human rights will not be sufficient to effectively meet the challenges of our age that create and sustain global health inequity.

References

Asian Human Rights Commission (1998). Asian Human Rights Charter: A People's Charter. Declared in Kwangju, South Korea, May 17, 1998.

Backman, G., Hunt, P., Khosla, R., et al. (2008). Health systems and the right to health an assessment of 194 countries. *Lancet* **372**(9655), 2047–2085.

Bakker, S., Van Den Berg, M., Duzenli, D., & Radstaake, M. (2009). Human rights impact assessment in practice: the case of the Health Rights of Women Assessment Instrument (HeRWAI). *Journal of Human Rights Practice* **1**(3), 436–458.

Baxi, U. (2002). *The Future of Human Rights*. Oxford, UK: Oxford University Press.

Benatar, S. (2016). Politics, power, poverty and global health: systems and frames. *International Journal of Health Policy and Management* **5**(10), 599–604.

Chapman, A. (2017). *Global Health, Human Rights, and the Challenge of Neoliberal Policies*. Cambridge, UK: Cambridge University Press.

Chapman, A., & Russell, S. (2002). *Core Obligations: Building a Framework for Economic, Social and Cultural Rights*. Antwerp: Intersentia.

Council of Europe (1965). European Social Charter (529 U. N.T.S. 89), entered into force February 26, 1965.

Cranston, M. (1973). *What Are Human Rights?* London: Bodley Head.

Constitutional Court of Latvia (2000), Case No. 2000–08-0109, cited in Stronks et al., 2016: 49.

De Cock, K. M., Mbori-Ngacha, D., & Marum, E. (2002). Shadow on the continent: public health and HIV/AIDS in Africa in the 21st century. *Lancet* **360**, 67.

de Sousa Santos, B. (2002). *Toward a New Legal Common Sense: Law, Globalization and Emancipation*, 2nd ed. London: Butterworths Lexis Nexis.

Easterly, W. (2009). Human rights are the wrong basis for healthcare. *Financial Times* (online). Available at www .ft.com/content/89bbbda2-b763-11de-9812-00144feab49a (accessed July 25, 2020).

European Court of Human Rights (2004). *Oneryildiz v. Turkey*, (GC), No. 48939/99), November 30.

First International Conference on Health Promotion (1986). Ottawa Charter for Health Promotion. WHO/HPR/HEP/95.121, November 21, Ottawa, Canada.

Ferraz, O. (2009). The right to health in the courts of Brazil: worsening health inequities? *Health and Human Rights Journal* **11**, 33–45.

Finnemore, M., & Sikkink, K. (1998). International norm dynamics and political change. *International Organizations* **52**(4), 887–917.

Forman, L. (2011). Making the case for human rights in global health education, research and policy. *Canadian Journal of Public Health* **102**(3), 207–209.

Forman, L. (2013). What contribution have human rights approaches made to reducing AIDS-related vulnerability in sub-Saharan Africa? Exploring the case-study of access to antiretrovirals. *Global Health Promotion* **20**(1), 57–63.

Forman, L. (2014). A rights-based approach to global health policy, in Brown, G., Yamey, G., & Wamala, S. (eds.), *The Handbook of Global Health Policy*. West Sussex, UK: Wiley-Blackwell, pp. 459–482.

Forman, L. (2019). Is the right to medicines a canary in the human rights coalmine? Humanity Online Symposium. Available at http://humanityjournal.org/author/lisa-forman/ (accessed July 25, 2020).

Forman, L., & Bomze, S. (2012). International human rights law and the right to health: an overview of legal standards and accountability mechanisms, in Backman, G., & Fitchett, J. (eds.), *The Right to Health: Theory and Practice*, 1st ed. Lund: Studentlitteratur AB, pp. 33–72.

Forman, L., & MacNaughton, G. (2014). Moving theory into practice with human rights impact assessment of trade-related intellectual property rights. *Journal of Human Rights Practice* **7**(1), 109–138.

Free Legal Assistance Group and Others v. Zaire. (1995). *African Human Rights Law Reports* **74**.

Garrett, L. (1995). *The Coming Plague: Newly Emerging Diseases in a World Out of Balance*. London: Penguin Books.

Gauri, V,, & Brinks, D. M. (2008). *Courting Social Justice: Judicial Enforcement of Social and Economic Rights in the Developing World*. Cambridge, UK: Cambridge University Press.

Glendon, M. A. (2002). *A World Made New: Eleanor Roosevelt and the Universal Declaration of Human Rights*. New York: Random House.

Gloppen, S. (2008). Litigation as a strategy to hold governments accountable for implementing the right to health. *Health and Human Rights* **10**(2), 21–36.

Griffin, J. (2010). On human rights. *Legal Studies* **30**(1), 151–160.

Goodman, T. (2005). Is there a right to health? *Journal of Medicine and Philosophy* **30**, 643–662.

Gostin, L. O. (2007). A proposal for a framework convention on global health. *Journal of International Economic Law* **10**(4), 989–1008.

Government of Canada (2009). A healthy, productive Canada: a determinant of health approach. Final report of Senate Subcommittee on Population Health, Government of Canada (online). Available at https://sencanada.ca/content/sen/committee/402/popu/rep/rephealth1jun09-e.pdf (accessed July 24, 2020).

Government of Canada (2018). Canada's National Housing Strategy: a place to call home. Government of Canada (online). Available at https://assets.cmhc-schl.gc.ca/sf/project/placetocallhome/pdfs/canada-national-housing-strategy.pdf (accessed July 24, 2020).

Hopgood, S. (2014). *The Endtimes of Human Rights*. Ithaca, NY: Cornell University Press.

Hogerzeil, H. V., Samson, M., Casanovas, J. V., & Rahmani-Ocora, L. (2006). Is access to essential medicines as part of the fulfillment of the right to health enforceable through the courts? *Lancet* **368**(9532), 305.

Holmes, S., & Sunstein, C. R. (2000). *The Cost of Rights*. New York: W.W. Norton.

Hunt, P. (1996). *Reclaiming Social Rights: International and Comparative Perspectives*. Aldershot, UK: Dartmouth Publishing.

Hunt, P. (2009). Missed opportunities: human rights and the Commission on Social Determinants of Health. *Global Health Promotion* **1757-9759** (Suppl. 1), 36–41.

International Conference on Primary Health Care (1978). Declaration of Alma-Ata. Alma-Ata, USSR, September 6–12.

Jorge Odir Miranda Cortez et al. v. El Salvador (2000). Case 12.249, Report No. 29/01, Inter-American Commission on Human Rights, Annual Report 2000, OEA/Ser./L/V/II.111, Doc. 20, Rev. 200.

Kapczynski, A. (2019). The right to medicines in an age of neoliberalism. *Humanity: An International Journal of Human Rights, Humanitarianism, and Development* **10**(1), 79–108.

Kenyon, K. H., Forman, L., & Brolan, C. E. (2018). Deepening the relationship between human rights and the social determinants of health: a focus on indivisibility and power. *Harvard Health and Human Rights Journal* **20**(2), 1–9.

Kemp, D., & Vanclay, F. (2013). Human rights and impact assessment: clarifying the connections in practice. *Impact Assessment and Project Appraisal* **31**(2), 86–96.

Koh, H. H. (1997). Why do nations obey international law? *Yale Law Journal* **106**(8), 2599–2659.

Klein, N. (2007). *The Shock Doctrine: The Rise of Disaster Capitalism*. New York: Picador.

Krieger, N., Northridge, M., Gruskin, S., et al. (2003). Assessing health impact assessment: multidisciplinary and international perspectives. *Journal of Epidemiology and Community Health* **57**(9), 659–662.

Lamprea, E. (2014). Colombia's right to health litigation in a context of health care reform, in Gross, A., & Flood, C. (eds.), *The Right to Health in a Globalized World*. Cambridge, UK: Cambridge University Press.

Lyon, B. (2003). *Discourse in Development: A Post-Colonial Theory "Agenda" for the UN Committee on Economic, Social and Cultural Rights* (Villanova Public Law and Legal Theory Working Paper Series, Working Paper No. 2003–9). Villanova University School of Law, Philadelphia.

Malawi African Association and Others v. Mauritania (2000). Communication 155/96. *African Human Rights Law Reports* **149**, 1–17.

Mariela Vicenconte v. Ministry of Health and Social Welfare (1998). Case No. 31.777/96, Buenos Aires, Argentina.

Mann, J., Gruskin, S., Grodin, M. A., & Annas, G. J. (eds.) (1999). *Health and Human Rights: A Reader*. New York: Routledge.

Marmot, M. (2015). *The Health Gap: The Challenge of an Unequal World*. London: Bloomsbury Press.

Minister of Health and Another v. Treatment Action Campaign and Others (2002). South African Constitutional Court, 5 S.Afr.L.R. 721.

Moestad, O., Rakner, L., & Motta Ferraz, O. L. (2011). Assessing the impact of health rights litigation: a comparative analysis of Argentina, Brazil, Colombia, Costa Rica, India and South Africa, in Yamin, A. E., & Gloppen, S. (eds.), *Litigating Health Rights: Can Courts Bring More Justice to Health?* 1st ed. Cambridge, MA: Harvard University Press, pp. 273–303.

Moyn, S. (2018). *Not Enough: Human Rights in an Unequal World*. Cambridge, MA: Belknap Press of Harvard University Press.

Organization of African Unity (OAU) (1986). African (Banjul) Charter on Human and Peoples' Rights, OAU Doc. CAB/LEG/67/3 rev. 5, 21 I.L.M. 58, adopted June 27, 1981, entered into force October 21, 1986.

Organization of African Unity (OAU) (1999). African Charter on the Rights and Welfare of the Child, OAU Doc. CAB/LEG/ 24.9/49 (1990), entered into force November 29, 1999.

Organization of American States (OAS) (1999). Additional Protocol to the American Convention on Human Rights in the Area of Economic, Social and Cultural Rights, "Protocol of San Salvador." OAS Treaty Series No. 69 (1988), entered into force November 16, 1999.

Orend, B. (2002). *Human Rights: Concept and Context*. Peterborough, ON, Canada: Broadview Press.

Pickett, K., & Wilkinson, R. (2009). *The Spirit Level*. London: Bloomsbury Press.

Rajagopal, B. (2003). *International Law from Below: Development, Social Movements and Third World Resistance*. Cambridge, UK: Cambridge University Press.

Rights and Democracy (2007). *Human Rights Impact Assessment for Foreign Investment Projects: Learning from Experiences in the Philippines, Tibet, the Democratic Republic of Congo, Argentina, and Peru*. Montreal, QC, Canada: International Centre for Human Rights and Democratic Development.

Risse, T., Ropp, S. C., & Sikkink, K. (eds.) (1999). *The Power of Human Rights: International Norms and Domestic Change*. Cambridge, UK: Cambridge University Press.

Siegel, R. B. (2004). The jurisgenerative role of social movements in United States constitutional law. Paper presented to the Latin American Seminar on Constitutional and Political Theory 2004 on the Limits of Democracy, June (on file with author).

Singh, J. A., Govender, M., & Mills, E. J. (2007). Do human rights matter to health? *Lancet* **370**(4), 521–527.

Stronks, K., Toebes, B., Hendriks, A., Ikram, U., & Venkatapuram, S. (2016). *Social Justice and Human Rights as a Framework for Addressing Social Determinants of Health: Final Report of the Task Group on Equity, Equality and Human Rights Review of Social Determinants of Health and the Health Divide in the WHO European Region*. Copenhagen: WHO.

Social and Economic Rights Action Centre and the Centre for Economic and Social Rights v. Nigeria (2001). Communication No. 155/96, African Commission on Human and Peoples' Rights, Banjul, Gambia.

South African Department of Health (2014). Joint Review of HIV, TB and PMTCT Programmes in South Africa. Available at www.health-e.org.za/wp-content/uploads/201 4/04/who-final-report-of-joint-hiv-tb-pmtct-main-report.pdf.

Toebes, B. C. A. (1999). *The Right to Health as a Human Right in International Law*. Antwerp: Intersentia.

Trout, L., Kramer, C., & Fischer, L. (2018). Social medicine in practice: realizing the American Indian and Alaska Native right to health. *Harvard Health and Human Rights Journal* **20**(2), 19–30.

Truth and Reconciliation Commission of Canada (2015). Honouring the truth, reconciling for the future: summary of the final report of the Truth and Reconciliation Commission of Canada (online). Available at http://nctr.ca /assets/reports/Final%20Reports/Executive_Summary_Eng lish_Web.pdf (accessed July 14, 2020).

United Nations (UN) (1945). Charter of the United Nations. 59 Stat. 1031, June 26, entered into force October 24, 1945.

United Nations (UN) (1946). Constitution of the World Health Organization, signed June 22, 1946.

United Nations (UN) (1948). Universal Declaration of Human Rights, G.A. Res. 217A (III), U.N. Doc A/810 at 71.

United Nations (UN) (1969). International Convention on the Elimination of All Forms of Racial Discrimination, G.A. Res. 2106 (XX), Annex, 20 U.N. GAOR Supp. (No. 14) at 47, U.N. Doc. A/6014 (1966), 660 U.N.T.S. 195, entered into force January 4, 1969.

United Nations (UN) (1976a). International Covenant on Economic, Social and Cultural Rights, G.A. Res. 2200A (XXI), 21 U.N. GAOR Supp. (No. 16) at 49, U.N. Doc. A/6316 (1966), 993 U.N.T.S. 3, entered into force January 3, 1976.

United Nations (UN) (1976b). International Covenant on Civil and Political Rights, G.A. Res. 2200A (XXI), 21 U.N. GAOR Supp. (No. 16) at 52, U.N. Doc. A/6316 (1966), 999 U.N.T.S. 171, entered into force March 23, 1976.

United Nations (UN) (1979). Convention on the Elimination of All Forms of Discrimination Against Women, G.A. Res. 34/180, 34 U.N. GAOR Supp. (No. 46) at 193, U.N. Doc. A/34/46 (1979), entered into force September 3, 1981.

United Nations (UN) (1989). Convention on the Rights of the Child, G.A. Res. 44/25, Annex, 44 U.N. GAOR Supp. (No. 49) at 167, U.N. Doc. A/44/49 (1989), entered into force September 2, 1990.

United Nations (UN) (1994). International Conference on Population and Development, Programme of Action, U.N. Doc. A/CONF.171/13, September 5–13.

United Nations (UN) (1995). Beijing Declaration and Platform for Action, Fourth World Conference on Women, U.N. Doc. A/CONF.177/20 & Add.1, September 4–15.

United Nations (UN) (2000). General Comment No. 14 (2000): The Right to the Highest Attainable Standard of Health (Article 12 of the International Covenant on Economic, Social and Cultural Rights), U.N. Doc. E/C.12/2000/4, August 11.

United Nations (UN) (2007). Declaration on the Rights of Indigenous Peoples, Resolution adopted by the United Nations General Assembly on September 13, A/61/ 295.

United Nations (UN) (2008). Convention on the Rights of Persons with Disabilities, G.A. Res. 61/106, Annex I, U.N. GAOR, 61st Sess., Supp. No. 49, at 65, U.N. Doc. A/61/49 (2006), entered into force May 3, 2008.

United Nations General Assembly (2008). Optional Protocol to the International Covenant on Economic, Social and Cultural Rights, Res. A/RES/63/117, 10, December.

UNAIDS (Joint United Nations Programme on HIV/AIDS) (2017). *South Africa Country Factsheet*. UNAIDS (online). Available at www.unaids.org/en/regionscountries/coun tries/southafrica (accessed July 25, 2020).

Wilkinson, R., & Pickett, K. (2018). *The Inner Level*. London: Penguin Press.

World Health Organization (WHO) (2008). *Closing the Gap in a Generation: Health Equity Through Action on the Social Determinants of Health: Final Report of the Commission on Social Determinants of Health*. Geneva: WHO

World Health Organization (WHO) (2011). *Rio Political Declaration on Social Determinants of Health*. Geneva: World Health Organization. Available at www.who.int/sdh conference/declaration/en/ (accessed July 24, 2020).

World Health Organization (WHO) (2018). *World Health Statistics 2018: Monitoring health for the SDGs*. Geneva: WHO.

World Conference on Human Rights (1993). Cairo Declaration on Human Rights in Islam, U.N. GAOR, World Conference on Human Rights, 4th Sess., Agenda Item 5, U.N. Doc. A/CONF.157/PC/62/Add.18, August 5, 1990.

Yamin, A. E., & Gloppen, S. (2011). *Litigating Health Rights: Can Courts Bring More Justice to Health?* Cambridge, MA: Harvard University Press.

Yamin, A. E., & Parra-Vera, O. (2009). How do courts set health policy? The case of the Colombian Constitutional Court. *PLoS Medicine* **6**(2), 148–150.

Responsibility for Global Health*

Allen Buchanan and Matthew DeCamp

Introduction: Growing Concern about Global Health

Global health is becoming a fashionable term among scholars, human rights activists, state officials, leaders of international and transnational organizations, and others.[1] Until recently, health as a matter of collective concern largely implied national health. When the health problems of people in other countries became a public issue, it was usually within the confines of the notion of disaster relief, short-term responses to acute health crises caused by natural disasters or wars. Global health is a relatively new category of moral concern, empirical investigation, and institutional action.

There are several reasons for the current prominence of global health issues. First, there is a widening recognition that some major risks to health are global in three senses: their adverse impact on health is potentially worldwide, the conditions for their occurrence include various transnational dependencies that are lumped together under the rubric of globalization, and an effective response to them requires cooperation on a global scale. Examples of health risks that are global in each of these three senses include emerging infections, pollution of the oceans, depletion of the ozone layer, global warming, nuclear terrorism, and bioterrorism. Second, because of the revolution in information technologies and the emergence of transnational epistemic communities equipped with powerful empirical methodologies for measuring and explaining health and disease, we now know more about the health problems of people

in other countries than ever before. We also now have greater institutional resources, both within wealthier states and through international and transnational organizations, for applying this new knowledge to ameliorate global health problems. Finally, human rights discourse and, more generally, the articulation of a cosmopolitan ethical perspective provide a normative basis for taking global health seriously as a moral issue.[2]

An Inadequate Response: Duty Dumping

Having reliable information about the nature and causes of global health problems, the capacity to ameliorate them, and a cosmopolitan ethical perspective that regards the need to ameliorate them as urgent is not sufficient, however. It is also necessary to move from the judgment that these problems must be addressed to concrete conclusions about who should do what to solve them. Call this the *problem of concrete responsibilities*.

One response to the problem of concrete responsibilities is what might be called *duty dumping*. To "dump" a duty in global health means to ascribe obligations to individuals or institutions, holding them accountable for the adverse health effects of their policies, without offering adequate justification for why particular obligations should be imposed on particular individuals or institutions. The mistake might be that the putative obligation is too onerous or that it has been assigned to the wrong entity. In either case, duty dumping occurs when critics assign

---

* An earlier version of this work has appeared: Buchanan, A., & Decamp, M. (2006). Responsibility for global health. *Theoretical Medicine and Bioethics* 27(1), 95–114.

[1] *International organization* here means an organization in which states are the primary participants. *Transnational organization* refers to an organization that encompasses individuals or groups across state borders and in which states may not be the primary participants.

[2] A cosmopolitan ethical perspective is one that takes individual human beings – regardless of where they happen to reside and independently of what national or ethnic group they are members of – as the fundamental objects of moral concern. Of course, the cosmopolitan perspective may not be the only possible normative basis for taking global health to be an important moral issue. On its most plausible reconstruction, however, the contemporary conception of human rights is a cosmopolitan conception.

duties or obligations without good – or sometimes without any – reason. However, we do not use duty dumping to signify *only* a mistake in assigning duties; in the complex area of global health, such errors might be expected. Instead, we reserve the term for errors of a particularly egregious sort that would be easily rejected in other contexts. Duty dumping is both morally unjustified and potentially counterproductive for the overall goal of improving global health.

A prominent example of duty dumping is the claim that pharmaceutical companies that produce antiretroviral HIV/AIDS drugs have a duty to supply these drugs to all who could benefit from them at prices they can afford. The claim here is not just that it would be a good thing for drug companies to do this, nor simply that they have a moral obligation to do *something* to make their medicines more affordable to the worst off. Instead, those who criticize these private corporations often imply something much stronger: that the companies are acting wrongly if they do not do *whatever* it takes to make the drugs affordable to all who need them. In this case, the assigned obligation seems too demanding. Analogously, two decades ago in the United States, it was often said that for-profit hospitals ought to provide free care for the medically indigent and that if they did not do so, they were guilty of acting unjustly (Gray, 1986).[3] Duty dumping seems to proceed on something like a "can implies ought" principle or a principle to the effect that the producers of healthcare goods or services have a determinate obligation to provide them to those who cannot pay. But such a principle cannot withstand scrutiny. There is no more reason to believe that drug companies are responsible for providing drugs to all who need them or that for-profit hospitals are to provide care to all who need it than there is to believe that grocers have an obligation to ensure that no one goes without sufficient food.

Duty dumping may be an effective political strategy, but it is unprincipled, evasive, and in the end most likely counterproductive. It may well be true that drug companies ought to do something to make their drugs more affordable. In the language of traditional moral theory, perhaps they have an imperfect duty of beneficence – a moral obligation to do something to help some of the needy. Whether they should

do this by lowering their drug prices or by engaging in some other form of beneficence (say funding scholarships to train people from poor countries to become doctors or scientists) is another matter.

Duty dumping is not only morally unjustifiable, but it is also a powerful mechanism for the evasion of responsibility. The analogy with the problem of securing access to care for the indigent in the United States is illuminating: The obligation to make basic healthcare affordable in the United States is a societal obligation; therefore, the lack of affordable basic healthcare is a moral failing of the citizens of the United States. To pretend that for-profit hospitals are the villains conveniently diverts attention from our failure to fulfill our obligations. Similarly, to focus exclusively or even primarily on the supposed obligations of drug companies is to divert attention from a whole range of responsibilities for responding to the HIV/AIDS crisis. From a cosmopolitan moral standpoint, all of us, as individuals, whether we happen to be leaders of corporations or not, have a moral obligation to help ensure that all persons have access to institutions that protect their basic human rights (Buchanan, 2003: chapters 1–3). From the perspective of the principle of humanity or benevolence, we also have an obligation to relieve the sufferings of others. From either of these vantage points, we might all have moral obligations for responding to the HIV/AIDS crisis. This includes the major multinational pharmaceutical companies, but it is substantially different because it recognizes our collective obligation rather than dumping this obligation solely on those companies (as if only they were responsible for the HIV/AIDS crisis). It is one thing to say that an appropriate collective effort to ensure that HIV/AIDS medications are affordable will include specific obligations on the part of drug companies; it is quite another to pretend that such specific obligations already exist.

Because of their own lack of resources and inability to participate effectively in political processes, however, many individuals are not in a position to do much to act on this obligation. Those of us who are fortunate enough to have resources beyond what we need for a decent and fulfilling life, and who have the freedom to organize with others to influence political processes, have many opportunities to fulfill our obligations regarding human rights and benevolence. Perhaps most important, we have the capacity – if we can muster the will – to work together to create an effective specification of responsibilities.

---

[3] For a further account of why for-profit healthcare organizations do not have determinate obligations to provide access to the indigent, see Brock and Buchanan (1986).

Duty dumping is also a short-sighted and inherently conservative response to global health problems. The problem is not simply that it leaves the root causes of both illness and lack of access to healthcare untouched, though this is bad enough. In addition, by focusing arbitrarily on unpopular private organizations (such as big drug companies), it gives political cover to institutions that do have determinate responsibilities for health and which are failing to fulfill them. Chief among these, we shall argue, are states.[4]

A satisfactory account of determinate responsibilities for ameliorating the most serious global health problems will have to do three things. First, it should correctly identify whatever reasonably determinate responsibilities for health already exist in our world (rather than simply foisting imagined determinate responsibilities on whatever resource-rich agents are conveniently at hand – duty dumping). Second, it should recognize *responsibility gaps*; that is, it should acknowledge that, in many cases, determinate responsibilities will have to be *created* through the development of new institutions or by modifying existing institutions. Third, it must make clear that the responsibility for holding powerful agents accountable for the determinate responsibilities they already have, and for creating institutions that assign new determinate responsibilities, lies with all of us – but especially with those who have surplus personal resources and political clout.

We have noted that from a cosmopolitan standpoint, there are two sources of moral concern about global health: the obligation to help ensure that every person has access to institutions that protect their basic human rights (including the human right to health and other rights, such as rights against discrimination, which have implications for health) and the so-called imperfect obligation of humanity, or benevolence. Both of these moral obligations are indeterminate – taken by themselves, they provide insufficient guidance for ameliorating the complex problems of global health. Taking them seriously requires a commitment to collective action to construct a moral division of labor that is both fair and effective. In most cases, successful collective action requires institutions.

Consider first the imperfect obligation of humanity, or benevolence. Because of the impact of health status on human well-being, those who act from the duty of humanity will naturally be concerned about improving health, whether by efforts to help ensure that the sick receive medical care or through the amelioration of social and economic conditions that adversely affect health. However, if they act alone, individuals cannot do much to alleviate large-scale health problems. Instead of continuing to act independently and inefficiently, they can and should create institutions for healthcare research and for the provision of services, thereby coordinating their efforts and achieving great efficiencies of scale, as well as the benefits of the division of labor. Such institutions will assign various determinate duties to a range of individuals occupying various institutional roles; they will create determinate duties, not simply identify preexisting determinate duties.

How is this different from duty dumping? Consider again the case of HIV/AIDS medications. We have already noted that it is a mistake to assume that drug companies already have determinate obligations to ensure that such medicines are available to all who could benefit from them. It might be possible, however, to create determinate obligations on the part of drug companies. For example, one way might be to modify existing intellectual property (IP) rules. As a condition of receiving drug patents – a form of IP right of particular import to the pharmaceutical industry – drug companies might be required to contribute a certain percentage of future sales to a global fund for subsidizing purchases of medications by the health services of poor countries. This hypothetical example is not offered as a policy proposal but rather as an illustration of the difference between the unprincipled attribution of determinate responsibilities (duty dumping) and a collective effort – in this case, new legislation regarding IP rules to create determinate obligations.

Acting conscientiously on the obligation to help ensure that all have access to just institutions also requires collective *institutional* action for at least two reasons. First, in some cases, institutions are needed to give determinate shape to abstract principles of justice, through legitimate processes for selecting particular "justice-regimes" from among a range of feasible alternatives. For example, even if it is true that justice requires some form of private property, there are many alternative private property rights regimes.

---

[4] Onora O'Neill argues against states as the primary agents of global justice; her view is at least partly based on the failure of states to accomplish justice beyond their borders in the past. This does not necessarily mean that states do not have, or are ill suited to carry out, at least some of the determinate responsibilities we describe. See O'Neill (2004).

Yet, to reap the benefits a property rights regime can produce, a society must have some way of settling on one particular arrangement, and the process of choosing a particular arrangement must itself accord with principles of justice. Within the constraints of a constitution, democratic institutions are needed to specify a particular property rights regime as one important element of the establishment of justice.

Second, institutions are needed to create or collect resources needed for the provision of justice and for ensuring that the costs of providing justice are distributed fairly (Buchanan, 1984). For example, if a particular society, through its institutional processes, recognizes that all its members have a right to a "decent minimum" or "adequate level" of healthcare, it will also need institutions for raising the revenues needed to secure this right for all and for ensuring that the costs of doing so are distributed fairly. Finally, institutions are often needed to enforce the fulfillment of the duties that institutions create.

Once these various roles of institutions are understood, it becomes clear that whenever human needs are not fulfilled, this need not be the result of someone's failure to fulfill a determinate duty; it could be primarily a failure of collective action. To revert to an earlier example, the fact that millions of people are dying whose lives could be prolonged by antiretroviral drugs does not necessarily show that any particular party has failed to perform a determinate duty. Instead, it may indicate a deeper failure of many people to undertake collective action to establish the sorts of institutions that make the ascription of determinate duties both morally justifiable and efficacious.

In the next section, we begin the task of identifying the most important existing determinate responsibilities regarding global health by outlining some of the main responsibilities of states. On our view, it is important to begin with the responsibilities of states both because state behavior plays a larger role in the burden of disease than is usually recognized and because, at present, states are the primary agents of distributive justice. Then, in the following section, we consider, also in a preliminary way, the responsibilities of some of the most important nonstate actors, including global corporations and certain types of global governance institutions, such as the World Trade Organization (WTO) and the World Bank.

Our inquiry will focus on responsibilities for ameliorating the most serious health problems of the world's worst-off people. Apart from the fact that this is literally a life and death matter, and for that reason morally urgent, there is another reason to concentrate on the most serious health problems of those who have the least resources for addressing them. This commitment can be seen as the focus of an "overlapping consensus" among quite disparate views of justice ranging from strict egalitarianism to an extreme prioritarianism, according to which only the well-being or resources of the worst off count from the perspective of distributive justice. This is a signal advantage because it allows us to make some progress on the problem of concrete responsibilities without having first to determine which of a number of competing conceptions of justice is correct (Sreenivasan, 2002).

The Responsibilities of States

The recognition that some health problems occur globally and may require supranational responses should not blind us to the fact that, in our world, states are not only the primary agents of justice but also the institutions that have the greatest impact on the health of individuals. Even if it were true, as libertarian political theorists argue, that there are no positive general moral rights, states would still have significant responsibilities for ameliorating health problems that are caused by the injustices they commit or support – responsibilities that they are not now fulfilling.

Justice and Membership in the State System

The first responsibility of states regarding global health is to avoid committing acts of injustice that have health-harming effects. This general obligation implies more determinate obligations. Among the most important of these are the obligation to refrain from fighting unjust wars abroad and using violence for oppression at home. In addition, states have a moral obligation to put an end to the common practice – especially among some of the wealthiest countries – of equipping and training the military forces of states that are likely to use this power unjustly, whether against their own people or others.

Another important source of rather determinate obligations of states is their participation in the state system. A key aspect of participation in the state system is the practice of recognizing the legitimacy of other states. States routinely contribute to massive health problems in other countries by recognizing the legitimacy of governments that either fail to fulfill their responsibilities regarding the health of their citizens or deprive them of the resources they might otherwise use for securing healthcare or the better living conditions that are essential for health.

Under the current state system, international recognition of the legitimacy of a government confers two eminently abusable rights: the right to dispose of the country's natural resources and the right to borrow from individual countries or international agencies such as the World Bank.[5] The first right enables corrupt government officials to enrich themselves with wealth that properly belongs to the people and could be used by them to ameliorate their health problems, in part, by raising their standard of living. The second right enables state leaders to incur crushing national debts that make it harder for their people to lift themselves from poverty and reap the health benefits of a higher standard of living.

The traditional criterion for legitimacy in the state system is normatively vacuous. The *principle of effectivity* asserts that the basis for conferring the rights of sovereignty, including the right to dispose of resources and the right to borrow, is simply the ability to exercise control over a relatively stable population within a given territory (cited in Buchanan, 2003: chapter 6). On this criterion, human rights–violating kleptocratic regimes that pillage their peoples' resources and exacerbate their poverty by incurring debts to fund projects that benefit only the ruling elite are legitimate so long as they achieve control. Furthermore, until recently, the recognition of legitimacy has largely been an all-or-nothing affair because sovereignty has been regarded as indivisible. However, both the normatively vacuous conception of sovereignty and the assumption that sovereignty is unitary are now being challenged (International Commission on Intervention and State Sovereignty, 2001).

States have a moral responsibility not to be accomplices in injustices by conferring predictably abusable rights on bad governments. The question is whether effective international institutions can be devised that reward responsible governments with the full range of sovereign rights and withhold certain rights from governments that seriously abuse them. If the effective fulfillment of this responsibility requires the creation

of new international institutions that "unbundle" the rights of sovereignty and confer rights only when they can be expected to be exercised responsibly, then states have a higher-order responsibility to contribute to their creation.

If more states did a better job of fulfilling their obligations to refrain from committing injustices and from supporting states that commit injustices, the positive impact on health would be enormous. Consider only the obligation not to engage in unjust wars and not to supply weapons and training to states that are likely to engage in unjust wars or use their military forces unjustly against their own people. From 1998 to 2004, approximately 3.9 million people died in the Democratic Republic of Congo (DRC) as a result of the war raging there. It is estimated that for every violent death in DRC's war zone, there are 62 "nonviolent" deaths – from starvation, disease, and exposure (Lacey, 2005). This is only one instance of the devastating direct and indirect health effects of war.

To summarize, even if there were no such thing as positive human rights (such as the right to an adequate standard of living, the right to basic healthcare, the right to basic education), states would still have rather determinate moral obligations to act in ways that would greatly ameliorate the health problems of the world's worst-off people. Simply by refraining from unjust violence and from supporting unjust governments, states could do much to improve global health.

Primary Guarantors of Their Own Citizens' Human Rights

So far we have made the case that states have determinate responsibilities whose fulfillment would do much to ameliorate some of the most serious threats to health simply by appealing to relatively uncontroversial standards of justice. Once we expand the moral framework to include states' responsibilities for protecting the human rights of their own citizens, the scope of their responsibilities increases considerably.

The primary addressees of human rights claims are states (Nickel, 1987). This is so not only because historically states have been the major violators of human rights but also because, for better or worse, they are best equipped to specify and apply determinate human rights norms and to achieve the conditions of distributive justice upon which the effectiveness of individuals' rights depends.

---

[5] Thomas Pogge has rightly emphasized the role that the recognition of these two rights plays in global poverty (Pogge, 2002: 22–23, 117, 153, 162–166, 238, 258, 264, 266).

International and regional human rights institutions have a valuable role to play in specifying the minimal human rights standards that all states should meet – and in providing venues and frameworks of discourse in which domestic and transnational forces can exert pressure on states to live up to them.

Unfortunately, the connection between human rights and health, though important, has not received the attention it deserves from moral theorists. There are at least two ways in which the connection might be made. On the one hand, a right to health could itself be included among the human rights. On the other hand, one could think of health as a precondition for the enjoyment of various human rights. Let us consider each approach briefly and try to ascertain their implications for the problem of concrete responsibilities.

The Idea of a Human Right to Health

Human rights are best understood as high-priority minimal moral entitlements of all persons and as implying both fairly determinate obligations on the parts of states (their primary addressees) and more indeterminate obligations on individuals to work with others to promote the protection of these rights, if they have the opportunity and resources to do so.[6] In order to integrate global health issues into the human rights framework, the first question to ask is whether the human right in question is a right to healthcare or to health. The attraction of focusing on a right to health rather than to healthcare is obvious: Health depends on many factors, healthcare being only one of them and – in the larger scheme of things – not the most important of them.

However, the idea of a right to health is not without difficulties. First, there is the problem of settling on a defensible definition of what health is. Among the most basic sources of disagreement here is the division between more "objectivist" and more "social constructivist" conceptions of health and disease. Second, if the notion of health is understood too ambitiously, satisfying the right to health for all will not be possible simply because there are some people whose health is so poor that they

could not be made healthy even if cost were not an issue. The third difficulty is that cost *is* an issue. However, if the right to health as a human right is to be understood, it must – as with other human rights – be understood as a moral minimum, not a maximum. Health is not the only good. For one thing, there are other human rights. and protecting them requires that not all of our resources be used to satisfy the right to health. In addition, as most moral theories recognize, there are limits on what we owe to others. For these reasons, any approach to global health that relies on the idea of a human right to health must first develop a defensible conception of the limited character of the right. Unless this is done, it will not be possible to make headway on the problem of determining specific responsibilities for seeing that all enjoy the right, if only because the whole idea will be dismissed as unrealistically demanding or as imposing unacceptable restrictions on individuals' freedom and property rights.

Nonetheless, the lack of a fully developed theory of the human right to health is not such a serious problem if our focus is on the most serious health problems of the world's most vulnerable people. Their health problems are undeniable and severe, regardless of which of a broad range of competing conceptions of health and disease one adopts. Furthermore, whatever the full content of the human right to health turns out to be, it is clear that many states are not ensuring that this right is enjoyed by all their citizens.

At present, the most significant mechanisms for ensuring compliance with human rights standards are domestic. More specifically, individual states that ratify human rights conventions increasingly incorporate them into their domestic legal systems over time, thereby giving individuals and groups standing to appeal to the courts when they believe their rights are being infringed upon.

However, as long as the idea of a human right to health is left vague and therefore subject to the charge that it implies ever-expanding obligations, there is little hope that it will be incorporated in a meaningful way into domestic legal systems. This pitfall can only be avoided by building a broad international consensus on a conception of the human right to health that is sufficiently determinate to allay the worry about an overexpansive entitlement while avoiding an overly specified right that would not do justice to cultural

---

[6] For a lucid articulation and defense of this *entitlements plus* conception of human rights, see Nickel, cited in Buchanan (2003: chapters 1 and 2). For the view that there are certain rights that are preconditions for the enjoyment of all other rights, see Shue (1980).

differences and differences in the resources available to various states.[7]

One way of achieving this goal would be to articulate a minimal conception of the human right to health that consists mainly of two elements. The first is a set of operationalizable standards for what might be called the *negative* right to health, a specification of the responsibilities of states to remove barriers to access to existing healthcare resources, to eliminate discrimination in health services, and to ensure that the health needs of all citizens are taken into account both in the development of health services and in the pursuit of policies of economic development that can have serious health effects. The second is a set of operationalizable standards for ensuring that all citizens enjoy a core set of *positive* health entitlements, including, for example, such relatively uncontroversial items as clean drinking water, basic sanitation, and shelter, as well as access to basic perinatal care and immunization for the most serious infectious diseases. In both cases, the standards must be operationalizable in the sense that appropriate international and transnational organizations must be able to make publicly defensible judgments as to whether states are complying with them. The chief responsibility for seeing that this two-pronged strategy is successfully executed lies with the leaders of international and transnational human rights organizations and with individuals who are in a position to work with others to influence their own governments to cooperate with these organizations.

Health as a Precondition for the Enjoyment of Human Rights

On some accounts, health is not a human right but rather something that is nonetheless of critical moral importance because it is a necessary condition for the enjoyment of human rights. To advocate human rights without making a commitment to achieving all the conditions for their effective exercise is morally incoherent.

To a large extent, this second approach to global health converges with that according to which health is a human right. Ensuring that the burden of disease does not undercut the effective exercise of human rights does not require equality of health (however

that might be defined) nor that all health needs must be met. Instead, it requires a collective effort to forge an international consensus on a core set of health entitlements (both negative and positive) that generally protect individuals against the most serious health problems and that are sufficiently concrete to allow states to be held accountable for providing them, either through their own judicial institutions or through formal or informal pressures from international and transnational organizations.

In some cases, states will not be capable of achieving these basic health entitlements for some or even most of their citizens. The most extreme example is that of literally "failed states," in which civil order no longer exists and there is no government capable of providing any services, including those that are important for health. In other cases, there may be a minimally functioning state, but it lacks some capacities that are critical for providing adequate levels of the core public health and healthcare services. When this occurs, the people of wealthier states have an obligation to work together to provide aid to help every state discharge its obligations regarding the health of its citizens.

The effective fulfillment of this obligation will generally require the world's wealthier people to act through the institutions of their own states by pressuring their political leaders to create international institutions that fairly distribute the burden of providing aid, devising benchmarks for progress, and providing incentives for donors to carry through on pledges of support. An example of this type of international institution might be the Global Fund to fight AIDS, tuberculosis, and malaria.

The Responsibilities of Nonstate Actors

An Obligation Not to Cause Harm?

We argued earlier that states have rather direct and relatively uncontroversial obligations that would, if fulfilled, avoid serious harms to health. It might be thought that every organization, whether private or public, has an obligation not to act in ways that are harmful to people's health. However, the notion of acting in ways that are harmful to people's health is so all-encompassing as to be incapable of providing moral guidance. It covers both cases where the causal connection is sufficiently clear and robust to warrant

---

[7] For a valuable contribution to the solution of this problem, see Hessler (2001). See also Hessler and Buchanan (2002).

the attribution of responsibility and those in which it is not.

Where the agent in question is itself a significant causal factor in the production of the harm, the attribution of responsibility may be unproblematic. In some cases, there clearly are obligations not to cause harm that nonstate actors violate with disastrous consequences for the health of some individuals. For example, a company may dump large quantities of toxic chemicals into a major river, causing death or serious illness not just in one country but in several.

However, in morality, as in the law, merely making a contribution to the production of a harm is not sufficient for the attribution of responsibility. One difficulty is that some harms result from the cumulative effects of the actions of many individuals, none of whom can reasonably be held responsible for the harm. Thus, when global health problems, such as the pollution of the oceans, result from the cumulative effects of the actions of millions of agents, including individuals, corporations, and governments, the attribution of concrete responsibilities on the basis of causality is not possible. Although much more could be done and ought to be done to hold corporations and governments legally liable for harms to health when appropriate standards for liability apply, it is a mistake to rest the case for addressing global health problems on the reduction of moral responsibility to the obligation not to cause harm. To do so not only requires an indefensible understanding of the relationship between causality and responsibility but also overlooks the responsibility of a wide range of actors to work together to develop institutions that create morally defensible assignments of concrete responsibilities.

Accordingly, in the discussion of the responsibilities of nonstate actors that follows, we focus chiefly on grounds for responsibility other than the more obvious cases in which an agent's actions play an important and direct role in the causation of health-related harms.

Global Governance Institutions

Like the term *global health*, the phrase *global governance institutions* is currently in vogue. It is used to refer to a quite heterogeneous collection of different international organizations, from "government networks" comprised of high-level bureaucrats from many nations (including judges and regulators networks; Slaughter, 2004) to the WTO and the United Nations Security Council. Because there are such great differences among these organizations, we should not expect them all to have the same causal role in global health nor the same responsibilities. For this reason, we do not attempt even to begin the daunting task of providing a theory of responsibility for all global governance institutions. Instead, we only aim to articulate some of the different grounds for attributing responsibilities regarding global health to them.

Consistency with the Public Goals of the Institution

In some cases, global governance institutions expressly or tacitly assume responsibilities for global health. One example is the World Health Organization (WHO). Less obviously, the WTO recognizes the importance of its activities for global health and welfare in several of its formal statements. A brief tract intended to explain the functions of the organization to the general public states that the WTO's "goal is to improve the welfare of the peoples of its member countries" (WTO, 2003), and in a joint report with the WHO, the WTO affirms human health as "important in the highest degree" (WHO & WTO Secretariat, 2002: 11).

Consider the WTO's Agreement on Trade-Related Aspects of Intellectual Property (TRIPS), which was negotiated and agreed upon in the Uruguay Rounds of 1986–1994 (WTO, 1994). A strong case can be made that this agreement, far from promoting health as being of "the highest-importance," in fact creates a new obstacle to the amelioration of some global health problems by raising the prices and slowing the introduction of generic drugs in developing countries. When an organization acts in ways that are inconsistent with its own public commitments to global health, the attribution of responsibility is relatively unproblematic.

Of course, it might also be argued that whether or not it explicitly includes health concerns within its public mission statement, the WTO has come to have responsibilities for health in the process of pursuing its primary goal of liberalizing trade. If the predictable consequences of liberalized trade in certain contexts include working conditions that endanger the health of workers, thereby endangering their human rights, then the organization that is the chief instrument for liberalizing trade is obligated to take these consequences into account in its policies and to cooperate with other actors to ameliorate them. Unlike the simple appeal to special responsibilities for health that organizations sometimes assume, this argument requires much more in terms of elaborating responsibility in the complex causal web connecting liberalized trade policies with the endangering of human rights at the individual level. Given that there can be disagreement about the facts that are relevant to the attribution of responsibilities, a credible identification of the special responsibilities of particular organizations may require reliance on the expertise of *epistemic communities*, mobilized through the operation of international organizations such as the International Labour Organization (ILO) or various transnational human rights organizations.

Global Corporations

The responsibilities of global corporations for global health fall into three main categories: (1) obligations to avoid actions and policies that in themselves are significant causal factors in harms to health, (2) obligations not to support governments engaged in unjust activities that are harmful to the health of their citizens or others, and (3) obligations not to impede the health-promoting efforts of states, labor organizations, and legitimate international and transnational organizations that have more direct responsibilities regarding global health. As we have already noted, the moral basis of the first class of obligations is relatively straightforward. The main problem is not the attribution of responsibility but rather how to achieve accountability. In developing countries, the state regulatory agencies charged with holding global corporations responsible for their harms are often too inadequately resourced to be effective. In more developed countries, they are often staffed by people who previously worked in, and still have connections with, the very industries they are supposed to regulate. Or the agencies are ordered to go soft on enforcement by higher government officials who seek political support from powerful corporations.

The second class of obligations is extremely important. Like states, global corporations can and often do help corrupt governments stay in power, with disastrous effects on the health and general welfare of individuals. And like states, global corporations can have powerful incentives to provide such support. However, as the case of apartheid South Africa demonstrates, under certain conditions, these incentives can be countered by a sustained global campaign to expose the role of corporations in supporting unjust governments and mobilize public pressure and state action against it.

When corporations explicitly embrace a role in helping to ameliorate a global health problem, as some drug companies have done, they assume new responsibilities and ought to be held accountable for fulfilling them. Apart from such self-assigned responsibilities, the extent to which global corporations have obligations to promote health is debatable. However, it is much less difficult to argue that they at least have the obligation not to impede the efforts of others to ameliorate the most serious health problems of the world's worst off. For example, a global corporation violates this obligation when it blocks the formation of labor unions committed to ameliorating hazards in the workplace. Similarly, even though it is problematic to say that drug companies have an obligation to provide essential medicines at prices that even the poorest people can afford, it is clear that they have an obligation not to exert pressure on governments to ratify IP agreements that increase their profits at the expense of preventing poorer countries from having access to less expensive generic drugs.

Conclusion

Global health is increasingly becoming the object of interdisciplinary empirical research, institutional action, and moral concern. If this convergence of factors is to result in a significant amelioration of the most serious health problems of the world's most vulnerable people, the abstract commitment to "improving global health" must be translated into concrete responsibilities for action. We have argued that the needed work of specification requires a systematic understanding of the different roles and capacities of a broad range of private and public institutions, with a sensitivity to the different grounds for attributing responsibility. One important result of our inquiry is that the responsibilities of states are much more extensive than is usually assumed. Instead of focusing only on the obligations of wealthier states to transfer resources to poorer ones, we should recognize the full range of state activities – from making war to according legitimacy to corrupt governments – that are harmful to health and prevent individuals from achieving a standard of living that makes better health possible.

Acknowledgments

The authors are grateful for research support for this paper from Duke University's Center for Genome Ethics, Law and Policy, part of the Duke Institute for Genome Sciences and Policy.

References

Brock, D. W., & Buchanan, A. (1986). Ethical issues in for-profit health care, in Gray, B. H. (ed.), *For-Profit Enterprise in Health Care*. Washington, DC: National Academy Press, pp. 224–249.

Buchanan, A. (1984). The right to a decent minimum of health care. *Philosophy & Public Affairs* **13**, 55–78.

Buchanan, A. (2003). *Justice, Legitimacy, and Self-Determination: Moral Foundations for International Law*. New York: Oxford University Press.

Gray, B. H. (ed). (1986). *For-Profit Enterprise in Health Care*. Washington, DC: National Academy Press.

Hessler, K. (2001). A theory of interpretation for human rights. Ph.D. dissertation, University of Arizona, Phoenix.

Hessler, K., & Buchanan, A. (2002). Specifying the content of the human right to health care, in Rhodes, R., Battin, M., & Silvers, A. (eds.), *Medicine and Social Justice: Essays on the Distribution of Health Care*. New York: Oxford University Press.

International Commission on Intervention and State Sovereignty (2001). *The Responsibility to Protect*. Ottawa, ON, Canada: International Development Research Centre.

Lacey, M. (2005). Beyond bullets and blades. *New York Times*, March 20, 2005, Section 4, p. 1.

Nickel, J. (1987). *Making Sense of Human Rights*. Berkeley: University of California Press.

O'Neill, O. (2004). Global justice: whose obligations?, in Chatterjee, D. K. (ed.), *The Ethics of Assistance: Morality and the Distant Needy*. New York: Cambridge University Press, pp. 242–259.

Pogge, T. (2002). *World Poverty and Human Rights*. Cambridge, UK: Polity Press.

Shue, H. (1980). *Basic Rights: Subsistence, Affluence, and U.S. Foreign Policy*, 2nd ed. Princeton, NJ: Princeton University Press.

Slaughter, A.-M. (2004). *A New World Order*. Princeton, NJ: Princeton University Press.

Sreenivasan, G. (2002). International justice and health: a proposal. *Ethics and International Affairs* **16**, 81–90.

World Health Organization (WHO) & World Trade Organization (WTO) Secretariat (2002). *WTO Agreements and Public Health*. Geneva: WTO.

World Trade Organization (WTO) (1994). Agreement on trade-related aspects of intellectual property rights. Available at www.wto.org/english/docs_e/legal_e/27-trips.pdf (accessed March 25, 2005).

World Trade Organization (WTO) (2018). *The WTO in Brief*. Geneva: WTO.

Bioethics and Global Child Health

Avram Ezra Denburg and Denis Daneman

Introduction

As many of the chapters in this volume document, we continue to bear witness to – and often create and perpetuate – wide disparities in global health outcomes. These inequalities extend to the health and well-being of children worldwide. Globally, more than 25,000 children under five years of age die every day, the vast majority of them in low-income countries (LICs). Under-five mortality is, on average, 14 times higher (69 versus 9 per 1,000 live births) in the world's LICs than in the industrialized world. Of note, however, under-five mortality decreased by 58% globally between 1990 and 2017, with a goal for all countries to reach a level below 25 per 1,000 live births by 2030 (Global Health Observatory [GHO], 2019).

The contributions to this collection also provide a compelling case for the role of a *global* bioethics in interrogating and combatting the root causes of such inequalities. But why inquire into global bioethics for children as a specific subgroup? What is unique about children or childhood – both biologically or socioculturally – that warrants discrete ethical inquiry? In this chapter, we argue that children are different and seek to lay the foundations for the development of a global child health ethics. Our argument is not an uncritical apology for pediatric exceptionalism but rather an effort to highlight some of the differentiating biological and normative dimensions of childhood to arrive at a more nuanced conception of how prevailing bioethical principles apply to children in a global context. To this end, we attempt to sketch the ethical and legal realities of global child health, with specific attention to collective rights and responsibilities in relation to the health of children. We begin by highlighting children and adolescents as separate groups from adult and aging populations and examine evolving moral conceptions of children, focusing on the three sentinel overlapping ideas that have fundamentally changed our views on the status of children: the best interests of the child, children's autonomy, and

the rights of the child. Focusing on the latter, we examine the role of current child rights law and scholarship in establishing and defending international responsibilities for the promotion and protection of child health globally. Finally, we consider a set of core principles for global health ethics – equity, freedom, and solidarity – and their specific application to child health, exploring potential synergies between global health ethics and child rights through the lens of early childhood development (ECD). A key finding of this work is that the moral language for addressing children's health and well-being globally remains underdeveloped – particularly in regard to collective responsibilities for policy and action. We hope our work demonstrates that important synergies result from the integration of global health ethics and human rights paradigms in defining the contours of these responsibilities.

Children Are Different: Normative Foundations

The evolution toward a specific focus on bioethics for children has been predicated on three emerging and interrelated concepts: *best interests, autonomy,* and *rights.* The best interests criterion emerged as a moral yardstick to measure the need for, and justify interventions to enhance, child protection and well-being. It is predicated on a striking shift away from regarding children as property to one that recognizes the child as an object of protection. The concept itself has roots in English feudal law and relates to the doctrine of *parens patriae*: the king as father of his people. Initially employed to legitimate sovereign wardship over "natural fools and idiots," it was gradually expanded to include state duty toward the protection of children. The best interests standard has come to serve, in most liberal democracies, as a bulwark against historically unfettered parental possessory rights and provides the legal right to a minimal threshold of care

(Shah, 2013). A child's best interests have become an elemental facet of legal decisions – and popular sensibility – regarding the protection and well-being of children in society. In the realm of health, the best interests standard is today the dominant standard of pediatric decision-making, best evidenced by the frequency of its use in legal analyses at local, national, and international levels.

Closely related to the best interests standard is mounting recognition of children's autonomy, which has challenged the medical decision-making role of parents, alternate caregivers, and healthcare professionals (Kenny et al., 2008). Scholarship related to the role of the child in healthcare decision making recognizes that children have evolving and very different levels of capacity and accords autonomy in degrees accordingly. Support for three levels of decision making has emerged from parental consent for those lacking any real decision-making capacity, to parental consent combined with child assent for those with developing capacity, to child consent in the context of established capacity (Canadian Paediatric Society & Bioethics Committee, 2004). There is also provision for surrogate decision makers when parents or usual caregivers are at odds with what is deemed the acceptable standard of best interests. Tensions often surface in the interpretation and practical instantiation of this standard, sometimes pitting involved stakeholders – including healthcare professionals, child protection authorities, and caregivers – against one another in determining a child's best interests and ensuring his or her health and well-being accordingly.

Finally, emergence of the concept of the child as a distinct moral agent invested with rights has revolutionized ethical and legal paradigms governing the health and well-being of children (United Nations Convention on the Rights of the Child [UNCRC], 1998; Bensimon & Zlotnik Shaul, 2015). Building on developing notions of autonomy, discourse on the rights of children has gained steady momentum since the 1980s, fostering recognition of the child as an autonomous and self-determining agent rather than an adult-in-waiting. The ratification and progressive adoption of the United Nations Convention on the Rights of the Child (UNCRC) has dramatically increased the volume and changed the tenor of scholarship, policy, and legislation on children's rights. The construct of *the competent child* has emerged, an image focused on the child as a rights-bearing individual –

one with legitimate needs and preferences, the right to voice them, and the right to participate in decisions about how to meet them. Notably, rights discourse introduces issues of policy process: the participatory rights of children and the inclusion of their voice in policy decisions impacting them are fundamental concerns. This discourse strains traditional notions of the child as a passive, incomplete, and ultimately incompetent vessel in need of protection and edification.

Important synergies are evident between child rights, best interests, and well-being. A telescopic view of conceptions of children's best interests in academic discourse captures their evolution from ideas related to the protection of the most vulnerable in the nineteenth and early twentieth century to expansive ideas about well-being as related to, and couched in, the universal rights of children, culminating in UNCRC. The justification for the best interests standard gradually evolved from one founded in charity to one premised on entitlement. The prominence and broad acceptance achieved by UNCRC have irrevocably tied notions of children's well-being to achievement of their social, cultural, economic, civil, and political rights and have tempered culturally relativistic renderings of children's interests and well-being through reference to universal conceptions of the rights of the child.

A parallel narrative centered on participation has emerged in law and scholarship on children's rights that sets in relief the role of rights in evolving conceptualizations of a child's best interests. Changing mores about children, founded in changing models of the young child, influence ideas about the legitimacy and necessity of involving children in policy decisions that affect them. Child rights, as enshrined in UNCRC, are one of the principal loci and drivers of changing societal perceptions. Relatedly, recent insights in the field of early childhood development studies have contributed to major changes in conceptual models of the young child, with corresponding implications for, and impacts on, ideas about involving children in policy decision making. Scholars have identified three dominant models of the young child – the child as possession, the child as subject, and the child as qualified participant – and have elaborated a new model of the child as social actor, founded in novel theory and evidence from a diverse array of disciplines. UNCRC principles and jurisprudence buttress this model: United Nations General Comment No. 7 elaborates an explicit accounting of a child's right to expression in "the development of policies and services, including through research and consultations." The upshot has been a progressive, if fraught, incorporation of ideas of autonomy and participation into the best interests standard: in policy domains as diverse as predictive genetic testing, sexuality and sexual health, child welfare, public health, and research involving children and in forms as varied as a seat at the policy table, proxy communication through identified advocates, and the incorporation of research evidence on children in policymaking.

These three dominant conceits – best interests, autonomy, and rights – form the basis of a unique bioethical lexicon for child health and well-being. However, their application in scholarship and policy has remained largely at the level of discrete persons or polities, with little elaboration to supranational or global spheres of health governance. The need for a distinct paradigm of global bioethics for children remains – one that recognizes the particular biological and sociocultural dimensions of childhood and reckons with our obligations to protect and promote them in an increasingly globalized world. In what follows, we examine advances in child rights law and scholarship that seek to address international duties toward children; then we turn to consider a set of bioethical principles that can support and extend rights-based arguments for collective obligations to improve the health and well-being of children globally.

Global Child Health Rights: UNCRC and International Obligations Toward Children

The right to health of children, as enshrined in UNCRC, has received broad acceptance by UN member states. However, the child's right to health functions mainly within the realm of the sovereign state; the duty to "protect, respect, and fulfill" this right has not typically crossed political boundaries. However, the legal contours of this map have begun to shift over the past two decades. The normative backdrop of UNCRC, coupled with the evolving concept of a right and duty to international assistance and cooperation for health (IAC-H), serves as a broad and durable canvas for the protection of global child health rights.

Its unique scope, acceptance, and substance set UNCRC apart in this regard. UNCRC is the most widely ratified human rights treaty in existence

(UNCRC, 1998). It is also the only human rights treaty that incorporates civil, political, social, and economic rights (Detrick, 1999). Substantively, UNCRC contains perhaps the most detailed and specific articulation of the right to health of any human rights document. It gives particular emphasis to the health issues of children in developing countries and contains an explicit recognition of international obligations thereto (UNCRC, 1998: 24.4; see also Box 10.1). UNCRC is thus the only international human rights document that formally confers a duty on states to help realize the right to health beyond their political borders. The plain force of article 24 obviates the need to derive a basis for IAC-H in subsequent jurisprudence. This confers significant power on the child's right to health: because the duty of IAC-H was crafted and agreed on directly by states parties, its legitimacy is not contingent on legal interpretation – and therefore not subject to political question.

BOX 10.1 UNCRC Articles Relevant to International Assistance and Cooperation for Health

Preamble: Recognizing the importance of international cooperation for improving the living conditions of children in every country, in particular in the developing countries. . . .

Article 4: States Parties shall undertake all appropriate legislative, administrative, and other measures for the implementation of the rights recognized in the present Convention. With regard to economic, social and cultural rights, States Parties shall undertake such measures to the maximum extent of their available resources and, where needed, within the framework of international co-operation.

Article 23.4: States Parties shall promote, in the spirit of international cooperation, the exchange of appropriate information in the field of preventive health care and of medical, psychological and functional treatment of disabled children, including dissemination of and access to information concerning methods of rehabilitation, education and vocational services, with the aim of enabling States Parties to improve their capabilities and skills and to widen their experience in these areas. In this regard, particular account shall be taken of the needs of developing countries.

Article 24.4: States Parties undertake to promote and encourage international co-operation with a view to achieving progressively the full realization of the [right of the child to the highest attainable

---

standard of health]. In this regard, particular account shall be taken of the needs of developing countries.

Article 28.3: States Parties shall promote and encourage international cooperation in matters relating to education, in particular with a view to contributing to the elimination of ignorance and illiteracy throughout the world and facilitating access to scientific and technical knowledge and modern teaching methods. In this regard, particular account shall be taken of the needs of developing countries.

Moreover, jurisprudence on UNCRC by the Committee on the Rights of the Child tends to interpret its provisions holistically. In assessing the obligations and actions of states parties, the committee treats distinct articles as mutually dependent and reinforcing (Doek, 2001). Consequently, it considers the health ramifications of all UNCRC articles. Uniquely, however, a number of these articles – such as those on education (28 and 29) and children with disabilities (23) – contain explicit admonitions about the need for international cooperation[1] (see Box 10.1).

Though UNCRC leaves the substance of international obligations to evolve through praxis and interpretation, the specific application of IAC to health, education, and disability sets it apart. Taken together, these rights have a multiplicative effect on the obligation of states parties to realize the right to health of children globally. Arguably, therefore, the right to health contained in UNCRC is more robust than that in the other signal human rights covenants, including the Covenant on Ethical, Social and Cultural Rights (CESCR), even without the added weight of committee interpretation. Consequently, the legal claim to real international obligations to ameliorate health disparities among children – both within and beyond national borders – is particularly compelling. The explicit links made between health, disability, and education are notable in this context. Lamentably, as with other human rights legislation and jurisprudence, much of the substance of children's right to health articulated in UNCRC remains aspirational, given the difficulties associated with

Table 10.1 Synergies Between Bioethics and Human Rights for ECD Policy Analysis

Dimension of ECD	Bioethics	Human Rights
Epigenetics and heredity	Luck egalitarian conceptions of of *equality of opportunity* to address the ethical implications of blurred social-biological boundaries	Human rights as a priori *determinants of health*: state-level obligation to remediate socially mediated hereditary disadvantage
Sensitive periods	Positive and negative forms of *liberty*, liberal theory on capacities for positive freedoms	Focus on needs of the *vulnerable* gives primacy to protection from harm where damage would be greatest
	Sufficiency theories of justice applied to critical junctures in human development and impact on essential dimensions of well-being	*Indivisibility* of rights as legal instantiation of justice founded on protection of well-being
(Trans) national disparities	Critical attunement to institutional *power* relations	International human rights law on *rights in early childhood*

Source: Modified from Denburg (2015).

implementation of states parties' duties in an anarchical global system – especially in terms of obligations to realize the health and well-being of those countries not our own.

Synergies Between Global Child Health Ethics and Child Rights: Focus on Early Childhood Development

A global child health ethics paradigm can bolster and broaden the justificatory framework for theory and law on child rights in important ways (Powers & Faden, 2006). It can attune the right to health to institutional power relations, help confront tensions between individual and collective spheres of protection, and advance claims to collective responsibilities for action to redress violations of the right to health

---

[1] Though it does not explicitly mention assistance, the phrase *international cooperation* is commonly construed in international law to include a duty to assist. In addition, article 45(b) refers explicitly to "technical advice and assistance" in response to state party need or request (Detrick, 1999).

(Nixon & Forman, 2008). Crucially, bioethics can serve to correct the widespread neglect of correlative duties in human rights discourse. An emphasis on duties recalibrates debate to an accounting of "who must do what," necessitating discussion of social realities, inadequacies, and responsibilities (Chapman, 1996; Benatar et al., 2003).

We highlight here three foundational principles – *equity*, *freedom*, and *solidarity* – that furnish a rich and stable grounding for discourse on global child health ethics. An exploration of these principles and their potential synergy with rights-based arguments in the realm of policy on early childhood development (ECD) provides a potent illustration of the distinct value of a global health ethics for children, one that extends the traditional ambit of pediatric bioethics – predicated on best interests, autonomy, and rights – to a collective responsibility for global child health (Table 10.1).

Equity: Early Experience and the Social Determinants of Child Health

The manifest links between variations in social, political, and economic conditions and disparities in child health outcomes have not, to date, received adequate attention in ethical terms. Key issues include which inequalities are inequitable, where responsibility for ameliorating these disparities lies, and how to accommodate disparate conceptions of health and equity across different societies (Anand et al., 2004).

A number of scholars have marshaled extant models of social justice to relate equity to health inequality. Norman Daniels and Fabienne Peter both draw on John Rawls' theory of justice (Rawls, 1971) to mount an ethical appraisal of health inequalities. Rawls develops the basis for a social contract that rests on a "fair system of cooperation" between people: it justifies not only shared basic liberties but also the choice of terms that will protect and improve the lot of the least fortunate. Rawls' notion of "justice as fairness" endeavors to limit social inequalities that obviate "fair equality of opportunity."[2] Daniels et al.

(2004) extend Rawls' notion of equality of opportunity to encompass health and its social determinants as a means of safeguarding a social contract that seeks to minimize health inequalities. Peter, by contrast, charts an "indirect" approach to health equity: rather than treat health as a distinct and superior good, she construes health equity as a component part of broader social justice goals. In this view, health disparities are unjust when, and insofar as, they stem from injustice in the "basic structure" – namely the political, economic, and social institutions – on which society rests (Peter, 2004). Thomas Pogge augments equity-oriented perspectives on justice by adding a "relational" element to their typically "distributional" grain. He argues that appraisals of distributional justice – that is, assessments of the allocation of goods against an ethical standard – are often causally naive. A "relational justice" perspective demands inquiry into the causes of allocative disparities. In short, our judgments about the equity of outcomes are incomplete without attention to the conditions and actions responsible for them (Pogge, 2004). For Pogge, this applies equally to international disparities, and the institutions that abet them, as to national ones. Insofar as wealthy countries have reaped the benefits of globalization, they should have a corresponding responsibility to attend to the costs (Pogge, 2002).

Global child health would benefit greatly from ensuring equity a place of primacy in health policy. Equity is a complex notion, with contested substance and scope. For all that, it naturally trains a lens on health inequalities and brings an emphasis on the social determinants of health to bear on health policy decisions. Discussions about equity could lead to a hardier right to health, extending notions of fairness beyond civil and political liberties to safeguards for equitable social and economic life. Rawls' fairness principle and elaborations thereon are not only consonant with a rights-based approach to health but also enhance it considerably. Framed by mounting evidence of the links between social inequality and disease, works by thinkers such as Daniels and Peter interpret equity in health as a function of justice in our social contract (Daniels et al., 2004; Peter, 2004). This enlarges rights-based renderings of "equality of opportunity" well beyond negative liberties to positive social and economic protections. It thus provides a fundamental justification for policies to mitigate socioeconomic disparities in defense of the right to

---

[2] Rawls permits social inequality to the degree that it conforms with a "Difference Principle" that recognizes that no one would contract to terms that minimized inequality at the expense of well-being. However, he subjugates his difference principle to equality of opportunity, thereby rigorously limiting the extent of ethically acceptable inequality in a given society (Rawls, 1971).

health. Pogge's efforts to give this social contract global jurisdiction could add weight and shape to evolving IAC-H duties (Pogge, 2004).

These principles are uniquely resonant in the realm of child health. Strong evidence has emerged demonstrating causal relationships between experience in early life and subsequent health and social outcomes. At the biological level, evidence of environmentally driven changes to brain architecture and function during critical periods of neural development continues to emerge. Recent evidence from the field of epigenetics – the study of heritable changes in gene function that occur without alterations to DNA sequence – suggests that the social environment has a profound impact on gene expression. Notably, early experience exerts a crucial and sustained influence on neuronal maturation, suggesting the potential for environmentally mediated changes to the developing brain (Knudsen, 2004).

Compelling data demonstrate the impact of interventions beginning before conception and progressing through pregnancy, labor, and delivery and into the early childhood years on brain development and hence physical and intellectual functioning. On the population level, both ecological and interventional trials have demonstrated links between socioeconomic inequalities and gradients in health, behavior, and cognitive development across the lifespan (Mustard, 2007; Denburg & Daneman, 2010a). Interventions to attenuate developmental risks in vulnerable groups of children have consistently cataloged developmental gains. Studies in diverse experimental settings, including Jamaica, Cuba, Romania, and the United States, have demonstrated sustained linguistic, cognitive, and behavioral benefits from early childhood development interventions (Commission on Social Determinants of Health [CSDH], 2008). Taken together, the biology and epidemiology suggest that social and physical well-being is radically contingent on experience in early childhood, which, in turn, hinges on determinants of child health, including maternal health, fetal and neonatal nutrition, and nurturing. The return on investment of early childhood interventions is often multifold greater than interventions at later developmental stages (Doyle et al., 2009).

Deeper understanding of the interaction between our environment and our epigenome in early life alters paradigms of thought about child health and human development. The knowledge that the social world influences gene expression is transformational. Lifelong and cross-generational patterns of illness and social inequality may originate and embed during critical periods of brain development. New and adapted modes of ethical inquiry are needed to make sense of this sea change in evolutionary biology (Schrey et al., 2012). Competing conceptions of equality of opportunity enable us to consider the interdependence of the social and the biological from various angles. The contrast between luck egalitarian and Rawlsian conceptions of equality of opportunity are illuminating in this regard. Luck egalitarians, who make no moral distinction between socially and biologically engendered forms of disadvantage, would interpret the potential heritability of socially determined patterns of ill-health as proof of the need to redress any inequality beyond one's control. The luck egalitarian notion of natural disadvantage fits easily with knowledge of the epigenome. Rawls' "fair equality of opportunity principle" (FEO), by contrast, does distinguish between social and natural inequalities, finding only the former inequitable. FEO necessitates mitigating social disadvantage to ensure equal life chances for those with similar natural endowments. Insofar as epigenetics blurs the boundaries between natural and social disadvantage, it challenges the classic Rawlsian conception of FEO as applied to ECD. This arguably demands a reformulation of FEO, one that accommodates inequalities stemming from social class "including when social class operates via natural endowments" (Loi et al., 2013: 150).

However, the epigenetics and social determinants of ECD also complicate luck egalitarian conceptions of equality through their challenge to notions of responsibility. Luck egalitarianism – specifically, its prioritarian incarnation – places moral emphasis on the degree of responsibility borne by an individual for his or her health state (Arneson, 2000). The mechanisms and temporal characteristics of key determinants of ECD trouble assessment of equality of opportunity founded on individual responsibility for health and social outcomes. Recklessness in parental health behaviors may translate not only into greater initial risk of disadvantage for offspring but also into perpetuation of the risk behaviors themselves – both throughout the life course and across generations. ECD science thus demands new account of responsibility for health opportunities and outcomes.

Theory on the coupling of disadvantages breaks ground in this regard. Madison Powers and Ruth Faden describe "densely woven, systematic patterns of disadvantage" that arise from the interaction of deprivation or adverse effects in discrete social determinants of health (Powers & Faden, 2006: 71). Social justice, in their formulation, is contingent on sufficiency in each of six composite elements of well-being: health, security, reasoning, respect, attachment, and self-determination. The resonance of these principles in light of the emergent science of ECD is immediately apparent. The degree to which sensitive-period experience in early life constitutively shapes physical, neurodevelopmental, and psychosocial development gives credence to their conception of well-being and the corollary demands for sufficiency in these domains as a prerequisite for social justice. Such empirically grounded, nonideal theory provides a coherent foundation for ECD policy, applicable at both the state and supranational levels. Where disparities in childhood development are evident at the community or population level, a focus on equity and the social determination of health can help make moral sense of inequality through attunement to institutional power relations and systems of political economy (Rogers, 2006; Benatar & Brock, 2011). There is, therefore, a strong empirical and ethical case to be made for policies that attend to disparities in opportunity by reducing differential risk in early childhood environments (Denburg & Daneman, 2010b).

Freedom: Rights, Capabilities, and Development

Various attempts at a global health ethic have sought to ground their logic in appeals to the inherent value and necessity of freedom. Amartya Sen's "capability" approach has proved influential in this regard (Sen, 1999). Drawing on Aristotelian notions of "capacity," Sen argues that one's "capabilities" – namely "the substantive freedoms he or she enjoys to lead the kind of life he or she has reason to value" – are of both intrinsic and instrumental worth and fundamental to human development (Sen, 1999: 87; see also Nussbaum, 1988). Others have extrapolated health-specific paradigms from Sen's model. Weaving together Sen's notion of freedom with Aristotelian conceptions of capacity, Jennifer Prah Ruger posits a model of "human flourishing" that places health at its ontological center (Ruger, 1998). The capability to ensure a baseline level of good health, through freedom from preventable disease and death, is construed as essential and irreducible (Ruger, 2006a). In this view, health is the sine qua non of human functioning, a kind of higher-order capability: without health, one could exercise no other freedoms (Gostin, 2008). Health deprivations are thus deemed unjust insofar as they limit the capacity for human agency and thus "human flourishing" (Ruger, 2006b). These first principles begin to establish a firm ethical footing for the analysis of global health disparities.

The notion of freedom meshes seamlessly with rights- and duties-based approaches to child health. Sen's capability framework is not only consonant with a right to health but also provides deeper justification (Sen, 1999). It would give health a place of primacy in child rights, focusing policy efforts on child survival and improved health as primary duties in international efforts to advance development. In addition, its emphasis on basic requirements for freedom dovetails well with the minimum core obligations of international human rights law. This could provide a way to gauge fidelity to UNCRC that is not compromised by the vague demands of "progressive realization."

The unique developmental needs of children give added value to this synergy. The fluid and complementary nature of a capability approach and the emphasis on child development in UNCRC[3] are readily apparent. Their natural confluence is fed by a unique vulnerability: the durable impact of developmental insults in early childhood on subsequent physical, psychological, and social functioning. Early childhood development is a quintessential and irreducible capability. The long-range effects of epigenetic changes to early brain development, both across the lifespan and to subsequent generations, demonstrate that our chances "to lead the kind of life we have reason to value" is radically contingent on our early environment. Inequalities therein lead to disparities in the freedoms necessary for full human development. This confers a special duty to protect child health globally, one justified on grounds distinct from those relevant to adult health.

The indivisibility of child rights likewise takes on added relevance and force in the context of ECD. Human rights are understood to protect imbricated

---

[3] UNCRC alludes to the centrality of rights to development in its emphasis on diminishing infant mortality [article 24.2 (a)] and, more explicitly, on achieving a standard of living "adequate for the child's physical, mental, spiritual, moral and social development" (article 27.1).

and mutually dependent dimensions of physical and social life. Inadequate protection of any one right risks compromise to the realization of others. In this vein, jurisprudence on the right to health has framed it as part and parcel of an integrated approach to human development, one that attends to both distal and proximal determinants of health (Covenant on Ethical, Social and Cultural Rights [CESCR], 2000). Rights indivisibility thus adds legal weight to conceptions of social justice – like that articulated by Powers and Faden – founded on the protection of well-being. Closely related to this is the growing recognition that human rights themselves constitute a priori determinants of health. This coheres with a scientific blueprint of human development as dependent on stable early childhood foundations, where multiple domains of biological and social life are implicated.

Finally, and crucially, the fact that the locus of responsibility for protecting human rights as clearly specified can serve as a conduit between ethics and policy on ECD. Seen in the light of emerging ECD science, states' duties to realize the health of citizens imply a state role in redressing socially mediated disadvantage, including its heritable forms. This duty has taken explicit form in international human rights regimes. UNCRC provides strong legal footing for a rights-based approach to ECD with corollary state duties (United Nations, 1989). In recognition of the unique developmental needs and vulnerabilities that characterize the early years, General Comment 7, "Implementing Child Rights in the Early Childhood" (GC:7), details the specific application of UNCRC to young children. Its implementation is buttressed by a set of GC:7 indicators that assist states parties in tracking, reporting, and assessing their ECD policies and programs in light of UNCRC principles. The framework includes sets of indicators on civil, political, social, and economic rights that mirror UNCRC articles and is based on UNCRC's structured reporting guidelines; it serves as a guide for the preparation of state party reports to the Committee on the Rights of the Child (ECD Indicators Group, 2010). In keeping with the precept of indivisibility, and in line with ECD science, the committee treats distinct articles as interdependent and mutually reinforcing when interpreting the obligations of states parties (Doek, 2001). This is arguably the most transparent and institutionalized method currently available to hold states to account for their ECD policies in the community of nations. Though the capacity for supranational enforcement of UNCRC principles – as with all human rights – remains weak, their instantiation in an international human rights regime lends the sort of political credence that bioethical theory often lacks.

Furthermore, as noted earlier, the case for transnational action to remediate global health inequalities – and, by extension, disparities in ECD outcomes – arguably finds its clearest articulation in UNCRC. The health and developmental concerns of children in developing countries are afforded specific attention, and international obligations to assist and cooperate in their protection are made explicit (UNCRC, 1998: 24.4). UNCRC is thus the only international human rights document that formally extends the ambit of the right to health and its corollary duties beyond national borders. The capability paradigm strengthens the collective dimensions of child rights obligations. Its emphasis on the social and economic structures necessary to support "human flourishing," including robust public health systems and minimum living standards, trains policy lenses firmly on these issues, providing a much-needed corrective to biases toward "rights individualism" and biomedical solutions. In addition, a focus on capabilities helps right the balance in international advocacy between civil and political rights, which have predominated, and social and economic rights, which have suffered a degree of neglect (Farmer, 2008). The conception of freedom inherent in a capabilities approach thus strengthens the normative and legislative case to translate extensive evidence on the social determinants of health – the inextricable links between poverty, education, food and shelter security, sense of belonging, and life-course health outcomes – into national and international policies that specify the substance of and obligations to children's right to health.

Solidarity: ECD, Interdependence, and IAC-H

Solidarity has been cited as a core principle of global health ethics. Solidarity in global health emphasizes the moral significance of an irreducible human connection and the role of health in defining and defending it. It ascribes foundational value to our deepest relational impulses: identification with and empathy for the other, familial and social character, group attachment, and association. These facets of our nature operate within and between us at multiple levels of social interaction – whether the nucleus of the family, the embrace of the community, national consciousness, or beyond. Solidarity as an ordering principle furnishes a strong alternative, or complement, to pure rights-based approaches to global health.

The moral import of human solidarity is given different expression in distinct philosophical, cultural, and political traditions (Benatar et al., 2003). Western political systems give primacy to liberal streams of thought, gathering moral and legal worth around the individual. By contrast, solidarity is given primacy in many African and aboriginal cultures. The concept of *ubuntu*, derived from the traditional Zulu aphorism "*Umuntu ngumuntu ngabantu*" ("A person is a person through other persons"), serves as a core social ordering principle in many African communities (Louw, 2006). It implies not only respect and compassion for others but also a sense that the full realization of purpose and justice in society is ultimately communal (Teffo, 1994; Sindane, 1995; Louw, 2006).[4] The Canadian First Nations concept of "justice as healing" understands justice as a process of communal reckoning; it embeds personal healing in community healing, locating the source of our moral river in this current of solidarity (Sa'ke'j Youngblood Henderson & McCaslin, 2005). Philosophical and religious renderings of solidarity also provide a moral corrective to naked individualism. Communitarian schools of thought place preeminent value on the "good society," searching out the character virtues that would constitute it; diverse philosophical traditions, including Platonic, Aristotelian, and Neo-Confucian, have cast social harmony as an essential goal of human life (Bloom, 1991; Roberts & Reich, 2002). Postmodern philosophy also grapples with solidarity. Richard Rorty distills the intuitive elements of solidarity and the emotional disposition required to realize it. He emphasizes the importance of humility in a process of identification, and ultimately empathy, with the other (Rorty, 1989). Elements of Rorty's thinking echo themes in Buddhist metaphysics. *Pratītyasamutpāda*, the doctrine of "dependent origination," holds that all things arise and exist because of each other, threads in an all-encompassing spatial and temporal web. *Anatta*, the concept of "non-self," breaks down

illusive barriers between autonomous "selves." The Mahayana focus of *śūnyatā* builds on these principles, emphasizing not only the lack of self-essence but also existential relativity and interdependence: all things exist only in relation to each other; they form an unbroken and unified reality, beyond identity (Rémon, 1980). Judeo-Christian thought also evinces communitarian themes. The Jerusalem Talmud likens the Jewish spiritual polity to an organic body: injury to any part is felt as pain throughout (Guggenheimer, 2005: Jerusalem Talmud, Nedarim 9:4). The centrality and universality of Christ's suffering, and the concomitant emphasis on compassion and assistance for vulnerable members of society, fill a strong vein of solidarity in Christian moral theology (Hollenbach, 2003).

Serious attempts to articulate and entrench a current of solidarity in local and global health policy could effect marked improvements in child health outcomes. Solidarity holds singular relevance for policy on ECD. It highlights the role of social context in the development of personhood, stressing the need to create social conditions that promote healthy ECD. In light of evidence on the critical effects of childhood experience on subsequent health and social functioning, solidarity also binds equality of opportunity to conceptions of the "good society." Emerging science on childhood development has demonstrated that the health of our societies rests in large part on our commitment to children during critical early stages of brain development (Denburg & Daneman, 2010a). Commonality of purpose in this regard implies attempts to damp experiential risk during early life in order to level the field for subsequent opportunity.

Like freedom and equity, solidarity complements human rights paradigms. Indeed, its incorporation with rights-based frameworks would build on existing, if immature, appeals to solidarity in international law and policy (Nixon & Forman, 2008). International legal scholars have construed solidarity as an intrinsic component of the right to development. Bedjaoui bases international solidarity on "the interdependence of nations," which is itself predicated on (1) a globalized economy, (2) the universal duty of states to develop this economy, and (3) the preservation of the human species (Bedjaoui, 1991: 1184–1187).

The use of solidarity as an ethical ordering principle thus would give rigor and a wider range to policies on development aid and humanitarian assistance, with both direct and indirect bearing on the

---

[4] As with unmitigated individualism, there are obvious dangers associated with extremes of subjection to group identity, not least of which are collective violence and minority oppression (Mbigi & Maree, 1995).

health of populations. This could help harness and organize the erratic momentum of current humanitarian and aid endeavors into consistent international policies. In this vein, it would strengthen the justification for IAC-H and, in so doing, galvanize action to realize it. Moreover, fidelity to solidarity in global health policymaking as a community-oriented right (Bedjaoui, 1991) would redouble the focus on accountability to people and populations in the developing world, privileging consultation and cooperation above donor priorities (African Rights, 1994). The place of solidarity in international human rights law remains contested and its substance underdeveloped. A system of global health ethics that emphasizes solidarity could give form and clarity to international legal duties to attenuate disparities in child health and underwrite policies to this end.

Conclusion

We have argued that there is something unique about children that warrants distinct bioethical language and inquiry. We have described the normative foundation on which much of pediatric bioethics rests and have proposed that the established principles remain necessary but insufficient to an accounting of, and reckoning with, global child health disparities. We have proposed a set of ethical principles that broadens the justificatory framework for child health and well-being to address global concerns and obligations and have explored complementarities between global child health ethics and human rights in the analysis of ECD science and policy.

A key finding of this chapter is that the moral language for addressing children's health and well-being globally remains underdeveloped – particularly in regard to collective responsibilities for policy and action. We hope that our work has also demonstrated that important synergies result from the integration of global health ethics and human rights paradigms in defining the contours of these responsibilities. Notions of justice as sufficiency of well-being are buttressed by rights indivisibility; the right to health is given further specificity through exposure to varied conceptions of equality of opportunity; liberal theory on capabilities reinforces the ontological priority of a right to health. These and allied synergies hold similar promise for mapping the ethical landscape of varied child health and social policy domains and for grappling with the social, economic, and political dynamics that condition the well-being of children within and beyond traditional borders.

Above all, we must seek to articulate and apply a global child health ethics that protects and promotes the health of all children, independent of conventional and restrictive labels – among them, gender, religion, geography, and income level. This represents an enormous challenge, given both the variation in sociocultural mores and the vicissitudes in identity and belonging wrought by global migration. Though the task of achieving global consensus on what children are owed, and how to realize it, remains daunting, there is much too much at stake to abandon the effort.

References

African Rights (1994). *Humanitarianism Unbound*. London: African Rights.

Anand, S., Peter, F., & Sen, A (eds.) (2004). *Public Health, Ethics and Equity*. Oxford, UK: Oxford University Press.

Arneson, R (2000). Luck egalitarianism and prioritarianism. *Ethics* **110**, 339–349.

Bedjaoui, M (1991). The right to development, in Bedjaoui, M. (ed.), *International Law: Achievements and Prospects*. Dordrecht: Martinus Nijhoff Publishers, pp. 1177–1202.

Benatar, S. R., & Brock, G (eds.) (2011). *Global Health and Global Health Ethics*. Cambridge, UK: Cambridge University Press.

Benatar, S. R., Daar, A. S., & Singer, P. A. (2003). Global health ethics: the rationale for mutual caring. *International Affairs* **79**(1), 107–138.

Bensimon, C., & Zlotnik Shaul, R. (2016). Pediatric bioethics through a global lens, in ten Have, H. (ed.), *The Encyclopedia of Global Bioethics*. New York: Springer.

Bloom, A (1991). *The Republic of Plato*, 2nd ed. New York: Basic Books.

Canadian Paediatric Society & Bioethics Committee (2004). Treatment decisions regarding infants, children and adolescents. *Paediatric Child Health* **9**, 99–103.

Chapman, A. (1996). Reintegrating rights and responsibilities, in Hunter, K., & Mack, T. (eds.), *International Rights and Responsibilities for the Future*. Westport, CT: Praeger, pp. 3–28.

Commission on Social Determinants of Health (CSDH) (2008). *Closing the Gap in a Generation: Health Equity Through Action on the Social Determinants of Health. Final Report of the Commission on Social Determinants of Health*. Geneva: WHO. Available at www.who.int/social_determinants/final_report/en/ (accessed May 1, 2019).

Covenant on Ethical, Social and Cultural Rights (CESCR) (2000). CESCR General Comment No. 14: The Right to the Highest Attainable Standard of Health (E/C.12/2000/4). Office of the United Nations High Commissioner for

Human Rights (online). Available at www.unhcr.org/ref world/publisher,CESCR,GENERAL,,4538838d0,0.html (accessed August 5, 2018).

Daniels, N., Kennedy, B., & Kawachi, I (2004). Health and inequality, or, why justice is good for our health, in Anand, S., Peter, F., & Sen, A. (eds.), *Public Health, Ethics and Equity*. Oxford, UK: Oxford University Press.

Denburg, A. E. (2015). A sensitive period: bioethics, human rights, and child development. *Health and Human Rights* **17** (1), 19–30.

Denburg, A. E., & Daneman, D. (2010a). The link between social inequality and child health outcomes. *Healthcare Quarterly* **14**, 21–31.

Denburg, A. E., & Daneman, D. (2010b). Pascal's wager: from science to policy on early childhood development. *Canadian Journal of Public Health* **101**(3), 235–236.

Detrick, S. (1999). *A Commentary on the United Nations Convention on the Rights of the Child*. The Hague: Kluwer Law International.

Doek, J. (2001). Children and their right to enjoy health: a brief report on the monitoring activities of the Committee on the Rights of the Child. *Health and Human Rights* **5**(2), 155–162.

Doyle, O., Harmon, C. P., Heckman, J. J., & Tremblay, R. E. (2009). Investing in early human development: timing and economic efficiency. *Economics and Human Biology* **7**, 1–6.

Early Childhood Rights Indicators Group (2010). *Manual for Early Childhood Rights Indicators (Manual of the Indicators of General Comment 7): A Guide for State Parties Reporting to the Committee on the Rights of the Child*. New York: UNICEF (online). Available at https://download.popdata.bc.ca/Manual_DRAFT3-AS+JB_16.12.2010.pdf (accessed May 10, 2019).

Farmer, P. (2008). Challenging orthodoxies: the road ahead for health and human rights. *Health and Human Rights* **10** (1), 1–15.

Global Health Observatory (GHO) (2019). Under-five mortality. Available at www.who.int/gho/child_health/mortality/mortality_under_five_text/en/ (accessed May 31, 2019).

Gostin, L. (2008). Meeting basic survival needs of the world's least healthy people: toward a framework convention on global health. *Georgetown Law Journal* **96**, 331–392.

Guggenheimer, H. W. (ed.) (2005). *The Jerusalem Talmud: Translation and Commentary*. New York: Walter de Gruyter.

Hollenbach, D. (2003). *The Global Face of Public Faith: Politics, Human Rights and Christian Ethics*. Washington, DC: Georgetown University Press.

Hillman, D., Kapoor, S., & Spratt, S. (2006). Taking the next step: implementing a currency transaction development levy. Stamp Out Poverty, Leading Group on Solidarity Levies to Fund Development (online). Available at www.innovativefinance-oslo.no/recommendedreading.cfm (accessed November 10, 2008).

Kenny, N., Downie, J., & Harrison, C. (2008). Respectful involvement of children in medical decision making, in Singer, P. A., & Viens, A. M. (eds.), *The Cambridge Textbook of Bioethics*. Cambridge, UK: Cambridge University Press, pp. 121–126.

Knudsen, E. (2004). Sensitive periods in the development of the brain and behavior. *Journal of Cognitive Neuroscience* **16** (8), 1412–1425.

Loi, M., Del Savio, L., & Stupka, E. (2013). Social epigenetics and equality of opportunity. *Public Health Ethics* **6**(2), 142–153 (see p. 150).

Louw, D. (2006). The African concept of *ubuntu* and restorative justice, in Sullivan, D., & Tifft, L. (eds.), *The Handbook of Restorative Justice: A Global Perspective*. New York: Routledge.

Mbigi, L., & Maree, J. (1995). *Ubuntu: The Spirit of African Transformation Management*. Johannesburg: Sigma Press.

Mustard, J. F. (2007). Experience-based brain development: scientific underpinnings of the importance of early child development in a global world, in Young, M. E. (ed.), *Early Child Development from Measurement to Action*. Washington, DC: World Bank.

Nixon, S., & Forman, L. (2008). Exploring the synergies between human rights and public health ethics: a whole greater than the sum of its parts. *BMC International Health and Human Rights* **8**(2), 1–9.

Nussbaum, M. C. (1988). Nature, function, and capability: Aristotle on political distribution, in von Gunther Patzig, H. (ed.), *Aristotele's Politik*. Lanham, MA: Rowmand & Littlefield, pp. 312–341.

Peter, F. (2004). Health equity and social justice, in Anand, S., Peter, F., & Sen, A. (eds.), *Public Health, Ethics and Equity*. Oxford, UK: Oxford University Press, pp. 93–106.

Pogge, T. (2002). *World Poverty and Human Rights*. Cambridge, UK: Polity Press.

Pogge, T. (2004). Relational conceptions of justice: responsibilities for health outcomes, in Anand, S., Peter, F., & Sen, A. (eds.), *Public Health, Ethics and Equity*. Oxford, UK: Oxford University Press, pp. 135–162.

Powers, M., & Faden, R. (2006). *Social Justice: The Moral Foundations of Public Health and Health Policy*. Oxford, UK: Oxford University Press.

Rawls, J. (1971). *A Theory of Justice*. Cambridge, MA: Harvard University Press.

Rémon, J. P. (1980). *Self and Non-self in Early Buddhism*. New York: Walter de Gruyter.

Roberts, M. J., & Reich, M. R. (2002). Ethical analysis in public health. *Lancet* **359**, 1055–1059.

Rogers, W. (2006). Feminism and public health ethics. *Journal of Medical Ethics* **32**, 351–354.

Rorty, R. (1989). *Contingency, Irony, and Solidarity.* Cambridge, UK: Cambridge University Press.

Ruger, J (1998). Aristotelian justice and health policy: capability and incompletely theorized agreements. PhD dissertation, Harvard University, Cambridge MA.

Ruger, J. (2006a). Toward a theory of a right to health: capability and incompletely theorized agreements. *Yale Journal of Law and the Humanities* **18**, 273–326.

Ruger, J. (2006b). Ethics and governance of global health inequalities. *Journal of Epidemiology and Community Health* **60**, 998–1002.

Sa'ke'j Youngblood Henderson, J., & McCaslin, W. (2005). Exploring justice as healing, in McCaslin, W. (ed.), *Justice as Healing: Indigenous Ways.* St. Paul, MN: Living Justice Press.

Schrey, A., Richards, C., Meller, V., et al (2012). The role of epigenetics in evolution: the extended synthesis. *Genetics Research International* **2012**, 286164. Available at http://dx .doi.org/10.1155/2012/286164 (accessed April 12, 2019).

Sen, A. (1999). *Development as Freedom.* Oxford, UK: Oxford University Press.

Shah, S. (2013). Does research with children violate the best interests standard? An empirical and conceptual analysis. *Northwestern Journal of Law and Social Policy* **8** (2), 121–173.

Sindane, J. (1995). *Democracy in African Societies and Ubuntu.* Pretoria: Human Sciences Research Council.

Teffo, J. (1994). *The Concept of Ubuntu as a Cohesive Moral Value.* Pretoria: Ubuntu School of Philosophy.

United Nations Convention on the Rights of the Child (UNCRC) (1989). G.A. Res. 44/25. Available at www2.ohchr.org/english/law/crc.htm (accessed April 1, 2019).

11

Trade and Health
The Ethics of Global Rights, Regulation, and Redistribution

Meri Koivusalo

Concerns about health are not new aspects of trade policies and have long been part of trade negotiations. It is also known that failures in public health policies can substantially and adversely affect trade. The economic costs of global epidemics have been increasing, but more important is that prevention of epidemics requires both functional public health measures at national borders and functional health systems.[1] Whereas health policies and trade policies have mutually compatible and strengthening aspects, they are marred by important conflicts of interests. In this chapter, I outline ethical issues and questions that relate to these conflicts and the importance of considering trade policies not merely as transnational policies but also as a component of global legal development and governance in relation to rights, redistribution, and regulatory measures. These have consequences not only across countries and among international organizations and actors but also for the balance between public policies and interests and those of national and increasingly global corporate actors and interest groups.

In assessing the implications of trade for health policies, three different components can be observed. The first is the impacts of trade on determinants of health and health outcomes. The core issue here relates to the *magnitude of flows of goods, services, people, or capital*, with positive and negative implications being assessed in relation to these flows and their influence on both health outcomes and how national health systems function. The second and often less clearly articulated influence of trade on health is through *policy space*, and how decisions are made and priorities are set in the sphere of trade will affect the regulatory scope and measures applied in health policies and national health systems. I have earlier addressed this

feature of trade policies as *trade creep* (Koivusalo, 1999) and (with Labonté and Schrecker) have defined *policy space* as the freedom, scope, and mechanisms that governments choose to design and implement public policies to fulfill their aims (Koivusalo et al., 2009). Although policy space is used mostly in relation to national policies, it can also be used to address the issue of policy space for health in regional and global-level regulatory and policy work. The third component applies to illegal trade and human trafficking and includes a number of profound ethical issues.

Two Cross-Cutting Issues

There are two important cross-cutting issues concerning the ethics of trade and health policies.

How Decisions and Policies Regarding Health and Trade Are Made

Concerns regarding the governance and politics of health and trade relate to where decisions are made and to the legitimacy and accountability of such decisions and those who make them. Health- and trade-related concerns have, for example, become heated issues under World Health Organization (WHO) auspices: on action on noncommunicable diseases and infant feeding and in relation to innovation and intellectual property (IP) rights. While health, trade, and human rights issues have in particular been considered in the context of access to medicines, crucial and substantially broader governance questions relate to trade and health at both national and global levels in relation to rights, regulation, and redistribution in the context of public policies as a result of trade policy priorities and obligations arising from trade agreements.

In terms of redistribution, the issue is not merely whether and how trade affects distribution of resources and sharing of risks within a country but also how

---

[1] An earlier version of this work has appeared: Koivusalo, M. (2006). The impact of economic globalisation on health. *Theoretical Medicine and Bioethics* 27(1), 13–34.

more systemic implications that result from trade policies and regulatory measures set the conditions of overall availability and use of public resources for health and how trade relates to social inequalities. Included here are systemic issues in relation to equity aspects of health and health systems, as well as implications of trade policies for social inequalities, social security, social rights, and regulation within countries.

Globalization and global trade policies have been promoted under the assumption that "globalization is good for the poor," but both the basis of this claim and the implications of trade policies on social equity have come under criticism. Birdsall (2006) has emphasized the inherent unequalizing impact of global markets. The current process of globalization and promotion of trade liberalization and protection of IP rights needs to be considered in the context of distribution of resources, impacts on social interventions or poverty-reduction measures, and the need for stronger global governance to coordinate social policy measures and interventions.

There are many concerns about the negotiation of so-called new-generation trade agreements between high-income countries or larger trading blocks, such as the Trans-Pacific Partnership (TPP) agreement and its later formally signed, slightly changed version of the Comprehensive and Progressive Agreement for Trans-Pacific Partnership (CPTPP), the Comprehensive Economic and Trade Agreement (CETA) between the European Union and Canada, negotiations on the Transatlantic Trade and Investment Partnership (TTIP) between the European Union and the United States, and negotiations on the Trade in Services Agreement (TiSA). These negotiations have all focused on more than tariffs, and whereas some of them have remained unfinished, they represent how trade negotiations and agreements are currently evolving. Although new-generation trade agreements are often named as free-trade agreements, tariffs are not the main focus of negotiations. Rodrik (2018) has described this discrepancy well, emphasizing the importance of what trade agreements actually do and contain rather than relying on assumptions of free trade. The importance of national trade interests has also emerged more prominently as part of international trade debates as a result of the changing US emphasis on trade. It is important, however, to separate health-related trade issues from simply protectionist policy stances because trade agreements that well serve local industries and commercial policy interests may still be problematic for public health policies. We cannot thus reduce health and trade issues merely to questions among global, transnational, and national interests but need to consider them as more systemic public policy interests at different levels of governance.

The WHO has legitimacy on the grounds of its constitutional obligations and mandate and in relation to successful negotiations on international health regulations (IHRs) and the Tobacco Framework Agreement experience to take a more proactive role in global public health law so as to ensure that health considerations remain high on the global agenda (WHO, 2007). Areas of ongoing concern with respect to governance for health include pharmaceutical policies, research and innovation for health needs, control of epidemics, antimicrobial resistance, health workforce recruitment practices, and public policies to regulate and guide consumption of unhealthy foods and drinks, including alcohol.

What Can Be Traded and How?

The second cross-cutting issue deals with more traditional public health issues, such as what should be tradable and how to deal with trade on products that are hazardous to health. One example of ethically problematic trade is organ trafficking. Anthropological studies have initially documented the nature and extent of trade and trafficking (Scheper-Hughes, 2000), and a formal United Nations (UN) and European Council (EC) study has placed the issue on the UN agenda with a call for a new binding international treaty to prevent trafficking in organs, tissues, and cells (OTCs), protect victims, and prosecute offenders. A distinction can be made between so-called more widespread transplant tourism, on the one hand, and trafficking of humans for this purpose, on the other hand, while calling for the prohibition of financial gain from the human body or its parts as the basis of legislation on organ transplants (Caplan et al., 2009). However, the line between more acceptable commercialized body enhancement and surgery and that of human cloning, transplants, or more ethically problematic areas of trade is likely to be thin. This applies in particular to surrogacy and services related to artificial insemination and human reproduction. The expansion of what is and can be tradable draws further attention to the need to address trade issues in a broader context than business interests alone.

A traditional concern with respect to trade in goods is the spread of infectious diseases. Here IHRs set the context of interaction between health and trade (Fidler, 1997). This is also the most traditional and historical context of health and trade relations. However, infectious diseases are not the only concern. Contamination of consumer products and inclusion of substances dangerous to health into products have been of concern in relation to trade in consumer goods, such as toothpaste and toys, where prospects for domestic regulation could become increasingly complex because of international production chains (Ofodile, 2009). In pharmaceuticals and other health-technology products, this issue is further complicated by the dangers of not including the correct substances or selling of otherwise substandard products. The large difference between sales price and production cost makes pharmaceuticals an increasingly attractive area for counterfeiters. However, counterfeiting has also been emphasized in the context of patent and trademark infringements and enforcement (Sell, 2008). The common statement by US President Donald Trump and President of the European Commission Jean Claude Juncker also emphasized addressing IP "theft" in trade negotiations between the European Union and the United States (EU & US, 2018). Trade agreements are important for industry interests in protection of IP rights, but they can also set limits on how governments can regulate. Because trade agreements seek to engage with regulatory cooperation and coherence, this comes with an emphasis on self-regulation and the increasing role of standardization within more corporate-driven contexts. Whereas standardization and industry-driven harmonization of technical standards can seem efficient under commercial policies, they are not without risks if commercial rather than safety priorities prevail. Medical devices, artificial intelligence, and personalized care are likely to require further ethical consideration, whereas global markets and exchanges of surrogacy, fertility, and reproductive health–related services and trade and exchange in human organs, blood, and tissue will continue to require ethical and regulatory attention.

Impact of Trade Flows in Goods, Services, and Capital on Health Outcomes

The general assumption in the sphere of economic and trade policies has been that as long as globalization increases economic growth, it will improve well-being and health. An increase in average income is expected to provide better access to food and care. This assumption remains at the core of claims that economic globalization is beneficial to health. However, the real implications of such expectations depend on whether economic growth takes place, how it is distributed within society and what implications it has for existing public policies, and the scope for regulatory measures on health and social determinants of health.

The impact of trade policies on the health status of populations differs from the impact of health policies on health systems. In practice, a large share of impacts on health takes place outside health systems through influence on the social determinants of health. Food security, access to food, and quality of food are all influenced by trade policies, although impacts of trade policies depend on how food production is governed and regulated in the first place.

Two main ethical concerns can be distinguished. The first ethical concern involves those emphasizing insufficient or partial liberalization of trade in agricultural products (including inequities related to unfair trade practices such as unfair use of agricultural subsidies). Second, there are ethical concerns about (a) the impact of the trade liberalization process on agricultural products and food security, (b) the power and roles of commercial interests in the field, and (c) the relative position and roles of consumers, types of farmers, and the food industry in a more liberalized trade regime. Trade policy proponents tend to assume that liberalization brings benefits, but in reality, the assessments of the consequences of the liberalization of trade range from more positive views (Anderson & Martin, 2005) to critical assessments of winners and losers in more liberalized markets of agricultural products (Food and Agriculture Organization [FAO], 2003). The global food and economic crises have also contributed to the reiteration of rights to food and the social security aspects of food security and to efforts to improve global governance on food policy (FAO, 2009).

Food security is an essential concern in light of an emerging focus on malnutrition and hunger as a result of crises in terms of availability, access to, and prices of basic food commodities (FAO, 2009). However, in food policy, changes in agricultural subsidies or policy reforms are not the only areas with trade implications. Powerful transnational actors often benefit more from liberalized trade because they can reap the benefits of substantial capital investments in technology and other measures that increase output and lower prices. One example is the presence of large agribusiness actors with their bargaining power and influence on lowering producer prices and accumulating profits higher up in the value chain of the final products (Fitter & Kaplinsky, 2001; FAO, 2003).

The role of global food industries has become more pronounced in relation to sustainable development and tackling of obesity and noncommunicable diseases. The complex relationship between trade liberalization and dietary transition is not only an issue of market responses to consumer needs but is also mediated through the impact on influence and growth of global transnational food industry, supply chains, and public policies as well as the role of advertising and promotion of processed and particular types of foods. (Lang, 2004) Whether and to what extent within a country or population transition takes place toward less healthy diets also depends on the initial quality of diets and on social and public policies at local, national, and global levels that shape access to food and nutritional contents of diets within societies (Swinburn et al., 2019).

Increasing mobility of goods tends to include goods of a hazardous nature – in particular, alcohol, tobacco, and products with high fat and sugar contents or low nutritional value. Empirical findings support the expectation of increased domestic consumption of tobacco as a result of increased trade and suggest that less wealthy countries may be more vulnerable than wealthier countries to the impact of trade liberalization (Bettcher et al., 2000).

Impact of Trade Policies on Health Policy

The impact of globalization on health policy is not the same as on health outcomes, because the former includes the scope and nature of regulatory measures that governments can impose, as well as the implications for costs and availability of health services and treatments. The more individualized and market-led health policies are, the less likely it is that health policies will become restricted by trade policies. Thus, the impact of globalization on national health policies strongly depends on the extent to which such policies regulate or restrict interests and priorities of commercial actors or markets in a more general sense.

Even in a more liberalized and individualized context, there remains a role for public regulation in standard-setting and labeling of products to promote consumer choice. However, trade-related concerns over legislation in other countries with respect to health-related issues have been raised in the Committee on Technical Barriers to Trade. For example, EC, US, and Australian delegations raised their industries' concerns over labeling requirements on certain snack foods proposed by the Ministry of Public Health of Thailand to prevent malnutrition among children with poor eating habits (World Trade Organization [WTO], 2006, 2008). The United States has raised trade-related aspects of policies promoting breast-feeding as part of reporting on technical barriers to trade in commentary on El Salvador and Hong Kong (US Trade Representative [USTR], 2018).

The impact of trade policies on health policies further depends on three main channels: (1) how health-related standard-setting and health-based regulatory measures outside the health sector are affected, (2) the regulatory implications for resources and service use within the health sector, and (3) access to knowledge and costs of innovation. The realization of these channels depends in part on the ways in which different national interests and trade policy priorities are dealt with in relation to commercial export interests and the willingness to use provisions of trade agreements or limit the scope of these agreements to allow policy space for health. Examples of this type of effort with respect to IP rights and the TRIPS agreement under the World Trade Organization (WTO) would include using flexibilities of the agreement to enable access to medicines as well as interpreting the agreement in favor of public health measures. In trade in services, this type of measure would include caution with trade and investment agreements that could exclude health services or limit the extent that health services, health insurance services, and respective aspects of state aid or government procurement are included in such agreements.

Health-Related Regulation and Standard Setting

The most traditional context for the implications of trade policy is within health-related arguments and standard-setting, and there are several settlement cases between countries under dispute. The General Agreement on Tariffs and Trade (GATT) covers international trade in goods and includes measures to protect public health. However, the basis for how these policies can be achieved is regulated by the Agreement on Sanitary and Phytosanitary (SPS) Measures (1994). A crucial issue in these disputes is whether measures taken are legitimate and necessary or "protectionism in disguise." It is not surprising that disputes concerning the use of public health provisions have also arisen between Europe and North America – for example, in the case of contesting hormone use in cattle raising or the European ban on asbestos. There are also lines of dispute in settlement cases concerning tobacco and alcohol. Although restriction of availability and taxation are known to be effective strategies to reduce consumption of products that are hazardous to health, these strategies tend to be more vulnerable to trade disputes than in more individualized or less market-restrictive interventions. Another related issue is the role and relevance of the Agreement on Technical Barriers to Trade (TBT), which covers all industrial and agricultural products and has implications for domestic regulation of quality of products such as toys. There are also broader implications of trade agreements for the implementation of domestic measures, for example, if a country restricts or bans imports of goods from particular countries or producers on the grounds of health and quality concerns (Ofodile, 2009).

While the role of the SPS Agreement in tackling domestic health protection interests has been emphasized in light of the potential hijacking of domestic health-related regulatory measures by national interest groups (Epps, 2008), there still remains a broader concern over the influence of transnational industries, how to regulate production practices, and how to address issues with scientific uncertainty or disagreement, as reflected in the dispute-settlement case on use of hormones in meat production (WTO, 1998).

Veggeland and Borgen (2005) have highlighted these problems in the context of the work of the Codex Alimentarius Commission, a joint WHO and Food and Agriculture Organization (FAO) food standard-setting organization to which two WTO agreements refer, as national and commercial trading interests have become reflected more strongly in government stands in Codex since the establishment of the WTO. The question is thus also to what extent strong trading interests have become reflected in the context of national positions and processes with respect to standard-setting. We also need to ask to what extent there might be other conflicts of interests in standard-setting and how standards are defined. This perspective is of importance in relation to the role of the International Organization for Standardization (ISO)[2] as a global standard-setting authority, especially if it expands its work further in services, environment, and occupational health and safety. In health, attention has already been drawn to the role of the tobacco industry in standard-setting for their products within the ISO (Bialious & Yach, 2001).

Health Systems and Regulation of Health Services

The General Agreement on Trade in Services (GATS) is of most importance in the field of services negotiations under WTO. In terms of health services, the impact of GATS has not yet been as visible or as important as the movement and migration of health professionals that have taken place as part of a broader globalization process and agenda. In Thailand, for example, external migration of health professionals has occurred without major influence by GATS (Wibulpolprasert, 2004). However, it is clear that this is considered a potential area where services trade could be further liberalized, with arguments by proponents of liberalization of services discussing, for example, how in the United States health insurance policies impede trade in health services and the potential savings from sending patients abroad for treatment (Mattoo & Rathindran, 2006).

Whereas the mobility of workforces from poorer countries to rich countries can be seen as a trading opportunity with positive implications for national economies in the form of remittances, the consequences of reduced professional workforces resulting from external and internal "brain drains" can be devastating to health systems, in particular, in poorer and less resourced areas. A study by the International Labour Organization (ILO) has drawn attention to the role of global recruitment agencies in the process (Kuptsch, 2006). Although the limits of ethical and practice guidelines on their own for retaining workforce in developing countries are known (Willet &

---

[2] The ISO is in many ways a hybrid organization that can also be seen as part of global private-sector governance with close engagement with business and industries. Its members are national standard-setting agencies, which can be public service agencies or formed by member associations, including companies or representatives of particular industries.

Martineau, 2004), the WHO (2010) Global Code of Practice on the International Recruitment of Health Personnel has provided global-level guidance.

Interest in further liberalization of services is now focused on health tourism[3,4] and the mobility of health professionals, in particular, provision of services by individuals temporarily in the country.[5] The interest in these areas is currently greater in developing countries, with commercial interests in both health tourism and sending health professionals abroad. Health tourism is enabled by the portability of health insurance benefits to other countries, as well as the scope for more commercialized services (such as cosmetic surgery) at the margins or outside the obligations of national health systems. Unless there is substantial oversupply of health professionals within a country, health tourism tends to draw professionals away from where they are needed and can lead to shortages of those with specific skills because these are in demand in the more commercialized health sector.

Another area of interest is cross-border trade in services as new technologies allow images and data to be transferred through various telemedicine or e-health channels such as the World Wide Web or email. This sector includes selling services in processing and interpretation of scans, x-rays, or laboratory samples and specimens. The shifting of clinical trials to developing countries may contribute financial resources and capacities to those countries but can draw skilled health personnel away from other clinical work. Whereas proponents of the liberalization of trade in health services welcome such developments as a way that developing countries can generate income and the developed world can cut research costs, this process creates both systemic and ethical concerns when health systems become increasingly driven or influenced by the commodification and commercialization of healthcare.

Services chapters in trade agreements and trade agreements on services (e.g., GATS and TiSA) can have relevance to domestic policies, including on regulation, rights, and redistribution within health systems. In GATS, implications to domestic regulation depend on whether a member state has included the services sector within its commitments (Fidler et al., 2003). It has been pointed out, for example, that cost containment may not be considered to be a sufficient ground for government intervention to limit patient choice (Luff, 2003). Concerns over subsidies and, in particular, equity aspects of health systems have also been raised. Although trade in health services is often promoted as a means for more effective health services, a more likely direct consequence is cost escalation as a result of increasing administrative costs, more constrained scope for national regulation, and limitations to scope for cost containment within health systems. The portability of health insurance is one example where there are pressures to change the basis of reimbursement practices to enable trade (Mattoo & Rathindran, 2006).

New-generation trade agreements, such as CETA, TiSA, and CPTPP, have continued negotiations on services further from GATS and have introduced new, more overarching elements. For example, in CETA, governments are to list which services they wish to exclude, in contrast to those they wish to include in GATS. The changing context of negotiations raises ethical questions because anything that has not been explicitly excluded is included under the agreement. Furthermore, investment chapters are often based on a different logic and general inclusion of all services under investment protection. Thus, even when a government would have explicitly excluded health services from services chapters, investment-protection provisions could still apply.

Investment Protection and Liberalization

Investment chapters have emerged under the new-generation trade agreements. The key ethical concern with investment agreements is the way in which these strengthen the position and interests of transnational investors and industries not only through obligations but also as a result of claims for compensation.

Investment protection has created substantial criticism with a number of ethical concerns because it allows investors to claim for compensation from legitimate public regulatory and policy measures and creates new rights for investors (Bonnitcha et al., 2017). The increasing number of cases that corporations have lost against high-income countries has been seen as an example of using investment arbitration claims against regulation to achieve so-called regulatory chill (Pelc, 2017).

---

[3] The latest draft code is available as an annex to WHO Executive Board Document EB 126/8, available from the WHO website: http://apps.who.int/gb/ebwha/pdf_files/EB126/B126_8-en.pdf.

[4] In GATS Mode 2, Consumption of Services Abroad.

[5] In GATS Mode 4, Movement of Natural Persons from One Country to Provide a Service in Another Country.

Investment protection gained wider attention as result of Philip Morris' complaints against Uruguay's and Australia's plain packaging legislation (Permanent Court of Arbitration [PCA], 2017; *Philip Morris v. Uruguay*, 2016). On medicines, Eli Lilly has made a complaint against Canada on patentability (*Eli Lilly v. Canada*, 2017). In the European Union, Slovakia was taken into arbitration when it removed profiteering from its publicly funded healthcare (*Achmea v. Slovakia*, 2012). The pattern of claims supports articulation of claims as means to seek "chill." In addition, closely related cases have concerned permissions to waste sites, water, occupational health and safety, mines, and regulation of chemical products.

Investment protection has been under growing criticism on the ground of individual cases but also in terms of a system moving power from public courts to less transparent private-sector arbitration (Koskenniemi, 2017; Howse, 2017). In addition, UN Special Rapporteur on Human Rights A. Zayas (UN, 2016) has called for a moratorium on investment protection negotiations on the ground of concerns with respect to human rights.

IP Rights

IP rights and their relationship to pharmaceutical policies have been perhaps the most discussed health policy aspect of trade policies globally, and they raise various ethical concerns, including with respect to human rights.[6] This is reflected in the focus of human rights advocates and special rapporteurs on the terms of particular trade agreements (Hunt, 2006) and in relation to access to medicines in developing countries (UN, 2009a). In October 2009, the Human Rights Council unanimously adopted a resolution on access to medicines (UN, 2009b). Another issue is how enforcement of IP rights as private rights – as recognized in the Preamble of the Trade-Related Aspects of Intellectual Property Rights (TRIPS) Agreement – has become an issue within public policies and in the allocation of public resources. In general, three main concerns can be raised with respect to health policies and protection of IP rights. The first emphasizes transparency and access to knowledge and information, the second focuses on the pricing of new innovations, and the third centers on incentives that international agreements provide for innovation and, in particular, innovation on the

basis of health needs. These are issues that affect health policies in all countries.

Whereas concerns of developing countries have become more legitimate in relation to the TRIPS Agreement, bilateral agreements have further changed the ground for debates in introducing provisions and measures that were not considered as part of multilateral negotiations (Fink & Reichenmiller, 2005; Roffe & Spennemann, 2006). Ethical issues at the core of both health and trade policies have also been dealt with as part of the WHO Intergovernmental Working Group (IGWG) negotiations on IP rights and innovation (WHO, 2008).

The protection of IP rights has become reflected also in measures against counterfeiting and theft of IP. At the core of these considerations is how and what are understood to imply counterfeiting. This issue is not new, and the WHO has been engaged with it since the 1980s, but it has gained more importance because of negotiations affecting enforcement of IP rights. Although no one denies the problem of substandard and false medicines, there remains a broad disagreement in terms of appropriate measures and focus of action, particularly because a significant number of health concerns relate to legitimate but substandard products in developing countries (Caudron et al., 2008). The balance between interests of rights holders and those of consumers is likely to be reflected more prominently on the trade and health agenda of all countries in the future. Particular attention has been drawn to the high prices of cancer medicines globally (WHO, 2018). Furthermore, the failure of current incentive system to support research and development of new antimicrobials is gaining increasing traction because of broader, more systemic risks.

IP rights provisions were also at the core of investment arbitration claims concerning tobacco plain packaging. IP rights thus relate to wider public health policy issues than medicines only.

Governance

Global governance on trade and economic policies has implications for health and social policies as well as for the scope and nature of measures that can be implemented at a national level. Global trade agreements regulate measures that governments can take without impeding trade and measures they are required to take to protect commercial rights. While trade agreements such as GATS do recognize governments' right to regulate, this is complemented by the

---

[6] In GATS Mode 1, Cross-Border Trade in Services.

requirement that regulatory measures fit within the scope of given agreements, which, while not limiting regulation as such, implies a modification in *how* governments can regulate.

The shift from trade in goods to trade in services and investment defines how risks are shared between corporate and public actors both within and between countries, with implications for national policies in all countries. This issue is reflected in the *Report of the Commission of Experts of the President of the United Nations General Assembly on Reforms of the International Monetary and Financial System* (UN, 2009b) assessment on capital and financial markets liberalization, GATS, and developing countries, stating:

> Capital and financial market liberalization, pushed not only by the IMF [International Monetary Fund], but also within certain trade agreements, exposed developing countries to more risk and has contributed to the rapid spread of the crisis around the world. In particular, trade-related financial services liberalization has been advanced under the rubric of the WTO's General Agreement on Trade in Services (GATS) Financial Services Agreement with insufficient regard for its consequences either for growth or stability. Externalities exerted by the volatility in the financial sector have severe negative effects on all areas of the economy and are an impediment to a stable development path.
>
> *(United Nations, 2009b: 103, paragraph 89)*

Whereas member state commitments in GATS can be changed, these changes need to be compensated by extending others. This "locking-in" feature has drawn criticism toward GATS in restricting the regulatory scope of governments in sectors they have included in the agreement and making it more difficult or costly to change this. The problem of locking in also applies to new-generation trade agreements because agreements of large trading blocs make changes more difficult.

The implications of broader global economic governance for global health policies are important because they affect how social determinants of health are shaped and what kinds of overall public policies are possible. If trade policies and agreements enable conditions where financial and economic crises are more probable with consequent government indebtedness and austerity measures, this can have major impacts on national health systems and policies. Furthermore, they do not settle issues where major

conflicts of interests remain between particular corporate policies and health policy interests, for example, between the interests of commercial health services providers or between the pharmaceutical industry and government health policy priorities. By contrast, the relevance and scope for taking into account global health policy considerations may be much greater within the WTO context than has been assumed. Pauwelyn (2003) has argued that because WTO agreements are framework agreements, their provisions may need to give way to, for example, more specific global agreements in particular areas, such as health or the environment.

In principle, a case can be made for strengthening global regulatory frameworks for health and rights to regulate for health and health policy interests and concerns beyond the traditional focus on epidemics and public health to include, for example, alcohol, pharmaceutical policies, nutritional contents of food, recruitment of a health workforce, and ensuring risk and resource sharing in health systems in the context of global health policies. The Tobacco Framework Convention and the IHRs remain the primary examples of implementing a legal public health framework globally. However, there is further scope to strengthen global governance for health through human rights and negotiation of international agreements for health (Gostin et al., 2011; Koivusalo & Pereduhoff, 2018).

Impact of Governance on Health

In terms of health more specifically, three aspects of governance and policymaking can be disentangled where more specific arguments and implications can be revealed. First, global trade policies and regulation affect the grounds on which, and how, health-related standards are set that affect trade and policies in other sectors, both at national and at global levels. Furthermore, trade interests and increasingly global trade policy interests in standard-setting enhance the tendency to shift decision making toward more corporate-driven bodies and arrangements that are not appropriate for regulatory decisions for health and consumer concerns.

Second, trade policies and decisions made in the sphere of trade increasingly affect health policies, as well as resources and national regulatory policy space within the health sector. This "creeping" impact of economic and trade policy priorities to govern and shape policies in other sectors on the basis of global or regional agreements is of particular importance in areas where national governance is decentralized or regionalized, making it more difficult to observe and recognize "national regulatory interests" in the area. Trade creep in health policies has also been cushioned by ignorance, assumed nonrelevance, and the fact that healthcare reforms have changed the more traditional organization of healthcare within many countries. Governance issues herein relate not only to prospects and the potential of ministries of health to engage more with trade negotiations but also affect politics and pressures at the global level and in relation to the competence of different international organizations.

The third aspect relates to trade negotiation practices and democratic decision making. This is of importance regarding lack of clarity both with respect to more specific implications of these agreements and with respect to implications from overall negotiation processes. Whereas agreements are considered to be single undertakings, where nothing is agreed on until all aspects are agreed on, the scope for "horse trading" across a number of these issues and sectors makes clarity and accountability difficult. Yet it is essential to democratic accountability that informed decisions are made understanding the extent and nature of commitments made, in particular, whether these commitments are enforceable and difficult to renegotiate later. Furthermore, the inclusion of investment protection, regulatory cooperation, and more overarching services and investment liberalization increases complexity and shifts accountability toward the commercial sector and foreign investors.

Whereas GATS provides leeway for governments in terms of deciding the sectors they wish to include and time-bound exceptions, in relation, TRIPS policy space needs to be sought for exceptions and provisions made for flexibility, for example, in the form of compulsory licensing. The Doha Declaration on public health was useful in confirming the scope for compulsory licensing and removing more narrow interpretations, but it did not change provisions or solve more systemic concerns. In GATS, the classification of services has been sufficiently unclear to cause unanticipated commitments, as was shown in the dispute-settlement case on gambling, where the United States did not interpret gambling and betting services as included with other recreational services in the GATS Agreement (WTO, 2005). The so-called public services exception in GATS on exclusion of services supplied in the exercise of governmental authority is expressed narrowly and

would not, on the basis of current interpretations of the treaty, include publicly funded but outsourced services (Fidler et al., 2003; Krajewski, 2003). Yet these types of exceptions are still used in negotiations of new-generation trade agreements (Koivusalo, 2014).

In addition to interpretational issues and lack of clarity regarding what is implied, trade negotiations also tend to use mechanisms that may deliberately lead to more extensive commitments than would have been sought otherwise. Whereas such practices have also been promoted in the context of multilateral negotiations of GATS, they are more obvious in the field of bilateral negotiations and new-generation trade agreements. Bilateral and plurilateral negotiations may use different structures and provisions, making it harder to understand how commitments have changed in comparison with GATS. This has been the case, for example, with respect to the EU–CARIFORUM partnership agreement (EU–CARIFORUM, 2008). The EU–Mexico Free Trade Agreement is an example of expansion of commitments because it also covers government procurement and investment and commits the European Union and Mexico not to enact legislation that would be more trade restrictive than is presently in force in their service sectors (EU–Mexico FTA, 2001). Furthermore, the new negotiation proposal includes investment protection as part of the investment chapter (EU–Mexico FTA, 2018). The legal language and nature of provisions often make it hard for ministries of health to understand particular implications of trade agreements with a higher probability of making more extensive commitments than intended. This is the case, in particular, for provisions that do not change current legislation but affect future regulatory policy space. These inadvertent inclusions in trade agreements "outside own priority setting" can be called *OOPS commitments* because the scope and extent of commitments are not realized by those to whom they will accrue at the time when they are made (Koivusalo et al., 2009).

Conclusion

In this chapter, I have tracked matters concerning trade and health and sought to raise issues that are of importance to the relationship between trade and health, in particular where there are conflicts of interests or priorities. Trade-related requirements may push countries toward compliance and enhance public health aims when regulatory capacity in health is nonexistent, inadequate, overwhelmed, or captured by strong national industries. However, these situations tend to reflect the failure of health policies to gain sufficient ground in the first place. The real challenge for health and trade policies is the extent to which trade interests and policies sought in the name of these interests may – intentionally or unintentionally – systemically undermine health-related regulatory priorities and practice. Furthermore, the realization of the benefits of economic growth and interconnectedness between countries is not independent of public policies and the ability to implement them.

The required emphasis on the ethics of public policies is too often displaced by a more narrow discussion of medical ethics, which is limited to the context of individuals and professional practice. There is therefore failure to address the following ethical dilemmas of public policies:

1. The ethical consideration of interrelationships between current global policies concerning commercial rights, on the one hand, and realization of human and social rights, on the other. This includes (a) cases where trade-related interests of particular interest groups differ or can be in conflict with health policy priorities; (b) the ethical aspects of the promotion of public or population health; and (c) broad notions of health protection and human security.

2. The ethical basis of current trade policies and expansion of commercial law globally and its relationship to national or regional capacities to address socioeconomic inequalities and vulnerability, including measures affecting the social determinants of health, and the ethical basis for the relationship between health and trade policies and governance, legitimacy, and accountability.

3. The ethical dilemmas associated with the implications of trade agreements for the cost-containment and equity aspects of health systems and on their organization and financing and the implications of trade policies for private and public sectors and how risks, responsibilities, administrative burdens, and burden of proof are shared between the public and private sectors.

The emphasis on public policies and international aspects of ethical concerns also raises crucial questions about global policy priorities in the context of trade and health and why a better balance between different aims and priorities needs to be sought. Why should IP rights be more important than rights to access to treatment? If health policy concerns would be paramount in pharmaceutical policies, what would this imply for research and development? Are IP rights the appropriate incentives for problem-based research and development? Why should the fair treatment of corporate actors within health services globally be more important than ensuring fair treatment of people within health systems? Why should all products or providers of services be treated similarly if, in practice, this favors global actors over local ones or undermines environmental and labor conditions of production? To what extent are health regulations "hijacked" by important interest groups? What kinds of health and public policy assumptions are taken as given in trade policies? Why has investment protection been included as part of trade agreements?

The recognition of conflicts of interests between trade and health policies is not a call for unrestricted protectionism but for better global governance on health and trade and recognition of the systemic implications, conflicting interests, country-specific concerns, and most important, a willingness to act on the challenges at all levels of governance.

References

Achmea v. Slovakia (2012). Final Award, December 7, 2012. Available at www.italaw.com/sites/default/files/case-documents/italaw3206.pdf.

Anderson, K., & Martin, W. (2005). *Agricultural Trade Reform and the Doha Development Agenda*. Washington, DC: World Bank.

Bettcher, D. W., Yach, D., & Guindon, G. E. (2000). Global trade and health: key linkages and future challenges. *Bulletin of the World Health Organization* **78**, 521–531.

Bialious, S. A., & Yach, D. (2001). Whose standard is it anyway? How the tobacco industry determines the International Organisation for Standardisation (ISO) standards for tobacco and tobacco products. *Tobacco Control* **10**, 96–104.

Birdsall, N. (2006). *The World Is Not Flat: Inequality and Injustice in Our Global Economy*. Helsinki: World Institute for Development Economics Research.

Bonnitcha, J., Poulsen, L. S., & Waibel, M. (2017). *The Political Economy of the Investment Treaty Regime*. Oxford, UK: Oxford University Press.

Caplan, A., Dominguez-Gil, B., Matesanz, R., & Prior, C. (2009). *Trafficking of Organs, Tissues and Cells and Trafficking in Human Beings for the Purpose of the Removal of Organs* (Joint Council of Europe/United Nations Study). Strasbourg: Directorate General of Human Rights and Legal Affairs, Council of Europe.

Caudron, J.-M., Ford, N., Henkens, M., et al. (2008). Substandard medicines in resource-poor settings: a problem that can no longer be ignored. *Journal of Tropical and International Health* **13**, 1062–1072.

Comprehensive Economic Trade Agreement (CETA) (2017). *Comprehensive Economic and Trade Agreement (CETA)*. Available at http://ec.europa.eu/trade/policy/in-focus/ceta/ceta-chapter-by-chapter/.

Epps, T. (2008). *International Trade and Health Protection: A Critical Assessment of the WTO's SPS Agreement.* Cheltenham, UK: Elgar International Economic Law.

EU–CARIFORUM (2008). Economic partnerships agreement between the CARIFORUM states, of the one part, and the European Union, on the other part. *Official Journal of the European Union* 30.10.2008, L 289/I/3.

EU–Mexico FTA (2001). European Union–Mexico Free Trade Agreement. Available at www.worldtradelaw.net/fta/agreements/eftamexfta.pdf.

EU–Mexico FTA (2018). Agreement in Principle. Available at http://trade.ec.europa.eu/doclib/press/index.cfm?id=1833.

Fidler, D. (1997). Trade and health: the global spread of disease and international trade. *German Yearbook of International Law* **40**, 300–305.

Fidler, D., Correa, C., & Oginam, A. (2003). *Legal Review of the General Agreement on Trade in Services (GATS) from a Health Policy Perspective* (Globalisation, Trade and Health Working Paper Series). Geneva: WHO.

Fink, C., & Reichenmiller, P. (2005). *Tightening TRIPS: The Intellectual Property Provisions of Recent US Free Trade Agreements* (Trade Note No. 20). Washington, DC: World Bank.

Fitter, R., & Kaplinsky, R. (2001). *Who Gains from Product Rents as Coffee Market Becomes More Differentiated.* Brighton, UK: Institute of Development Studies.

Food and Agriculture Organization (FAO) (2003). *Trade Reforms and Food Security: Conceptualising the Linkages.* Rome: FAO.

Food and Agriculture Organization (FAO) (2009). *The State of Food Insecurity in the World.* Rome: FAO.

Gostin, L. O., Friedman, E. A., Ooms, G., et al. (2011) The Joint Action and Learning Initiative: towards a global agreement on national and global responsibilities for health. *PLoS Medicine* **8**(5), e1001031. https://doi.org/10.1371/journal.pmed.1001031.

Howse, R. (2017) Designing multilateral investment court: issues and options. *Yearbook of European Law* **2017**, 1–28.

Hunt, P. (2006). The human right to the highest attainable standard of health: new opportunities and challenges.

Transactions of the Royal Society of Tropical Medicine and Hygiene **100**, 603–607.

Eli-Lilly v. Canada (2017). *Eli Lilly and Company v. Government of Canada.* Nations Commission on International Trade Law, ICSID Case No. UNCT/14/2. Available at www.italaw.com/cases/1625.

Koivusalo, M. (1999). *WTO and Trade-Creep in Health and Social Policies* (GASPP Occasional Papers No. 4). Helsinki: National Research and Development Centre for Welfare and Health.

Koivusalo, M., Labonté, R., & Schrecker, T. (2009). Globalization and policy space for health and social determinants of health, in Labonté, R., Schrecker, T., Packer, C., & Runnels, V. (eds.), *Globalization and Health: Pathways, Evidence, and Policy.* New York: Routledge.

Koivusalo, M. (2014). Policy space for health and trade and investment agreements. *Health Promotion International* **29** (Suppl. 1), i29–i47. https://doi.org/10.1093/heapro/dau033.

Koivusalo, M., & Pereduhoff, K. (2018). What future for global health governance and right to health in the era of new generation trade and investment agreements? *Global Health Governance* **XII**(1), 116–125.

Koskenniemi, M. (2017). It's not the cases, it's the system. *Journal of World Investment and Trade* **18**, 343–352.

Krajewski, M. (2003). Public services and trade liberalisation: mapping the legal framework. *International Journal of Economic Law* **6**, 341–367.

Kuptsch, C. (ed.) (2006). *Merchants of Labour.* Geneva: International Labour Organization.

Lang, T. (2004). *Food Industrialisation and Food Power: Implications for Food Governance* (IIED Gatekeeper Series No. 114). London: International Institute for Environment and Development.

Luff, F. (2003). Regulation of health services and international trade law, in Mattoo, A., & Sauve, P. (eds.), *Domestic Regulation and Service Trade Liberalisation.* New York: World Bank and Oxford University Press.

Mattoo, A., & Rathindran, R. (2006). How health insurance inhibits trade in health care. *Health Affairs* **25**, 358–368.

Ofodile, U. (2009). Import (toy) safety, consumer protection and the WTO Agreement on Technical Barriers to Trade: prospects, progress and problems. *International Journal of Private Law* **2**, 163–184.

Pauwelyn, J. (2003). *Conflict of Norms in Public International Law. How WTO Law Relates to Other Rules of International Law.* Cambridge, UK: Cambridge University Press.

Permanent Court of Arbitration (PCA) (2017). *Philip Morris Asia Limited (Hong Kong) v. The Commonwealth of Australia.* Available at www.pcacases.com/web/view/5.

Pelc, K. (2017) What explains the low success rate of investor–state disputes? *International Organization* **71**(3), 559–583. https://doi.org/10.1017/S0020818317000212.

Philip Morris v. Uruguay (2016). *Philip Morris Brands Sàrl, Philip Morris Products S.A. and Abal Hermanos S. A. v. Oriental Republic of Uruguay (formerly FTR Holding SA, Philip Morris Products S.A. and Abal Hermanos S. A. v. Oriental Republic of Uruguay).* ICSID Case No. ARB/ 10/7, July 8. Available at www.italaw.com/sites/default/files/ case-documents/italaw7417.pdf.

Rodrik, D. (2018). What do trade agreements really do? *Journal of Economic Perspectives.* **23** (2), 73-90. Available at https://j.mp/2EsEOPk

Roffe, P., & Spennemann, C. (2006). The impact of FTAs on public health policies and TRIPS flexibilities. *International Journal of Intellectual Property Management* **1**, 75–93.

Scheper-Hughes, N. (2000). The global traffic in human organs. *Current Anthropology* **41**, 191–208.

Sell, S. (2008). The global IP upward ratchet, anti-counterfeiting and piracy enforcement efforts: the state of play. Available at www.twnside.org.sg/title2/intellectual_ property/development.research/SusanSellfinalversion.pdf.

Swinburn, B., Kraak, V., & Allenden, S. (2019) The global syndemic of obesity, undernutrition, and climate change: The Lancet Commission report. *Lancet* **393**, 791–846

United Nations (2009). Access to Medicine in the Context of the Right of Everyone to the Enjoyment of the Highest Attainable Standard of Physical and Mental Health, resolution adopted by the Human Rights Council. A/ HRC/ RES/12/24. Available at https://ap.ohchr.org/documents/all docs.aspx?doc_id=16180.

United Nations (2009b). *Report of the Commission of Experts of the President of the United Nations General Assembly on Reforms of the International Monetary and Financial System.* New York: United Nations.

United Nations (2016). *Report of the Independent Expert A de Zayas on the Promotion of a Democratic and Equitable International Order.* A/HRC/33/40. Available at https://do cuments-dds-ny.un.org/doc/UNDOC/GEN/G16/151/19/P DF/G1615119.pdf?OpenElement.

US Trade Representative (USTR) (2018). *National Trade Estimate Report on Foreign Trade Barriers.* Washington, DC: Office of USTR.

Veggeland, F., & Borgen, S. O. (2005). Negotiating international food standards: the World Trade Organization's impact on the Codex Alimentarius Commission. *Governance: An International Journal of Policy, Administration and Institutions* **18**, 675–708.

Wibulpolprasert, S., Pachanee, C., Pitayarangsarit, S., & Hempisut, P. (2004). International service trade and its implications for human resources for health: a case study of Thailand. *Human Resources for Health* **2**, 10. https://doi.org /10.1186/1478–4491-2-10.

Willetts, A., & Martinea, T. (2004). *Ethical International Recruitment of Health Professionals: Will Codes of Practice Protect Developing Country Health Systems?* Version 1.1, January. Available at www.liv.ac.uk/lstm/research/docu ments/codesofpracticereport.pdf.

World Health Assembly (WHA) (2008). Global Strategy and Plan of Action on Public Health, Innovation and Intellectual Property (Resolution 61.21, Annex). Geneva: WHO.

World Health Organization (WHO) (2007). *World Health Report.* Geneva: WHO.

World Health Organization (WHO) (2010). WHO Global Code of Practice on the International Recruitment of Health Personnel (WHA 63), May 16. Geneva: WHO. Available at www.who.int/hrh/migration/code/code_en.pdf?ua=1.

World Health Organization (WHO) (2018) Access to medicines, vaccines and pharmaceuticals. pricing of cancer medicines and its impacts. Technical report. Geneva: WHO.

World Trade Organization (WTO) (1998). EC measures concerning meat and meat products (hormones). Appellate body report, WT/DS26AB/R, January 16. Geneva: WTO.

World Trade Organization (WTO) (2005). United States: measures affecting the cross-border supply of gambling and betting services. WT/DS285/ AB/R, April 7. Geneva: WTO.

World Trade Organization (WTO) (2006). Committee on Technical Barriers to Trade. Notification, G/TBT/N/ THA/ 215, October 10, 2006. Geneva: WTO.

World Trade Organization (WTO) (2008). Committee on Technical Barriers to Trade. Minutes of the meeting of 9 November, G/TBT/M/43, January 21. Geneva: WTO.

Debt, Structural Adjustment, and Health

Jeff Rudin and David Sanders[*]

Introduction

The debt narrative is encapsulated in the conundrum of why postapartheid South Africa chose to cripple itself with debts that it could so easily have repudiated. Nelson Mandela described the apartheid debt as "the greatest single obstacle to progress in this country." He explained further:

> We are limited in South Africa because our democratic government inherited a debt, which we were servicing at the rate of 30 billion rand a year. That is 30 billion we did not have to build houses, to make sure our children go to schools and to ensure that everybody has the dignity of having a job and a decent income.
>
> *(Malala, 2003; Action for South Africa [ACTSA],*
> *2003)*

Given that debt accumulated by the apartheid system is a striking example of odious debt, the new democratic South Africa had compelling legal and ethical reasons for disowning it[1] (Rudin, 1999, 2002).

Rather than disown the odious debt, the government actively sought to undermine Jubilee South Africa, the campaign founded to repudiate the apartheid debt (*Business Report Sunday* (SA), November 6 and 22, 1998).

Moreover, it is arguable that few governments or other creditors would have insisted on Mandela's South Africa repaying odious apartheid debts at the expense of the newly liberated black majority. Additionally, South Africa is far from being a poor country. These considerations put South Africa in a

far stronger position to resist the debt burden than most other peripheral countries.

Before attempting to make sense of this conundrum of South Africa's debt, a few preliminary comments are apposite.

Our understanding of the world is of a global economic system characterized by interactions between countries of grossly uneven economic development and political power such that the system can be described as having a "core" or center comprising the most developed and powerful countries and a "periphery" made up of all the others.[2] This typology is preferred to geographic terms that are either anachronistic (the *West*) or inaccurate (*North/South*). The idea of a *third world* is also anachronistic, whereas *developed/developing* suggests that countries that are not "developed" are "developing," even when they are either stagnant or moving backwards mainly as a result of their historical and current position in the global economic architecture. For the purposes of this chapter, the principal core countries are the United States, Canada, the European Union (EU) countries of Western Europe, and Japan – but it should be noted that cores and peripheries also exist within countries.

Numbers That Don't Add Up

To appreciate the magnitude of current debt, a comparison should be made with the Marshall Plan, the grants provided by the United States that contributed significantly to the post–World War II reconstruction of Europe. In today's terms, the Marshall Plan provided aid of some $100 billion. By comparison, in 2007, the total external debt for countries of the periphery was estimated to be $3,360 billion. Between 1970 and 2007, this debt increased 4,800%, and the amount repaid during this period – $7,150 billion – was 102 times greater than what was owed in 1970. In

---

[*] David Sanders died on August 30, 2019.

[1] The *doctrine of odious debt* reverses normal international law, in which incoming governments unconditionally honor the debts incurred by their predecessors. The doctrine applies to debts incurred by illegitimate regimes for purposes of defending and/or enhancing their illegitimacy when, additionally, such illegitimacy is known, or ought to have been known, by the creditors.

[2] The terms *center*, *core*, and *periphery* derive from Frank (1967, 1969).

2007, the latest year for which information is available, the countries of the periphery repaid $520 billion, of which $198 billion was public debt.[3] In the same year, the governments of countries in the periphery received $169 billion in new public loans. This translates to a net loss of $29 billion to the countries supposedly benefiting from the very loans that give rise to the debt repayments.

In addition to noting that this difference amounts to a profit of $460 billion to the foreign creditors, this outward flow forces a critical examination of what is universally described as "aid" in its various forms. Official development aid (ODA) from the core and the countries immediately around the center totaled $104 billion in 2007. In the same year, the countries of the periphery spent $800 billion servicing – paying off the amount originally loaned plus interest charges – their external and internal debt (Toussaint & Millet, 2009: 18, 34, 101–109).

Between 1970 and 2007, Sub-Saharan Africa, the poorest region in the world, repaid $350 billion in debt. It owed $190 billion in 2007 and repaid $17 billion. The $190 billion owed was more than the total gross domestic product (GDP) of Africa's 36 poorest countries combined, whereas the $350 billion that has been repaid is larger than South Africa's 2009 GDP; it is also larger than the combined GDPs of 50 of Sub-Saharan Africa's 53 countries. In 2000, Mozambique's per capita external debt was almost seven times the GNP per capita, Angola's was almost four times, and Tanzania's and Zambia's debts were twice their per capita GDP (Toussaint & Millet, 2009: 102, 107, 108; *Business Report* (SA), August 8, 2000). Clearly, debt of this magnitude undermines economic and other development.

These numbers should be contrasted with the almost $13,000 billion the US government alone has made available with its various emergency measures during the 2008–2009 economic crisis (Bloomberg. com, March 31, 2009).

We understand debt to be the result of corporate and geopolitical imperatives. However, most individuals associated with debt are probably unaware of the harm they were causing. But there are others who have lost all sense of decency and who are keenly aware of what they do and who seemingly care little about the consequences for others.

---

[3] *Public debt* is defined as money (or credit) owed by any level of government, either central government, federal government, municipal government, or local government.

The Etiology of Debt and Its Morbidity

Too Much Money

How did we get to the position conveyed by the above-mentioned data? In recounting the history of poor country debt, we will say nothing about the debt crises of the nineteenth and early twentieth century or deal in any depth with what form remedies may take today for the now-acknowledged debt crisis. Rather, we shall provide a highly condensed summary of the origins of today's debt debacle with only passing references to how these origins link to the present. Our main focus is on the perversity of debt and the ways in which its effects impact health (see also George, 1988).

The background causes of the debt crisis of the early 1980s are largely uncontroversial. By the beginning of the 1970s, Europe was awash with money seeking profitable outlets. The previously mentioned Marshall Plan aid had locked a large number of dollars into Europe – the eurodollars. These were followed in 1973 by the "petrodollars" placed in US and European banks by Middle Eastern oil potentates following the superprofits from the then-huge increase in the price of oil. This "surplus" money was offered at preferential and exceedingly low rates to countries of the periphery, many of which had only recently become independent and were eager to commence with the development denied them during colonialism.

It was only in 1979 when the United States began a major policy shift, cemented in 1981 by the election of Ronald Reagan, that US nominal interest rates were increased sharply to attract foreign investment into the United States. Real interest rates (i.e., minus inflation) jumped from –1% in 1978 to +9% in 1982 (Hanlon, 2000: 877). From a nominal rate (i.e., with inflation) of about 5% in 1973, they shot up to 18.9% in 1981. European banks followed suit to counter what would have otherwise been a US competitive advantage.

Countries of the periphery were adversely affected by two factors. First, interest rates on their foreign debt increased from about 4%–5% in the 1970s to 16%–18%. Second, because most of their loans were in hard currencies earned by exports, the collapse of commodity prices, especially oil in 1981, led to a debt crisis in Mexico, a major oil exporter. In August 1982, Mexico was the first country unable to meet its debt obligations. Argentina and Brazil followed in quick succession. All indebted countries in Africa and Latin

America and several Asian countries met the same fate (all interest rates quoted are from Toussaint & Millet [2009: 53–55]).

The Banks Come First

Faced with defaulting debtors, the banks – principally the International Monetary Fund (IMF) and the World Bank, which took over many of the loans made by commercial banks – did what banks always do, regardless of whether their client is a country or a person: they took steps to protect their money. Besides either rolling over the debt or making a further loan to make repayment on the original one possible, these institutions set a number of preconditions before any rescue could happen. To earn the hard currency required for their debt repayment, the banks insisted on priority being given to exports. The banks also insisted on what for them was prudent practice through (1) reducing government expenditure by minimizing budget deficits and hence the need for government borrowing and (2) cutting government's social expenditures by removing subsidies on basic foods, introducing user charges for services previously provided for free, and freezing civil service pay along with reducing the number of public servants – and all this in order that more could be spent on servicing the debt. The ensuing "fiscal discipline" would additionally address inflation, which had become another concern.

The banks, eager to find new investment outlets and accepting the then-prevailing Reagan/Thatcher antipathy toward the public sector, with its alleged inefficiencies and predilection to corruption, added privatization to their conditions for helping governments in crisis with their debts. The claimed efficiencies, together with the business practices and ethos of privatization, would supposedly create jobs and ease poverty, with the former resulting in greater tax revenue and the latter in reduced government expenditures on the poor; both would enhance the government's ability to repay its debt. Moreover, privatization would attract foreign investment, which would, in turn, further stimulate the economy and thereby facilitate debt repayment. However, a precondition for foreign investment was the ending of controls on capital to facilitate its free flow across the globe. Finally, loans to the defaulters or the countries in trouble with their debt repayments would be paid only in installments, after verification that the banks' requirements were being met.

These conditions are all perfectly explicable in terms of the financial institutions, seeking, not unreasonably, to protect their loans and accordingly placing seemingly reasonable conditions on defaulting governments. The governments, like defaulting individuals, remained at all times free to reject the banks' conditions. All this is standard banking practice. There was no necessary conspiracy involved or ill-will intended.

These various banking requirements are the conditionalities associated with what became known as *structural adjustment programs* (SAPs) designed to reduce debt to a level repayable by each country. It should be noted that SAPs never addressed questions about development, poverty, health, or postwar reconstruction, and few were concerned with the ethical implications associated with their implementation. As with any business, the ethics of SAPs were focused on the bottom line.

SAPs: The Wrong Medicine

Over time, the conditionalities associated with SAPs were incorporated into a range of other programs: the Enhanced Structural Adjustment Program (ESAP), the Heavily Indebted Poor Countries Initiative (HIPC), the Multilateral Debt Relief Initiative (MDRI), Poverty Reduction Strategy Papers (PRSP), and the Poverty Reduction and Growth Facilities (PRGF). The conditionalities themselves have remained essentially unchanged right up to the present day.

What has been the overall effect of these conditionalities? SAPs, in whatever form, have failed to reduce the debt burden. All the creditors and their supporting governments recognized this failure, but only implicitly. Explicitly having acknowledged that the debts could not be paid in full, they have offered to "forgive" part of the debt subject to further formalities. These formalities are SAPs dressed in updated clothing. As Detief Kotte, of the UN Conference on Trade and Development (UNCTAD), said of the HIPC in 2002:

> The IMF & World Bank have changed the words, changed the acronyms, changed their methods of consultation, but they have not changed an iota of their creed.

The failure to ameliorate – let alone cure – the "debt disease" is inherent in the remedy, something that ought to have been apparent at the birth of SAPs in 1982. The main SAPs requirement was then (as now) for each country to prioritize exports. The colonial background of most of the countries of the periphery, however, meant that most of those countries were economically backward, mining and agriculture being the basis of their economies.

The requirement to concentrate on exports meant that the peripheral countries would suffer three clearly predictable outcomes: (1) the market would be flooded, (2) they would unavoidably end up competing amongst themselves, and (3) prices would fall – as a result of the first two outcomes. Falling export prices meant economic disaster for poor countries – and a deeper debt trap. In the absence of money to pay off their debt, countries got deeper into debt because they had to borrow new money to pay off old debts.

The data confirm these predictions: between 1977 and 2001, there was a net fall in the price of all raw materials, dropping about 2.8% annually. Minerals and metals were also affected, with an annual average fall of 1.9%, whereas the prices of silver, tin, and tungsten dropped by more than 5%. Being so dependent on external markets gravely exposed commodity exporters to the vagaries of what was happening in other countries. Thus, between 1997 (the year when Southeast Asia's financial crisis resulted in large-scale economic collapse) and 2001, commodity prices fell by 53% in real terms. Sub-Saharan Africa's debt crisis of the 1980s was significantly precipitated by a 30% fall in commodity prices between 1980 and 1985 (UNCTAD, 2003a, 2003b; Hanlon, 2000: 882).

These examples do not, however, convey the depth of human suffering that lies behind the data. Zambia provides egregious examples of the consequences of both enforced privatization and the more direct human effects of the conditionalities. Copper mining is the Zambian economy. A major test of Zambia's commitment to meet HIPC conditionalities, and thereby have some of its debt forgiven, required Zambia to privatize its copper mines. In early 2000, it sold ZCCM, the company producing 70% of its copper, to the South African corporate giant Anglo-American. This privatization was also intended to unlock bilateral loans, principally £20 million from Great Britain, which had been delayed pending the sale. The privatization resulted in large-scale retrenchment of workers (30% of the workforce, according to the trade union) in a country with already huge unemployment.

Although this forced privatization was to receive debt relief, the World Bank made a further loan available to the Zambian government to finance the workers' layoff. ZCCM had paid for most social services on the copper belt and for Zambia's spending on education and healthcare. Anglo-American refused to take on any ZCCM-funded local schools and hospitals. For its part, Great Britain withheld the promised bilateral loan after the privatisation, saying that it then expected Zambia to root out corruption before it would advance the £20 million loan. Shortly after buying ZCCM, Anglo-American changed its mind because the slump in world copper prices made its involvement unprofitable. ZCCM, sold to Anglo-American at a bargain price, had to be sold again, this time for even less, along with other incentives. Besides a low tax rate, the mines (which use 80% of Zambia's electricity) were guaranteed a fixed price for electricity, at a cost that was 50% below actual cost and for an extended period. A few years later, the price of copper on the world market went sharply upward, but Zambia was still obliged to provide subsidized electricity to the profitable mines (*Business Report* (SA), March 3, 2000, June 4, 2000, July 4, 2000, February 6, 2000; *Mail & Guardian*, July 4, 2000; see also Zulu, 2007).

Noting that Zambia's debt servicing exceeding its annual spending on health, welfare, education, and sanitation projects combined, South Africa's then Finance Minister Trevor Manuel stated in 1999:

> For every dollar that Zambia is able to raise from the Bretton Woods institutions [the IMF and World Bank] they pay out $1.30 in debt settlement. There is something fundamentally wrong with the whole system.
>
> *(G7 has failed in debt relief – Manuel, Reuters, September 20, 1999)*

The IMF suspended Zambia from its HIPC relief program in 2003 because the government had overspent on its 2003–2004 budget. This forced Zambia to increase income tax to 40% and impose a pay freeze. The pay freeze was especially difficult for the nearly half-million public service workers because, besides inflation of 17.2%, the government had been unable to honor its 2003 wage agreement.

As with so many parts of Africa, one worker supports up to 10 other people. In 2004, three-quarters of Zambia's population of 11 million lived below the World Bank's poverty threshold of $1 a day. Before the HIPC, the figure was 50% (in 1990; *Business Report* (SA), October 23, 2000).

Education was also affected by the "prudent financial management and fiscal discipline" required by the World Bank as a condition of Zambia's partial debt forgiveness. Not only were workers not paid, but the budget ceiling imposed on Zambia meant that some 9,000 trained teachers were unemployed while Zambian schools were in desperate need of 9,000 extra teachers! Zambia spent $221 million on education in 2004. In the same year, it spent $247 million on debt servicing (Reuters, 1999; South African Press Association–Agence France Presse (SAPA-AFP), February 5, 2004, February 7, 2004, February 14, 2004, February 19, 2004; *Business Report* (SA), October 23, 2000; Oxfam Press Release, October 1, 2004). Table 12.1 provides some comparative statistics.

In many low-income, highly indebted countries, the low level of spending on social services is explained not only by the high proportion of the budget committed to debt servicing but also by constraints on gaining revenue through taxes and managing a government's budget (fiscal space), usually as a conditionality of debt relief, and the low levels of national wealth, which reflect *inter alia* countries' colonial histories and current positions in the global economy. For instance, only a few years ago, Ethiopia was spending 22% of its national budget on health and education, but this totaled only US$1.50 per capita on health. Even if Ethiopia spent its entire budget on healthcare, it would still not reach the WHO target of US$30–$40 per capita, the amount needed for a basic "package" of health services. Indeed, 31 African countries had annual per capita health expenditures of $20 or less in 2001.

Table 12.1 Portion of Budget Allocated to Basic Social Services and Debt Servicing for the Period 1992–1997

Country	Social services	Debt servicing
Cameroon	4.0 %	36.0 %
Côte d'Ivoire	11.4 %	35.0 %
Kenya	12.6 %	40.0 %
Zambia	6.7 %	40.0 %
Niger	20.4 %	33.0 %
Tanzania	15.0 %	46.0 %
Nicaragua	9.2 %	14.1 %

Source: United Nations Development Program (UNDP), 2000 Poverty Report.

Killing the Patient: SAPs' Health Consequences

The evolution of debt and the resulting macroeconomic reforms have been associated with significant reversals in welfare and health. These impacts have been exhaustively documented in the Report of the Commission on Social Determinants of Health (CSDH) (Commission on Social Determinants of Health [CSDH], 2008). As the CSDH showed, these factors operate at local, national, and, increasingly, global levels.

Historical and contemporary experiences have shown that there is a definite but complex relationship between economic growth and health (see Chapter 1). In general, sustained economic growth leads to improved health and nutritional status: in the now-industrialized countries, large and sustained declines in mortality, morbidity (disease), and malnutrition paralleled economic growth and largely preceded any effective medical interventions. However, improved income distribution – even at low income levels – can accelerate improvements in health – China, Sri Lanka, Costa Rica, and Cuba being examples (Halstead, Walsh, & Warren, 1985). The short-term interrelationship is even more complex. Countries with high (but unequal) growth have been associated with a decline in health status, as reflected by such indicators as infant mortality (e.g., Brazil in the 1970s). There are also cases where economic decline has been associated with significant improvements in health status (e.g., Chile and Tanzania). A detailed understanding of these relationships requires study of the circumstances in which economic changes take place and the context within which health status is determined. However, issues of provision of services and social equity are of primary importance (CSDH, 2008).

Although health-sector inputs may be the most obvious proximal determinants of health status, the effects of upstream and more distal non-health-sector inputs are probably more important. Whereas it is relatively easy to achieve rapid improvements in health, as measured by standard quantitative indicators such as infant mortality rates, sustained improvements in the quality of life are more difficult to produce and measure. For instance, certain indicators, such as infant and young-child mortality rates, may be rapidly improved by selective primary health-care interventions (e.g., immunization) targeted at these high-risk groups. There is, however, little evidence to suggest that improved nutrition levels, for example, can be maintained by the application of such technical packages in the absence of more general improvements in access to resources.

Further, different time frames apply to the appearance of changes in both sets of indicators. For example, whereas changes in food prices and health service utilization rates may occur quite quickly and be readily assessed and documented, changes in mortality and morbidity rates, as well as in nutritional status, are both more problematic to monitor and often become evident only in the medium to long term; short-term changes thus may reflect processes operating before the implementation of imposed conditionalities. Another major problem in assessing the impact of SAPs on health is the poor quality and often unavailability of data on mortality, morbidity, and nutritional status, especially in the poorest countries, where economic decline has often been most severe and debt most debilitating. Finally, especially in Sub-Saharan Africa, it is extremely difficult to disentangle the effects of general economic decline and HIV/AIDS from those of SAPs – although there are analyses that also link the spread of HIV/AIDS in several Sub-Saharan African countries to economic crisis and SAPs (De Vogli & Birbeck, 2005).

Given the foregoing, assessing the impact of structural adjustment on health status requires analyzing the impact of factors operating both within and beyond the health sector, and a range of health indicators must be examined over both the short and long term. These methodological complexities challenge the attribution of health changes to the SAPs themselves and have been invoked in controversies surrounding the welfare effects of these policies. Several studies conducted in the 1980s showing an association between reversals in welfare and health were questioned (Cornia, Jolly, & Stewart, 1988); it was suggested that other contextual factors could explain these phenomena and even that such reversals might have been more dramatic had such economic reforms not been applied (the *counterfactual* argument). A review of the impact of SAPs on child health therefore suggested that future research in this area should use alternative methodologies, including longitudinal study design, to monitor factors likely to have an impact on health (Costello, Watson, & Woodward, 1994).

In 1991, Zimbabwe embarked on a structural adjustment program. The reform package contained the typical elements of World Bank/IMF economic strategies, including trade liberalization, reduction in social expenditure, and devaluation of the currency. In the health sector, user fees were introduced. Concerns were soon expressed that this package would have damaging health impacts because of reduced access to healthcare and growing poverty at the household level. The assertion that previous studies had lacked methodological rigor, together with the opportunity offered by Zimbabwe being a "late" adjuster, prompted the initiation of a carefully designed long-term longitudinal study.

Approximately 600 households, equally divided between a rural area and a high-density working-class periurban suburb, were enrolled in a longitudinal household study in 1993 and reinterviewed in 1994, 1995, 1996, and 1998. Information was gathered on household economic activity, use of health services, and nutritional status of under-five-year-olds. Data based on serial follow-ups suggested that households responded to growing economic hardship by greatly diversifying means of income generation; however, these multiple sources of income did not protect households from growing poverty. Rural areas experienced more hardship than urban areas, and there was evidence of significantly increased income inequality even within relatively homogeneous communities. Health service use was adversely affected by the introduction of user fees, a disturbing increase in childhood malnutrition, and suggested deterioration in the quality of healthcare (Bassett, Bijlmakers, & Sanders, 1997, 2000; Bijlmakers, Bassett, & Sanders, 1999).

Notwithstanding the difficulty in separating the effects of structural adjustment from other variables, the weight of research emphasizes that it often preceded increased disparities in health while exerting both short- and long-term effects on health systems (Labonté et al., 2007).

A Canadian study on Tanzanian health systems found that "[t]he era of structural adjustment may be over, but the effects of earlier damage continue to cast a long shadow" (de Savigny et al., 2004: 56).

A WHO commission, providing the most comprehensive review on structural adjustment and health in Africa, stated:

The majority of studies in Africa, whether theoretical or empirical, are negative towards structural adjustment and its effect on health outcomes.

(Breman & Shelton, 2001)

The final word on the health effects of debt is fittingly linked to the most devastating pandemic in human history. The eminent founding executive director of United Nations Programme on HIV and AIDS (UNAIDS) Peter Piot noted that Africa spends more on debt servicing each year than on health and education – the building blocks of the AIDS response (Piot, 2004).

Making Sense of It All

Everyone Agrees But …

SAPs, in whatever form, have remarkably few supporters. The early comments cited herein emphasize the long-recognized problem of the debt of periphery countries.

In 1969, Nelson Rockefeller alerted the US president of problems accumulating in Latin America:

> Many of the countries are, in effect, having to make new loans to get the foreign exchange to pay interest and amortization on old loans, and at higher interest rates. (Toussaint & Millet 2009: 56)

In the same year, the US General Accounting Office (GAO) warned:

> Many poor countries have already incurred debts past the possibility of repayment. (Ibid.)

Robert McNamara, then president of the World Bank, noted as early as 1972:

> This situation could not go on indefinitely. (Ibid.)

In 2000, the Meltzer Commission (the US Congress on international financial institutions' advisory committee) informed the president:

> The IMF [has] a degree of influence over member countries' policymaking that is unprecedented for a multilateral institution. … These programmes have not ensured economic progress.
> (Toussaint & Millet, 2009: 81)

In 2000, Canadian Prime Minister Paul Martin urged the IMF and World Bank to limit the conditionalities. It "is absurd!" he commented (*Cape Times* (SA), September 26, 2000), to require 160 policy actions by Sao Tome, the nation of 140,000 people, to obtain debt relief.

In 2001, the UN special rapporteur was especially forthright:

> Increasing malnutrition, falling school enrolments and rising unemployment have been attributed to

the policies of structural adjustment. Yet these same institutions continue to prescribe the same medicine as a condition for debt relief, dismissing the overwhelming evidence that Structural Adjustment Programmes have increased poverty.
> (Toussaint & Millet, 2009: 208)

The UN Conference on Trade and Development (UNCTAD) remarked:

> On any objective assessment of two and half decades of standardised packages of "stabilization, liberalisation and privatization", the right kind of growth has simply failed to materialise. (Ibid.)

The Economist, in its Christmas 1999 edition, asked of the just announced enhanced version of the HIPC:

> Who believes in fairy tales?
> (Toussaint & Comanne, 2000)

Susan George, author and long-time campaigner against debt, merits the last word. She observed in 2000:

> If I put forward a hypothesis in physics which is proved wrong by an experiment, I must question the theory. … In economics, you can undermine the existence of millions of people, but none of that human evidence will affect the ideology of structural adjustment. (Toussaint & Millet, 2009: 82)

Given this unanimity of well-informed consensuses on SAPs' unworkability, the obvious question to ask is why the debt burden is still with us? Why has it not been canceled outright, a long time ago? Or, at least, why has most of the debt of most countries not been recognized as unpayable? Why, in other words, is there still need for a chapter such as this one in a book published in 2020? There are three parts to our answer: economic, political, and the status of countries of the periphery.

Moral Hazard

Before addressing these issues, it is necessary to dispose of the argument that debt cannot be canceled because of *moral hazard*. In this view, letting debtors off is an offense against morality and sets a bad precedent. The tortuous invoking of morality is displayed by Horst Kohler, then managing director of the IMF:

> I doubt that simply writing off debt is the best medicine because it could create a nice and cosy feeling that "we are now better off" and reduce the awareness

of African countries (of the need) to tackle their own problems.   (Cape Times (SA), September 10, 2000)

So the debt can't be written off, according to the IMF's leader, because to do so would blind African countries to their own problems. The poor must be tortured for their own good!

However, this issue can be easily disposed of by two considerations. First, core country banks ignored moral hazard when they accepted huge bailouts to prevent their own bankruptcy during the 2008–2009 financial crisis. Second, moral hazard has not prevented debt cancellation, given political will. Core countries have canceled all or large parts of the debt of at least five countries, for example Poland in 1991.

The concept of moral hazard highlights the double standards that plague international debt. Making creditors responsible for their loans is not part of bankers' morality!

SAPs as a Business Opportunity

In 1994, responding to huge pressure from the major transnational corporations (TNCs) of the core countries, the World Trade Organization (WTO) was founded. The WTO, ostensibly created to provide international trade with clear rules, greatly extended the meaning of trade to include investment and services (the latter through the General Agreement on Trade in Services [GATS]). The WTO's real purpose, known to all its members but seldom openly acknowledged, is twofold: to maintain the uneven trade system and to promote a decidedly one-sided understanding of "free trade." More specifically, this means (especially through GATS) liberalization, privatization, and the free flow of capital.

The symmetry and synergy between the WTO and SAPs are striking. Whereas it is arguable that SAPs were initially a straightforward banking response to debt-defaulting countries, its wider "benefits" would soon have become manifest. The enormous growth of finance to its present dominant position within the world economy gives a special importance to SAPs, one that could not have been anticipated in the early 1980s. It would make little sense for the banks to give away, via debt cancellation, what they are struggling to achieve via the WTO and, more especially, GATS. The conclusion is unavoidable: business has a vested interest in perpetuating the debt trap that fuels SAPs and economic liberalization.

The Not So Benign Bankers

The London Agreement of 1953 between Germany and its creditors provides a striking example of what is possible (Rudin, 2003). Germany was responsible for the death and destruction of two world wars. Moreover, unlike the people now being burdened by debt, the German electorate, having voted for Hitler, were directly accountable. Yet the contrast between the London Agreement and the HIPC couldn't be starker:

- Germany was required to pay a maximum of 3.06% of its annual export income on repaying its debt. For the poorest countries on earth, the HIPC requires them to use between 20% and 25% of their export income on debt servicing.
- To qualify for consideration for debt-relief opportunities under the HIPC, a country's total external debt must be on the order of 160% of its GDP. The *debt ratio* is usually considered problematic if it is anything between 80% and 100%, that is, if the debt is equivalent to between 80%–100% of what a country generates annually in its own currency from all economic activities. Germany's debt ratio in 1953 was a mere 21.2%.
- To qualify for consideration under the HIPC, a country's foreign debt must be at least 280% larger than its national budget. Germany's *fiscal debt ratio* in 1953 was 4.9%.
- A HIPC candidate country has three years in which to introduce its particular conditionalities. It then has a further three years in which to demonstrate its good behavior before receiving very limited debt relief. The London Agreement placed no similar conditionalities on Germany.
- What the London Agreement did instead was to place significant conditionalities on the creditors. The London Agreement required three major benefits from creditors. First, creditors had to promote German exports because the debt payments were made entirely from trade surpluses. No trade surplus meant no debt payments; reduced trade surpluses meant reduced debt servicing. Second, the absence of a balance of trade surplus with any of the debtor countries gave Germany the option of imposing import restrictions.
- Finally, creditors had no sanctions against Germany in the event of any German infringement of the agreement. The most that the

177

creditors could expect was the convening of direct negotiations with the option of seeking advice from an appropriate international organization. The HIPC is without even these limited options.

The London Agreement shows that SAPs could be very different. The HIPC, which in any event applies only to a tiny number of countries and even fewer people when compared with the population of the countries of the periphery, testifies to economic and political interests trumping the needs of the people of the periphery.

The Even Less Benign IMF and World Bank

Politics shape debt as much as finance. The IMF and World Bank make this clear. As the previously mentioned Meltzer Commission observed in its 2000 report:

> The G7 governments, particularly the United States, use the IMF as a vehicle to achieve their political ends.

Robert Zoelick, who became president of the World Bank in 2007, but speaking as the then US trade representative, was no less forthright:

> Countries seeking free trade agreements with the United States should meet criteria beyond those of an economic and commercial nature. At the very least, those countries should cooperate with the United States in its external policy and its national security objectives.

Debt, a highly advantageous lever, made possible the US's abuse of the World Bank and IMF; whereas the undemocratic governance structures of both the IMF and the World Bank made these institutions perfect instruments of core country – especially US – control (Toussaint & Millet, 2009: 39–43, 67–73, 99).

Political Control

Africa was debt free before the 1960s. This was because Sub-Saharan Africa was under colonial rule, except for Ethiopia. Core countries learned that debt was a most useful mechanism of control over nominally independent countries. This much is alluded to in the preceding two quotations.

The threat of the Soviet Union – and now China – added enormously to the political value of creating and maintaining dependency, via debt. Indonesia provides an early example of how that dependency is

created and the connection between dependency and dictatorships, especially when large loans are involved. In August 1965, Indonesia withdrew from the IMF and World Bank. Shortly afterward, the army overthrew the president and massacred 750,000 communists. Under the new president, General Haji Mohammad Suharto, Indonesia rejoined both bodies. In December 1966, Suharto was rewarded with a four-year moratorium on all debt servicing, followed by the renewal of payments limited to less than 6% of export earnings and 0.7% of GDP.

As Joseph Stiglitz, chief economist of the World Bank from 1997 to 1999, noted:

> In many cases, the loans were used to corrupt governments. ... The issue was not whether the money was improving a country's welfare, but whether it was [meeting] the geopolitical realities of the world.
> *(Hanlon, 2000: 885; Toussaint & Millet, 2009: 38)*

Governments Willing to Be Corrupted

Why, regardless of country and continent, of race or religion, and as a constant since independence, should there be a never-ending supply of political and economic leaders willing to be corrupted? Greed is too simple an answer, unless one posits a highly problematic "human nature." A more developed answer is required, especially when leaders, as in postapartheid South Africa, include many who readily risked their lives and made great sacrifices in liberation struggles without any expectation of material reward.

One explanatory factor is the structural position of countries of the periphery: they are the marginal parts of a world system. This subsidiary structural position profoundly shapes how the bourgeoisie, the elites within the peripheral countries, think, feel, and act. This second factor is best captured by Franz Fanon in his classic of 1961 book:

> The national middle-class discovers its historic mission: that of intermediary. Seen through its eyes, its mission has nothing to do with transforming the nation; it consists, prosaically, of being the transmission line between the nation and a capitalism, rampant though camouflaged, which today puts on the mask of neo-colonialism. The national bourgeoisie will be quite content with the role of the Western bourgeoisie's business agent. ... But this same lucrative role, this cheap-Jack's function, this meanness of outlook ... symbolize[s] the incapability of the middle class to fulfil it historic role ... [of national

transformation. Instead] the spirit of indulgence is dominant … and this is because the national bourgeoisie indentifies itself with … the decadence of the bourgeoisie of the West. … [The national bourgeoisie] is in fact beginning at the end. It is already senile before it has come to know the petulance, the fearlessness, or the will to succeed of youth.

(Fanon, 1963: 152–153)

How does being a "business agent" become "lucrative"? How does it feed "the spirit of indulgence" other than through the rent-collecting of bribery?

The "historic mission" of the peripheral bourgeoisie that makes them prematurely "senile" explains why governments of the periphery accept SAPs in all their odious forms. Core countries often provide the (legal) pay and perks of peripheral politicians and public officials (Hanlon, 2004). The readiness of the Zambian government to meet the conditionalities of the HIPC, regardless of the consequences for the majority of Zambians, is readily explicable when one realizes that almost half its national budget comes from foreign "aid."

The Psychopaths?

As stated earlier, most of the people dispensing aid, including loans, and devising SAPs are probably well intentioned. There are, however, a smaller number for whom the ethics of decent human relationships seem not to count (Bakan, 2005; Perkins, 2005). Most of them, however, including a core of policy advisers in the World Bank, the IMF, the Pentagon, and similar institutions, would claim to be driven by higher – though still moral – considerations involving the national interest or ideologies in which difference (e.g., communism, socialism, Islam) is seen as dangerous.

There are, however, a few people who make a living buying, at discounted prices, that part of debt that even SAPs recognize as being unpayable and then squeezing the indebted countries to pay up the full debt. Yet this unconscionable behavior is perfectly legal. Its name within the financial industry is revealing: *vulture funds*.[4] This suggests that these human vultures, although reprehensible, hold up a mirror to the rest of us. What system and what ethical theories or values tolerate such living off the weak and

desperate in far-away countries? Being the ultimate form of debt collection, vulture funds in their various forms force the rest of us to question our humanity and our society's ethics.

The Way Forward

Rights-Based Debt Repudiation

Human rights have long been enshrined in both national and international law. More recently, social and economic rights complement the established civil and political ones (see Chapter 7). Debt clashes most directly with social and economic rights. Health rights clearly compete with debt servicing.

All countries of the periphery can calculate the cost of meeting their still outstanding socioeconomic rights. These costs ought to have unquestioned priority over debt servicing. The predictable cry from the creditors that they could not afford the cost of putting human rights first rings hollow when set against the almost $13 trillion the United States alone was spending saving its selfish and greedy bankers (Bloomberg. com, March 31, 2009).

Although the moral argument is unassailable, ethics seems to count for little in such matters. The issue is political. However, a rights-based approach could provide the ethical, legal, and ultimately the political grounds for uniting the peoples of both the core and periphery of our single world. Their united mobilization might enable a challenge to the governments, bankers, and peripheral bourgeoisie. The message is a simple one. People come first. Repudiate the debt to make this happen. Ecuador has recently done so.

Postrcript

It is now South Africa's turn. Our chapter, to which this is the postscript, began, "The debt narrative is encapsulated in the conundrum of why postapartheid South Africa chose to cripple itself with debts that it could so easily have repudiated." Nine years after we first invoked debt repudiation as the ethical and health-appropriate way forward, the South African government is again being urged to invoke odious debt – this time to repudiate its debt of $3.75 billion to the World Bank.

In what follows, I draw heavily on Cannard (2019). The World Bank loan of 2010 was granted to finance Eskom's now-notorious Medupi coal-fired power station. The debt is odious in international law because it

---

[4] A vulture fund is a private equity or hedge fund that invests in debt issued by an entity that is considered to be very weak or dying…en.wikipedia.org/wiki/Vulture_funds

was incurred contrary to the needs of the population – a fact that was known to the World Bank.

The loan was contrary to the needs of the population for three main reasons. First, the South African government is signatory to all 24 agreements made since 1995 at the Conference of the Parties (COP), the United Nations' climate change body. Central to all these agreements is a commitment to transition away from coal (and other fossil fuel–based energy sources) as the primary source of the greenhouse gas causing climate change. Medupi is designed to be one of the largest coal-fired power stations in the world. This makes it, self-evidently, contrary to the best interest of the population. Second, coal directly kills people: both coal miners and others are forced to breathe coal-polluted air. Both these groups have also to suffer the nonlethal but serious respiratory and other adverse health effects of coal. Third, debt repayment to the World Bank severely reduces resources for social subsidies to poor South Africans for electricity and other basic needs. This, in turn, contributes to the shack fires which kill large numbers of people and leave even larger numbers homeless.

The World Bank, itself the publisher of climate change research, is aware of coal mining and use being a primary cause of climate change. Even if it were not aware, it could not claim ignorance. Demonstrations against the loan occurred in various parts of the world, including the United States and South Africa.

Finally, there is corruption. Even though the World Bank did not know this at the time, it does know it now. Hitachi, the boiler supplier, has already paid a fine in the United States for its collusion with the African National Congress (ANC). It is an ANC government that made the loan agreement with the World Bank.

Successful use of the doctrine of odious debt remains a long-awaited aspiration, particularly in the context of erosion of ethical commitments to reducing inequalities in the world, since the first edition of this book. Despite huge advances made in the science and technology of health and enormous growth of global wealth, millions of people lack access to even basic medical services, let alone many of the new life-enhancing medical treatments.

References

Action for South Africa (ACTSA) (2003). Southern Africa calls for reparations for apartheid. August.

Bakan, J. (2005). *The Corporation: The Pathological Pursuit of Profit and Power*. London, Constable.

Bassett, M., Bijlmakers, L., & Sanders, D. (2000). Experiencing structural adjustment in urban and rural households of Zimbabwe, in Turshen, M. (ed.), *African Women's Health*. Trenton, NJ: Africa World Press, pp. 167–191.

Bassett, M. T., Bijlmakers, L. A., & Sanders, D. M. (1997). Professionalism, patient satisfaction and quality of health care: experience during Zimbabwe's structural adjustment programme. *Social Science and Medicine* **45**(12), 1845–1852.

Bijlmakers, L., Bassett, M., & Sanders, D. (1999). Socioeconomic stress, health and child nutritional status in Zimbabwe at a time of economic structural adjustment: a three-year longitudinal study. Research Report No. 105. Nordiska Afrikainstitutet, Uppsala.

Breman, A., & Shelton, C. (2001). Structural adjustment and health: a literature review of the debate, its role players and the presented empirical evidence. WHO Commission on Macroeconomics and Health Working Paper WG 6:6. WHO, Geneva.

Cannard, J. (2019). Cancel Eskom's odious debt to the World Bank, August 19. Available at https://mg.co.za/article/2019–08–19–00-cancel-eskoms-odious-debt-to-the-world-bank.

Commission on Social Determinants of Health (CSDH) (2008). *Final Report: Closing the Gap in a Generation: Health Equity Through Action on the Social Determinants of Health*. Geneva: WHO.

Cornia, G., Jolly, R., & Stewart, F. (eds.) (1988). *Adjustment with a Human Face: Ten Country Case Studies*. Oxford, UK: Oxford University Press.

Costello, A., Watson, F., & Woodward, D. (1994). Human face or human facade? Adjustment and the health of mothers and children. Occasional paper. Institute of Child Health, London.

de Savigny, D., Kasale, H., Mbuya, C., & Reid, G. (2004). Fixing health systems: Ottawa. International Development Research Centre, cited in Labonté, R., Blouin, C., Chopra, M., et al. (2007). *Towards Health-Equitable Globalisation: Rights, Regulation and Redistribution* – Final Report of the Globalization Knowledge Network. Geneva: WHO Commission on Social Determinants of Health.

De Vogli, R., & Birbeck, G. L. (2005). Potential impact of adjustment policies on vulnerability of women and children to HIV/AIDS in Sub-Saharan Africa. *Journal of Health Population and Nutrition* **23**(2), 105–120.

Fanon, F ([1961]1963). *The Wretched of the Earth*. New York: Grove Press.

Frank, A. G (1967). *Capitalism and Underdevelopment in Latin America: Historical Studies of Chile and Brazil*. New York: Monthly Review Press.

Frank, A. G (1969). *Latin America: Underdevelopment or Revolution – Essays on the Development of*

Underdevelopment and the Immediate Enemy. New York: Monthly Review Press.

George, S. (1988). *A Fate Worse than Debt: A Radical New Analysis of the Third World Debt Crisis*. London: Pelican Books.

Halstead, S. B., Walsh, J. A., & Warren, K. (eds.) (1985). *Good Health at Low Cost*. New York: Rockefeller Foundation.

Hanlon, J. (2000). How much debt has been cancelled? *Journal of International Development* **12**(6), 877–901.

Hanlon, J. (2004). *How Northern Donors Promote Corruption*. Manchester, UK: Cornerhouse Publications.

Labonté, R., Blouin, C., Chopra, M., et al. (eds.) (2007). *Towards Health-Equitable Globalisation: Rights, Regulation and Redistribution – Final Report of the Globalization Knowledge Network*. Geneva: WHO Commission on Social Determinants of Health, p. 56. Available at www.global healthequity.ca/electronic%20library/GKN%20Final%20Ja n%208%202008.pdf.

Malala, J. (2003). Mandela: apartheid debt paralysed ANC. *This Day*, October 9.

Oxfam (2004). Undervaluing teachers: IMF policies squeeze Zambian education system. Press release, Global Campaign for Education, Oxford, UK, October 1.

Perkins, J. (2005). *Confessions of an Economic Hit Man*. London, Ebury Press.

Piot, P. (2004). Plenary address for closing ceremony, in XV International AIDS Conference: Getting Ahead of the Epidemic (Bangkok, July 16, 2004). Cited in Schrecker, T., Labonté, R., & Sanders, D. (2007). Breaking faith with Africa: the G8 and population health

post-Gleneagles, Chapter 12 in Cooper, A. F., Kirton, J. J., & Schrecker, T. (eds.), *Governing Global Health: Challenge, Response, Innovation*. Aldershot: Ashgate, pp. 181–251.

Reuters (1999). G7 has failed in debt relief – Manuel. September 20.

Rudin, J. (1999). *Apartheid Debt: Questions and Answers*. Johannesburg: Jubilee South Africa.

Rudin, J. (2000). *Odious Debt Revisited*. Johannesburg: Jubilee South Africa.

Rudin, J. (2003). Forgive us this day our odious debt. *Mail & Guardian*, February 21.

Toussaint, E., & Comanne, D. (2000). *Debt Relief: Much Ado about Nothing*. Brussels: Committee for the Abolition of Third World Debt.

Toussaint, E., & Millet, D. (2009). *60 Questions, 60 Answers on Debt, IMF and World Bank*. Brussels, Committee for the Abolition of Third World Debt, pp. 18, 34, 101–109.

United Nations Conference on Trade and Development (UNCTAD) (2003a). *Economic Development in Africa: Commercial Results and Dependence on Commodities*. Geneva: UNCTAD.

United Nations Conference on Trade and Development (UNCTAD) (2003b). *Commodity Yearbook*. Available at http://rO.unctad.org/infocomm.

World Health Organisation (WHO) (2006). *Harmonization for Health in Africa: An Action Framework*. Geneva: WHO.

Zulu, M. (2007). Multi-stakeholder consultation on "Financing Access to Basic Utilities for All." Unpublished, Lusaka, Zambia, pp. 23–25.

The International Arms Trade and Global Health

Jonathan Kennedy, David McCoy, and Joseph Gafton

Introduction

War, armed conflict, and other forms of collective violence are incompatible with health, especially when we use the World Health Organization's (WHO, 2006) conceptualization of health as a state of complete physical, mental, and social well-being, a fundamental human right, and the responsibility of the state. In addition to their obvious direct physical and psychological effects, wars, conflict, and collective violence damage health through a variety of indirect channels, including: the destruction of healthcare and undermining of the broader determinants of health by, for example, disrupting food, water, and sanitation systems; displacing large numbers of people; polluting and degrading the environment; and damaging the economy (Weinberg & Simmonds, 1995). There is an enormous opportunity cost. The Institute for Economics and Peace (2018) estimates that violence cost the global economy US$14.76 trillion in 2017 (12.4% of world gross domestic product [GDP]). This is more than the amount of money spent on healthcare – 9.9% of world GDP in 2017 (World Bank, n.d.) – and a hundred times the total official development assistance given by the Organisation for Economic Co-operation and Development (OECD, n.d.) countries.

There are social costs associated with "militarism" and the incorporation into civilian life of ideas, behaviors, and language aimed at legitimizing the use of force to address political problems, expanding the power of military actors in society, and creating support for military spending (Williams & McCleary, 2009; Wiist et al., 2014). The use of military power to undermine democracy is one concern. It may be conspicuous in countries such as Myanmar and North Korea, where military oppression is overt, or more subtle, as in the United States, where the military-industrial complex spends vast amounts of money to buy political influence (Center for Responsive Politics, 2013). In low-income countries, militarization is associated with greater inequity in access to healthcare and education, as well as higher levels of corruption (Institute for Economics and Peace, 2015). Other data show that militarism is positively correlated with authoritarianism and negatively correlated with human rights, tolerance of dissent, and sympathy for the poor (Williams & McCleary, 2009). In contrast, the constitutional demilitarization of Japan after World War II was accompanied by significant and rapid social and economic benefits in the ensuing years (Williams & McCleary, 2009).

It is for good reason, then, that the World Health Assembly affirmed in 1981 that "the role of physicians and other health professionals in the preservation and promotion of peace is the most significant factor for the attainment of health for all" (quoted in Wiist et al., 2014: e35). Over the past century, health professionals have played an impressive role in preventing armed conflict and mitigating its effects. This is apparent from the number of health organizations that have received the Nobel Peace Prize: International Committee of the Red Cross (ICRC) on three occasions (1917, 1944, and 1963); International Physicians for the Prevention of Nuclear War (IPPNW) in 1985 for spreading information about the catastrophic consequences of atomic warfare; Doctors Without Borders (MSF) in 1999 for providing medical care in humanitarian crises and raising awareness of potential humanitarian disasters; and International Campaign to Abolish Nuclear Weapons (ICAN) – which was launched by IPPNW in 2017 for its work on nuclear disarmament. If health professionals are to continue to work to prevent, resolve, and mitigate the effects of armed conflict, it is necessary to understand the nature of contemporary armed conflict, the role of the arms trade in fueling collective violence, and the devastating impact they have on health.

This chapter begins with a brief description of recent historical trends in the prevalence and nature of armed conflict. The next section describes the international arms industry, including patterns of military expenditure and trade in weapons. The third section discusses the threat posed by weapons of mass destruction, particularly nuclear weapons. The fourth section focuses on efforts to prevent war and armed conflict. The final section considers how artificial intelligence (AI) might shape future armed conflict and considers the implications for health.

Armed Conflict and Violence: Recent Trends

The numbers of people killed by armed conflict are staggering. The Uppsala Conflict Data Programme (UCDP) estimates that since 1989, there have been 1.4 million battle-related deaths – that is, people killed by guns, bombs, and other weapons (UCDP, 2018a). In 2014, the number of fatalities (104,769) was higher than at any point since the end of the Cold War. The annual total has fallen steadily since then, standing at 68,969 in 2017. It should be noted that UCDP figures are believed to underestimate the true number of

battle-related deaths by a factor of at least three because they are compiled from news reports, and journalists are not always present in conflict zones (Obermeyer et al., 2008). Moreover, such figures do not include the far larger number of people who die as a result of the indirect impact of war, such as conflict-exacerbated disease and malnutrition. The UCDP reports that there were 68,027 battle-related deaths in Iraq between 2004 and 2017, whereas a retrospective mortality survey estimates that there were 654,965 excess deaths between 2003 and 2006 (Burnham et al., 2006). Even more remarkably, the UCDP reports 18,360 battle-related deaths in the Democratic Republic of Congo between 1996 and 2017, whereas a retrospective mortality survey estimated that there was a total of 5.4 million direct and indirect deaths between 1998 and 2007 (International Rescue Committee, 2007).

The UCDP defines an armed conflict as "a contested incompatibility that concerns government and/or territory where the use of armed force between two parties, of which at least one is the government of

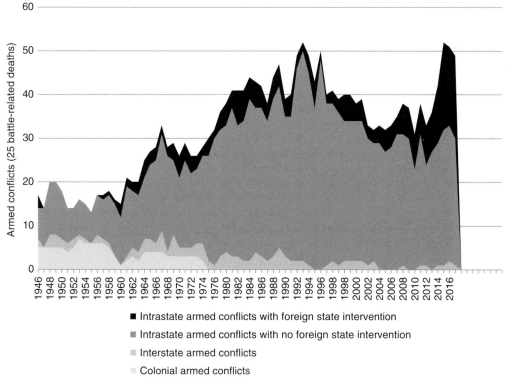

Figure 13.1. Number of armed conflicts by type, 1946–2017 (25 battle-related deaths per year)
Source: UCDP Armed Conflict Dataset.

a state, results in at least 25 battle-related deaths in one calendar year" (UCDP, n.d.). Using this definition, there have been a greater number of armed conflicts in the last few years than at any point since World War II, with the exception of the period immediately after the collapse of the Soviet Union (UCDP, 2018b) (see Figure 13.1). When a threshold of 1,000 battle-related deaths is used, the current number of armed conflicts is at its highest for two decades. It is also important to note how the nature of armed conflict has changed. Most conflict-related deaths in the first half of the twentieth century were caused by a handful of catastrophic interstate wars, in particular World Wars I and II. Now the vast majority of armed conflicts are between states and one or more nonstate actors. UCDP data show that intrastate conflicts accounted for 90.2% of battle-related deaths during 1989–2017 and 99.9% since 2010. One interesting feature is that the number of intrastate armed conflicts involving foreign state intervention increased over the last few years: they accounted for 34.2% of fatalities between 1989 and 2017, but the proportion has increased in recent years, and in 2017 the figure was 88.8%. Such armed conflicts include Syria, Iraq, Afghanistan, and Yemen, which together account for 77.1% of global battle-related deaths in 2017.

Intrastate conflicts pose specific challenges for global health. To understand how, it is useful to consider the distinction between "old wars" and "new wars" (Kaldor, 1999). Old wars are fought between states represented by uniformed armies on the battlefield, whereas new wars are fought between the state and nonstate actors. Because nonstate actors are militarily weaker, they tend to avoid direct engagement, instead using a strategy of guerrilla warfare to control territory and build base areas (Kaldor, 1999; Kalyvas, 2006). In such situations, the nonstate actors' prospects are determined by the support of the local population, and both the state and nonstate actors use a combination of sanctions and incentives to win civilian support. As such, intrastate conflicts are fought "*through* the people" often resulting in high levels of civilian casualties and violations of international law (Kalyvas, 2006: 91). Kaldor (1999) estimates that at the start of the twentieth century, the ratio of combatants killed in armed conflict to noncombatants was roughly 8:1; by midcentury, it was 1:1 and was 1:8 in the 1990s. Several recent conflicts have had a catastrophic impact on civilians. The Syrian Civil War is notable for violence against civilians and the displacement of half the population (Human Rights Watch, 2018). In Yemen, the bombardment and blockade of rebel-controlled areas by a Saudi-led military alliance left 22 million people in need of humanitarian assistance and resulted in outbreaks of cholera and diphtheria (Kennedy, Harmer, & McCoy, 2017).

Since 1945, few conflicts have occurred in Europe and the Americas, whereas most have been in Africa, Asia, and the Middle East. The increase in the armed conflicts and battle-related deaths in the past few years is largely driven by war in the Middle East, with the region accounting for 63.7% of all battle-related deaths in the 2010s (UCDP, 2018a). Historically, the vast majority of armed conflicts were in poor countries, but this is changing. In the 1990s, 75% of battle-related deaths occurred in low-income countries according to the World Bank's classification, but in the 2010s, 77% of battle-related deaths occurred in middle-income countries (Kennedy et al., 2019a).

Notwithstanding the focus on armed conflicts in this chapter, it should be noted that most violent deaths occur outside of war zones. According to the Small Arms Survey, interpersonal and collective violence claimed the lives of 560,000 people around the world in 2016 (McEvoy & Hideg, 2017). This works out at about 1% of all the people who died in the world that year (WHO, 2018). "Only" 18% (99,000) of these were casualties of war, whereas 78% (385,000) were homicides. About 38% of all these violent deaths (210,000) were caused by firearms, including about a third of those who died in armed conflicts. Six countries account for over half the gun deaths in the world – the United States, Brazil, Mexico, Colombia, Venezuela, and Guatemala (Global Burden of Disease, 2018). With the exception of Colombia, none of these have been affected by significant armed conflicts in recent times, but Latin America has the highest murder rates of any region in the world – to a large extent as a consequence of organized crime (Muggah & Tobón, 2018).

The International Arms Industry

By far the biggest purchasers of weapons and military equipment are national governments. World military expenditure was estimated at US$1,739 billion in 2017, making up 2.2% of global GDP and the equivalent of US$230 per person (Stockholm International Peace Research Institute [SIPRI], 2018). Levels of military expenditure have plateaued over the last decade, following a rise in spending since 1999. Global military expenditure is highly concentrated. The United States accounts for 35% of worldwide military expenditure. The second biggest spender is China (13%), and the next eight countries account for a further quarter of the global total (see Figure 13.2).

It is impossible to get a complete and accurate description of the international arms trade. Large segments of the trade in weapons are illicit and hidden, whereas data on many official transactions are not adequately captured by information systems, particularly in relation to small arms and light weapons (SALWs). The UN's Register of Conventional Arms (UNROCA) was designed to record all conventional arms transfers involving member states. It was established as a voluntary reporting system but is now mandatory for the 100 states that have ratified and adopted the international Arms Trade Treaty (UN, 2019). However, the UNROCA database suffers from considerable incompleteness – three of the four biggest arms producers, the United States, Russia, and China, do not participate. It is also inaccurate, as it is not uncommon for recipient states to deny arms imports that have been declared by exporting states (Wezeman et al., 2011).

It is, nonetheless, possible to paint a reasonably detailed picture of the licit trade in "major weapons" – a category that includes aircraft, armored vehicles, ships and missiles, but not SALWs. SIPRI uses government documents, industry publications, and media reports to collate data on the production and transfers of major weapons. According to SIPRI, the sector is dominated by a relatively small number of companies based in the United States and Western Europe, with 66 of SIPRI's list of top 100 companies (measured by monetary value in sales, including to their own states) in 2017 coming from these two regions (Fleurant et al., 2018). Of the top 10 companies, which accounted for 50% of total arms sales, all came from the United States or Western Europe, except for one Russian company – the first from outside these two regions to make the top 10. This marks the growing role of Russia as an arms-producing nation. Among the top 100 arms companies, the total sales of British companies were second only to those of US companies from 2002 to 2016. In 2017, Russia displaced the United Kingdom as the second largest in 2017, mainly due to Russia's increased procurement of arms for its own military. SIPRI's top 100 list does not include Chinese companies because of lack of access to reliable and comparable data. However, the limited available information suggests that three Chinese arms companies would probably be listed in the top 10 (Fleurant et al., 2018).

The volume of *international transfers* of major weapons grew by about 10% between 2008–2012 and 2013–2017 (Wezeman et al., 2018), with about 80% of such transfers since 2008 being directed to countries in the Global South (Theohary, 2016). The five largest importers between 2013 and 2017 were India, Saudi Arabia, Egypt, the United Arab

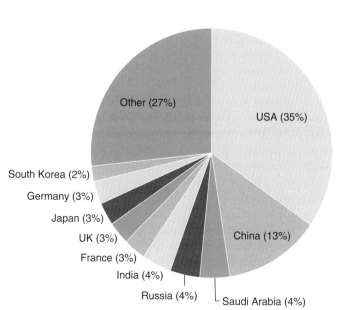

Figure 13.2. Global military expenditure in 2017 by country
Source: SIPRI, 2018.

Emirates, and China, with most of the supply of major arms coming from the United States, Russia, China, France, and the United Kingdom – the five-member permanent members of the UN Security Council – as well as Germany (Wezeman et al., 2018). With 42% of global imports from 2013 to 2017, Asia and Oceania constitute the largest importing region, followed by the Middle East, which accounts for 32% of global imports. From 2008–2012 to 2013–2017, while arms imports into Asia and Oceania increased by 1.8%, imports to the Middle East increased by 103% (Wezeman et al., 2018). This reflects the fact that over the last decade, the Middle East accounted for a large and increasing proportion of armed conflicts and battle-related deaths.

The Oxford Research Group's Sustainable Security Index analyses the proportion of arms exported to "internally repressive" states or states with a history of "illegal annexation/occupation, militarisation of territorial disputes and foreign military interventions not authorised by the UN" (Larsson & Reeve, 2018). Russia scored worst overall, but five Western democracies (United Kingdom, France, Netherlands, United States, and Switzerland) were also listed in the worst 10 because of "their willingness to sell to repressive regimes" (Larsson & Reeve, 2018). For example, from 2016 to 2017, 75% of arms exported by the United Kingdom went to internally repressive states – mainly Saudi Arabia and Oman – and 46% of US exports went to internally repressive states including Egypt, the United Arab Emirates, China, Saudi Arabia, and Uzbekistan. Israel is conspicuous by its absence from this list despite being a major market for US arms exports (Wezeman et al., 2018). The exclusion is the result of Oxford Research Group's use of Freedom House's classification, which codes Israel as "free" – a claim that would surely be contested by the Palestinian inhabitants of Gaza and the West Bank. The repressive and genocidal regime in Myanmar acquires 68% of its arms from China and 15% from Russia (Wezeman et al., 2018).

The Small Arms Survey attempts to document the international trade in SALWs, which encompasses sporting shotguns and rifles, as well as their parts, accessories, and ammunition. The trade is estimated to be worth at least US$5.7 billion in 2015 – roughly 1.5% of the total spent on major weapons sales. As with major weapons, a relatively small number of countries dominate this trade, with 21 countries known to have exported at least US$100 million worth of SALWs in a single year between 2001 and 2015 (Small Arms Survey, n.d. [a]). The import and purchase of SALWs is also unevenly spread across the world. For the period 2001–2014, seven countries (Australia, Canada, France, Germany, Saudi Arabia, United Kingdom, and United States) routinely imported SALWs worth US$100 million or more per year (Small Arms Survey, n.d.[b]). A significant amount of trade in SALWs is illicit, mainly occurring in areas affected by conflict, violence, and organized crime. Illicit arms trafficking fuels civil wars – which account for almost all contemporary armed conflicts – and contributes to violent crime (Small Arms Survey, n.d.[c]). Large and well-organized intercontinental shipments of SALWs account for only a small fraction of illicit transfers. Instead, the most important form of illicit trafficking is the so-called "ant trade," consisting of numerous shipments of small numbers of weapons that, over time, result in the accumulation of large numbers of illicit weapons by unauthorized end users (Small Arms Survey, n.d.[d]). For example, many of the firearms in Mexico were purchased in small numbers in the United States and smuggled over the border.

The design, manufacture, and supply of weapons are shaped by many factors, including the way that the arms industry is structured. The arms industry involves a symbiotic relationship between private companies and the state. Many arms negotiations and deals occur through intergovernmental forums, brokered by politicians, diplomats, and civil servants, as well as corporate agents (Feinstein, 2011). A "revolving door" operates between the arms industry and government. For example, a 2010 investigation found that between 2004 and 2008, 80% of retiring US generals went on to work in the arms industry as either consultants or executives (Bender, 2010). An interesting feature of the major weapons industry is the relative heterogeneity of arms companies. Most companies are either partly or, in the cases of Chinese firms, mainly state-owned. At the same time, some companies are clearly multinational and have connections to more than one country. BAE Systems (n.d.), for example, is a corporation with 85,800 employees in over 40 countries and major operations in the United Kingdom, United States, Saudi Arabia, and

Australia. BAE Systems is primarily an arms company, with 98% of its total sales consisting of arms sales, but some of the biggest arms companies are conglomerations that manufacture other items. For example, General Electric was the twenty-second biggest company in SIPRI's top 100 in 2017, but its arms sales represented only 3% of its total sales. Similarly, arms only make up 29% and 15% of all sales made by Boeing and Airbus, respectively (Fleurant et al., 2018).

Geopolitical factors also shape the arms trade. A key aspect of the Cold War was both Russia and the United States arming favorable regimes or rebel groups. Such behaviors have continued, as illustrated by the conflict in Syria, where the Assad regime receives military aid from Russia and Iran while the United States and Saudi Arabia supply Syrian rebel groups (Schanzer, 2012; Mazzetti & Apuzzo, 2016). Arms transfers can also be used to gain access to natural resources: China increasingly supplies African states with manufactured products, including arms, in exchange for access to natural resources (Conteh-Morgan, 2017). Similarly, the United States supplies Saudi Arabia and other Gulf states with weapons in exchange for secure access to oil (Bove et al., 2018). In some instances, arms transfers appear to proceed indiscriminately, with single suppliers selling arms to both sides of a conflict, such as US exports to both India and Pakistan and Russia and Ukraine supplying both sides in the Sudanese civil war (Campain Against Arms Trade [CAAT], 2003; SIPRI, 2009; Wezeman et al., 2011). This underlines the point that arms transfers are strongly influenced by commercial motives, including the military-industrial complex's imperative to generate a demand for weapons and military technologies by fostering armed conflict. Certain governments also contribute to the illicit trade by deliberately arming proxy groups involved in insurgencies against rival governments or non-state armed groups. In recent years, governments have covertly delivered tens of thousands of SALWs to various armed groups in Somalia despite a long-standing UN arms embargo (Small Arms Survey, 2012). Similarly, between 2006 and 2010, the UN embargo on moving military equipment into Darfur was repeatedly broken by Sudan using weapons supplied by Belarus, China, Russia, and Ukraine (Wezeman, Wezeman, & Béraud-Sudrea, 2011).

A key characteristic of the arms industry is that it is beset with systematic corruption. One particularly notorious example is the Al-Yamamah arms deal between BAE Systems and Saudi Arabia, which was worth around £40 billion and allegedly included around £6 billion of "unauthorized commissions" – effectively bribes – to members of the Saudi royal family (Feinstein, 2011; Wearing, 2018). A criminal investigation launched by the UK's Serious Fraud Office was shut down following pressure from erstwhile UK Prime Minister Tony Blair under the guise that it could jeopardize UK-Saudi relations and undermine cooperation on national security. Another example is a US$5 billion arms deal between BAE Systems and South Africa in the early 2000s, which was reported to have involved US$300 million of unauthorized commissions to South African officials to secure the deal ahead of other suppliers (Feinstein, 2011). This case draws stark attention to the opportunity cost involved in such arms deals, because South Africa's President Thabo Mbeki claimed simultaneously that the state could not afford antiretroviral drugs for the 5 million citizens suffering from HIV (Gilby, 2014). Feinstein (2011) argues that illicit activity in the arms industry has become the norm because it can be readily concealed through appeals to national security and because it is extraordinarily profitable for the relatively limited number of individuals involved.

Nuclear Weapons and Other Weapons of Mass Destruction

Nuclear weapons are perhaps the ultimate weapon of mass destruction. When a nuclear bomb is detonated, buildings are flattened, and temperatures reach several million degrees centigrade, vaporizing human tissue and producing a conflagration that consumes all oxygen and kills even those sheltering underground. Many initial survivors of the blast die from burns, internal bleeding, and injuries. The destruction of roads, buildings, and electricity supplies makes immediate humanitarian response futile (ICRC, 2013a). Survivors who have been exposed to high radioactive doses will suffer from acute radiation syndrome and die in the ensuing days and weeks. Those who do not die will be at heightened risk of cancer in the future (ICRC, 2013b). There are also long-term psychological effects: many survivors of

Hiroshima and Nagasaki experienced post-traumatic stress disorder for the rest of their lives, and some also suffered from the effects of forced migration and stigmatization (owing to unfounded fears of contamination).

Multiple nuclear detonations would produce even more catastrophic effects (Helfand, 2013). Nuclear war between India and Pakistan involving only 1.5% of the world's total stockpile would throw enough dust and soot up into the atmosphere to dim the sunlight for months or years, producing what has been termed a *nuclear winter*. Food production would decline to such an extent that up to 2 billion people could die of starvation (International Physicians for the Prevention of Nuclear War [IPPNW], n.d.; Robock & Toon, 2010; Helfand, 2013). A full-scale nuclear war between the United States and Russia may result in a new ice age, imperiling the future of humanity (ICRC, 2013a).

The majority of the world's stockpile of 9,000 nuclear bombs is held by Russia and the United States. Seven other nations also possess nuclear weapons (France, China, United Kingdom, Israel, Pakistan, India, and North Korea), and a further 32 countries incorporate nuclear weapons into their national defense policies (e.g., the NATO countries, Australia, New Zealand, and South Korea). Nearly 1,800 warheads are on alert and ready for use at short notice, and China, France, Russia, United Kingdom, and the United States are actively upgrading their weapons systems as part of a continuing nuclear arms race (Blair, 2011). The United States and Russia also have a large number of retired nuclear warheads awaiting dismantling, which pose a risk in terms of their radioactivity and the potential for plutonium to be stolen to build a *dirty bomb* (a bomb packed with radioactive material that is detonated conventionally and which then spreads highly toxic radioactive material) (Helfand et al., 2002).

Some people argue that the fear of "mutually assured destruction" restrains the nuclear powers from full-scale armed conflict with each other. Such an approach to maintaining world peace, however, is a high-risk gamble. Safety measures designed to prevent the accidental or mistaken launch of nuclear weapons are not completely failsafe, and it cannot be taken for granted that trained and disciplined personnel will be in charge of nuclear weapons. There have been several occasions when the world

has come close to catastrophe because of accidents and mistakes (Schlosser, 2013; Lewis et al., 2014). The possibility of an unintended nuclear weapons launch will only increase with further nuclear proliferation and increasing international tension, combined with risks posed by cyberwarfare (Abaimov & Ingram, 2017). In recent years, there has been a strong push to challenge this conventional wisdom and to make the case that disarmament is absolutely necessary given the existential threat posed by nuclear weapons. In early 2019, the Bulletin of Atomic Scientists (2019: 3) noted "the global nuclear order has been deteriorating for many years" and warned that the risk of a nuclear catastrophe is as great as it has ever been. There are several potential nuclear flashpoints in the world, notably in Eastern Europe, the Indian subcontinent, and around the South and East China Seas, as well as worries about a new Cold War emerging between the West and Russia.

There are other forms of weapons of mass destruction, including chemical and biological weapons. Following the use of poisonous gas in World War I, the 1925 Geneva Protocol banned asphyxiating, poisonous, or other gases and bacteriological methods of warfare. The fact that neither chemical nor biological weapons were used by the main belligerents in World War II indicates that the protocol established a clear norm (ICRC, 2013c). This was reinforced by further bans in 1972 and 1993 on the development, production, stockpiling, and transfer of chemical or biological weapons. There have been a handful of high-profile violations with chemical weapons – for example, in 1988 Iraqi warplanes dropped chemical agents on the Kurdish town of Halabja and in 2013 the Syrian Army used sarin against opposition-controlled Ghouta (Üzümcü, 2013). These cases resulted in widespread international criticism. Similarly, the use of biological weapons has been limited, with the most recent notable incident being in 2001, when an unidentified attacker in the United States sent anthrax-contaminated letters that killed five people. However, there are concerns that technological advancements are increasing the risk posed by biological weapons, particularly from nonstate actors. For example, clustered regularly interspaced short palindromic repeats (CRISPR) gene editing could be used to create lethal infectious microbes using unregulated technology ordered online for less than US$200 (Thompson, 2018).

Arms Control and the Prevention of War

The United Nations was established after World War II, with two of its prime functions being to prevent international conflict and mitigate their humanitarian consequences. The Security Council is the United Nations' most powerful body. In theory, it has the tools to prevent and resolve armed conflict or reduce its humanitarian impact because it can issue legally binding resolutions supported by sanctions, peace-keepers, or military force. It is interesting to consider why it has failed to do this in many recent conflicts. The permanent members of the UN Security Council are the victors of World War II: the United States, United Kingdom, France, Russia, and China, which are also some of the world's major arms exporters. There is no permanent representative from South Asia, Africa, and the Middle East, the regions most affected by armed conflict. Permanent members of the UN Security Council have the power of veto. This makes it difficult to pass resolutions, particularly because foreign states are increasingly interfering in intrastate conflicts. Russia has used its veto 14 times since the beginning of the Syrian civil war – sometimes on issues as uncontroversial as condemning chemical weapon attacks and expressing concern about human rights violations (BBC, 2018a) – whereas the United States has consistently vetoed resolutions that would have ameliorated the suffering of Palestinians at the hands of the Israeli state (Campos, 2018).

Intrastate conflicts are particularly problematic for an international organization such as the United Nations. This is because, in part, new wars tend to result in greater violence against civilians as they are fought *through* civilian populations (Kalyvas, 2006; Kaldor, 1999). But civil wars also create governance problems. As the nonstate actor exerts control over territory, it undermines the state's exclusivity of juris-diction, creating a situation of dual or multiple sover-eignty (Kalyvas, 2006). This is problematic for the United Nations, which is responsible for leading and coordinating the response to conflict-related humani-tarian emergencies but is also mandated to respect its member states' sovereignty (Kennedy & Michailidou, 2017). For example, in the Syrian conflict, the internationally recognized government and its allies have been largely responsible for creating and sustain-ing the humanitarian emergency by attacking civilians in rebel-controlled areas and restricting their access to aid, but UN agencies were obliged to work closely with the state to address the crisis (Kennedy & Michailidou, 2017).

The Geneva and Hague Conventions define the obligations of nation-states engaged in armed conflict (ICRC, n.d.). For example, the Fourth Geneva Convention requires warring parties to refrain from targeting civilian populations and protects health and humanitarian workers. This legal regime was codified in the nineteenth and twentieth century when the main concern was so-called old wars that were fought between states represented by armies on battlefields (Kaldor, 1999). New wars create a different set of problems. Unlike in old wars, the civilian population is crucial to the outcome of the conflict. Consequently, the civilian population is much more likely to be targeted in contravention of international law. In addition, nonstate actors play an important role in new wars, but they are not signatories to intergovernmental treaties and conventions (Kennedy et al., 2019b). However, as noted earlier, even when international law is broken by a state actor – in Syria and Yemen, for example – the accused is not brought to account if it is protected by at least one Security Council permanent member.

The United Nations (and its predecessor, the League of Nations) is the main platform for the estab-lishment of international laws designed to limit the impact and control the proliferation of weapons and prevent the use of weapons of mass destruction. There are a number of international treaties and conven-tions aimed at inhibiting the development, distribu-tion, and use of weapons that cannot discriminate between civilians and enemy combatants. However, the adoption of these treaties is not universal, and even among the states that have ratified them, com-pliance is patchy. Moreover, nonstate actors are not party to these agreements. Mechanisms for disciplin-ing states and enforcing adherence are often weak or even absent. For example, the use of chemical weap-ons in Syria in 2013 illustrates the many difficulties in preventing chemical weapons proliferation. In add-ition to Russia vetoing Security Council efforts to condemn the attacks, leaked US government cables and other sources show that Syrian procurement agents may have targeted firms in countries including

China, Greece, India, Italy, South Korea, and Switzerland (Martin et al., 2013).

New Technologies and the Future of War

About one-third of the US$600 billion that the United States spends on defense each year is assigned to research, development, and procurement of new weapons systems (Clark, 2018). In an environment of rapid technological development, it is difficult to predict the future by extrapolating from past trends. Notwithstanding, it seems likely that armed conflict will be increasingly influenced by AI. Indeed, it has been argued that the impact of AI might rival that of nuclear weapons (Allen & Chan, 2017). The Pentagon is investing billions of dollars in what it calls "algorithmic warfare" (Tarnoff, 2018). In new wars, in which frontlines are blurred and the enemy is not wearing a uniform, a major issue is deciding who to kill. Target identification becomes much more labor intensive because the enemy could be anywhere, but AI can help to overcome this issue. For example, the first phase of US military's Project Maven uses machine learning to scan drone video footage and identify people, vehicles, and buildings to attack. Ultimately, AI has the potential to transform the nature of warfare into "battlefield robots waging constant war, algorithms that determine who to kill, face-recognition fighting machines that can ID a target and take it out before you have time to say 'Geneva conventions'" (Chan, 2019).

Military planners argue that the application of AI to armed conflict will enable more precise identification of targets and reduce civilian casualties. We should, however, approach such claims with skepticism. First, with the development of autonomous ground and aerial robots, fewer or no ground troops will be needed to fight wars (Allen & Chan, 2017). This will lower the political costs of war for militarily stronger countries, which may lead to an increase in the number of armed conflicts. Drones have already achieved this to some extent: for example, over the last decade and a half, the United States has fought as an undeclared war with drones in the Federally Administered Tribal Areas of Pakistan (Kennedy, 2017). Second, algorithms are created by humans working for institutions; they reflect their masters' and mistresses' prejudices. For example, algorithms have been shown to reinforce racial bias in policing

and criminal sentencing (Angwin, 2016). It is worrying that similarly faulty algorithms could be used to decide who to kill. An insight into what might happen is the US military's use of so-called signature strikes in Pakistan, where drone attacks targeted individuals whose identities are unknown but who displayed "signatures" as imprecise as being military-aged males in a particular area (Heller, 2013). Third, it will expand the number of powerful businesses that make money from armed conflict. We noted earlier that arms companies play an important role in driving armed conflict, but "algorithmic warfare will bring big tech deeper into the military-industrial complex," giving it incentives for finding enemies and waging war (Tarnoff, 2018). This is particularly concerning when we consider tech firms' ability to control and manipulate information of various kinds.

Profound concerns have been expressed about the potential impact of AI on armed conflict. Google pulled out of Project Maven after thousands of its employees objected to the company's involvement (BBC, 2018b). More than 250 research and academic institutions and 3,000 prominent people have called for a ban on the use of autonomous robots in war (Chan, 2019). Similarly, the Campaign to Stop Killer Robots advocates the global prohibition of any kind of autonomous weaponry, arguing that the best method to achieve this is an international treaty. Nevertheless, AI creates specific challenges for those who want to restrain its use in military operations. Unlike with nuclear weapons, development of AI is in large part driven by the commercial sector, making the use of AI in the military sphere more difficult to control (Cummings, 2017). Moreover, whereas nuclear weapons require input of large amounts of money, resources, and scientific knowledge, code and digital data tend to be cheap or even freely available (Allen & Chan, 2017). Consequently, it is plausible that nonstate combatants will be able to develop this technology, making it much harder to control.

In China, the state uses algorithms to monitor and control minority groups such as the Uighers in Xinjiang Province in what it terms a "people's war on terror" (Byler, 2019). It scans digital communications in order to identify suspicious patterns of behavior, which can be religious speech or even "lack of fervor in using Mandarin." Suspects can be apprehended using facial-recognition software and sent to detention centers.

Conclusion

The promotion of peace and the avoidance of armed conflict are vital and legitimate public health pursuits. Such a public health agenda would include providing humanitarian care and protection to civilians on the front line of war and armed conflict in a manner that is impartial and in accordance with international law; taking active measures to monitor, document, and publicize breaches of international law; and describing the full impacts of war and armed conflict, including all long-term intergenerational effects. Away from the front line, it should also include advocating for reform of international law, not only to bring it up to date in an era where the majority of armed conflicts occur within states and have a devastating impact on civilian populations but also to preempt the increasing role that will be played by AI in the future, advocating for stronger legal and democratic controls over the military-industrial complex, and ending the excessive profiteering of the arms trade, which encourages violence and armed conflict. It can also be argued that the health community has a professional duty to examine and challenge militaristic approaches to defense and national security that fail to emphasize international diplomacy, tolerance, and other determinants of peace, such as social and economic justice within and between countries. This is all the more so given the impotence of military might in the face of new threats to national security such as cyber-attacks, which have become increasingly alarming because of our reliance on globalized systems of information and communication (Sanger, 2018). Health professionals can use their social mandate and public health expertise to promote a more holistic conception of human security that highlights health, social security, and environmental protection while countering cultural practices that celebrate and legitimize violence and aggression.

References

Abaimov, S., & Ingram, P. (2017). *Hacking UK Trident: A Growing Threat*. Available at www.basicint.org/publications/stanislav-abaimov-paul-ingram-executive-director/2017/hacking-uk-trident-growing-threat.

Allen, G., & Chan, T. (2017). *Artificial Intelligence and National Security*. Available at www.belfercenter.org/sites/default/files/files/publication/AI%20NatSec%20-%20final.pdf.

Angwin, J. (2016). Make algorithms accountable. *New York Times*, August 1. Available at www.nytimes.com/2016/08/01/opinion/make-algorithms-accountable.html.

BAE Systems (n.d.). Where we operate. Available at www.baesystems.com/en/our-company/about-us/where-we-operate.

British Broadcasting Corporation (BBC) (2018a). Syria: Does Russia always use a veto at the UN Security Council? Reality Check team. Available at www.bbc.co.uk/news/world-43781954.

British Broadcasting Corporation (BBC) (2018b). Google "to end" Pentagon artificial intelligence project. Available at www.bbc.co.uk/news/business-44341490.

Bender, B. (2010). From the Pentagon to the private sector. Available at http://archive.boston.com/news/nation/washington/articles/2010/12/26/defense_firms_lure_retired_generals/.

Blair, B. (2011). World nuke spending to top $1 trillion per decade. *Time Magazine*. Available at http://time/2pSsHVc.

Bove, V., Deiana, C., & Nisticò, R. (2018). Global arms trade and oil dependence. *Journal of Law, Economics, and Organization* 34(2), 272–299.

Bulletin of the Atomic Scientists (2019). A new abnormal: it is still two minutes to midnight. Available at https://thebulletin.org/doomsday-clock/2019-doomsday-clock-statement/.

Burnham, G., Lafta, R., Doocy, S., & Roberts, L. (2006). Mortality after the 2003 invasion of Iraq: a cross-sectional cluster sample survey. *Lancet* 368(9545), 1421–1428.

Byler, D. (2019). China's hi-tech war on its Muslim minority. *The Guardian*, April 11. Available at www.theguardian.com/news/2019/apr/11/china-hi-tech-war-on-muslim-minority-xinjiang-uighurs-surveillance-face-recognition.

Campain Against Arms Trade (CAAT) (2003). Fanning the flames: how UK arms sales fuels conflict. Available at www.caat.org.uk/campaigns/fanning-the-flames/ftf-6-page-briefing.pdf.

Campos, R. (2018). US vetoes UN resolution denouncing violence against Palestinians. Reuters. Available at www.reuters.com/article/us-israel-palestine-un-vote/u-s-vetoes-u-n-resolution-denouncing-violence-against-palestinians-idUSKCN1IX5UW.

Center for Responsive Politics (2013). *Defense Influence and Lobbying*. Available at www.opensecrets.org/industries/background.php?cycle=2014&ind=D .

Chan, M. (2019). The rise of the killer robots: and the two women fighting back. *The Guardian*, April 8. Available at www.theguardian.com/world/2019/apr/08/the-rise-of-the-killer-robots-jody-williams-mary-warehan-artificial-intelligence-autonomous-weapons.

Clark, C. (2018). This is a reality, not a threat. *New York Review of Books*, November 22). Available at www.nybooks.com/articles/2018/11/22/future-war-reality-not-threat/.

Conteh-Morgan, E. (2017). China's arms sales in Africa. Oxford Research Group. Available at www.oxfordresearchgroup.org.uk/Blog/chinas-arms-sales-in-africa.

Cummings, M. (2017). *Artificial Intelligence and the Future of Warfare*. London: Chatham House.

Feinstein, A. (2011). *The Shadow World: Inside the Global Arms Trade*. London: Hamish Hamilton.

Fleurant, A., Kuimova, A., Tian, N., et al. (2018). The SIPRI top 100 arms-producing and military services companies, 2017. SIPRI Fact Sheet. Available at www.sipri.org.

Gilby, N. (2014). *Deception in High Places: A History of Bribery in Britain's Arms Trade*. London: Pluto Press.

Global Burden of Disease (2016). Global mortality from firearms, 1990–2016. *Journal of the American Medical Association* **320**(8), 792–814.

Helfand, I. (2013). *Nuclear Famine: Two Billion People at Risk*. Cambridge, MA: International Physicians for the Prevention of Nuclear War.

Helfand, I., Forrow, L., & Tiwari, J. (2002). Nuclear terrorism. *British Medical Journal* **324**(7333), 356–359.

Heller, K. (2013). "One hell of a killing machine": signature strikes and international law. *Journal of International Criminal Justice* **11**(1), 89–119.

Human Rights Watch (2018). Syria. Available at www.hrw.org/world-report/2018/country-chapters/syria.

International Committee of the Red Cross (ICRC) (2013a). Climate effects of nuclear war and implications for global food production. Available at www.icrc.org/eng/assets/files/2013/4132-2-nuclear-weapons-global-food-production-2013.pdf.

International Committee of the Red Cross (ICRC) (2013b). Humanitarian assistance in response to the use of nuclear weapons. Available at www.icrc.org/eng/assets/files/2013/4132-3-nuclear-weapons-humanitarian-assistance-2013.pdf.

International Committee of the Red Cross (ICRC) (2013c). Chemical and biological weapons. Available at www.icrc.org/en/document/chemical-biological-weapons.

International Committee of the Red Cross (ICRC) (2015). Long-term health consequences of nuclear weapons: 70 years on Red Cross hospitals still treat thousands of atomic bomb survivors. Available at www.icanw.org/wp-content/uploads/2015/08/Hiroshima-and_Nagasaki-ICRC-Info-Note-final.pdf.

International Committee of the Red Cross (ICRC) (n.d.). The Geneva Conventions and their additional protocols. Available at www.icrc.org/en/war-and-law/treaties-customary-law/geneva-conventions.

Institute for Economics and Peace (2015). *Global Peace Index 2015: Measuring Peace, Its Causes and Its Economic Value*. Available at http://visionofhumanity.org/app/uploads/2017/04/Global-Peace-Index-Report-2015_0.pdf.

Institute for Economics and Peace (2018). *Global Peace Index 2018: Measuring Peace in a Complex World*. Available at http://visionofhumanity.org/app/uploads/2018/06/Global-Peace-Index-2018-2.pdf.

International Physicians for the Prevention of Nuclear War (IPPNW) (n.d.). *The Humanitarian Impact of Nuclear Weapons*. Available at http://ippnw.org/catastrophic-consequences.html.

International Rescue Committee (2007). Mortality in the Democratic Republic of Congo: An ongoing crisis. Available at www.rescue.org/sites/default/files/document/661/2006-7congomortalitysurvey.pdf.

Kaldor, M. (1999). *New and Old Wars: Organised Violence in a Global Era*. Cambridge, UK: Polity.

Kalyvas, S. (2006). *The Logic of Violence in Civil War*. Cambridge, UK: Cambridge University Press.

Kennedy, J. (2017). How drone strikes and a fake vaccination program have inhibited polio eradication in Pakistan: an analysis of national level data. *International Journal of Health Services* 47(4), 807–825.

Kennedy, J., & Michailidou, D. (2017). Civil war, contested sovereignty and the limits of global health partnerships: a case study of the Syrian polio outbreak in 2013. *Health Policy and Planning* 32(5), 690–698.

Kennedy, J., Harmer, A., & McCoy, D. (2017). The political determinants of the cholera outbreak in Yemen. *Lancet Global Health* 5(10), e970–e971.

Kennedy, J., Abouzeid, M., Jabbour, S., & McCoy, D. (2019a). Armed conflict trends and the implications for public health. Unpublished manuscript, Barts and the London School of Medicine and Dentistry, Queen Mary University, London, UK.

Kennedy, J., McCoy, D., Abouzeid, M., & Jabbour, S. (2019b). Militaries and global health. *Lancet* 394(10202), 916–917.

Larsson, O., & Reeve, R. (2018). Sustainable security index: research note on arms exports. Oxford Research Group. Available at https://web.archive.org/web/20190802102454/www.oxfordresearchgroup.org.uk/sustainable-security-index-research-note-on-arms-exports.

Lewis, P., Aghlani, S., & Pelopidas, B. (2014). *Too Close for Comfort: Cases of Near Nuclear Use and Options for Policy*. Chatham House. Available at www.chathamhouse.org/publications/papers/view/199200#sthash.k7C1RdHx.dpuf.

Mazzetti, M., & Apuzzo, M. (2016). US relies heavily on Saudi money to support Syrian rebels. *New York Times*, January 24. Available at www.nytimes.com/2016/01/24/world/middleeast/us-relies-heavily-on-saudi-money-to-support-syrian-rebels.html.

Martin, S., Salisbury, D., & Takacs, D. (2013). Chemical weapons and trade: preventing the next Syria. Available at https://theconversation.com/chemical-weapons-and-trade-preventing-the-next-syria-19997.

McEvoy, C., & Hideg, G. (2017). Global violent deaths 2017: time to decide. Available at www.smallarmssurvey.org/fileadmin/docs/U-Reports/SAS-Report-GVD2017.pdf.

Muggah, R., & Tobón, K. A. (2018). Citizen security in Latin America: facts and figures. Igarapé Institute Strategic Paper No. 33. Available at https://igarape.org.br/wp-content/uploads/2018/04/Citizen-Security-in-Latin-America-Facts-and-Figures.pdf.

Obermeyer, Z., Murray, C. J., & Gakidou, E. (2008). Fifty years of violent war deaths from Vietnam to Bosnia: analysis of data from the world health survey programme. British Medical Journal 336(7659), 1482–1486.

Organisation for Economic Co-operation and Development (OECD) (n.d.). Development aid stable in 2017 with more sent to poorest countries. Available at www.oecd.org/development/development-aid-stable-in-2017-with-more-sent-to-poorest-countries.htm.

Robock, A., & Toon, O. (2010). Local nuclear war, global suffering. Scientific American 302, 74–81.

Sanger, D. E. (2018). The Perfect Weapon: War, Sabotage and Fear in the Cyber Age. New York: Crown Publishing Griup.

Schanzer, J. (2012). Saudi Arabia is arming the Syrian opposition. foreighpolicy.org. Available at https://foreignpolicy.com/2012/02/27/saudi-arabia-is-arming-the-syrian-opposition/.

Schlosser, E. (2013). Command and Control: Nuclear Weapons, the Damascus Accident and the Illusion of Safety. London: Penguin Books.

Stockholm International Peace Research Institute (SIPRI) (2009). SIPRI Yearbook 2009: Armaments, Disarmament and International Security. Available at www.sipri.org/sites/default/files/2016-03/SIPRIYB09summary.pdf.

Stockholm International Peace Research Institute (SIPRI) (2018). SIPRI Yearbook 2018: Armaments, Disarmament and International Security. Available at www.sipri.org/sites/default/files/2018-06/yb_18_summary_en_0.pdf.

Small Arms Survey (2012). Small Arms Survey 2012: Moving Targets. Cambridge, UK: Cambridge University Press.

Small Arms Survey (n.d.[a]). Exporters. Available at www.smallarmssurvey.org/weapons-and-markets/transfers/exporters.html.

Small Arms Survey (n.d.[b]). Importers. Available at www.smallarmssurvey.org/weapons-and-markets/transfers/importers.html.

Small Arms Survey (n.d.[c]). Transfers. Available at http://www.smallarmssurvey.org/weapons-and-markets/transfers.html

Small Arms Survey (n.d.). Illicit Trafficking. Available at www.smallarmssurvey.org/weapons-and-markets/transfers/illicit-trafficking.html.

Tarnoff, B. 2018. Weaponised AI is coming. Are algorithmic forever wars our future? www.theguardian.com/commentisfree/2018/oct/11/war-jedi-algorithmic-warfare-us-military.

Theohary, C. (2016). Conventional Arms Transfers to Developing Nations, 2008–2015. Washington, DC: Congressional Research Service.

Thompson, L. (2018). The threat of biological warfare is increasing, and the US isn't ready. Forbes, April 9. Available at www.forbes.com/sites/lorenthompson/2018/04/09/biowar-a-guide-to-the-coming-plague-years/#50edaac25fe5.

United Nations (2019). United Nations Office for Disarmament Affairs: Arms Trade Treaty. Available at www.un.org/disarmament/convarms/arms-trade-treaty-2/.

Uppsala Conflict Data Programme (UCDP) (n.d.). Definitions. Available at www.pcr.uu.se/research/ucdp/definitions/.

Uppsala Conflict Data Programme (UCDP) (2018a). Battle-Related Deaths Dataset. Available at https://ucdp.uu.se/downloads/#d8.

Uppsala Conflict Data Programme (UCDP) (2018b). Armed Conflict Dataset. Available at http://ucdp.uu.se/downloads/#d3.

Üzümcü, A. (2013). Working together for a world free of chemical weapons, and beyond. Nobel Peace Prize Lecture OPCW. Available at www.nobelprize.org/uploads/2018/06/opcw-lecture.pdf.

Wearing, D. (2018). AngloArabia: Why Gulf Wealth Matters to Britain. Hoboken, NJ: Wiley.

Weinberg, J., & Simmonds, S. (1995). Public health, epidemiology and war. Social Science and Medicine 40(12), 1663–1669.

Wezeman, P., Wezeman, S. T., & Béraud-Sudrea, L. (2011). Arms flows to Sub-Saharan Africa. SIPRI Policy Paper. Available at www.spiri.org.

Wezeman, P., Fleurant, A., Kuimova, A., et al. (2018). Trends in international arms transfers, 2017. SIPRI Fact Sheet. Available at www.spiri.org.

World Health Organization (WHO) (2006). Constitution of the World Health Organization. Available at www.who.int/governance/eb/who_constitution_en.pdf.

World Health Organization (WHO) (2018). The top 10 causes of death. Available at www.who.int/news-room/fact-sheets/detail/the-top-10-causes-of-death.

Wiist, W., Barker, K., Arya, N., et al. (2014). The role of public health in the prevention of war: rationale and competencies. *American Journal of Public Health* 104(6), e34–e47.

Williams, B., & McCleary, D. (2009). Sociopolitical and personality correlates of militarism in democratic societies. *Peace Conflict* 15(2), 161–187.

World Bank (n.d.). Current health expenditure (% of GDP). Available at https://data.worldbank.org/indicator/SH .XPD.CHEX.GD.ZS.

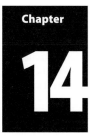

Chapter 14

Allocating Resources in Humanitarian Medicine

Samia A. Hurst, Nathalie Mezger, and Alex Mauron

Introduction

Allocating resources in humanitarian medicine is a vitally important and cruelly difficult exercise. In the huge disconnect between severe human needs and limited resources, even asking how allocation can be fair can seem harsh. Do those involved in humanitarian medicine not simply do all they *can*?

Daunting as the questions regarding how to allocate resources fairly and legitimately in humanitarian medicine may be, they are gaining in importance for at least three identifiable and related reasons. First, one of the primary motivating factors for humanitarian medicine is the rule of rescue, "the imperative people feel to rescue identifiable individuals facing avoidable death" or other plights invoking a shock or horror reaction "without thinking about the costs too much" (Jonsen, 1986; McKie & Richardson, 2003). As humanitarian medicine successfully raises awareness of urgent health-related needs in poverty-stricken regions of the world, the number of such identifiable victims increases. Without a vast increase in the resources available to humanitarian medicine, this makes it likely that the identified needs will remain greater than the available means as long as there are both pressingly needy sick persons and advocates raising awareness of their plight. One usual implication of the rule of rescue is that an identifiable, immediate victim should have priority over distant "statistical" lives. From the perspective of a humanitarian organization, persons in need are indeed identifiable, and giving aid to them is saving real, not "statistical," lives. As the number of such identifiable victims and the diversity of their needs increase, so does the complexity of allocation decisions. This makes allocation decisions more important but also harder to think through. Another difficulty is that part of the rule of rescue is that we should not think about the costs involved. This means that even asking how to allocate

resources in humanitarian medicine can seem problematic. If humanitarian medicine "must do *something*" about each crisis, then allocating resources away from any of them could seem intrinsically wrong. Asking how to allocate resources could seem to reflect a lack of moral concern. Although it could seem obvious that humanitarian medical organizations must, and should, make choices between competing situations of need, this point nevertheless needed formal defense (Wikler, 2003). This would seem to confirm the difficulty of thinking through allocation when faced with different situations where the rule of rescue could apply.

Second, one of the reasons why many find humanitarian advocacy convincing is an ongoing – though admittedly controversial and incomplete – shift from a charity view to a rights-based view of international health (Hendriks & Toebes, 1998; Katz, 2004). Such a view makes the claim for help more compelling. Humanitarian medical organizations usually originate from the financially richer part of the world, although not all individual humanitarians do. On a rights-based view, it would thus be all the more convincing to assign a share of the duty to fulfill such a right to these organizations. Exactly how much the rich are required to help the poor is controversial. Very generous answers, such that we owe until the need becomes smaller than our own, have been criticized as too altruistic to be required (Scheffler, 1992). But it has also been argued that we do have a collective duty to maximize beneficence to those in need (Murphy, 2000) or that such duties arise in rich countries from shared responsibility in maintaining global rules that harm the global poor (Pogge, 2005) or from a collective duty to rescue that nongovernmental organizations enable us to fulfill (Nagel, 2005). Under such views, the basic problem becomes practical: most people do not do their share. Even so, we may not be required to do more than our own share (Murphy, 2000). So *how much* humanitarian medicine would be required under this obligation remains unanswered.[1] Any claim to a right to health – for example, to ensure fair equality of opportunity (Daniels, 1985) on a global scale (Caney, 2001) or to fulfill a human right (United Nations, 1948) – would be likely to lead to an increase in the number of those recognized as requiring assistance compared with charity-based views. The importance of fair allocation consequently would be increased as well as the need for fairness and the strain on resources both increased. Indeed, this would be the case even if we were to take a more modest view. Minimally, humanitarian medical organizations should offer help when they are the only, or one of the few, that are on the spot and able to offer help or make the emergency known to others, as in the duty to rescue: if you can save someone at no excessive cost to yourself, then you should (McIntyre, 1994). Nevertheless, this would still mean that as the breadth of their activities increased, so would the number and scope of the situations with which they would be expected to deal and, with it, the importance of fair resource allocation.

Third, partly as a consequence of increased recognition of rights-based claims to healthcare, an increasing number of the situations faced by humanitarian medicine are protracted rather than acute "crises." Such protracted crises simultaneously increase the difficulty and the importance of fair allocation.

In war or natural disaster, humanitarian medicine intervenes to minimize the effect of the crisis on human health through medical intervention (Birch & Miller, 2005). In acute crises, this is often understood to mean "through any means available at the time." In such situations, the kind of response that can be set up is limited by the severity of the emergency. The crisis is usually limited in time. Finally, although these situations are sadly not rare, they are perceived as exceptional. They are violently different from ordinary life, even when ordinary life is set in precarious circumstances. Even if "the best possible intervention" is far from perfect, humanitarians are indeed doing "the best they possibly can" under very obvious and specific circumstances. They are not allocating resources away from

anyone, nor are they setting a precedent or sending a message that the limits used would in any way be appropriate under more normal circumstances.

Increasingly, however, humanitarian medicine's actions extend to more protracted crises (Rougemont, 1995; Michael & Zwi, 2002), such as access to antiretroviral drugs in Sub-Saharan Africa or responses to recurring epidemics of Ebola. These situations give rise to different technical challenges (Hendrickson, 1998). They also pose different ethical challenges. The kinds of harm they risk inflicting differ. Acute interventions risk diminishing self-sufficiency in specific ways (such as wiping out local food markets, for example; Redmond, 2005). Interventions of a more chronic kind have raised concerns about "propping up repressive and irresponsible governments" (Michael & Zwi, 2002). The importance of consulting communities in order to understand their needs and show them respect also becomes more visible in protracted crises (Palmer, 1999; Diallo et al., 2005).

Protracted crises also differ from acute crises with regard to resource allocation. The available time frame no longer quasi-automatically constrains the available resources. Deliberate choices more clearly control the amount of resources that will, in fact, be made available. Defining "the best we can possibly do" becomes fuzzier, and resources will sometimes be allocated away from other situations of need. Furthermore, situations of chronic need are not always distinct from everyday life. They are part of the daily routine for much of humanity. This is a crucial difference: decisions made in exceptional circumstances do not constitute appropriate precedents for normal life. A degree of double standard will set times of acute crisis apart from normal times, and this can be justified by exceptionally strained circumstances. However, the ethical picture changes when that double standard becomes part of everyday life. We may then become used to it. It may even seem to provide an unfortunate justification to an ethically unacceptable situation. Whereas "crisis standards of care" may be acceptable in acute crisis (Hodge, Hanfling, & Powell, 2013; Leider et al., 2018), this may not be the case when a disaster situation has become a part of everyday life. Protracted crises can lower our moral thresholds regarding a range of values we usually deem important in medicine (Civaner, Vatansever, & Pala, 2017), thus inflicting lasting damage on local medical practice and communities. Making resource-allocation decisions responsibly is both more difficult and more important in protracted crises.

---

[1] An approach based on nonideal theory does point to one avenue where further enquiry could suggest a threshold, both for the duty of humanitarian medicine, and for the resources that it ought to have. Additionally, since some may do their own share by giving resources to humanitarian medicine, and inasmuch as many people currently do not do their share, this could mean that humanitarians could claim, up to a point, that others could fulfill their share by giving them more resources than they currently do.

This chapter invites further examination of several challenges specific to resource allocation in humanitarian medicine and proposes one strategy to improve distributive fairness in this context.[2] Because experience regarding actual allocation decisions in humanitarian medicine is not widespread, the next section briefly outlines examples. Following that, we describe some of the difficulties in allocating resources fairly and legitimately that are either increased in humanitarian medicine or specific to its international context. All these issues would benefit both from theoretical exploration on specific application to humanitarian medicine and from empirical research on the impact of different strategies. We then propose that some headway could be made by adapting existing frameworks of procedural fairness for practical use in humanitarian organizations. The penultimate section presents Daniels and Sabin's (1997) "accountability for reasonableness," an influential approach to resource allocation, and the limits to its application to humanitarian medicine. Finally, we propose adaptations that could address some of these limits.

A Few Examples

Allocation decisions in humanitarian medicine can take several forms. Some choices will involve weighing different programs against each other. This was the case in 2005 when the Swiss section of Doctors Without Borders (DWB) took a very painful decision not to respond to the Pakistani earthquake. At that time, the huge emergency nutritional crisis in Niger was already occupying a large portion of the organization's human resources, as were other difficult crises such as Darfur. The annual budget for departures had already been doubled that year. Responding to this new medical crisis would clearly have led to serious neglect of other missions and might have pushed the organization over the brink. In this case, priority was given

to the more stable missions. Backup was offered to other DWB sections on site, conditions were defined under which a greater response would have been initiated, and the situation was regularly reevaluated.

Some choices will address the scope of an organization more generally. An example is the choice of whether to consider HIV a worldwide neglected emergency. Until this choice was made, DWB usually provided treatment for acute, medical, often neglected problems and only dealt with chronic diseases such as diabetes and cardiovascular diseases on a case-by-case basis.

Such choices regarding which disease to treat also directly lead to choices between individuals. Strict admission criteria in hospitals can mean that, as a doctor, you may have to send back a young patient complaining of clear inaugural diabetic symptoms. The treatment he or she needs is obvious (insulin), yet you cannot offer it even though you know that the patient will not find it elsewhere either. Although selection on the basis of the disease a patient suffers from is usually viewed as a public health rather than as an individual criterion in resource allocation, this can be – and in practice often is – understood as choosing one individual over another on the criterion of their diagnosis.

Challenges to Fair Allocation in Humanitarian Medicine

In cases such as these, and in addition to the difficulties attached to resource allocation in any context (Coulter & Ham, 2000), fair allocation in humanitarian medicine raises specific ethical difficulties regarding nonideal fairness, the scope of global solidarity, legitimacy in nongovernmental institutions, and the potential for conflicts of interest.

Fairness in an Unfair World

Fair access to medical treatment can be understood in a variety of ways, but sufficientarian, egalitarian, and prioritarian views all lead to the same initial conclusion regarding the international context of humanitarian medicine: it is more difficult. If fair access to healthcare is usually understood to mean that everyone has access to some basic response to their health-related needs (sufficientarian), perhaps even the same access (egalitarian), and that the worse off get at least some priority (prioritarian), how should we face the choice between practicing medicine to a lower standard to share out resources among more people or

---

[2] We recognize that normative controversy could focus on the very existence of humanitarian medicine. For the purposes of this chapter, however, we will accept the premise that its existence is justified so as to examine the more specific issue of fair resource allocation in its context. This assumption is reasonable. Despite its suggested negative effects, humanitarian medicine saves many lives and improves others, is mostly welcome by its recipients, garners enough support to owe its continued existence to funding by individuals, and more generally exists to help those in the sort of physical need we readily recognize as a valid claim for help. The skeptical reader may perhaps find the empirical premise – that humanitarian medicine actually does exist – sufficient to read on.

refusing this change and treating fewer people, all of whom are, by the way, equally needy and certainly among the worse off globally with regard to their health-related needs? Generic antiretroviral therapy, used with simplified follow-up protocols, made treatment available to tens of thousands who would otherwise not have had access to it in poor countries (Calmy et al., 2004). The effectiveness of these drugs can be similar to that of others used in industrialized countries (Laurent et al., 2004), but the degree of safety afforded by simplified surveillance may not be the same. This led to heated debate (Dyer, 2004). In addition to the difficulty of either allowing a greater degree of risk or allowing more people to go without treatment, both these solutions still leave many patients without access to lifesaving drugs. Thus, it could be said that neither outcome is fair. How does one identify a fair decision in such a context? One of the aspects this controversy reveals is that in most circumstances we count on some degree of fairness already existing in the group where issues of resource allocation arise. Humanitarian medicine faces the problem of having to be as fair as possible in an unfair world.

Equity Without a Community

Health systems usually exist to support a common endeavor to care for everybody's health. We are accustomed to thinking of equity within defined groups, where reciprocity forms the basis for accepting unified standards in access to healthcare. Humanitarian medicine faces the problem of finding equitable solutions where no community supports reciprocity. Humanity itself could theoretically form such a circle of solidarity, in that there is no presently identified intrinsically insurmountable obstacle to such a situation. However, in practice, it is currently clearly not a cohesive group or even a group united with regard to reciprocity in healthcare. It has been argued that "the extension of economic and cultural relationships beyond national borders" gives us reason for international solidarity or even social contracts (Beitz, 1975) and that global distributive justice ought to be egalitarian (Hinsch, 2001), at least with regard to minimum conditions for a decent human life (Beitz, 2001). Despite our increasingly rights-based view of international health, which grounds itself in the emergence of a human right not only to the conditions of health (United Nations, 1948) but also to health itself (Hendriks & Toebes,

1998; Katz, 2004), such common standards do not extend to how to allocate health resources fairly. Humanity currently supports neither a system of reciprocity for healthcare nor common standards of equity in allocating healthcare resources. Thinking about fairness and equity in the context of humanitarian medicine is harder.

In the context of antiretroviral therapy to face the HIV/AIDS pandemic, Macklin (2003) proposed definitions of equity based on priority to those likely to benefit the most, to reducing disparities in health or in access to healthcare, to the worse off, or to some form of reciprocity. Each of these principles is problematic in some circumstances, and they can conflict with one another. For example, the utilitarian principle can result in our ignoring claims on the part of the most vulnerable or the worse off. It is beset with difficulties regarding how to weigh medium- and long-term consequences against one another (see, e.g., Granich et al., 2018). Giving unlimited priority to the worse off can result in our pouring resources into situations where we help but little and ignoring situations where more effective help can be offered. Giving in return to those who have contributed – one form of reciprocity – can sometimes favor the best off, those capable of contributing in the first place, who are likely to be less needy. A consequence of these problems is that none of these principles seems to be a likely candidate to substitute straightforward application of a theory of justice for the sort of social contract that is lacking.

Legitimacy

Although we may be more likely to accept allocation decisions as legitimate if they are fair, legitimacy in humanitarian medicine poses a distinct problem. First, how is the question of what makes a decision legitimate to be understood in this context? The actions of humanitarian medicine do not represent "coercively imposed collective authority" (Nagel, 2005), so if we are asking about the sort of legitimacy a state requires, any requirement for legitimacy could be questioned upfront. Nevertheless, the extent of humanitarian organizations' actual role in decisions that affect the basic conditions of a decent life, especially "where states are weak" and where "a diversity of agents and agencies . . . can contribute to justice," is compelling (O'Neill, 2001: 194). So questions usually linked to state legitimacy may not be entirely inappropriate here. Minimally, under what conditions can decisions regarding the allocation of international healthcare resources be considered legitimate when made by nongovernmental organizations? The nature and extent of a duty to provide humanitarian medicine may shape questions regarding legitimacy. If we view humanitarian medicine as charity and base decisions on which plight we find most poignant, it is not clear that we need to give any further reasons. If, however, we have a duty to provide help, including humanitarian medicine, for example, because we share responsibility in maintaining international rules that harm the global poor (Pogge, 2005) and their health (Pogge, 2002), this could affect not just what our duty is but also how it should be fulfilled. If "the extension of economic . . . relationships" gives us reason to share resources internationally (Beitz, 1975), this too will affect what legitimacy in humanitarian medicine might look like. Recognizing a right to healthcare for any reason has a similar effect. Consequently, the same development from charity-based to rights-based claims to health should be expected to affect the issue of legitimacy as well. A more rights-based approach will require stronger legitimacy in allocation decisions and would also tend to shift the target of accountability from donors to include beneficiaries (Asgary & Waldman, 2017; Scarnecchia et al., 2017).

The second difficulty is that just about any claim for legitimacy in allocating resources in humanitarian medicine seems bound to be incompletely fulfilled. We may, for example, think that those affected by allocation decisions should have the possibility of understanding and critiquing them (Forst, 2001). This, however, might include all populations who need the assistance of humanitarian medicine, as well as donors and those who would implement these decisions: a difficult logistical problem. Fulfilling minimal claims for legitimacy, such as those based on the view that humanitarian medicine is strictly supererogatory charity work, does seem more feasible[3] but does not make such a view any more convincing.

Although procedural fairness could represent some beginning toward greater legitimacy (see following sections), allocation decisions in humanitarian medicine may ultimately never be entirely legitimate under current international circumstances. In any case, philosophical analysis of legitimacy in humanitarian intervention has tended to focus primarily on legitimacy to transgress negative rights in the context of decisions regarding whether or not any intervention was justified.[4] Humanitarian medicine, however, raises issues of legitimacy in resource allocation for positive rights, such as the right to health or healthcare and allocation within existing programs, in decidedly nonideal circumstances. These issues would benefit from further exploration.

Conflicting Goals and Interests

Justifications used by DWB for allocation decisions are not limited to a single goal or even to principles of equity (Fuller, 2006). This shows that something richer is going on but also makes a potential for goal conflicts apparent. One example is the potential for conflict between the goals of *témoignage* – speaking out regarding human tragedies – and care. At first sight, these two goals seem very similar. They arise from the same kinds of motivations and circumstances: being there and able both to help and to speak out when no – or few – others are. Indeed, *témoignage* may sometimes take up where the possibility of other actions stops. An action remains possible when we are otherwise powerless.

There are, however, two potential tensions there. First, for humanitarians, "doing the best they can" in an imperfect world can involve "cutting corners" in individual actions to do the most good overall. For example, using simplified follow-up protocols for antiretroviral treatment has enabled scale-up of programs to reach more patients, but possibly at the cost of a small degree of safety to individuals because some side effects will be detected later than would have been the case with more intensive laboratory testing. Such expediency, however, should not be perceived as the norm (Harding-Pink, 2004). Second, conducting advocacy and care simultaneously can also lead to conflicts of interest. Speaking out regarding a human tragedy can also be in the interest of the organization itself, at the cost of vulnerable individuals who, for example, might be identified on posters in a victim role that could be detrimental to them individually. In theory, the most important points may be to protect consent and confidentiality in advocacy and to ensure that the goal of benefiting the victims is always

---

[3] Legitimacy may then require truthfulness toward donors as to the use of funds but little else.

[4] For example by intruding on the independence of a state, through force, to protect its citizens from human rights abuses – see, for example, Buchanan, (1999).

present, avoiding situations where a campaign might be purely self-serving. Nonetheless, the implementation of strategies to regulate conflicts of interest could be difficult to verify in self-regulating organizations serving disenfranchised individuals.

Although this set of issues does not aim to be comprehensive, careful and creative thoughts on any of these points could contribute to better strategies for allocating resources in humanitarian medicine, based on more robust ethical argumentation than could be the case otherwise. The development of more robustly argued ethical conclusions has been called for regarding public health in general (Ashcroft, 2008). At least some specific approaches are likely to be needed in the international nongovernmental setting of humanitarian medicine. Although we agree with this call for more substantive solutions, in the following sections we propose that some headway could nevertheless be made by adapting existing frameworks of procedural fairness for practical use in humanitarian organizations. The application and specification of principles of procedural fairness to this context point to a number of areas where governance, but also distributive fairness, could be improved despite the specific difficulties faced there.

Accountability for Reasonableness and Its Limits in Humanitarian Distribution

Because reasonable people will disagree about where the limit ought to be, and about what correct criteria might be, discussion of resource allocation has increasingly shifted from searching for guiding principles to outlining processes for fair decision making (Coulter & Ham, 2000). One influential process put forward for this purpose, Daniels and Sabin's "accountability for reasonableness" (Daniels & Sabin, 1997), starts by recognizing that we have no generally accepted principles for setting limits in healthcare. This poses a problem both for fairness and for legitimacy, the latter being especially problematic in instances where democratic control is lacking, such as limitation decisions made by private insurance companies in the United States. It should be noted here that although the context addressed by these authors is very different from humanitarian medicine, the absence of a participative democratic process is a crucial similarity. In their seminal paper, Daniels and Sabin critique three prevalent views regarding fair distribution. First, the market is subject to too many failures to function as a fair limit-

setting mechanism (Arrow, 2001) and should not be expected to function to provide us with positive rights (such as the right to healthcare; Daniels, 1985) but only with goods that we have a liberty right that no one should prevent us from acquiring (such as cars). Second, moral philosophy cannot be simply applied to allocation dilemmas that present us with unresolved issues (Daniels, 1994). Third, democratic decision making is not the only feasible option. The authors present a process that, so they argue, is able to offer procedural fairness – and with it conditions of legitimacy for these decisions – in resource allocation.

The idea is to make decisions about limits legitimate by accepting that both "winners" and "losers" in allocation decisions will have valid claims and following a fair process using the following four elements:

1. *The publicity condition.* Decisions regarding both direct and indirect limits to care and their rationales must be publicly accessible.
2. *The relevance condition.* A rationale will be reasonable if it appeals to evidence, reasons, and principles that are accepted as relevant by fair-minded people who are disposed to finding mutually justifiable terms of cooperation.
3. *The revision and appeals condition.* There must be mechanisms for challenge and dispute resolution regarding limit-setting decisions and, more broadly, opportunities for revision and improvement of policies in the light of new evidence or arguments.
4. *The regulative condition.* There is either voluntary or public regulation of the process to ensure that conditions 1–3 are met.

In addition to more robust allocation decisions, the authors hope to foster the development of a corpus of argued decisions from which a basis could be drawn for future situations: a sort of case law that could help to refine decisions through time. Through the second condition, they aim to recognize that all have an interest in having justifications acceptable to all. The third and fourth conditions aim to connect the process to broader deliberative processes in society.

Using this framework in humanitarian medicine poses specific difficulties. In applying the publicity condition, reaching the beneficiaries of humanitarian medicine with the relevant information is likely to be particularly difficult. The revision and appeals condition will be similarly difficult to apply because the affected populations are often disenfranchised and less able than most to defend their own interests. Indeed, this is often precisely why they need humanitarian aid. Identifying "evidence, reasons, and principles that are accepted as relevant" could be more difficult across cultural barriers. Lack of public regulation, which sometimes places humanitarian organizations in situations where they assume state duties without state legitimacy or checks and balances, also limits the ways in which the regulatory condition can be applied. The additional goals pursued by the authors, which form a part of their approach's appeal, also seem more difficult in a humanitarian context. Connection to broader deliberative processes requires a community within which such processes exist. Our common interest in having justifications that are acceptable to all is strongly grounded in reciprocity. Even more pragmatically, where would a corpus of similar decisions be kept? How would it be accessible? Given the tension between distribution in humanitarian medicine and the "rule of rescue," could humanitarian organizations fear that keeping such a corpus would make them seem callous, thus endangering their funding?

Adaptations for Use in Humanitarian Medicine

Some of these obstacles may not be surmountable, at least at present. The first requirement in attempting to adapt accountability for reasonableness to humanitarian medicine is recognizing that doing better is a valid goal, even if problems remain. This should be no surprise. In our unjust world, aiming directly at ideal fairness could be daunting to the point of immobilization. It is already crucial that a lesser goal does not leave us lacking criteria for fair distribution. In other words, immobilization is unnecessary: making a situation fairer is worthwhile even if complete fairness is inaccessible. Neither does fair distribution require that everyone get what they have a valid claim to: it requires that what is available be distributed without discounting anyone's claims. As long as, say, the decision to use generics rather than brand-name drugs to treat HIV avoided such discounting, then it was a fair decision. Our incapacity to make the world globally fair does not make concerns for fairness moot. We can still judge decisions according to whether they make things *fairer*, even if they cannot make them *fair*. Similarly, increasing fairness in allocation decisions is a valid goal even if a perfect process cannot be implemented.

An adapted version of accountability for reasonableness could at least complement other mechanisms in doing so.

Some possible adaptations are outlined in Table 14.1. Despite the difficulty in reaching beneficiaries, the publicity condition would at minimum be a requirement for internal explicitness. As one member of a humanitarian organization put it, there are things that we cannot do if we must acknowledge them in writing. Although these examples are purely fictitious, such "things" might include giving priority to a personal friend in a program with limited treatment spots, keeping a program open at the expense of a more urgent one to avoid admitting failure, or siding with individuals belonging to one of several warring factions in allocation decisions. In any case, according to this comment, even strictly internal publicity could sometimes represent an improvement. Attempting to fulfill the publicity condition could also include publicity to donors. Humanitarian organizations depend on their reputation to raise funds from private donors. This could not legitimately replace, but might complement, accountability to beneficiaries themselves. Although such solutions would remain imperfect, decisions could also be made accessible at least to local staff, community leaders, and governments. Reasons for allocation decisions would also have to be accessible to any beneficiaries with whom it happened to be easy to come into contact. For example, individual patients who might ask why a local program was being terminated should receive a frank answer.

The relevance condition poses a particular problem because different understandings of equity can lead to contradictory conclusions and different considerations might be deemed more or less relevant across cultural settings. If we admit that there will be no single principle of fairness applicable to all situations, however, we can retain consistency in our decisions by examining all the plausible principles accessible to us and systematically choosing the "least worse" option *on each principle's own terms*. On this model, decision makers would first attempt to optimize the amount of good that could be obtained with the available resources, for example, by optimizing the use of existing resources (Timble et al., 2013), drawing on local knowledge and networks (Bealt & Mansouri, 2018), and limiting possible harms and tradeoffs as much as possible. Then they would examine the conclusions predicted by sufficientarian, prioritarian, egalitarian,

Table 14.1 Adapting Frameworks

Daniels and Sabin's "accountability for reasonableness"	Publicity condition	Relevance condition	Revision and appeals condition	Regulative condition
	Decisions regarding both direct and indirect limits to care, and their rationales, must be publicly accessible.	A rationale will be reasonable if it appeals to evidence, reasons, and principles that are accepted as relevant by people who are disposed to finding mutually justifiable terms of cooperation.	There must be mechanisms for challenge and dispute resolution regarding limit-setting decisions and, more broadly, opportunities for revision and improvement of policies in the light of new evidence or arguments.	There is either voluntary or public regulation of the process to ensure that conditions 1–3 are met.
Obstacles in humanitarian medicine	Reaching beneficiaries is difficult.	Different understandings of equity and no opportunity to discuss them	Disenfranchised populations	No public regulation
Adaptation to practice	Internal explicitness, publicity to donors, local staff, community leaders, and governments and readiness to explain reason to beneficiaries who are reached	Consistent reasoning strategy to weigh these different views in specific situations	Advocacy within the organization on behalf of those populations	Regulation must be internal and should itself be publicly accessible.

Source: Daniels & Sabin, 1997.

or utilitarian criteria for reaching the specific allocation decision they faced. They would then estimate how great each available transgression would be. This smallest degree of wrong would not be determined according to yet another principle but internally, based on the severity of each transgression *on the basis of the principle that it transgressed.* When attempting to make a fair choice based on considerations of equity, we would first evaluate what conclusion each definition of equity would point to. Then we would assess how severe the transgression of the other principles would be with each of these conclusions (Hurst & Danis, 2007). When HIV programs were first included within humanitarian medicine, for example, a recurrent dilemma at DWB was when and where to start such programs in unstable regions, where the organization may not stay long. Figure 14.1 illustrates how evaluative judgments regarding different parameters of such cases (here infrastructure stability and the population's need for the program) could be expressed. In the example presented here, country A is needier than country B, so in a prioritarian framework it is likely to be preferred on grounds of fairness as the target of

an intervention. However, its infrastructures are also slightly less stable, making an intervention there less likely to be sustainable and decreasing long-term utility to beneficiaries compared with an intervention in country B. Such comparisons are rarely straightforward, but they are routinely made. So far, so good. If we apply prioritarian – or egalitarian – principles and start a program in country A, we will thus get a little less benefit because the situation will be less stable in the long term. On utilitarian grounds, and all other things being equal, there will be a degree of wrong involved. If, however, we apply a utilitarian principle and go to country B, we will be disregarding the greater need of the citizens of country A. On prioritarian grounds, there will again be a degree of wrong involved. Inasmuch as each of these principles allows for the existence of greater or lesser wrongs, the respective degree of wrong in each case can be estimated. Comparing them will identify which is the smallest available wrong, as assessed according to the principle being transgressed. In this case, then, the transgression to prioritarianism would be worse if humanitarian medicine used a utilitarian approach and gave priority

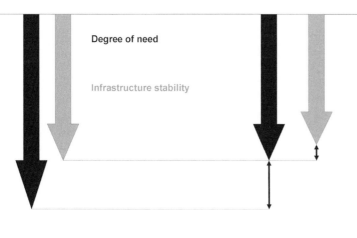

Figure 14.1. Choosing the smallest degree of wrong when evaluating two specific situations (arrows represent two countries, A [darker arrow] and B [lighter arrow]).

Degree of need

Infrastructure stability

to the country with the more secure context. Therefore, country A should have priority. This is not the same as choosing the best consequences, which could lead to the opposite conclusion. This approach is limited because different principles may well be incommensurable. Data on which to assess consequences – or need – may be lacking (Colombo & Checchi, 2018). Nevertheless, moral judgment is still necessary in such cases, and reasons must be given where possible. Whereas these evaluations and judgments cannot be spelled out in detail, humanitarian organizations currently do make them: they may often be able to explain why, in a specific case, problems linked to unsustainable infrastructures, say, are minor while the needs at stake are extreme. Although the reasons that can be given on this basis will often underdetermine such choices, the exercise in reflective equilibrium that we propose does delimit the sorts of choices more likely to be justifiable by setting each principle relevant in a given situation as a partial constraint on the others.

Difficulties linked to the revision and appeals condition would be increased by the very vulnerability of the populations requiring humanitarian assistance. Those affected by allocation in humanitarian medicine are often disenfranchised and less able than most to defend their own interests. Here, however, the increased scope of humanitarian medicine's actions could provide a partial alternative. Given enough competing projects, decisions could be challenged by members of the organization itself. This would require that humanitarians act as advocates for the people they are helping "on the ground" – a form of internal *témoignage*.

Given the absence of public regulation of humanitarian allocation decisions, the regulative condition

would have to be met voluntarily, or at least through internal regulation. In order to bolster this condition, enforcement mechanisms could themselves be subject to the publicity condition.

The aim to improve fairness in allocating decisions thus could be furthered by using an adapted form of Daniels and Sabin's "accountability for reasonableness" framework in humanitarian medicine. This application would require internally explicit decisions and rationales; publicity to donors as well as local staff, community leaders, and governments; frank answers to any beneficiary – or potential beneficiary – who asked for clarification of decisions and their rationale; a consistent reasoning strategy to weigh conflicting views of equity in specific situations; advocacy within the organization as a mechanism for revision and appeals; and internal regulation according to publicly accessible mechanisms.

The additional goals pursued by the authors to connect such decisions to broader deliberative processes fulfill our common interest in having justifications that are acceptable to all, and initiating a corpus of similar decisions probably could also be reached in an adapted form, at least in part. Given organizations with a strong deliberative tradition or that are challenged to explain their motives publicly, connection to broader deliberative processes could happen either internally or externally. It could increasingly take place internationally as the number of such organizations increases and they confront their choices and motivations. With regard to the requirement to "do the most good" with available resources, the "effective altruism" movement has made some headway in making at least one kind of justification internationally transparent. Potential disincentives to keeping a corpus of similar decisions could also have a pragmatic solution. Because harms to the reputation of humanitarian organizations would mostly accrue in comparisons, a common decision to keep a pooled corpus of allocation decisions could partly address this concern. This would have the added benefit of increasing the size of the corpus available to each organization. Risks to the reputation of humanitarian medicine as a whole could be addressed by visible enhancement of fair allocation decision making.

Clarity about the needs to make allocation decisions and to accept imperfect solutions, as well as about the process used to reach such decisions, helps to fulfill the "duty of mind" – the requirement for sound ethical decision making even under conditions of physical and emotional exhaustion prevalent in humanitarian situations (Ryus & Baruch, 2018). It would be important in forming an evolving base for refining resource-allocation decisions in humanitarian medicine. Clarity about these points would also serve an additional purpose. Becoming habituated to making do with very little and coming to perceive this as morally acceptable in general is a very real risk in humanitarian medicine (Harding-Pink, 2004). It should remain clear that such expediency, including the use of imperfect allocation strategies, is only morally acceptable *as long as there is no morally better alternative available*. This kind of clarity must, for example, be fostered if humanitarians are to speak out against unequal treatment, attempt to make treatment *fairer* by sometimes applying a double standard themselves, and avoid the impression that they are accusing themselves of unfairness in the process.

Conclusion

Allocating resources is difficult in any context but raises specific ethical difficulties in humanitarian medicine. These difficulties are becoming more visible and have prompted the development of tools such as the one presented here, as well as general frameworks for ethics in humanitarian medicine (Clarinval & Biller-Andorno, 2014; Fraser et al., 2015) and public health emergencies (Barnett et al., 2009). Minimally, we believe headway could be made by adapting existing frameworks of procedural fairness for practical use in humanitarian organizations. Despite the difficulties in applying it to humanitarian medicine, Daniels and Sabin's "accountability for reasonableness" could be adapted to include internally explicit decisions and rationales; publicity to donors as well as

local staff, community leaders, and governments; frank answers to any beneficiary – or potential beneficiary – who asked for clarification of decisions and their rationale; a consistent reasoning strategy to weigh conflicting views of equity in specific situations; advocacy within the organization as a mechanism for revision and appeals; and internal regulation according to publicly accessible mechanisms. Clarity about the needs to make allocation decisions and to accept imperfect solutions, as well as about the process used to reach such decisions, would be important both to refine resource-allocation decisions and to bear in mind the difference between standards to advocate and standards that must currently be accepted. Importantly, the complexity of these challenges should encourage rather than hinder broader discussion on the ethical aspects of resource allocation in humanitarian medicine.

Acknowledgments

The authors wish to thank Bernard Baertschi, Alexandra Calmy, Maria Merritt, Ulrike von Pilar, Marinette Ummel, Ulrich Vischer, the participants of the ethics and policy workshops of the DWB HIV training programs of Geneva and Berlin, and the editors and anonymous reviewers for useful comments, as well as Christophe Fournier from DWB International, and Isabelle Segui-Bitz and Christian Captier from DWB Switzerland for allowing us to use real examples.

This work was funded by the Institute for Biomedical Ethics at the Geneva University Medical School and by the Swiss National Science Foundation (grant 3233B0–107266/1). This chapter is based on a background paper written in 2005 by one of the authors (SAH) for Doctors Without Borders as a contribution to the La Mancha deliberation process. The views expressed here are the authors' own and not necessarily those of the Geneva University Medical School, the Swiss National Science Foundation, or Doctors Without Borders.

Competing interests: NM was a member of the board of DWB Switzerland. SAH has given workshops for DWB Switzerland, DWB Germany, and DWB International.

References

Arrow, K. J. (2001). Uncertainty and the welfare economics of medical care. 1963. *Journal of Health Politics, Policy and Law* **26**(5), 851–883.

Asgary R., & Waldman R. J. (2017). The elephant in the room: towards a more ethical approach with accountability towards intended beneficiaries in humanitarian aid. *International Health* **9**(6), 343–348

Ashcroft, R. (2008). Fair process and the redundancy of bioethics: a polemic. *Public Health Ethics* **1**(1), 3–9.

Barnett, D. J., Taylor, H. A., Hodge, J. G., & Links, J. M. (2009). Resource allocation on the frontlines of public health preparedness and response: report of a summit on legal and ethical issues. *Public Health Reports* **124**(2), 295–303.

Bealt, J., & Mansouri, S. A. (2018). From disaster to development: a systematic review of community-driven humanitarian logistics. *Disasters* **42**(1), 124–148

Beitz, C. R. (1975). Justice and international relations. *Philosophy and Public Affairs* **4**(4), 360–389, p 388.

Beitz, C. R. (2001). Does global inequality matter? *Metaphilosophy* **32**(1–2), 97–112.

Birch, M., & Miller, S. (2005). Humanitarian assistance: standards, skills, training, and experience. *British Medical Journal* **330**(7501), 1199–1201.

Buchanan, A. (1999). The internal legitimacy of humanitarian intervention. *Journal of Political Philosophy* **7**(1), 71–87.

Calmy, A., Klement, E., Teck, R., et al. (2004). Simplifying and adapting antiretroviral treatment in resource- poor settings: a necessary step to scaling-up. *AIDS* **18**, 2353–2360.

Caney, S. (2001). Cosmopolitan justice and equalizing opportunities. *Metaphilosophy* **32**(1–2), 113–134.

Civaner, M. M., Vatansever, K., & Pala, K. (2017). Ethical problems in an era where disasters have become a part of daily life: a qualitative study of healthcare workers in Turkey. *PLoS ONE* **12**(3), e0174162.

Clarival, C., & Biller-Andorno, N. (2014). Challenging operations: an ethical framwork to assist humanitarian aid workers in their decision-making processes. *PLoS Currents* **23**(6) pii.

Colombo, S., & Checchi, F. (2018). Decision-making in humanitarian crises: politics, and not only evidence, is the problem. *Epidemiologia and Prevenzione* **42**(3–4), 214–225.

Coulter, A., & Ham, C. (2000). *The Global Challenge of Health Care Rationing*. Maidenhead, UK: Open University Press.

Daniels, N. (1985). *Just Health Care*. New York: Cambridge University Press.

Daniels, N. (1994). Four unsolved rationing problems: a challenge. *Hastings Center Report* **24**(4), 27–29.

Daniels, N., & Sabin, J. (1997). Limits to health care: fair procedures, democratic deliberation, and the legitimacy problem for insurers. *Philosophy and Public Affairs* **26**(4), 303–350.

Diallo, D. A., Doumbo, O. K., Plowe, C. V., et al. (2005). Community permission for medical research in developing countries. *Clinical Infectious Diseases* **41**(2), 255–259.

Dyer, O. (2004). Bush accused of blocking access to cheap AIDS drugs. *British Medical Journal* **328**, 783.

Forst, R. (2001). Towards a critical theory of transnational justice. *Metaphilosophy* **32**(1–2), 160–179.

Fraser, V., Hunt, M. R., de Laat, S., & Schwartz, L. (2015). The development of a humanitarian health ethics analysis tool. *Prehospital and Disaster Medicine* **31**(4), 412–420.

Fuller, L. (2006). Justified commitments? Considering resource allocation and fairness in Médecins Sans Frontières Holland. *Developing World Bioethics* **6**(2), 59–70.

Granich, R., Gupta, S., & Williams, B. G. (2018). HIV, 95-95-95 and the allocative efficiency fallacy: why treating everyone makes sense from a humanitarian, clinical, economic and disease control perspective. *Journal of the International AIDS Society* **21**(10), e25191.

Harding-Pink, D. (2004). Humanitarian medicine: up the garden path and down the slippery slope. *British Medical Journal* **329**(7462), 398–399.

Hendrickson, D. (1998). Humanitarian action in protracted crisis: an overview of the debates and dilemmas. *Disasters* **22**(4), 283–287.

Hendriks, A., & Toebes, B. (1998). Towards a universal definition of the right to health? *Medical Law* **17**(3), 319–332.

Hinsch, W. (2001). Global distributive justice. *Metaphilosophy* **32**(1–2), 58–78.

Hodge, J. G., Hanfling, D., & Powell, T. P. (2013) Practical, ethical, and legal challenges underlying crisis standards of care. *Journal of Law and Medical Ethics* **41**(Suppl 1), 50–55.

Hurst, S. A., & Danis, M. (2007). A framework for rationing by clinical judgment. *Kennedy Institute of Ethics Journal* **17**(3), 247–266.

Jonsen, A. R. (1986). Bentham in a box: technology assessment and health care allocation. *Law, Medicine and Health Care* **14**(3–4), 172–174.

Katz, A. (2004). The Sachs report: investing in health for economic development – or increasing the size of the crumbs from the rich man's table? *International Journal of Health Services* **34**(4), 751–773.

Laurent, C., Kouanfack, C., Koulla-Shiro, S., et al. (2004). Effectiveness and safety of a generic fixed-dose combination of nevirapine, stavudine, and lamivudine in HIV-1-infected adults in Cameroon: open-label multicentre trial. *Lancet* **364**(9428), 29–34.

Leider, J. P., DeBruin, D., Reynolds, N., et al. (2018). Ethical guidance for disaster response, specifically around crisis standards of care: a systematic review. *American Journal of Public Health* **107**(9), e1–e9.

Macklin, R. (2003). Ethics and equity in access to HIV treatment: "3 by 5"initiative. WHO. Available at www.who.int/ethics/en/background-macklin.pdf.

McIntyre, A. (1994). Guilty bystanders? On the legitimacy of duty to rescue statutes. *Philosophy and Public Affairs* **23**, 157–191.

McKie, J., & Richardson, J. (2003). The rule of rescue. *Social Science and Medicine* **56**(12), 2407–2419.

Michael, M., & Zwi, A. B. (2002). Oceans of need in the desert: ethical issues identified while researching humanitarian agency response in Afghanistan. *Developing World Bioethics* **2**(2), 109–130, p109.

Murphy, L. B. (2000). *Moral Demands in Non-ideal Theory.* Oxford, UK: Oxford University Press.

Nagel, T. (2005). The problem of global justice. *Philosophy and Public Affairs* **33**(2), 113–147.

O'Neill, O. (2001). Agents of justice. *Metaphilosophy* **32** (1–2), 181–195.

Palmer, C. A. (1999). Rapid appraisal of needs in reproductive health care in southern Sudan: qualitative study. *British Medical Journal* **319**(7212), 743–748.

Pogge, T. W. (2002). Responsibilities for poverty-related ill health. *Ethics and International Affairs* **16**(2), 71–79.

Pogge, T. W. (2005). Real World Justice. *Journal of Ethics* **9**, 29–53.

Redmond, A. D. (2005). Needs assessment of humanitarian crises. *British Medical Journal* **330**(7503), 1320–1322.

Rougemont, A. (1995). From humanitarian action to international health. *Soz Praventivmed* **40**(1), 3–10.

Ryus, C., & Baruch, J. (2018). The duty of mind: ethical cpacity in a time of crisis. *Disaster Medicine and Public Health Preparedness* **12**(5):657–662.

Scarnecchia, D. P., Reymond, N. A., Greenwood, F., et al. (2017). A rights-based approach to information in humanitarian assistance. PLoS Current **20**(9), pii.

Scheffler, S. (1992). *Human Morality.* Oxford, UK: Oxford University Press.

Timble, J. W., Ringel, J. S., Fox, D. S., et al. (2013). Systematic review of strategies to manage and allocate scarce resources during mass casualty events. *Annals of Emergency Medicine* **61**(6), 477–689.

United Nations (1948). Universal Declaration of Human Rights, Article 25. Available at www.un.org/Overview/rights.html.

Wikler, D. (2003). Why prioritize when there isn't enough money? *Cost Effective Resource Allocation* **1**(1), 5.

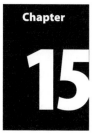

15

Development Assistance for Health
Trends and Challenges

Anthony B. Zwi

The patterns in health-related development assistance have changed markedly in recent years. This chapter seeks to provide an overview of both the value and the *underpinning values* that shape development assistance for health (DAH). The chapter is structured around four key elements: (1) motivations and influences on development assistance, (2) trends in development assistance for health, (3) debates and critiques of aid structures and approaches, and (4) ongoing challenges around more meaningful and equitable development assistance for health.

Background

In 2009, the Organisation for Economic Co-operation and Development (OECD), the "club" that represents many of the countries with leading economies, noted as "outrageous" the ongoing human tragedy of failed development: 9 million avoidable deaths in those under five years of age and 536,000 maternal deaths per year (OECD, 2009). Indeed, widespread acknowledgment of the limited achievements of international aid, a decade earlier, had led to agreement at the Millennium Summit to establish global targets for development, the Millennium Development Goals (MDGs). These comprised a set of eight interrelated development goals designed to close the poverty gap between rich and poor countries and to improve the health and well-being of over a billion people living on less than $1 per day (see www.un.org/millennium goals/). The MDGs reflected priority development concerns and included commitments to reduce poverty and gendered inequalities; improve access to education, water, sanitation, and healthcare; promote environmental sustainability; and enhance partnerships for development. Whereas all were intimately connected to health, three were explicitly focused on health goals and targets: MDG 4 (reducing child mortality), MDG 5 (reducing maternal mortality), and MDG 6 (tackling HIV/AIDS, tuberculosis, and malaria).

By the end of 2015, achievements in relation to the MDGs were patchy: both successes and failures had been reported, highlighting sectoral, geographic, and societal differences. Development advances against the MDGs were least evident across Sub-Saharan Africa, with widespread differences in the Asia-Pacific. China's development and growth achievements were impressive at many levels and helped secure global reductions in extreme poverty. However, widespread disparities and inequities remained, leaving major challenges not only between but increasingly within countries.

The MDGs were appropriately critiqued, including for establishing uniform rather than context-specific targets, for lack of attention to rights and inequalities, and for their focus on inputs rather than quality, effectiveness, outcomes, and impact. Concerns were raised that they contributed to excessive "Afro-pessimism" and stigmatized countries unable to meet global targets (Vandemoortele, 2009). The MDGs functioned as the core of the global development agenda, and as the 2015 endpoint approached, the next generation of ambitious development goals, targets, and indicators, the Sustainable Development Goals (SDGs), were framed and agreed for 2016–2030.

There is widespread recognition and extensive documentation of global inequity (unfair, unjust, remediable inequalities) in health and all the determinants of health, both within and between countries. It is clear that poverty at both individual and collective levels leads to ill-health and ill-health to exacerbating poverty. Breaking the vicious cycle between health and poverty and poverty and health and promoting health gain, both within and between countries, are broad social policy objectives, again widely agreed.

States play an important part in setting out health and social policies, along with articulating the underpinning values, mobilizing the resources, and leading the vision and implementation of services within coherent systems. Although other actors and organizations assist, and states alone, especially in some of the least-developed and low-income settings, are rarely able to address all the needs present, states remain central.

Inequities and poverty operate at a global level, where inequality is widening: Oxfam demonstrated in its "Even It Up" report (Oxfam, 2014) that eight men had as many wealth assets as 3.5 billion of the poorest people. Piketty (2014) demonstrated that wealth is increasingly concentrated among those who start off wealthy. Analyses in the United States similarly show that the wealthiest 0.1% of the population owns about 22% of all household-held assets in 2019 (*Financial Times*, November 13, 2019). The world is more and more challenging for those who have the least assets, and inequality widens despite more people being brought out of extreme poverty.

A recent report on global health expenditure revealed that the median per capita health spending was over $2,000 in high-income countries (and $5,000 or more in the top 10 wealthiest countries), whereas the bottom 10 countries spent less than $30 per person (Xu et al., 2018). These inequities have been much the same since 2000 and are likely widening.

Benatar (2005: 1208) highlighted the lack of "moral imagination" in addressing the "deplorable state of global health." He drew attention to how relatively low amounts but high-profile aid eclipses "recognition of the fact that financial, human and other material resources are continuously being extracted from developing countries by wealthy nations striving for their own ongoing economic growth," often in collusion with kleptocratic despots who use their power and control over national resources for personal gain.

Pogge (2008) critiques the notion that global development is about supporting those less fortunate; arguing instead that global inequities and poverty result from inequitable global macroeconomic and political structures and policies. He argues forcefully that the constraints to achieving development objectives in many under-resourced countries do not simply reflect poor domestic political choices and policies but rather global power imbalances. Pogge (2008) argues for a commitment not merely to providing official development aid (ODA) but for more fundamental reshaping of the global political economy.

Addressing Global Health Inequalities: Why Development Assistance for Health?

Selgelid (2008) sets out the arguments for why wealthy developed nations should promote health improvements in the Global South. Addressing these inequities and responding to them with development assistance support can be argued on moral, ethical, and pragmatic grounds. He identifies a range of reasons that can be summarized under four headings: egalitarian, utilitarian, libertarian, and self-interest. Each has its own rationale and proponents – but together they present a compelling case for addressing health problems in the Global South.

Egalitarian arguments seek to ensure that all people have equal opportunities, arguing that inequalities in well-being are undeserved and should be rectified, that the needs of those worst off should be addressed, and that the right to health should be fulfilled. Utilitarian arguments recognize that there are costs associated with addressing vast needs but that overall betterment of the human condition will be worthwhile as a result. Libertarian arguments stress that historical injustices need redress and that many of the benefits that have accrued to wealthy countries have resulted from the exploitation of less developed nations and peoples. Where these arguments are still insufficiently compelling, self-interest can be invoked: addressing health needs in the Global South reduces threats of emerging infectious diseases, enhances the potential for new markets and economic and social development, and reduces the costs associated with global health threats and promotes "health security."

In the decades after World War II, ODA increased substantially and continued to do so for decades. Although undoubtedly an important source of revenue for development processes, it is important to note that there are other, often more substantial contributions in low- and middle-income countries: private capital flows, remittances, and other investments (Figure 15.1).

Effective ODA can provide support to the political, economic, and social policy transformations that contribute to improving the lives and livelihoods of people across the globe. The SDGs focus on 17 goals and highlight the interdependence of different forms of investment across sectors; they need to work together to achieve optimal development outcomes.

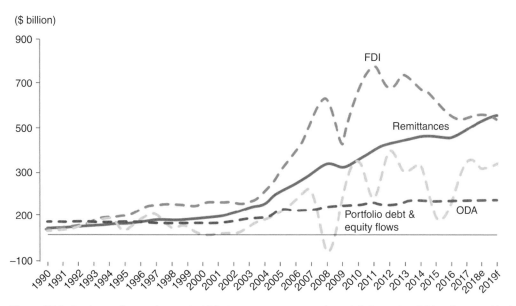

($ billion)

Figure 15.1. Remittance flows to low- and middle-income countries are substantially larger than ODA and more stable than private capital flows 1990–2019.
Source: OECD, 2019

Substantial improvements to health and eradicating poverty result from educating girls; both ODA and DAH can play a valuable role in promoting these linked objectives. The commitment within the SDGs to promote universal health coverage is an ambitious objective that will help promote equity in health and ensure that those most marginalized are not "left behind."

The UN Millennium Project found that only about 40% of the cost of achieving the MDGs could be met by low-income countries themselves, even after taking account of likely increases in domestic incomes and government revenue, and that ODA would be required to fill the gap. In 2002, the World Bank estimated that if countries improved their policies and institutions, the additional ODA required to achieve the MDGs by 2015 would have been US$40–60 billion a year (World Bank, 2002). In 2015, it was estimated that more than $189 billion was required to meet the MDGs in all countries. A recent estimate by the International Monetary Fund (IMF) and focused only on 49 of the least-developed countries suggested that US$520 billion per year would be required to achieve the more ambitious SDGs, with a focus on social and infrastructure developments. Although these different metrics are not directly comparable, they indicate the scale of the challenge

to national governments and the international community. Many countries are unable to mobilize the levels of funding proposed and ODA and DAH are required. The least-developed counties, for example, mobilized an average of only $9 per capita per year for healthcare costs of their citizens (Xu et al., 2018).

ODA levels "required" depend on many factors, including the predicted growth of economies in the Global South and national stability. Increased needs have resulted from global financial downturns, extreme weather events, conflicts and other crises such as the COVID-19 pandemic. Despite global efforts to secure increased development finance, contributions have flattened, and rising nationalism threatens cosmopolitan thinking and populist regimes exert pressure to reduce or seriously constrain government commitments to international development.

The Commission on Social Determinants of Health identified socioeconomic and political context, social position, material circumstances, and the healthcare system as all influencing the distribution of health and well-being. Development assistance for health can make a valuable contribution given poor health status, high levels of inequity, poor state capabilities, and the need for technical information, evidence, and support to promote appropriate interventions.

And while ODA and DAH have the potential to influence all the key determinants of health, the contribution they make will depend not only on the magnitude of aid but also on what vision, values, and processes underpin the formulation of priorities, the selection of intended beneficiaries, and the approach to implementation and assessing outcomes, among others.

Trends in ODA and DAH

ODA is extremely fickle, with large variations by donor, recipient countries, and sectors, year on year. At a macro level, ODA has in general risen in absolute amounts over the past decades, with troughs in the 1980s and 1990s, again after the financial crisis of 2008–2009, with a plateau more recently given the rise of populism.

Figure 15.2 reveals the plateau in ODA up to 2018. With further examination, ODA net flows declined in real terms from 2017 to 2018 by 3% to the least-developed countries, by 4% to countries of Africa, and by 8% for humanitarian aid (OECD, 2019). In 2018, seventeen OECD countries raised contributions, but 12 decreased ODA funding. ODA represented only 0.31% of the gross national income (GNI) of OECD member countries in 2018, well below the target of 0.7% of GNI. The number of countries contributing 0.7% of GNI or above was only five in 2018 (Denmark, Luxembourg, Norway, Sweden, and the United Kingdom), whereas major contributors such as the United States (0.17%) were way below target (OECD, 2019). Australia's contribution to development funding is currently at its lowest level for decades, is narrowly focused only on the Indo-Pacific, and

is increasingly stingy: only 0.2% of GNI. Real ODA from Australia has declined substantially, reflecting a conservative government being pulled further to the right by populist and nationalist interests.

Bensimon and Benatar (2006) drew attention to the difference between world military expenditure and ODA; in 2018, the divide remained massive. World military expenditure was $1,822 billion (excluding a handful of countries with notable expenditure, such as North Korea and Syria), 12 times more than ODA of that year ($153 billion).

Though proportions vary year on year, in 2017, about one-third of ODA from OECD countries was destined for the least-developed and other low-income countries, one-third for lower-middle-income countries, and one-third either unallocated or for upper-middle-income countries. The largest recipients of ODA in 2007–2008 were Iraq ($9.46 billion), Afghanistan ($3.48 billion), China ($2.6 billion), Indonesia ($2.54 billion), and India ($2.26 billion); the top five recipients received over 22% of ODA distributed by OECD countries in 2007–2008. In 2017, the top five country recipients of ODA differed substantially: Syria ($10.36 billion), Ethiopia ($4.12 billion), Afghanistan ($3.8 billion), Bangladesh ($3.74 billion), and Nigeria ($3.36 billion; OECD, 2019). The main components were humanitarian assistance, alongside bilateral development projects, programs, and technical cooperation, with lesser contributions to debt relief and multilateral agency activities.

The precise amounts allocated to global health are not clear but have been increasing. The World Bank cites a rise from US$2.5 billion in 1990 to almost

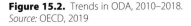

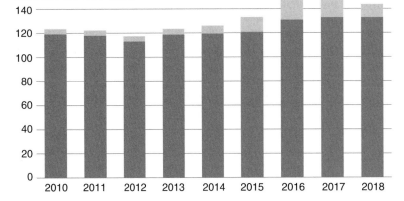

Figure 15.2. Trends in ODA, 2010–2018. *Source:* OECD, 2019

US$14 billion in 2005, a figure questioned by McCoy et al. (2009a), who draw attention to disbursements being substantially lower than public commitments. The Institute for Health Metrics Analysis in 2019 indicated that $US38.9 billion was allocated to DAH. The proportion of ODA directed to health was 5.3% of all ODA in 1980–1984 and 7.8% by 2002–2006 (Piva & Dodd, 2009).

Increased DAH reflected a range of influences: acceptance of the MDGs and SDGs as an overriding framework for ODA, recognition of the social determinants of health and their contribution to eradicating poverty, health as a core component of governance and nation building, concerns with emerging and reemerging infections and other health threats, the rising costs of healthcare, and anxieties about the threat of bioterrorism. The entry of a wide range of new actors, notably large-scale private and nongovernmental organization (NGO) investments in health and the establishment of new modalities for providing aid, such as the Global Fund Against AIDS, TB, and Malaria (GFATM), Global Alliance for Vaccines and Immunization (GAVI), Bill and Melinda Gates Foundation, and the US President's Emergency Plan for AIDS Relief (PEPFAR), contributed to further growth in DAH. In 2018, for example, the Bill and Melinda Gates Foundation contributed US$3.2 billion in DAH; this was 8.3% of global DAH and much more than the US$1.9 billion from all UN agencies combined.

Devastating outbreaks of Ebola viral disease in West Africa in 2014 and in the Democratic Republic of Congo (DRC; 2018–2019) drew attention to the vulnerabilities of countries in the aftermath (or presence) of conflict and highlighted the longer-term underfunding and underinvestment in systems and institutions, human resources, and management capacity. Reinforced by mistrust of authorities and, in the DRC, belligerent nonstate actors, communities suffer. The COVID-19 pandemic has further revealed vulnerabilities within systems and inequities within societies.

DAH is lumpy: much of the funding has been channeled to disease-specific interventions, notably HIV/AIDS, and has been critiqued for failing to build the structures and capacity of institutions or to assist states to act as guarantors for health advancement. Sustained benefits for general populations have not typically been achieved (Ravishankar et al., 2009).

High-profile initiatives attract available (rarely additional) funds and channel them in a way that satisfies donors that their investments are being managed "safely." This is apparent in the massive increases in support to HIV/AIDS, accounting for 32% of DAH from 2002 to 2006 (Piva & Dodd, 2009). In 2018, support for HIV/AIDS was still high (US$ 9.5 billion), amounting to 25.3% of all DAH. For the United States, HIV/AIDS was the target of over 60% of its direct disease control and health systems funding, highlighting its ongoing prioritization.

Whereas the delivery of healthcare is a major responsibility of national governments, there are many impediments to doing so, including constrained human and financial resources, poorly designed systems, and limited organizational and managerial capacity. External support has often neglected these systemic issues, undermining longer-term potential for health development.

The additional funds from private sources, notably the Bill and Melinda Gates Foundation, has stimulated key donors and institutions to exert more agency in shaping the global policy agenda; McCoy et al. (2009b) argue that this is implicitly promoted through widespread funding of key contributors to global health activity and thinking, including UN agencies, global health partnerships, the World Bank, NGOs, and universities (McCoy et al., 2009b). This funding footprint "give[s] the foundation (sic) a great deal of influence over both the architecture and policy agenda of global health" (McCoy et al., 2009b: 1650).

At a global level, ODA contributes only about 1% of total expenditure on health (Xu et al., 2018). The least-developed countries spent only about $9 per capita in 2016 and drew extensively on ODA for health expenditure support (Xu et al., 2018). Indeed, many countries, especially those categorized as least developed, are highly dependent on DAH, with more than 30 countries drawing at least 40% of their health funding from ODA (Reinikka, 2008), particularly among fragile and conflict-affected states. Moreover, these states demonstrate the least improvement in health and development outcomes, which remain a major priority, but often attract only limited support given the risk-averse stance of many funders (Bornemisza & Zwi, 2008).

A Critique of ODA with Emphasis on Global Health

Given the diversity of stakeholders operating within the global humanitarian and development systems, each has its own objectives and agendas and uses its power and influence to maximize benefits and minimize risk. Sumner & Tribe (2008: 25) argue that "values are central to disputes about the definition of development – what to improve, how to improve it and, especially, the question of who decides." Conceptually, development is informed by one of three main paradigms: development as a long-term process of structural and societal transformation, development as a short- to medium-term outcome of desirable targets, and development as a dominant discourse of Western modernity.

Kingsbury (2013: 3) asserts that there "remains no clear understanding or definition of what is meant when referring to 'development', not least of which is whether 'development' is a process or an outcome." This highlights questions not only about the role of external funds and ODA but also about the objectives, underpinning values, and vision of development.

A political economy perspective helps examine (and reveal) trends in the policy actions of development actors, unmasking underlying political and economic goals, and relates this to culture, institutions, power, and competing interests. Political economy analyses highlight three dimensions to ODA. They see aid as reflecting the economic interests of powerful groups (i.e., political parties, military, private companies, NGOs) within donor countries, aid as an effort to maximize donor benefits (diplomatic and trade interests and influence alongside promotion of cultural and other values) by working through bilateral or multilateral channels to enhance their influence in the international system, and aid as the outcome of bargaining (choices and compromises) among producers and consumers of aid (i.e., aid bureaucracies, multilateral agencies, and recipient countries [governments, officials, and sometimes civil society]) in order to maximize their own benefits. Donors may seek agreement with other nations on broad objectives, values, and approaches to conditions placed on aid recipients. The recipient countries, and the political and economic elites within them, seek to capture, or maximize, the value of ODA to support their own economic, political, and personal objectives while minimizing any imposed requirements.

ODA has historically been linked to conditionalities imposed by donors. Three of the biggest donors, the United States, Japan, and France, have all had noticeable biases in their patterns of aid: the United States typically targeted one-third of its aid budget to allies such as Israel and Egypt, with an emphasis on military not development assistance; France directed support to its former

colonies; and Japan favored countries that voted with it in the United Nations (McCormick, 2008). Emerging donors, too, such as China, require endorsement of foreign policy objectives such as the "one China policy" or tie ODA for infrastructure projects to implementation by Chinese companies (McCormick, 2008).

Political economy perspectives assist in understanding why weaknesses and failures in the development and aid system persist. It becomes apparent that much ODA is not intended to be transformative but to reinforces neoliberal and Western hegemonic approache. Maximizing the effectiveness of ODA, addressing poverty, and promoting equity may be side issues rather than the primary concern. Influence may be exercised through subtle means. The World Bank, for example, works through its role as a "knowledge bank," promoting use of "common language, rhetoric and discourse" that are internalized as ideas, norms, and constructs that reinforce the neoliberal paradigm (Das, 2009: 10).

Tandon (2009: 356) identifies three things wrong with the present aid and development architecture: the relationship between aid and development is not fully understood or "is deliberately fudged"; there is an assumption that both aid and development are "technical" despite their obvious political determinants; and the dominant conceptual framework hides "under the carpet" their "power-political" and historical dimensions.

In recent years, many countries have operated more explicitly in their own direct national interest (economically and politically; see Chapter 16) with respect to ODA. ODA has been used to reward or punish client states, to develop or exploit markets, to enforce diplomatic stances on particular issues, and to garner support locally. The content of ODA, such as support to sexual and reproductive rights, has been explicitly targeted under Trump as a reassertion of conservative, rights-opposing agendas in the United States and globally.[1] In 2017, President Trump reasserted the so-called global gag rule that sought to limit US-funded NGOs from providing counseling on,

---

[1] The Trump impeachment initiative of 2019 was in large part fueled by an even more personalized use of aid and trade: Trump proposed withholding military aid to Ukraine unless the government there publicly engaged with an internal US party and personal political agenda – a more extreme use of tying aid to conditions than usually comes to light.

referring to, or advocating around abortion services and laws. A valuable review of the impact of the set of conditionalities imposed shows a substantial negative impact not only on family planning delivery systems but also on HIV and AIDS services, maternal and child health, and advocacy and coalition space. These negative results resulted from "misunderstanding, miscommunication and chilling effects" of the policy. No impact on rates of abortion were observed, however (Mavodza, Goldman, & Cooper, 2019: 1).

Numerous assertions concerning the contribution of DAH to improved health outcomes have been made. However, the difficulties and complexities of assessing DAH should also be noted: (1) despite improvements, many countries still did not meet the MDGs, (2) the principal determinants of progress on health are domestic and include public policies and institutions, governance, levels of education, and the absence of conflict, and (3) enhancing aid effectiveness may improve the quality of DAH, but it remains difficult to measure the specific impact of interventions on health outcomes (OECD, 2009).

McCoy et al. (2009a: 407) asserted in 2009 that the "fragmented, complicated, messy and inadequately tracked state of global health finance requires immediate attention"; this is as true or perhaps even more so today. Three functions for global health funding were identified: provision, management, and expenditure. The providers of global health funding (i.e., governments, private foundations, individuals, and the corporate sector), those who manage these funds (including bilateral ODA agencies, intergovernmental organizations, global health partnerships, NGOs, private foundations, and the corporate sector), and those spending funds (including multilateral agencies, global health partnerships, NGOs, the private sector, and also low- and middle-income governments and their civil society) differ little in their approaches. Their activities and roles overlap; the fuzziness adds complexity and reduces transparency and accountability. This makes it difficult to assess efficiency, performance, and equity impact of activities.

Development assistance for health is inflated and imprecise (McCoy et al., 2009a), making it difficult also to track funding transfers and facilitate coordination and accountability, especially with intended beneficiaries. Data on private sources of global health funding are especially inaccurate, as are data from emerging donors, non-OECD governments such as China and India, and wealthy countries from the Middle East (Piva & Dodd, 2009). New sources of

data such as the Institute for Health Metrics and Evaluation (IHME) extend beyond the OECD and help provide a more complete picture of the patterns of ODA.

The securitization of ODA and development warrants close observation: countries such as Australia, the United States, and the United Kingdom have promoted close interaction between their foreign policy, defense, and overseas development activities, creating new structures to better coordinate the three "D's": development, diplomacy, and defense). In so doing, there has been an "almost unnoticed eclipse of the notion of 'human security' by more aggressive notions of 'security'" (Howell & Lind, 2009).

Seven Deadly Sins Associated with ODA

Birdsall (2008) ascribed "seven deadly sins" to ODA. She identified (1) "impatience" – with institution building and having a limited commitment to longer-term support; (2) "envy" – failure to effectively coordinate with one another in order to exert their own influence; (3) "ignorance" – and a failure to effectively evaluate development interventions; (4) "pride" – notably a failure to exit when appropriate; (5) "sloth" – sloppiness with concepts and their application and in particular pretending that participation is equivalent to developing-country ownership; (6) "greed" – characterized by unreliable and inadequate or, as Birdsall (2008) puts it, "stingy" transfers; and (7) "foolishness" – characterized by inadequate commitments to funding global and regional public goods. Each one of these is relevant to DAH and has been described more fully elsewhere (Zwi, 2011). The critique that follows draws on these ideas supplemented by other established critiques of ODA and DAH.

Impatience with Institution Building

Development can be conceptualized as a process of "creating and sustaining the economic and political institutions that support equitable and sustainable growth" (Birdsall, 2008). It should be inherently transformative if it is not to reproduce systems of control and power wielded by the Global North in its own interest (Kothari, 2005, republished in 2019).

In the effort to deliver specific services and promote lines of accountability to donors, the underlying health systems and state institutions have often been neglected, and the interface between external support and national development priorities has been poor. Delivering multiple public goods such as disease control, peace and security, and surveillance and information systems, as well as building local capacity, all depend on a functional health system with adequate infrastructure and human, material, and other resources, yet investment in these is often missing. Particular problems arise where states have undemocratic and/or poor leadership, poor institutions, low capacity, are "fragile" or conflict affected, or are in other ways hampered from exerting agency over their own development trajectory.

In conflict-affected and postconflict countries, initial surges in ODA are typically channeled through short-term emergency relief funding. The mobilization of development funding and the more sustained efforts required to build accountable and democratic institutions over the longer term are difficult to mobilize and sustain (Health and Fragile States Network, 2009).

Impatience for "results" may also lead to a focus on highly visible short-run projects where donors can claim successes and avoid the risk of being associated with institutional failures (Birdsall, 2008: 518). Donors often establish their own "vertical programs" – project implementation units operating outside government bodies, bypassing and, in some cases, undermining government systems. The emphasis on vertical and disease-specific programs (Zwi & Mills, 1995) reflects a failure, in health, to address long-term institutional constraints. Powerful donors such as the Bill and Melinda Gates Foundation often fund alongside, rather than to or through, emerging health systems. Impatience for results may lead to underinvestment in important areas that are less politically visible, such as human resources, management, and leadership development. The COVID-19 pandemic, however, powerfully reveals their importance and centrality.

Failure to Coordinate

Recipient countries deal with dozens of donors and a wide array of bilateral and multilateral agencies, foundations, NGOs, other civil society bodies, and the private sector. Despite changing language and discourse proposing a shift to engaging with "development partners," many remain "donors" who seek to maintain control in order to promote political and economic objectives rather than maximizing the value of coordinated aid on poverty reduction (Bigsten & Tengstam, 2015).

For public-sector staff in any low- or middle-income country, the range of agencies may be bewildering and burdensome, each requiring forms of engagement, hosting of missions, field visits, materials procurement, separate systems of monitoring and evaluation, and more. Grundy (2010), examining immunization programs in five Asian countries, highlighted their failure to support the "immunization system" itself.

Donors compete not only for visibility but also for local talent and skills – "poaching" staff from each other or from the public sector, at times weakening the institutions they ostensibly seek to support. Initiatives to bring donors together to better coordinate and reduce pressures on recipient governments may operate through agreement on broad health strategy and support for national plans or sector-wide approaches (SWAps) for health but are often resisted by powerful donors that seek bilateral arrangements outside these "common basket" approaches. Donors establish parallel structures for managing programs and projects despite the "evident savings and other benefits that would result from better coordination" (Addison and Tarp, 2015: 4).

New groups of nation-states such as the g7+ representing the least-developed and conflict-affected countries have begun to articulate how development assistance ought to be provided if it is to support rather than undermine national systems. The Busan Partnership for Effective Development Cooperation of 2011 (www.oecd.org/dac/effectiveness/49650173.pdf) set out the elements of good development practice and aid. It followed on a range of other OECD Development Assistance Committee guidance documents including the Paris Declaration on Aid Effectiveness (2005) and the Accra Agenda for Action (2008) and reasserted the importance of developing-country ownership of development priorities, a focus on results, inclusive development, partnerships, and transparency and accountability.

In recent decades, the engagement of a wider range of actors and organizations in development, alongside the more "traditional" OECD funders, has stimulated discussion of how development is both framed and achieved. The role of China in particular has been much critiqued as being self-interested, but Six (2009) and others argue that Chinese engagement has simply made explicit and transparent the expectations of those providing ODA. Chinese donors seek to frame development as solidarity with countries of the Global South, pursuing common development objectives, securing mutual benefits, and solidifying strategic interests (McCormick, 2008). These are also associated with promoting aid and trade, linking with

China's One Belt One Road initiative, and seeking to simultaneously secure Chinese access to resources and markets. Such activities also provide a focal point for securing diplomatic ("One China"), economic, and military or security objectives.

In the Pacific region, substantial efforts by China to build infrastructure and support resource extraction, trade, and services delivery fed into Australian (and other countries') anxieties about Chinese influence. This contributed to intensified efforts by Australia to focus its diminished ODA budget on the Pacific and to engage in larger-scale infrastructure projects, such as telecommunications, to avoid this sector being totally dominated by China. A 2019 conference of Pacific Island states was forced to modify its climate-change demands and to soften its stance against coal at the behest of Australia, a key donor and perceived "bully" in the region. The "green economy" and response to climate change are major thrusts of current development policies, yet some donors, such as Australia, have been reluctant to embrace them.

Failure to Evaluate

One of the most consistent and damning critiques of ODA is that it is poorly evaluated and that the same mistakes are made time and again. Policies and reforms are often proposed in the absence of good evidence. Whereas policy is unlikely to be entirely "evidence based," it should be transparently "evidence informed" (Bowen & Zwi, 2005) if accountability is to be promoted. Key health system reforms, such as the introduction of user fees, as promoted by the World Bank, were based on theoretical and ideological considerations; when the evidence was synthesized and assessed, benefits were limited and potential harms considerable.

Failure to evaluate may also, at some levels, be functional: it reduces the likelihood of exposing development flaws and weaknesses. Although recognizing limitations and failures is important, "according to the current perception, one risks undermining aid support if one admits failure" (Bigsten & Tengstam, 2015: 83). Careful evaluation is costly. Determining what contribution has been made is extraordinarily difficult given that so many factors, organizations, and actors may have played a part.

Fiszbein (2006) argued that development impact evaluation is an international public good, an issue echoed by policy and systems researchers, who have highlighted the importance of independent analyses and critique if we are to learn from experience rather than replicate systems of inequality and powerlessness (Storeng et al., 2018). Indeed, documenting weaknesses or even failures can be a powerful and important intervention to improve practice.

Donors are often reluctant to exit even in the absence of evident achievement. In some cases, countries have sought to broaden the scope for which funding can be "counted" as assistance for development, and national political pressures and populist concerns may seek not only to reduce development expenditure but also to channel it into more narrowly focused programs, including the control of migration or training of national security and police agencies. Furthermore, there may be reluctance to withdraw from programs that absorb large amounts of funding and satisfy certain domestic constituencies; closing them down and diverting funds elsewhere requires. i.e. requires energy, creativity, time, and political capital, all often in short supply.

Failure to Promote Genuine Ownership

Engagement is often top down and hierarchical – reflecting a biomedical and technocentric approach with limited local ownership, participation, or engagement. Davis (2009) suggests that donors talk about commitment to consultation, participation, and engagement, but their actions are limited. Meaningful engagement of communities and responding to voice and agency involve relinquishing some power to local actors and organizations and are typically resisted by donor countries.

A recent study indicated that DAH, if provided to government, appears to lead to concomitant reductions in government commitment to health expenditure, whereas if directed through civil society structures, it would leave government expenditure intact (Lu et al., 2010). Donors could usefully strengthen critical relationships among policymakers, providers, and clients (Reinikka, 2008). The recent examination of funding for health by Xu et al. (2018) also suggested that the least-developed countries diverted government expenditure to other sectors as external funds to health increased. The sample of countries was limited, the figures involved so low, and the pressures on least-developed countries so great that this deserves closer examination.

Stingy Contributions to ODA and DAH

Although total funding for global health has risen substantially, much funding continues in small, limited tranches that achieve little alone but require as much work (negotiation, transaction costs, reporting, and monitoring) as for much larger projects. Piva & Dodd's (2009) study of OECD DAH found 13,819 commitments for activities valued at under $0.5 million each – these small projects represented 67.5% of all DAH but accounted for only 3.6% of total health ODA. Large numbers of small projects are inefficient, exert high transaction costs in negotiating and reporting, require extensive additional monitoring and implementation capacity, and reflect high degrees of fragmentation of DAH.

There are "significant imbalances" in the allocation of aid that run counter to agreed principles of "effective aid" (Piva & Dodd, 2009: 930). Countries with comparable levels of poverty and health receive remarkably different levels of ODA, and there are considerable imbalances in relation to which sectors and, within health, which conditions attract attention. Some countries, some sectors, and some conditions (notably HIV/AIDS) attract a disproportionate level of funding. Xu et al. (2018) report that a poor relationship between HIV/AIDS funding and prevalence of the condition exists.

The OECD itself has recognized the inefficiencies and inequities that result from unequal commitment of aid to "aid darlings" and those who receive little DAH, the "aid orphans" (OECD, 2009). The vast majority of aid orphans are in Africa, where needs are often greatest. In only seven countries did attention to MDG-5 (improve maternal health) comprise more than 10% of health ODA (Piva & Dodd, 2009).

Important areas remain seriously underfunded: health system strengthening, mental health, and human resources development. Campaigners argue that health and economic gains for the "bottom billion" of the world's population would result from relatively modest investment in neglected tropical diseases (Hotez et al., 2009).

Foolishness: Underfunding of Regional and Global Public Goods

Around 25% of all DAH is associated with global and regional multicountry initiatives – considerably more than education-related ODA in the same period (2002–2006; Piva & Dodd, 2009). In part, this reflects the high proportion of funds allocated to HIV/AIDS (40% of global and regional multicountry initiatives) and global immunization programs.

In Malawi, in the middle to late 1990s, a "staggering" 10% of DAH was allocated to training (Reinikka, 2008). One of the rationales for this was to provide incentives and additional benefits to health workers with low wages, but at the same time, large training commitments meant that many health workers were away from their posts. If the same amount of funding were allocated to supporting salaries, health workers on average could have been paid 50% more that year (Reinikka, 2008).

The Bill and Melinda Gates Foundation has stimulated new technologies, devoting more than one-third (37%) of its funds to research and development or basic sciences research, but has risked underfunding core health system support. McCoy et al. (2009b) argued that the Bill and Melinda Gates Foundation promoted the growth of private provision of healthcare in low- and middle-income countries, further undermining an important role for public and government systems in shaping policies that set the context for health system development.

Funding for chronic and noncommunicable diseases has been inadequate. Gupta, Katz, and Swaminathan (2018) draw attention to the "anemic" funding for global chronic diseases, contrasting the US government spend of $US77 *million* on noncommunicable diseases in 2017 with the US$59 *billion* spend on HIV/AIDS in 2017. They argue for a more agile response through DAH to changing global epidemiological patterns.

General budget support amounted to only 6.4% of health ODA, and Piva and Dodd (2009: 937) draw attention to the lack of support for "systems issues" – management, logistics, procurement, infrastructure, and workforce development. They highlight the fact that these "areas may not appeal to donors," but "they will have to be tackled if current progress in disease control is to continue and if the quality and coverage of health services are to improve." Das Gupta and Gostin (2009) noted the absolute lack of attention to, and support of, public health systems and capacity in developing countries. Improvements may be emerging but are still inadequate, with approximately 14% of DAH associated with health system support in 2018.

McCoy et al. (2009b) critiqued the global health program of the Bill and Melinda Gates Foundation, drawing attention to the apparent inequities in how such resources are distributed. Significant amounts were allocated to a relatively small number of grantees (e.g., more than $1 billion to the Program for Appropriate Technology in Health [PATH]), large amounts were destined for US-based organizations, and granting decisions seemed to be "largely managed through an informal system of personal networks and relationships rather than by a more transparent process based on independent and technical peer review" (McCoy et al., 2009b: 1650).

Public–private partnerships have been promoted as a means for mobilizing additional resources and support for health activities and are widespread. Many focus on combating neglected diseases or on developing new drugs or vaccines. The United Nations and its agencies have sought to foster collaboration around global health and development in an effort to increase available resources and promote partnerships with civil society organizations, philanthropic foundations, governments, and the private sector. The World Bank suggests that such partnerships could help address specific cost and investment challenges, whereas the WHO hopes that engaging these wider groups of players will contribute to improving equity in access to essential drugs and to researching neglected diseases.

Concerns about the viability of public–private partnerships to improve global health equity revolve around several issues (Asante & Zwi, 2007). While seeking to be seen as socially responsible and to demonstrate "good corporate citizenship," they remain largely motivated by profit and return to their shareholders. Several multinational drug companies still engage in policies that restrict universal access to antiretroviral drugs. A number of "unhealthy habits" have characterized many global public–private partnerships: they skew national priorities, deprive national stakeholders of a voice in decision-making, are not accountable or transparent in relation to partner selection or grant disbursements, fail to compare the costs and benefits of public versus private systems of delivery, and do not adequately resource the transaction costs (Buse & Harmer, 2007). The SDGs explicitly call for private-sector engagement; this is not a bad thing in itself but an approach that brings complexity and reinforces the importance of understanding the range of stakeholders and their underpinning values and approaches.

The more traditional OECD donors have been complemented by an expanding number of increasingly influential countries such as India, China, Brazil, South Africa, and Indonesia. These "new" or nontraditional donors often have different viewpoints on how development should proceed and expected return on their investments. Their approach to providing ODA *without* engaging in local politics but ostensibly in solidarity with other countries of the Global South is a powerful counterbalance to long-standing but conditional support from OECD members. China, India, and others are actively engaged in a "silent revolution" in development assistance, weakening the bargaining position of Western donors and exposing standards and processes that are out of date or ineffectual while offering competitive and, in many ways, attractive alternatives (Woods, 2008).

Efforts spearheaded by the OECD to enhance the effectiveness of aid have included the Paris Declaration on Aid Effectiveness (2005) and the Accra Agenda for Action (2008), which aimed to address issues of ownership by recipient countries, to improve predictability of aid disbursements, and to ensure greater donor harmonization and alignment with national country priorities. The Busan Declaration (2011) responded to the concerns of some of the least-developed and conflict-affected countries and sought to recognize the particular challenges they faced.

Tan-Mullins et al. (2010: 857) argued that Chinese and Western donors "employ different ideologies and practices of governance to conceal their own interests and political discourses in the African continent." It remains important to scrutinize whose agendas lie at the foundation of agreed policies and strategies and whether coordination, harmonization, alignment, and country ownership occur in practice. The record to date has been poor.

Emerging Issues, Considerations, and Recommendations

The preceding discussion highlights numerous problems and weaknesses within the aid environment. Some of these are inherent given the political economy of aid and the desire for each of the stakeholders involved – donors, civil society, multilateral institutions, government, and service providers – to secure benefits for themselves and their clients. The diverse actors and organizations espouse different objectives and values, employ different methods, and seek different outcomes.

Better donor coordination, common-basket funding, and broad health system strengthening are required. The OECD (2009: 12) highlighted the degree of fragmentation present in the global health environment, arguing that the default position should be to "think twice" before establishing other initiatives related to DAH and that a "radical pruning" of the very long tail of small health projects was required.

There is, to some extent, greater recognition that ODA should be increased and that a substantial proportion of such funds should be devoted to the social sector – among which are health, education, water, and sanitation. The additional funds mobilized should make possible a far wider engagement and support for longer-term development of the health sector, as promoted by the UN High Level Meeting on Universal Health Coverage of September 2019.

Readers would agree with Ruger (2009) that it is unacceptable that a child born in Afghanistan should be 75 times more likely to die by the age of five than a child born in Singapore. Espousing a "global health justice" approach demands a commitment to promoting universal ethical norms and shared global and domestic responsibilities for health. Tandon (2009) argues that ODA should be based on solidarity, stating that the entire aid industry and its present architecture need to be thoroughly reformed in order to create "a more honest relationship" between donors and recipients. He argues that countries of the Global South are making "heroic efforts to disengage" from the "lock-in situation" through which their development was constrained by former colonial powers who continue to dominate the processes of globalization and the institutions of global governance. He suggests that not only are the well-documented structural adjustment programs major "shackles," but so too are new coordination and harmonization mechanisms that leave the powerful OECD countries in control.

The Bill and Melinda Gates Foundation and the Global Fund Against HIV/AIDS, TB and Malaria should not only be open to more scrutiny and accountability but should further reinforce their support to health systems worldwide in an effort to ensure delivery of appropriate, effective, and equitable services (Sidibe et al., 2006). Although new technologies are desirable, applying what is already known and ensuring that people gain access to effective preventive, promotive, and treatment services would make a massive difference to the global health situation.

Institutional development and capacity enhancement generally ought to be prioritized. An independent assessment of ODA activities would be valuable – allowing a range of independent agencies to participate in independent and accountable evaluation and monitoring activities. Greater investment in evaluations is required.

The future should have a much stronger rights-based approach; reasonable health and health services should be seen as the right of all people on the planet, and both their own governments and others further afield are duty bearers with a responsibility to address these needs and present inequities. Rights-based development should bring together the right to development with rights-based approaches, conceptualizing development as, in part, the attainment of economic justice (Davis, 2009).

Cometto et al. (2009) identify one of the structural constraints as being the privileging of financial sustainability from domestic revenues as a key consideration – employing Tandon's approach to solidarity and Pogge's identification of the responsibilities of wealthy countries would turn the tables substantially. Cometto et al. (2009) propose a focus on seeking measurable outcomes in all spheres that affect coverage, quality, equity, and access to services that influence health outcomes; that key bottlenecks in health system functioning and delivery should be overcome; that disbursements should go beyond the public health sector to other sectors that have an influence on health; that more budgetary support through grants not loans is necessary; and that these should be greater engagement of civil society, more transparent governance and accountability for major funding initiatives, and an independent mechanism for assessing proposals and presumably also monitoring outcomes.

In assessing the long-run contribution of ODA to growth and development, Arndt, Jones, & Tarp (2015: 15) conclude that aid has contributed to stimulating growth, promoting structural changes, improving social indicators, and reducing poverty. They caution that these effects are modest but accrue over the longer term and that "aid should not be considered a panacea or silver-bullet for stimulating growth and development."

Conclusion

This chapter has sought to situate DAH within a broader context. It has drawn attention to the opportunities resulting from the increased commitment and resources devoted to global health and to consider their implications. Trends in ODA were reviewed and the greater attention to global health issues highlighted. Major initiatives in keeping with public health approaches – concern with equity, justice, rights, national sovereignty, and accountability – are apparent. At the same time, however, countervailing pressures resulting from populist approaches, nationalist agendas, rising inequalities, xenophobia, and the "othering" of minorities pose significant challenges.

Key issues relate to the range of players and their interests and how political economy can help us understand performance, effectiveness, and failure within the global health environment. Political economy enhances understanding of differing interests and why and how these might arise. The chapter drew attention to Birdsall's "seven deadly sins"; it also considers their relevance to DAH. Differing perspectives on the purpose and definition of "development" influence whether, how, and how much ODA is provided. Recommendations regarding efforts to place human rights, social justice, civil society, and the interests of communities in low-income countries at center-stage have been made.

A fundamental shift away from blaming governments in low- and middle-income countries to acknowledging the responsibilities of wealthy countries and others for failed, incomplete, and uneven development is required. Development assistance for health is no panacea, but if operationalized effectively and in *solidarity* with those whose poor health most constrains their lives and livelihoods, it can make an important contribution to transformative development.

References

Addison, T., & Tarp, F. (2015). Aid policy and the macroeconomic management of aid. *World Development* **69**, 1–5.

Arndt, C., Jones, S., & Tarp, F. (2015). Assessing foreign aid's long-run contribution to growth and development. *World Development* **69**, 6–18.

Asante, A. D., & Zwi, A. B. (2007). Public-private partnerships and global health equity: prospects and challenges. *Indian Journal of Medical Ethics* **IV**(4), 176–180.

Benatar, S. R. (2005). Moral imagination: the missing component in global health. *PLoS Medicine* 2(12), e400.

Bensimon, C. M., & Benatar, S. R. (2006). Developing sustainability: a new metaphor for progress. *Theoretical Medicine and Bioethics* 27, 59–79.

Bigsten, A., & Tengstam, S. (2015) International coordination and the effectiveness of aid. *World Development*, **69**, 75–85.

Birdsall, N. (2008). Seven deadly sins: reflections on donor failings, in Easterly, W. (ed.), *Reinventing Foreign Aid*. Cambridge, MA: MIT Press, pp. 515–551.

Bornemisza, O., & Zwi, A. B. (2008). Neglected health systems research: health policy and systems research in conflict-affected fragile states. Alliance for Health Policy and Systems Research Issues 1, October. Available at www.who.int/alliance-hpsr/AllianceHPSR_ResearchIssue_FragileStates.pdf.

Bowen, S., & Zwi, A. B. (2005). Pathways to "evidence-informed" policy and practice: a framework for action. *PLoS Medicine* 2(7): e166. Available at https://doi.org/10.1371/journal.pmed.0020166.

Buse, K., & Harmer, A. (2007). Global health: making partnerships work. Briefing Paper No. 15, January. Overseas Development Institute, London.

Cometto, G., Ooms, G., Starrs, A., & Zeitz, P. (2009). A global fund for the health MDGs? *Lancet* 373, 1500–1502.

Das, T. (2009). The information and financial power of the World Bank: knowledge production through UN collaboration. *Progress in Development Studies*, 9, 209–224.

Das Gupta, M., & Gostin, L. (2009). How can donors help build global public goods in health? Policy Research Working Paper No. 4907. World Bank, Washington, DC.

Davis, T. W. D. (2009). The politics of human rights and development: the challenge for official donors. *Australian Journal of Political Science*, **44**(1), 173–192.

Fiszbein, A. (2006). Development impact evaluation: new trends and challenges. *Evidence & Policy* 2(3), 385–393.

Grundy, J. (2010). Country-level governance of global health initiatives: an evaluation of immunization coordination mechanisms in five countries of Asia. *Health Policy and Planning* 25, 186–196.

Gupta, V,, Katz, R., & Swaminathan, S. (2018). Reimagining development assistance for health. *New England Journal of Medicine* 379(20), 1891–1893,

Health and Fragile States Network (2009). Health systems strengthening in fragile contexts: a report on good practices and new approaches. Available at www.healthandfragilestates.org.

Hotez, P. J., Fenwick, A., Savioli, L., & Molyneux, D. H. (2009). Rescuing the bottom billion through control of neglected diseases. *Lancet* 373, 1570–1575.

Howell, J., & Lind, J. (2009). Changing donor policy and practice in civil society in the post-9/11 aid context. *Third World Quarterly* 30(7), 1279–1296.

Kothari, U. (ed.) (2005; republished 2019). *A Radical History of Development Studies: Individuals, Institutions, and Ideologies*. London, Zed Books.

Kingsbury, D. (2013). Introduction, in Kingsbury, D. (ed.), *Critical Reflections on Development*. Basingstoke, UK: Palgrave Macmillan, pp. 1–12.

Lu, C., Schneider, M. T., Gubbins, P., et al. (2010). Public financing of health in developing countries: a cross-national systematic analysis. *Lancet* 375, 1375–1387.

Mavodza C., Goldman R., & Cooper C. (2019). The impacts of the global gag rule on global health: a scoping review. *Global Health Research and Policy*, **4**, 26.

McCormick, D. (2008). China and India as Africa's new donors: the impact of aid on development. *Review of African Political Economy* **35**(115), 73–92.

McCoy, D., Chand, S., & Sridhar, D. (2009a). Global health funding: how much, where it comes from and where it goes. *Health Policy and Planning* **24**(6), 407–417.

McCoy, D., Kembhavi, G., Patel, J., & Luintel, A. (2009b). The Bill & Melinda Gates Foundation's grant-making programme for global health. *Lancet* **373**, 1645–1653.

Organisation for Economic Co-operation and Development (OECD) (2009). *Aid for Better Health: What Are We Learning about What Works and What We Still Have to Do?* An interim report from the Task Team on Health as a Tracer Sector. DCD/DAC/ EFF(2009)14, Millennium Development Project, www.un.org/millenniumgoals/.

Organisation for Economic Co-operation and Development (OECD) (2019). Development aid drops in 2018, especially to neediest countries. Available at www.oecd.org/develop ment/development-aid-drops-in-2018-especially-to-neediest-countries.htm.

Oxfam (2014). Even it up: Time to end extreme inequality. Available at www-cdn.oxfam.org/s3fs-public/file_attach ments/cr-even-it-up-extreme-inequality-291014-en.pdf .

Piketty, T. (2014). *Capital in the Twenty-First Century.* Cambridge, MA: Harvard University Press.

Piva, P., & Dodd, R. (2009). Where did all the aid go? An in-depth analysis of increased health aid flows over the past 10 years. *Bulletin of the World Health Organization* **87**, 930–939.

Pogge, T. W. M. (2008). *World Poverty and Human Rights: Cosmopolitan Responsibilities and Reforms*, 2nd ed. Cambridge, UK: Polity Press.

Ravishankar, N., Gubbins, P., Cooley, R. J., et al. (2009). Financing of global health: tracking development assistance for health from 1990 to 2007. *Lancet* **373**, 2113–2124.

Reinikka, R. (2008). Donors and service delivery, in Easterly, W. (ed.), *Reinventing Foreign Aid*. Cambridge, MA: MIT Press, pp. 179–199.

Ruger, J. P. (2009). Global health justice. *Public Health Ethics* **2**, 261–275.

Selgelid, M. J. (2008). Improving global health: counting reasons why. *Developing World Bioethics* **8**(2), 115–125.

Sidibe, M., Ramiah, I., & Buse, K. (2006). The Global Fund at five: what next for universal access for HIV/AIDS, TB and malaria? *Journal of the Royal Society of Medicine* **99**, 497–500.

Six, C. (2009). The rise of postcolonial states as donors: a challenge to the development paradigm. *Third World Quarterly* **30**(6), 1103–1121.

Storeng, K. T., Abimbola, S., Balabanova, D., et al. (2019). Action to protect the independence and integrity of global health research. *British Medical Journal Global Health* **4**(3).

Sumner, A., & Tribe, M. (2008). *International Development Studies. Theories and Methods in Research and Practice.* London: Sage.

Tan-Mullins, M., Mohan, G., & Power, M. (2010) Redefining "aid" in the China–Africa context. *Development and Change* **41**(5), 857–881.

Tandon, Y. (2009). Aid without dependence: an alternative conceptual model for development cooperation. *Development* **52**(3), 356–362.

United Nations (2019). Political Declaration of the High-Level Meeting on Universal Health Coverage "Universal Health Coverage: Moving Together to Build a Healthier World."

Vandemoortele, J. (2009). The MDG conundrum: meeting the targets without missing the point. *Development Policy Review* **27**(4), 355–371.

Woods, N. (2008). Whose aid? Whose influence? China, emerging donors and the silent revolution in development assistance. *International Affairs* **84**(6), 1–18.

World Bank (2002). The costs of attaining the Millennium Development Goals. Available at www.worldbank.org/htm l/extdr/ mdgassessment.pdf.

Xu, K., Soucat, A., Kutzin, J., et al. (2018). Public spending on health: a closer look at global trends (WHO/HIS/HGF/ HF Working Paper No. 18.3), WHO, Geneva. Available at http://origin.who.int/health_financing/documents/health-expenditure-report-2018/en/.

Zwi, A. B. (2011). International aid and global health, in Benatar, S., & Brock, G. (eds.), *Global Health and Global Health Ethics*. Cambridge, UK: Cambridge University Press, pp. 184–197.

Zwi, A. B., & Mills, A. (1995). Health policy in less developed countries: past trends, future directions. *Journal of International Development* **7**(3), 299–328.

Geopolitics, Disease, and Inequalities in Emerging Economies

Eduardo J. Gómez

In recent years, an international consensus has emerged claiming that developing nations must now, more than ever, merge the fields of foreign policy and health. To that end, in 2006, the Ministers of Foreign Affairs from Brazil, France, Indonesia, Norway, Senegal, South Africa, and Thailand established a ministerial accord agreement in Oslo, Norway, emphasizing that healthcare become an integral component of foreign policy (Amorim et al., 2006). Whereas improved diplomatic relations in health, also commonly referred to as *global health diplomacy*, have led to increased communication between nations, technical assistance, and disease preparedness (Long, 2011), unfortunately, they also have led to an increase in domestic healthcare inequalities and policy shortcomings. As I explain in this chapter, this shortcoming mainly has to do with how global health diplomacy has shifted politicians' focus away from prioritizing domestic healthcare needs.

This chapter introduces two inequality challenges associated with the turn to global health diplomacy. The first inequality is the use of bilateral aid in health to increase a nation's geopolitical influence and power – henceforth *geopolitical power in healthcare inequalities* – that may lead governments to overlook ongoing domestic healthcare needs, often to the detriment of the poor. The second is what I refer to as a nation's *geopolitical soft power in healthcare inequalities*, a diplomatic ambition that may lead governments to place an obsessive focus on diseases garnering a lot of international attention (e.g., HIV/AIDS), thus generating incentives to increase a nation's international reputation through more progressive domestic policy reforms. My concepts of geopolitical power and soft power in inequalities builds upon the soft power in foreign policy and global health diplomacy literature (Nye, 1990; Lee and Smith, 2011), which emphasizes the usage of policy norms and ideas to attract and persuade others into adopting a nation's foreign policy objectives, and the literature emphasizing how nations use healthcare policy to increase their international reputation in health (Gómez, 2018). Such soft-power focus has led some nations to emphasize domestic responses to HIV/AIDS and to overlook the need to simultaneously prioritize other diseases (e.g., those strongly associated with HIV/AIDS, such as tuberculosis) and health systems strengthening.

In this chapter, I argue that the first challenge, *geopolitical power in healthcare inequalities*, has been deployed in emerging economies through the provision of bilateral financial and technical foreign aid assistance, by, for example, Russia and the United States striving to rejuvenate their historical foreign policy traditions in leading the world in eradicating disease. Alternatively, the second challenge, *geopolitical soft power in healthcare inequalities*, has been more prevalent in the emerging economies of Brazil, China, and India. In line with these nations' foreign policy traditions, recent government leaders have consistently strived to focus more on responding to global priority diseases, such as HIV/AIDS, through more progressive domestic policy reforms in order to bolster their international reputation as nations capable of development and disease eradication. Building geopolitical soft power in health has also entailed engaging in multilateral cooperation in order to share successful policy experiences and shape international policy discussions based on these governments' policy success, often ensconced, as in Brazil, in normative human rights principles while providing financial and technical assistance to lesser-developed nations. When it came to HIV/AIDS, however, this soft-power focus resulted in less attention being paid to diseases and healthcare issues affecting the poor within Brazil, India, and China and thus contributing to broader health systems inequalities.

This chapter concludes by highlighting some key foreign policy lessons in health for the emerging economies. Whereas displaying foreign policy leadership in health can lead to greater international cooperation and assistance, these countries need to simultaneously deepen their commitments to domestic healthcare needs, particularly among poor and aging populations. Furthermore, international organizations should take steps to ensure that their own governments are achieving these domestic policy commitments before helping other nations achieve the same.

Geopolitical Power in Health: Lessons from Russia and the United States

Since the early nineteenth century, Russia and the United States have established firm foreign policy commitments to leading the world in the fight against disease. Both nations viewed providing bilateral assistance in combating infectious diseases, such as polio, smallpox, and yellow fever, as a way to bolster their international reputation for being advanced, industrialized nations, overcoming disease and developing other countries (Gómez, 2018, 2016). Furthermore, during the 1960s, in response to the smallpox outbreak in developing nations, Russia and the United States competed with each other over their financial contributions to the World Health Organization's (WHO) division on infectious disease, as well as bilateral contributions to developing nations (Henderson, 1988). It was a time, as Gómez (2018) claims, when both nations engaged in a Cold War race in global health (Henderson, 1988).

These deep foreign policy traditions shaped the rise of *geopolitical power in healthcare inequalities.* With the arrival of the HIV/AIDS epidemic several decades later, both nations built on their foreign health policy traditions to pursue foreign policies that focused on using bilateral and multilateral aid in health to embolden, in the case of the United States, and rejuvenate, in the case of Russia, their international leadership and policy influence. The first US effort to achieve this came with the George W. Bush administration's creation of the President's Emergency Plan for AIDS Relief (PEPFAR) in 2003. By far the largest US public health agency ever created for HIV/AIDS (perhaps even in the world), the goal was to facilitate the ability of the United States to provide antiretroviral medications (ARVs), with a focus on Africa, while stipulating that money only be used for treatment, not prevention programs – for example, funding for sex workers and drug addicts (Gómez, 2016). Much like the past, the Bush administration's focus was also to increase the global policy influence of the United States, shaping international policy decisions in favor of ARV treatment.

But these endeavors came at a significant cost. While the Bush administration was increasing spending abroad for HIV/AIDS, within the United States, many state governments lacked sufficient access to ARV medications. Major cities, such as New York City and Chicago, had long AIDS Drug Assistance Program (ADAP) waiting lists (McManus et al., 2013). Reports revealed that patients often died while waiting for ARV medications provided through ADAP (Hayes, 2013). What's more, federal funding for prevention programs, such as sex education in high schools and condom distribution, was not provided to the state health departments in need (Gómez, 2016). These domestic policy shortcomings contributed to a decrease in access to HIV/AIDS services, with the poor suffering the most from a lack of additional federal support. Meanwhile, the more affluent classes could rely on a steady supply of ARV medications through private health insurance. These inequalities in access to HIV/AIDS treatment also to a certain extent reinforced the ongoing racial divide in healthcare and HIV/AIDS treatment.

Russia also displayed a high degree of *geopolitical power in healthcare inequalities.* After 2005, when the Vladimir Putin administration finally decided to escalate the government's HIV/AIDS policy response, a series of concrete foreign policy steps was taken to bolster bilateral and multilateral aid contributions. Putin in fact viewed foreign aid in health as a way to rejuvenate Russia's geopolitical power and influence (particularly within Eastern Europe) yet at the detriment, as Celeste Wallander (2005) maintains, of leading the global community in response to HIV/AIDS while not working closely with the international community by taking policy advice from those nations successfully combating HIV/AIDS. Putin was so focused on providing foreign aid in health that by 2010, healthcare comprised nearly half the government's foreign aid budget (Gómez, 2018).

In addition to providing bilateral aid to several Eastern European, Asian, and African nations, the Putin administration also increased contributions to multilateral donor agencies. By 2012, Russia had become the largest contributor to the Global Fund to Fight HIV/AIDS, Tuberculosis, and Malaria, among the emerging BRICS (Brazil, Russia, India, China, and South Africa) economies (Sridhar et al., 2013).

Furthermore, Putin has demonstrated his global leadership role by proactively supporting his former minister of health, Dr. Tereza Kasaeva, as the WHO's new global tuberculosis director (Wheaton, 2018). This focus on global leadership in health led to a lack of sufficient political support for domestic healthcare

Table 16.1 BRICS' Contributions to the Global Fund (US$ millions, 2012)

Brazil	0.0
Russia	297.0
India	10.0
China	25.0
South Africa	10.3

Source: Sridhar et al., 2013.

needs. For example, there continues to be an ongoing shortage of funding for HIV/AIDS prevention and treatment programs (Goble, 2011; Gómez, 2018). Along with HIV, tuberculosis (TB) has also resurfaced as an epidemic, mainly within crowded prisons and among drug addicts and the poor. There has also been an insufficient amount of federal assistance to state health departments in need of funding treatment services (Stracansky, 2014). What's more, whereas the Putin administration has provided funding to neighboring countries for methadone treatment for drug addicts, an HIV prevention measure prescribed by the WHO since 1993 (incessantly pressuring Russia to adopt this policy since then), to this day, no methadone program exists in Russia. Embarrassingly, Moscow-based nongovernmental organizations (NGOs) have had to ask NGOs in neighboring countries for assistance to fund their methadone program – NGOs to which the Putin administration has provided bilateral assistance on this very policy endeavor (Gómez, 2018)! In a poll taken by the World Bank in 2010, many claimed that Russia was not in any position to provide foreign aid to other countries. This view mainly reflected the growing disdain within society toward the Putin's administration's focus on prioritizing needs in other nations before his own citizens (Brezhneva & Ukhova, 2013).

Both the United States and Russia also continue to see internal worsening access to not only effective HIV/AIDS treatment but also to healthcare in general. In both countries, the poor continue to rely on underfunded federal and state programs – in the United States, Medicare for the elderly and Medicaid for the poor, and in Russia, the federally state-provided "Guaranteed Package" in healthcare (Cook, 2015). In rural areas, the poor's access to public healthcare has worsened. For example, in Russia, from 2005 to 2013, the number of health facilities in rural areas fell by 75% (Epple, 2015). Although Russia does provide a constitutionally backed universal healthcare system through the Guaranteed Package, it has been repeatedly

underfunded (Cook, 2015), with major reductions in spending beginning in 2013, when the Putin administration decided to reduce the federal budget for healthcare in order to finance an increase in military spending.

Thus, in both the United States and Russia, the race to deepen their *geopolitical power in healthcare inequalities* contributed to ongoing domestic healthcare challenges and inequalities. But was this the case in other emerging economies?

Soft Power in Health: Insights from Brazil, India, and China

In contrast to the United States and Russia, Brazil's, India's, and China's historic foreign policy interests were rather different, in turn, shaping their long-term visions in global health diplomacy. Since the early twentieth century, neither of these governments aspired to lead the world with respect to providing healthcare funding and technical assistance (Gómez, 2018). Instead, they strove to work closely with international health organizations and other governments. This occurred either by working with the WHO in response to disease outbreaks, by receiving World Bank funding, or by engaging in close partnerships with major philanthropic institutions such as the Rockefeller Foundation. For example, during the first half of the twentieth century, the Rockefeller Foundation helped to build Brazil's largest federal center for malaria eradication in the Amazonian region (Griffing et al., 2015). What emerged from this type of global health engagement was a firm desire to establish a foreign policy commitment of multilateral cooperation in health, an unwavering commitment to learn from other nations, and never striving to lead the world, or their respective regions, in providing foreign aid assistance (Gómez, 2018).

Nevertheless, an alternative foreign policy tradition emerged throughout the nineteenth and early twentieth century: that is, the desire to elevate these nations' international reputations as effective disease combatants (Gómez, 2018).. Interestingly, in sharp contrast to what we saw in the United States and Russia, Brazil's, India's, and China's political leaders were incessantly worried about how the world perceived their nations when it came to health and development. While Brazil's political leaders during the 1930s and 1940s complained about Brazil's international reputation for constantly being perceived as "a huge, sick hospital," India's and China's leaders also vocalized their discontent for being constantly perceived as inept and underdeveloped in the areas of healthcare and social policy (Hochman, 2008; Gómez, 2018). To avoid this, China's political leadership would go so far as to create a phalanx of federal institutions focused on rebranding China's global image through the creation of several media centers that marketed China's social and political success while spreading its cultural influence through the creation of Confucius Institutes throughout the world (Chung Dawson, 2010).

Brazil

Similar types of foreign policy legacies and political interests shaped future responses to public health crises in Brazil. This was particularly noticeable when it came to the HIV/AIDS epidemic. Despite a substantial delay in the government's policy response – for a variety of reasons, stemming from fear of discrimination against the gay community – and in response to international criticisms and pressure in the late-1990s, the government substantially improved its response. Under the Fernando H. Cardoso administration (1994–2002), for example, after the World Bank and world-renowned scientists criticized the government for its lackluster response to HIV/AIDS, Cardoso began to delegate a considerable amount of policymaking autonomy to the National AIDS Program within the Ministry of Health (Gómez, 2018). In addition to a gradual increase in federal spending for the National AIDS Program (NAP), in 1993, the program signed a loan with the World Bank (the first of three) to fund several prevention programs, such as increased public awareness through media campaigns, as well as funding for NGOs working with high-risk groups. What's more, in 1996, the Congress created a federal law mandating that all in need of ARV medication receive this medication, couched in terms of the patient's human rights in health, a principle that was enshrined within Brazil's new 1988 democratic constitution (Paiva et al., 2006). By the mid-1990s and into the turn to the twenty-first century, the government was fully committed to bolstering its financial and political commitment to the HIV/AIDS epidemic.

Why was this the case? Similar to how the government responded to yellow fever, malaria, and smallpox outbreaks in the past, the government's improved policy response to HIV/AIDS aimed to bolster its international reputation in health. Two issues were at stake: on the

one hand, reassuring Western investors (e.g., Wall Street) that Brazil was safe to invest in and prosper, and, on the other hand, revealing the Cardoso administration's unwavering commitment to the international principle of access to healthcare as a human right, introduced by the WHO and enshrined through the 1976 Alma Ata Conference on primary healthcare. By strengthening the government's policy response, the government was capable of increasing its reputation in positively influencing these two areas, which were deemed critical for Brazil's ongoing prosperity and development (Gómez, 2018).

But it was under the Luiz Inácio "Lula" da Silva administration (2002–2010) that the government's *geopolitical soft power in healthcare inequalities* took flight. Motivated by his preexisting commitment to eradicate poverty and disease, Lula worked closely with the NAP to export Brazil's AIDS policy success through the provision of multilateral and bilateral assistance (Gómez, 2009). At the international level, Lula and the NAP traveled to several UN conferences, sharing their policy experiences and success, striving to help and inspire other nations to pursue similar kinds of HIV prevention and treatment programs, all in the name of "human rights in health" (Gómez, 2018). With respect to bilateral aid, Lula also worked closely with the NAP to provide technical assistance to several African nations, such as Mozambique and Angola, seeking to build their own pharmaceutical plants for the production of ARV medications (Gómez, 2009). In contrast to most nations, Brazil's bilateral assistance was not focused on providing money but rather on transferring technical skills and knowledge through worker training, which could provide African nations with the knowledge and experience needed to engage in ongoing, sustainable pharmaceutical production (Gómez, 2009). This capacity-building endeavor would also be important for improving African nations' bargaining power vis-à-vis those pharmaceutical industries seeking to impose high prices for ARV medications. That is, by threatening to issue compulsory licenses and produce and distribute generic versions of ARV medications at much lower prices themselves, these African countries could now, as had been the case in Brazil, credibly commit to do so (because of their new pharmaceutical production capacity) and thus successfully threaten pharmaceutical companies into lowering their drug prices.

Nevertheless, whereas Brazil was successful in positively influencing international institutions and developing nations in their struggle to eradicate disease, the government's obsessive focus on HIV/AIDS translated to a lack of sufficient attention to other diseases, even those closely associated with HIV/AIDS. Similar to what we saw in Russia, TB had also resurfaced in Brazil during the 1990s because of the HIV/AIDS epidemic (Gómez, 2013). And yet, despite a very high HIV–TB coinfection rate throughout the 1990s, the Ministry of Health never responded as effectively as it did to HIV/AIDS (Gómez, 2013). There simply were no geopolitical soft-power incentives to do so: the degree of international attention and pressures for an improved response to TB were essentially nonexistent during the 1990s. Few activists and researchers were interested in working on an old disease, thus failing to garner significant international and media attention and, consequently, not providing an opportunity to improve their career prospects (Gómez, 2013). The problem was that TB was mainly concentrated among the poor in congested urban areas, such as Rio and São Paulo (Gómez, 2013), a population that was desperately in need of ongoing medical attention and directly observed treatment (DOTS). Despite these needs, the National TB Program never received nearly the amount of government attention and financial support as the NAP (Gómez, 2013). At the same time, most NGOs and activists were working on AIDS, striving to obtain funding – and thus secure jobs – from international organizations and philanthropists.

But even under the Lula administration and subsequent Dilma Roussef administration (2010–2015), both of which were leftist governments dedicated to fighting poverty, the government did not increase its financial support for the universal healthcare system, Sistema Único de Saude (SUS). Federal funding for SUS essentially flat-lined under both administrations, whereas further cuts were planned under the conservative Michael Temer administration (2015–2018; Philips, 2016). In this context, SUS reinforced massive inequalities in access to reliable and effective healthcare treatment between the poor, who relied on SUS, and the rising middle- and upper-income classes, who relied mainly on private health insurance. At a time of impressive soft power in global health, there was no simultaneous commitment to addressing the innumerable financial and human resource needs of SUS and, needless to say, diseases mainly associated with the poor, such as TB.

China

Shortly after the arrival of the HIV/AIDS epidemic, as seen in Brazil, China's political leaders also confronted considerable pressures from international organizations such as the World Bank, the United Nations, and medical scientists. However, it was not until the SARS epidemic of 2003 that the government began to positively respond to these pressures. Similar to what was seen in Brazil, China's goal was to use new policy initiatives to bolster its international reputation as a state capable of eradicating disease (Gómez, 2018). This response was essentially built up on a rich foreign policy tradition of, as mentioned earlier, engaging in institution building and state-sponsored propaganda campaigns in order to sharpen China's international reputation (Zhang, 2008). But the goal was also to reassure financial investors and international economic organizations that the government could control the growth of disease and prosper.

Similar to what we saw in Brazil, China's *geopolitical soft power in healthcare inequalities* emerged through the use of progressive domestic institutional and policy reforms. Beginning in the mid-2000s, a phalanx of new laws, regulations, and public awareness HIV/AIDS prevention campaigns emerged (Knutsen, 2009). Impressively, the Comprehensive AIDS Response (CARES) program provided free medication for indigent city residents and the rural poor (Zhang et al., 2006). To further the government's international reputation and influence as a policy innovator, the government also began to provide bilateral assistance to countries in need. In Africa, for example, the Ministry of Health provided financial and technical assistance, with a focus on improving health systems capacity (Grépin et al., 2014). China has also joined the other BRICS nations in contributing money to the Global Fund to Fight HIV/AIDS, TB and Malaria (Sridhar et al., 2013).

The upshot with China's *geopolitical soft power in healthcare inequalities*, however, is that HIV/AIDS appears to have distracted the government from providing as much financial and political support for other diseases. As in Brazil, TB and even noncommunicable diseases (NCDs) such as obesity, type 2 diabetes, and heart disease have not received as much political attention and support (Gómez, 2018). In this context, a high level of geographic inequality has emerged, where the rural poor often do not have access to clinics and medications; this has been particularly problematic for type 2 diabetes, an NCD that has been burgeoning in rural areas yet has not been matched with adequate health system support (Wang et al., 2018). In contrast, the aforementioned CARES program for HIV/AIDS explicitly focuses on providing medications for the rural poor.

Perhaps with the exception of environmental health policy, such as reducing air pollution in congested urban areas, which, like HIV/AIDS, has garnered considerable international attention and, in turn, an opportunity for China to display its *geopolitical soft power in healthcare inequalities*, this has not been the case with other diseases and the healthcare system in general. Although several federal health insurance programs were created, beginning in the late-1990s, providing insurance coverage for the urban employed, rural poor, and government employees, there continues to be insufficient financial and human resources to ensure that these programs run effectively and that they meet the poor's needs. Recent studies in fact find that the inadequate funding and management of these programs has contributed to an increase in out-of-pocket and catastrophic expenses for the poor (Gómez, 2017). At the same time, however, those earning higher incomes have been able to purchase private health insurance, an industry that has been thriving in recent years. All together, then, and as seen in Brazil, China's *geopolitical soft power in healthcare inequalities* has contributed to placing too much attention on internationally popular diseases at the expense of ensuring that domestic health insurance programs work well and that they meet the poor's needs. Unless this is achieved, healthcare inequalities will continue and in the end potentially harm China's broader image in global health.

India

After several years of failing to adequately respond to the HIV/AIDS epidemic, India also joined Brazil and China in confronting increased international criticism and pressure for a delayed response to HIV/AIDS. Because of inadequate political support and funding, the National Committee on AIDS, first created in 1987, did not establish adequate prevention and treatment programs (Lieberman, 2009). Whereas another federal program was subsequently created in 1992, namely the National AIDS Control Organization (NACO), it was quickly viewed as a bureaucratic shell: empty, full of ideas, but no concrete action taken (Lieberman, 2009; Gómez, 2018). But as Lieberman (2009) correctly points out, increased international pressures presented a critical juncture in the government's interest in combating AIDS. These pressures provided a golden opportunity for India to build on its foreign policy tradition of increasing the government's international reputation as a modern, developed state capable of eradicating disease and prospering (Gómez, 2018).

The government's first visible attempt at *geopolitical soft power in healthcare inequalities* was with Sonia Gandhi's visitation to the 2003 International AIDS Conference in Thailand. In the presence of UN Secretary General Kofi Anan and other dignitaries, Gandhi took the podium to announce that her government was fully committed to eradicating AIDS (Gómez, 2018). As India had done in the past in response to smallpox, Gandhi also reaffirmed her commitment to working with other nations through the WHO, providing as well as receiving technical assistance. During this period, and similar to what we saw in Brazil and China, India's government started to invest more in its NACO programs while establishing new public awareness prevention programs, such as the Red Ribbon Express; this initiative provided a locomotive railroad train traveling throughout the states dispersing information about HIV (*Hindu*, 2009). Greater federal funding was also provided for ARV medications (Lieberman, 2009). In short, it was a time when the government saw investing in its AIDS program as a way to rejuvenate its international reputation as an effective disease combatant.

A key aspect of India's *geopolitical soft power in healthcare inequalities* was also providing bilateral assistance for HIV/AIDS. The Ministry of External Affairs (MEA), the government's primary agency responsible for foreign aid, achieved this by providing funding for AIDS prevention programs in several African nations (Morrison & Kates, 2006) while providing ARV medications to Mozambique and Angola – thus taking advantage of its pharmaceutical expertise (Ruger & Ng, 2010). Ironically, despite being the world's largest producer of ARV medications, the government never went as far as to guarantee a steady supply of medications to other nations, as exemplified by the US PEPFAR. What was even more ironic was that there was no federal legal commitment to universally distribute ARV medications to everyone in need in India (Gómez, 2018).

India's obsessive focus on HIV/AIDS did not, however, lead to a renewed commitment to combating other infectious diseases. In an increasingly decentralized context, where the state and local *panchayati raj* governments have become increasingly responsible for providing medical services, inadequate federal support has translated to lackluster public health services. This is especially the case in rural areas (Pahwa & Beland, 2013). What's more, even those diseases garnering more international attention and pressure, such as the NCDs of obesity and type 2 diabetes, have received insufficient federal support. As Gómez (2018) claims, in large part this has to do with the comparatively late arrival of these international pressures (relative to HIV/AIDS) to stimulate opportunities to bolster the government's international reputation and soft power through domestic policy innovations.

Moreover, the government's national healthcare system is poorly funded and supported. As Dréze and Sen (2013) explain, the Ministry of Health and Family Welfare's various public health and insurance programs, such as the Rural Heath Commission and the RSBY (*Rashtriya Swasthya Bima Yojana*) program for the poor, respectively, have not received sufficient financial and human resources support (Gómez, 2015). According to Dréze and Sen (2013), this problem is due to a lack of sufficient media attention, convincing data, and, consequently, a lack of sufficient political will. In this context, out-of-pocket (OOP) and catastrophic expenses for the poor have continued to increase (Gómez, 2015), in turn generating a high level of inequality in access to medical treatment. Conversely, higher-income families have benefited from private insurance programs and enrollment in more modern hospital facilities, excellent doctors, and flourishing medical staff. One must keep in mind that India is world famous for its thriving medical tourism industry (Suri, 2019).

Thus, similar to what was seen in Brazil and China, India's *geopolitical soft power in healthcare inequalities* appears to have led to a biased focus on particular diseases, such as HIV/AIDS, while neglecting to invest in other diseases and the healthcare system in general. Whereas eradicating HIV/AIDS should be a priority for all governments, this should not come at the expense of overlooking ongoing domestic healthcare needs. Ironically, focusing too much on a disease amid ongoing healthcare inequalities and public criticisms may tarnish the government's global health image.

Conclusion

In this chapter, I have highlighted the often-overlooked domestic healthcare challenges associated with global health diplomacy. While these diplomatic efforts are certainly necessary for sharing information and resources and avoiding global pandemic threats, they can come at a high cost if not balanced with strong domestic political commitments to other diseases and the healthcare system in general.

This chapter has introduced the concepts of *geopolitical power in healthcare inequalities*, as seen in Russia and the United Sates, and *geopolitical soft power in healthcare inequalities*, as seen in Brazil, China, and India; these are global health diplomacy strategies that appear to have impaired domestic healthcare systems while contributing to inequalities in access to healthcare. Whereas Russia and the United States have done a commendable job of providing foreign aid in health, both nations have continued to see a lack of government commitment not only to investing in domestic diseases (even those that these governments are providing foreign aid for, e.g., HIV/AIDS) but also to ensuring adequate domestic health insurance coverage and treatment. Alternatively, Brazil, India, and China's *geopolitical soft power in healthcare inequalities* has led to simultaneous improvements in domestic responses to HIV/AIDS and international cooperation and assistance, sharing policy lessons developed at the domestic level, while helping other nations overcome this dreadful disease. However, this *geopolitical soft power in healthcare inequalities* has favored internationally recognized diseases, such as HIV/AIDS, while neglecting other diseases, even those that have resurfaced as a result of HIV/AIDS, such as TB; moreover, for different political and economic reasons, none of these nations has displayed an ongoing government commitment to improving health insurance coverage and overcoming inequalities in access to healthcare between the rich and poor.

Several broader policy lessons emerge from this chapter. First, to truly bolster an emerging economy's international reputation in health, governments need to be equally committed to treating all types of diseases, especially those mainly found among the poor. Second, either a lack of domestic government response (Russia and the United States) or biased domestic responses (Brazil, India, and China) may impair a government's international reputation in health. Going forward, these responses may limit these nations' ability to shape international policy discussions, propose new policy ideas, and find international organizations and/or nation-states eager to work with them in eradicating disease. Finally, international funders, such as the WHO, the Global Fund to Fight HIV/AIDS, TB and Malaria, and the World Bank need to play a stronger role in monitoring nations' global health diplomacy activities and ensuring that governments are simultaneously addressing their own health-related poverty and inequality challenges; this can be achieved by potentially including this policy priority as an agreed-upon conditionality for future funding agreements.

References

Amorim, C., Douste-Blazy, P., Wirayuda, H., et al. (2006). Oslo ministerial declaration. Global health: a pressing foreign policy issue of our time. *Lancet* **6736**(7), 60498.

Brezhneva, A., & Ukhova, D. (2013). *Russia as a Humanitarian Aid Donor*. Oxford, UK: Oxfam Press.

Chung Dawson, K. (2010). Confucius Institutes enhance China's international image. *China Daily Online*, April 23. Available at www.chinadaily.com.cn/china/2010-04/23/content_9766116.htm.

Cook, L. (2015). *Constraints on Universal Healthcare in the Russian Federation: Inequality,Informality, and the Failures of Mandatory Health Insurance Reforms*. Geneva: UN Research Institute for Social Development.

Dréze, J., & Sen, A. (2013). *An Uncertain Glory: India and Its Contradictions*. Princeton, NJ: Princeton University Press.

Epple, N. (2015). Russian healthcare is dying a slow death. *Moscow Times*, April 16. Available at www.themoscowtimes.com/2015/04/16/russian-health-care-is-dying-a-slow-death-a45839 (accessed April 1, 2019).

Goble, P. (2011). Russia no longer to provide free treamtent for victims of tuberculosis. *KyivPost*, February 21. Available at www.kyivpost.com/article/opinion/op-ed/paul-goble-helping-putin-russify-non-russians-would-be-a-horrific-mistake.html.

Gómez, E. (2009). The politics of Brazil's commitment to combating HIV/AIDS in Africa: technological assistance, capacity building, and the emergence of a new donor aid paradigm. *Harvard Health Policy Review* **10**(2), 16–18.

Gómez, E. (2013). An inter-dependent analytical approach to explaining the evolution of NGOs, social movements, and government response to HIV/AIDS and tuberculosis in Brazil. *Journal of Health Politics, Policy & Law* **38**(1), 123–159.

Gómez, E. (2015). *Health Spending and Inequalities in the Emerging Economies: India, China, Russia, and Indonesia in Comparative Perspective*. Oxford, UK: Oxfam Press.

Gómez, E. (2016). *Contested Epidemics: Policy Responses in the United States and Brazil and What the BRICS Can Learn*. London: Imperial College Press.

Gómez, E. (2017). Democratic transitions, health institutions, and financial protection in emerging economies: insights from Asia. *Health Economics, Policy & Law* **12**(3), 309–323.

Gómez, E. (2018). *Geopolitics in Health: Confronting AIDS, Tuberculosis, and Obesity in the BRICS Emerging Economies*. Baltimore: Johns Hopkins University Press.

Grépin, K., Fan, V., Shen, G., & Chen, L. (2014). China's role as a global health donor in Africa. *Globalization & Health* **19** (84), 1–11.

Griffing, S., Tauil, P., Udhayakumar, V., & Silva-Flannery, L. (2015). A historical perspective on malaria control in Brazil. *Memórias do Instituto Oswaldo Cruz* **110**(6), 701–718.

Henderson, D. (1988). Smallpox eradication: a cold war history. *World Health Forum* **19**, 113–119.

Heys, J. (2013). Funding cuts hurt AIDS program: patients dying awaiting drugs. *Charleston Gazette*, August 28.

Hochman, G. (2008). *A era do saneamento: as bases da política de saúde pública no Brasil*. São Paulo: Editora Hucitect-Anpocs.

Knutsen, W. (2009). Resistance and radical shift: an institutional account of China's HIV/AIDS policy process from 1985–2020. *Politics and Policy* **40**(1), 161–192.

Lee, K., & Smith, R. (2011). What is global health diplomacy: a conceptual review. Global Health Diplomacy 5(1), 1–12.

Lieberman, E. (2009). *Boundaries of Contagion: How Ethnic Politics Have Shaped Government Responses to AIDS*. Princeton, NJ: Princeton University Press.

Long, W. (2011). *Pandemics and Peace*. Washington, DC: US Institute of Peace.

McManus, K., Wngelhard, C., & Dillingham, R. (2013). Current challenges to the United States' AIDS Drug Assistance Program and possible implications of the Affordable Care Act. *AIDS Research and Treatment* **2013**, 350169.

Morrison, S., & Kates, J. (2006). *The G-8, Russia's Presidency, and HIV/AIDS in Eurasia*. Washington, DC: Center for Strategic and International Studies.

Nye, J. (1990). Bound to Lead: The Changing Nature of American Power. New York: Basic Books Press.

Pahwa, D., & Beland, D. (2013). Federalism, decentralization, and health care policy reform in India. *Public Administration Research* **2**(1), 2–10.

Paiva, V., Pup, L., & Barboza, R. (2006). The right to prevention and the challenges of reducing vulnerability to HIV in Brazil. *Revista de Saúde Pública* **40**, S1–10.

Philips, D. (2016). Brazil senate approves austerity package to freeze social spending for 20 years. *The Guardian*, December 16. Available at www.theguardian.com/world/2016/dec/13/brazil-approves-social-spending-freeze-austerity-package.

Rugger, J., & Ng, N. (2010). Emerging and transitional countries' role in global health. *St Louis University Journal of Health Law and Policy* **3**(2), 253–289.

Sridhar, D., Brolan, C., Durrani, S., et al. (2013). Recent shifts in global governance: implications for the response to non-communicable disease. *PLoS Medicine* **10**(7), e1001487.

Stracansky, P. (2014). Outdated approaches fueling TB in Russia, says NGOs. Inter Press Service, July 14. Available at www.ipsnews.net/2014/07/outdated-approaches-fuelling-tb-in-russia-say-ngos/.

Suri, M. (2019). India wants to make medical tourism a $9 billion industry by 2020. CNN, February 15. Available at https://edition.cnn.com/2019/02/13/health/india-medical-tourism-industry-intl/index.html.

Wallander, C. (2005). The politics of Russian AIDS aolicy (PONARS Policy Memo No. 389). Center for Strategic and International Development, Washington, DC.

Wang, Q.,, Zhang, X., Fang, L., et al. (2018). Prevalence, awareness, treatment and control of diabetes mellitus among middle-aged and elderly people in a rural Chinese population: a cross-sectional study. *PLoS ONE* **6**, e0198343.

Wheaton, S. (2018). World's doctor gives WHO a headache. *Politico*, January 10. Available at www.politico.eu/article/tedros-adhanom-ghebreyesus-gives-who-a-headache/.

Zhang, F., Hsu, M., Yu, L., et al. (2006). Initiation of the national free antiretroviral therapy program in rural China, in Kaufman, J., Kleinman, A., & Saich, T. (eds.), *AIDS and Social Policy in China*. Cambridge, MA: Harvard University Asia Center, pp. 96–124.

Zhang, X. (2008). China as an emerging soft power: winning hearts and minds through communicating with foreign publics (Discussion Paper No. 35). University of Nottingham, Nottingham, UK.

Neoliberalism, Power Relations, Ethics, and Global Health[*]

Solomon Benatar, Ross Upshur, and Stephen Gill

Introduction

Spectacular progress, both intellectual and material, has been achieved through the Enlightenment notion of the centrality of the individual and the supremacy of science and technology in advancing health and healthcare practices. The modern Western belief system and its frames for global thinking that have now become powerful worldwide are succinctly characterized by an individualistic, self-determining, and rights-bearing concept of being; an epistemological framework that centers on abstract thinking, objectivity in observation, logical reasoning processes, verifiable knowledge, and a positivist version of the scientific method; and moral and political values of autonomy supportive of individual rights. Scientific and technological progress and diverse socioeconomic systems contributed to fostering great "accelerations" in the scale of production, consumption, communication, and transportation that in particular since 1945 have improved the duration and quality of life for many people. Since the collapse of Soviet communism, such progress has also been achieved through transformations driven principally by the power structures, geopolitical arrangements, and patterns of social and economic organization of world capitalism. In the past 30 years, an extreme form of capitalist and hypermaterialistic thinking and practice (neoliberalism) has come to pervasively dominate the practices and principles not only of healthcare systems but also of almost all aspects of social life, including education and the governance of nature and the biosphere, seeking to accelerate the transformation

of aspects of each into salable commodities in ways that have distorted some of the key Enlightenment principles noted earlier. It is the ethical, material, political, health, and ecological nature and consequences of this perspective that we critically address in this chapter. This is followed by suggestions for alternatives to enhance the health of people on a finite planet.

Neoliberalism

Neoliberalism is a particular form of capitalist ideology and a set of governance practices rather than simply an economic or policy framework. It comprises a range of transformations that are simultaneously economic and political, social, cultural, legal, and scientific. Characteristic features include liberalized re-regulation of economic and trade activities, enhanced privatization, reduced expenditure on public goods and social welfare, major tax reductions for the wealthy, and structural adjustment programs within a consumption-driven culture and a fossil-fuel-intensive economy (Gill, 2015; Birn et al., 2018). It is also characterized by a narrow conception of human rights, emphasis on possessive individualism and acquisitiveness, and freedom defined as "freedom to do" eclipsing "freedom from fear" and "freedom from want" (Hanlon & Christie, 2016).

Increasingly, this perspective has been coupled with an economic conception of healthcare. Neoliberal healthcare principles are connected to wider patterns and practices of the political economy and to a development model that drives energy-intensive, wasteful, consumerist, and ecologically myopic lifestyles within a capitalist-governed "market civilization" (Gill, 1995),[1] with the interests of

---

[*] Based on Benatar, S., Upshur, R., & Gill, S. (2018). Understanding the relationship between ethics, neoliberalism and power as a step towards improving the health of people and our planet. *Anthropocene Review* 2018, 1–22, and to a lesser extent on Benatar, S., Sanders, D., & Gill, S. (2018). The global politics of health care reform, in Lee, K., McInnes, C., & Youde, J. (eds.), *Oxford Handbook of Global Health Politics*. Oxford, UK: Oxford University Press 445–468 (with permission of SAGE publishers and Oxford University Press).

[1] The orthodoxies of its economic theory are considered by its adherents to be a science on a par with the physical sciences. Indeed, what is understood as the normal science in prevailing neoliberal economic policies and theories, by definition, excludes from consideration as "unscientific" any heterodox or critical perspectives on economic theory and any consideration of alternative ways of governing economic and social life.

particular patterns of human development overriding interests in the preservation of well-being and nature.

In societies that have enjoyed continuous economic growth over many decades, healthcare systems in some jurisdictions are understood not simply as public goods but also as commercial ventures providing highly successful, often costly personalized medical and surgical treatments As healthcare becomes increasingly subject to market forces and values, it is treated like a commodity that simply can be bought and sold for reasons of profit at the expense of conditions for healthy living and for delivery of healthcare. Despite all the adverse effects on the poorest, this dominant development model has been treated in public policy as an accepted "norm" and as a self-evident representation of progress, as well as a prerequisite for further progress.

It is the contradictory health effects, political consequences, and basic ethical questions raised by this perspective and model of development that form some of the foci of this chapter. We also suggest that neoliberalism needs to be seen in the context of a range of *belief systems* and ideologies that have (in part) driven progress or retrogression in human well-being over centuries. Such ideologies have also played a role in defining what is right or wrong in human relationships and in shaping how power is distributed geographically, socially, and across time. All belief systems and ideologies mobilize feelings and motivations through frames and symbols that work most powerfully when subliminal.[2]

What is believed becomes an important aspect of "reality," whether true or not, and this applies both to religious and secular belief systems. According to social constructivist ideas in psychology, how we know the world is not only determined by examining and testing hypotheses but also significantly based on knowledge derived from interactive relationships within the social, political, economic, and physical world in which we are situated (Gergen, 1985). This helps us to understand why despite the fact that there are many diverse ways of seeing and understanding the world, neoliberalism has taken hold in contemporary governance and ideology. It also enables us to point toward those ways of ethical, epistemological, and political thinking that might be premised on the health of both people and the planet – issues addressed later in this chapter.

Some Benefits, Costs, and Consequences of Neoliberalism

It is not surprising that the benefits and harms of neoliberal globalization over the past 40 years have been intensely debated. But what is more precisely at issue in the debates about neoliberalism, ethics and power? And what does this imply for the health of people and the planet?

Friedrich von Hayek (1944) claimed that a neoliberal paradigm is the only way out of the modern "road to serfdom," facilitating market efficiency and decentralized, distributed knowledge to produce more sophisticated outcomes than any form of planning. Indeed, proponents claim that *inter alia* it has opposed excessive inhibitory government controls, increased individual freedoms in all walks of life, stimulated economic growth, alleviated severe poverty, increased longevity for all, and reduced early childhood deaths. Moreover, in placing the highest political value on minimally restrained individual freedom, neoliberalism also insists on economic growth as *the* solution to poverty.

Many others continue to advocate this pattern of development as offering undeniable overall benefits of progress to humankind (see, e.g., Pinker, 2017). This is despite ecologically and socially significant adverse effects on the health and lives of the majority, associated with intense competition, endless consumerism, and incessant demands for ever-greater capitalist production.

Possessive individualism is associated with powerful social and economic forces promoting private patterns of healthcare. Opponents of neoliberalism argue that this undermines solidarity, civic citizenship, reciprocal obligations, and social justice as the ingredients of the good society. Some also indicate how this form of political economy contrasts with the Keynesian era of economic policies that, despite high marginal tax rates, enabled reconstruction of the global economy after World War II (Tooze, 2017). They also argue that it is a version of capitalist ideology adopted by the rich and powerful to enhance dominance of their own self-regarding economic considerations and

---

[2] *Frames* are mental structures with mostly subconscious reference points that determine automatically and repetitiously how knowledge is constructed and debated. They allow us to create what we take to be reality and to facilitate our most basic interactions with the world by structuring our ideas and concepts, shaping the way we reason and impacting on how we perceive and how we act. *Cognitive bias* refers to systematic patterns of deviation from norms of judgment, whereby inferences about other people and situations may be drawn through subjective perception of our own social reality. *Metaphors* are additional fundamental mechanisms of mind that through indirect comparisons subtly shape our perceptions and structure our most basic understandings of our experience and actions.

short-term interests in all aspects of life *inter alia* by giving greater rights to corporations to use their power to impair the freedom of individuals and communities (Garrido, 2003; Rowden, 2009; Stiglitz, 2015).

More recently, it has been cogently argued that distortions of Adam Smith's ideas of capitalism within the practices of those seeking to claim him as their inspiration, together with incremental displacement of public government by covertly private government, have disrupted the symbiosis of freedom and equality required to sustain democracy (Anderson, 2015). Others have also seen threats to the future of Western civilization from an excessive focus on freedom (for the powerful) that undermines the extent of equality needed to sustain democracies (Emmott, 2017).

It is against this background that the highly valued benefits of scientific/medical progress, impressive economic growth, and advances in healthcare have impacted mainly a minority of about one-third of the world's population in countries worldwide, bringing very significant advantages for only a small proportion of those who could potentially benefit. High costs have limited accessibility to medical treatments and other requirements for human flourishing, with consequent debilitating impacts on population health, particularly among the poor, as well as a massive increase in inequality both within and between nation-states (Alexander, 1996; Piketty, 2013; Atkinson, 2015; Stiglitz, 2015; see also Chapters 1 and 31). Consequent political anger and global instability are becoming evident in several tipping points with serious implications for future generations (Mishra, 2017).

Great Accelerations

Structural acceleration in post-1945 economic growth and patterns of production, transportation, and consumption, along with waste and spoliation of the oceans and nature by many countries with varied ideologies and agendas but underpinned most powerfully in recent decades by neoliberal policies, have aggravated loss of biodiversity and adversely impinged on the sustainability of the biosphere and the health of whole populations (Oreskses & Conway, 2013; McMichael, 2013; Rockstrom & Foley, 2009; Schlossberg, 2017). Accelerations in the depletion of nonrenewable resources (such as fresh water supplies and fossil fuel sources), deforestation, soil degradation, and the acidification and pollution of oceans

(undermining many of the sources of global food chains) have led to what is now referred to as the *sixth great extinction* of biodiversity with associated unsustainable transformations in the ecology and biosphere (Kolbert, 2014). The already visible effects have been most pronounced in the Global South.

The accumulation of wealth is now on an increasingly divergent path from the health/well-being of people and life of all kinds on our planet (Grantham, 2018). The privileged 20%, who have benefited maximally from recent economic growth, seem to be largely oblivious of (or in denial about) the adverse implications of their affluent lifestyles and large ecological footprints on the lives of the 80% less fortunate than themselves and, ultimately, on the health of all globally on a finite planet with reduced resilience to cope with endless demands.

The "Great Acceleration" must lead us to consider how we have reached a point at which all future life on our planet will be increasingly threatened by climate change, environmental degradation, the ongoing emergence and rapid spread of potentially fatal infections (Garrett, 1994), the relentless increase in antibiotic resistance, and other critical tipping points beyond which irreversible entropy will escalate (Benatar, 2001; Barnosky et al., 2012; Kopp et al., 2016).

We have elsewhere referred to these interconnected crises of economy, ecology, and social development, along with the ethical and political questions they raise, as parts of a *global organic crisis* that locates the world at a historical crossroads necessitating a significant change of sociopolitical-economic direction in order to make peaceful and sustainable progress (Gill, 2015). Before we address this question, we now outline other aspects of the neoliberal development model.

Inequalities, Health, and Ongoing Crises

Despite many of the benefits that have flowed from the impact of neoliberal economic policies, five negative social impacts are evident since the 1980s: rising wealth and health inequalities globally, even within wealthy countries; reduced value of wages and increased debt; redistribution of profits from nonfinancial companies to the finance sector; the growth of social and financial insecurity; erosion of social infrastructure with associated escalation of crime; and last but not least, the relentless commodification of more aspects and components of social life, including culturally specific life processes such as healthcare systems, education systems, and social values, with erosion of the ethos of the caring professions.

Moreover, there has been intensification of the long-standing tendency of humans to exploit fellow human beings, social processes, and nature, often involving incremental dispossession of communities of their basic and local means of subsistence and livelihood (Harvey, 2005), acceleration in the turnover time of the production and sale of commodities to generate more rapid accumulation of profits for firms and investors; and the restructuring or privatization of previously public institutions and public goods, including provisions for healthcare and education (Klein, 2008; Gill & Benatar, 2016; Monbiot, 2016). Associated valorization of disruption of such social systems undermines their wholeness and integrity.

The above-mentioned processes have been punctuated by frequent crises, often driven by financial breakdown, that most adversely affect the poorest and most vulnerable. The continued unfolding of the 2008 global financial crisis seriously damaged the poor worldwide and continues to do so as food prices rise, job creation lags behind needs, and corporations have freedom to move money around the world, evade taxation, and incrementally enclose the commons through privatization to preferentially favor corporate control and wealthy shareholders.

Africa has been most adversely affected in the past through the serial and incremental dehumanizing effects of slavery, colonization, and decolonization (with corruption fostered through collusion with "big men" (kleptocrats). More recently, adverse effects continue through the economic slavery emanating from neoliberal policies creating/sustaining debt, stultifying local food production, making jobs more precarious, and fostering high drug prices and ongoing extraction of vast resources to feed insatiable consumption patterns of East and West and, most recently, China (Caplan, 2008). Between 1980 and 1996, Sub-Saharan Africa paid twice the sum of its total debt in the form of interest yet still ended up owing three times more in 1996 than it did in 1980 (Monbiot, 2004).

The middle classes in the United States, the United Kingdom, Europe, and elsewhere (Standing, 2014; Welsh, 2016) have not escaped these ravages of economic crises, and even in the United States, millions of working-class families have lost their homes and become insolvent as well as dispossessed (DeGraw, 2010a, 2010b).

Financially driven crises have fostered widespread imposition of austerity measures since 2008 while bailing out banks and large corporations (Katz, 2011; Collins, 2015) in ways that have eroded the tax base of many countries, with resulting endemic fiscal crises. Many governments globally have cut back on health and other public services, with consequent unequal class-related and gendered effects through shedding public-sector jobs, hitting women the hardest (Cooper & Whyte, 2017).

Power Relations and Ethics

Military power has been increasingly replaced by material, epistemic, and moral modes of power that function through social structures or technical production and communication. These modes and functions, within varied forms of power relations, underlie how institutions operate to influence what we believe to be right and good. Nonetheless, power in many societies, past and present, is premised on unequal and hierarchical social relations (class based, gendered, and racialized).

In the particular case of today's capitalist societies, these social hierarchies are shaped by the enhanced power of capital under neoliberalism. The power of capital associated with giant corporations and financial firms such as those on Wall Street is reinforced by laws and regulations that sustain capitalist private property rights and other associated prerogatives. Indeed, neoliberalism – and its correlate, corporate power – involves more than economic policy. Its implications and impact extend into and pervade all walks of life and frames that influence what is deemed politically and economically possible (Gill, 1995, 2008, 2011; Birn et al., 2018; Gill & Benatar, 2019).

The power of capital under neoliberal governance is based on the privileged ownership, control, or access to both financial and physical assets in contrast to the bulk of the rest of society. It is reflected, for example, in the massive concentration of assets, including substantial control over the media and mechanisms of communication, by large corporations and wealth holders worldwide. Its scope is also reflected in the subordination of public policies of many nations to the imperative of economic growth based on the commodity form in ways that substantially influence the nature of society and its future possibilities.

Here it should also be noted that global institutions set up in the past to run the world in a democratic fashion are undemocratic in practice, and they reflect the policy preferences of corporate capital and financial interests of the most powerful corporations. For example, the UN General Assembly is far less influential than the International Monetary Fund (IMF) and World Bank, institutions that are, in turn, dominated by the G8 nations, which hold 49% of votes. Because all major decisions require an 85% majority and the United States possesses 17% of the votes, it can veto any decision it opposes, even those supported by every other country (Monbiot, 2004), although some change is now evident, for example, in the increasing influence of China. This constellation of features is antithetical to the ethical values of equity, human dignity, solidarity, and social justice.

Challenging the Dominant Belief System: Where to Go from Here, and How?

In the social world, there is no such thing as a "view from nowhere" or a single claim to truth, and there is a need for "reflexivity" about the origins of any epistemological perspective and its links to the actual exercise of structural or productive power (Shiffman, 2014). By contrast, the ideological strategies of neoliberalism seek to dismiss or marginalize other more critical epistemologies, which are treated as "unscientific" and not "universal," with the latter defined from a partisan and indeed a singular perspective that has a unilateral claim to "truth." Indeed, power influences the intellectual and moral frames that are used to constitute the "real." This is why the unequal power relations within the structure and function of the global political economy and society just noted remain central to how we perceive and evaluate the significance of disparities in wealth, health, and the ecological pressures that ultimately threaten us all, although some more than others.

However, this moment of reflexivity – and the associated claims that there is no monopoly on claims to truth – also helps to explain why the present conjuncture is generating conflict "from below" by those who lack hope for the future and feel powerless and silenced (Mishra, 2017). The result is diverse forms of political contestation and resistance from both right and left, as well as new forms of fascism and authoritarian, theocratic, and right-wing nationalist forces that are emerging throughout the world in response to the global organic crisis and the inability of

neoliberal leaderships to provide convincing exit strategies that are credible to a majority of the population. Yet many of these forces still lack coherence as an organized opposition offering real alternatives to the dominance of neoliberalism.

It remains the case that the quality of life and the ongoing expectations of the 20% of people in the world who consume 80% of the world's energy and resources are associated with a reluctance to admit that our current global ecological and health predicaments are to a considerable extent universal issues that are attributable to endless entitlements and wasteful consumption patterns, with free-riding on the environmental commons.

The dominant and dominating mind-set of the most privileged people in the world tends to lock us into our particular optimistic realms of thinking and action (Pinker, 2017) that must surely seem mysterious, untrustworthy, and irremediable to those whose lives remain severely restricted by socially constructed causes of poverty and lack of opportunities to flourish.

Such reluctance to admit to the errors of current ways of thinking and action is supported by the popular notion that more philanthropy and new technology should have the highest priority to overcome current crises (see Chapter 33). These features of the lives of the privileged and powerful also tend to generate neglect and denial of the need for the required paradigmatic change to restructure national and international taxation systems and power relations in ways that could achieve the financial means and consideration of practical solutions that are potentially within our grasp.

By contrast, the era in which we now live has been described "as resembling the end of classical antiquity, or the beginning of the modern era, that generates great stress" and that "calls for a fundamental transformation in the underlying assumptions and principles of our cultural world view" (Tarnas, 2006). Amid the debates and controversies that fill the intellectual arena, Richard Tarnas suggests that "several of our basic understandings of what is reality are in contention: the role of the human being in nature and the cosmos; the status of human knowledge; the basis of moral values; the dilemmas of pluralism, relativism, objectivity; the spiritual dimension of life; and the direction and meaning (if any) of history and evolution" (Tarnas, 2006).

It is thus legitimate to also imagine that very different political and ethical notions of global health could be influenced by alternatively constructed social systems, powerfully shaped by a broader set of beliefs associated with forgotten aspects of global history (Drayton & Motadel, 2018) and neglected aspects of international relations (Grice, 2016). Such contestation from without is of vital importance and should be explored and addressed. For example, the positive influences of more optimistic traditional belief systems with their own powerful heuristic influences, as discussed elsewhere, cannot be ignored (see Chapters 25 and 26). It is also possible that an interphilosophies dialogue methodology could facilitate a constructive tension capable of modifying the dominant perspective that seems increasingly out of touch regarding the limits of economic growth and other dangers at a time when human activity threatens sustainable life on our planet (Benatar et al., 2016) and chapter 27.

With such contestations and imaginaries in mind, we now selectively discuss some perspectives that might illuminate the ways forward.

The Challenge of Anticolonialism

Aimé Césaire (2001), an early critic of colonialism, highlighted the role of the West in perpetuating and enhancing the notion of the "other." Regarding the impact of colonialism on the colonized/colonizer/culture and the concept of civilization, he argued that "the instruments of colonial power rely on barbaric, brutal violence and intimidation, and the end result is the degradation of Europe itself" (Césaire, 2001: 9).[3]

His writings presaged a recent resurgence of protests, postcolonial discourses, and the rise in political anger in Africa, South Africa, and elsewhere (Mishra, 2017). Growing attention to Indigenous people in Canada has led to acknowledgment that they have been lied to, betrayed, and belittled, which, together with increasing delegitimization of colonizing forces and power structures, highlights the perfidy and falsity of so-called universal values, ways of life, and governance (Ralston Saul, 2014; Manuel & Derrikson, 2017; Talaga, 2018).

Lying at the heart of these critiques are reactions to lack of respect for human dignity and the devaluing of the lives of so many. Most who live well within the "Western" way of life or in the Global North feel that their lives and persons have some inherent dignity. Conversely, many who live deprived and exploited lives (most but not all in the Global South) have a deep sense of not being accorded equal basic human dignity, as eloquently described by Richard Wagamese (2008).[4]

"Power With" Rather Than "Power Over"

Notably and more constructively, there is also political mobilization on the left throughout the world, drawing on grassroots movements, trade unions, some socialist parties, and international forums such as the World Social Forum, seeking to develop more progressive alternatives that can speak in quite different ways to the ethics and politics of our global predicament (Pradella & Marois, 2015; Gill, 2008). Indeed, the power relations associated with radical democracy may potentially offer a more balanced distribution of power than that associated with the neoliberal era. The challenge might be viewed as the need to use creative intelligence and imagination to develop such democracy against the background of an increasingly technological world that alienates ordinary people from centers of power and decision making (Nettelford, 1995). What might be needed are forms of political society that are more clearly associated with the use of "power with" rather than "power over" and with concern for the emancipatory and collective interests of humans.

Consideration for the Health of Others: How We View Ourselves

How we view the widely disparate states of health across the world and other major threats that have become clearly manifest in the past decade depends on how we view ourselves, the world in which we live, and the kind of world we might want in the future. How we view global health also significantly influences our understanding of the appropriate research agenda for the pursuit of improved global health.

The Lancet–University of Oslo Commission on governance for global health has been critiqued as a prominent example of an insightful but incomplete and largely technical diagnosis of global health problems. Its failure to make appropriate recommendations for progress, inclusive of a majority of the

---

[3] Other civilizations can also justifiably be accused of such alienation of fellow humans

[4] "As an Ojibway man I have been marginalized, analyzed, criticized, ostracized, legitimized, politicized, dehumanized, downsized and Supersized. Struggling with my identity I've been, misinterpreted, misfiled, misjudged, misunderstood, and misguided. I have been misinformed, misdirected, mismatched, misstated, and misused. These days I am misgoverned and misrepresented."

world's people, can be explained by its intellectual framing (Gill & Benatar, 2016). The latter ignores the underlying economic and political structures, values, and social forces that shape the ideological, intellectual, and research frameworks of global health and its governance. Indeed, it could be argued that the global health discourse agenda has been captured and held hostage by those with the most power.

In contrast to the Oslo Commission, with its piecemeal recommendations for reform, we suggest that improving global health in the twenty-first century requires a willingness to implement new conceptions such as *developing sustainability* as a more apt metaphor than the twentieth-century notion of *sustainable development* (Bensimon & Benatar, 2006). We need to go beyond the belief that scientific and technological advances, economic growth, and current market practices can provide not only all the required solutions but also a sustainable perspective on the future. Appreciation is required of the multifactorial underpinnings and magnitude of the many interlinked global crises that constitute a complex planetary crisis that involves the modes and patterns of social and economic development as well as a crisis of political representation and leadership (Gill & Benatar, 2019).

Associated with this crisis is denial, including that of climate change, as the product of the public relations activities of large corporations associated with the lack of sociological and moral imagination regarding the future and the responsibility and role of the most privileged and powerful. One aspect of this denial is the refusal to acknowledge the increasingly inequitable net redistribution of global resources from the poor to the rich with resulting intensifying threats to global health, security, and democracy.

Our Choices at the Historical Crossroads?

Our current global predicament provides us with a choice – whether to continue on the current neoliberal trajectory, which in fundamental respects is unethical and unsustainable socially and ecologically, or to pursue globally constructive alternatives. It seems to us that we cannot hope for a more peaceful and secure world when conditions of life remain so inadequate for so many while we continue to consume almost exponentially without concern for the future.

Short-sighted and self-interested satisfaction with medical progress and neglect of what is being done for the poor, together with claims in an article entitled "Global Health 2035: A World Converging within a Generation" (Jamison et al., 2013), obstruct achievement of a much-needed twenty-first-century paradigm shift to the more complex framing of an ecological and systems conception of global social justice and global health, pursued through governance under more effective democratic control (Monbiot, 2004; Brock, 2009; Gill & Benatar, 2016).

We propose that at tipping points between sustainability and nonsustainability at the current historical crossroads, there is an imperative for another shift in the direction of thought and action about life and living to facilitate future advances in human and planetary health (Baudet, 2000; Westley et al., 2011; Oreskes & Conway, 2013; Waters et al., 2016; Emmott, 2017; Benatar et al., 2018; Gill & Benatar, 2019). Our perspective is in keeping with a proposal made 50 years ago for a major change in thinking and action toward framing global health in terms of a healthy planet (Potter, 1971).

We consider that rectifying humanly imposed harms requires ethical and ecological understandings of the impact of our transition from being a species dependent on nature for our survival, through striving to bring nature under our control, to processes that are now impairing planetary resilience by exceeding the renewability of natural resources (Rockstrom & Foley, 2009) and attempting to reinvent nature through potentially hazardous advances in synthetic biology (Kaebnick, 2013).

From an Anthropocentric Perspective to an Ecological Perspective

In addition to changes in the global political economy and attitudes toward progress, today's challenge is to replace the current meaning of "global health" with a concept of *global/planetary health*, long perceived as a more complex ecologically centered notion that includes acknowledgment of the upstream social and societal determinants of health, the lack of geographic or social barriers to the spread of infectious diseases, and the importance of the interconnectedness of all forms of life and human well-being on a threatened planet. The One Health Initiative is an admirable example of ecologically minded approaches to human health (One Health, http://onehealthinitiative.com/about.php). This perspective, related to the interdependency of health for all, within an increasingly threatened global ecological framework, has long remained beyond our horizons in an era of high-technology medicine, where progress is increasingly focused on genomics and personalized medicine. It is also arguably not possible to contemplate health or how health could be improved and how progress could be made, for example, toward what Albrecht (2016) has called the "Symbiocene," without insight into how the global political economy is structured and controlled, its ideological and cultural underpinnings, and what should and could be changed (Harvey, 2005; Atkinson, 2015; see also Chapters 18 and 38).

This might be a starting point for visionary research and ambitious intersectoral and transdisciplinary collaboration toward taking effective action to avert the tragedies looming on the horizon and already becoming manifest. Prominent values and frames within this system would include a deep sense of physical, moral, and spiritual interdependence with nature (i.e., animals, plants, and the ecological system) that sustains all life and a spirit of solidarity, cooperation, sharing, and social responsibility that respects the public commons and future generations.

These considerations point to the important role that ethics can play in reimagining possibilities for the future. An expansive and inclusive vocabulary and a set of concepts can be drawn from the traditions of interpersonal ethics, public health ethics, global health ethics, and environmental ethics. Elements of each, together with considerations of cosmopolitan global justice (Brock, 2009), could play a role in a higher synthesis and articulation of values that are identified as important in each domain.

Traditional concerns for respect for persons within interpersonal and medical ethics could be extended to communities and environments. Recognition of mutual dependence links into the importance of relational values such as reciprocity and solidarity that are prominent in public health ethics and global health ethics. Dynamic tension between dominant ethical theories and their political correlates reveals legitimate disagreement about the fundamental values that animate action toward the good. Such values need to be explicitly articulated and differences negotiated.

Creating, nurturing, and protecting the space to navigate across value-based differences in worldviews may be one of the preeminent challenges of the twenty-first century (Tomsons & Meyer, 2003; Benatar et al., 2016; Porter & Barry, 2016). The challenges we face in the twenty-first century are to explore these issues and understand the associated power relationship implications. New political processes could harness economic growth to human development, reduce global disparities in health, and promote peaceful coexistence premised on social justice and a truly global perspective on society, our ecological environment, and the future.

Neoliberalism, with its lack of credible ethical underpinnings, has not served us well collectively at a global level, and there is no idyllic paradigm to which to revert. We suggest that an alternative paradigm with space for genuine dialogue could help facilitate sustainable lives with recognition of the equal moral worth and dignity of all, preservation of freedom to achieve individual potential, solidarity with others, and collaborative participation in creating circumstances that foster such values and reduce inequities.

Conclusion

In our view, making progress toward a more sustainable and less unjust world with less suffering requires (1) acknowledging the distortions of prized values that underlie the dominant paradigm that has shaped and governed how we currently live, (2) acknowledging that compromised population health reflects profound systemic dysfunction, (3) accepting the discomfort of insights into how the structure of the global political economy, power relations, cultural complexities, pervasive corruption, and poor global leadership all perpetuate intractable and dehumanizing core/periphery disparities and threaten the lives of all, and (4) striving to enhance the sociological and moral imagination (including the ability of individuals and communities to empathize with others) to effect change through ethical and intellectual innovation that may promote a shift toward a global frame of mind and appropriate sociopolitical action.

Other steps forward should include the use of creative intellect and imagination to educate ourselves about the needs of increasingly diverse and complex societies, promote the social innovation that could revitalize public services and infrastructure within a reconceptualized idea of a good society, act as vigilant stewards for future generations, promote dialogue across different worldviews, valuing compassion and empathy as the "glue" that holds society together, and finally to rethink the logic of dominant affluent lifestyles and balance reasonable demands with appropriate supply.

Seeking to develop and maintain authentic means toward a better life for more people would also require global governance that includes responsibility for the ecology of the planet. The idea of "being" would not be focused on acquiring and having more, as in the market civilization and anthropocentric models, but rather on "being better people" within a more ecological conception of ethically sustainable life for all beyond mere first-order survival needs. These dimensions of global health and well-being are scarcely recognized as research or policy priorities in an era of high-technology medicine, where progress is instead being increasingly focused on genomics and personalized medicine.

Rectification cannot be achieved with outdated, highly individualistic ways of thinking. New paradigms of citizenship could reinforce the interconnectedness and mutual dependency of humans on each other and on nature. An expanded ethical discourse inclusive of ecological ethical considerations is required to encourage the paradigm shifts required to drive such progress.

While the current state of the world and the attitudes of some of the most powerful nations and people offer little prospect of making such progress, a modicum of hope should be retained. Some encouragement to achieve ambitious goals could be derived from the immensity of human scientific ingenuity (e.g., in exploring the genome and the universe) and the extent of philosophical insights into the ethical and sociopolitical requirements for peaceful progress. Such ingenuity, combined with deep reflexivity and sustained transdisciplinary, innovative social research on a scale equivalent to the innovative scientific quest for an HIV vaccine, could promote initiatives and develop policy options capable of facilitating a shift of the current damaging trajectory toward better and more sustainable lives for all.

Ultimately, however, such progress toward a sustainable relationship with our ecological system requires the transformation of political power and political economy, as well as policies that are grounded in ethical commitments. Moving toward the "development of sustainability" as a maxim of wisdom and praxis to promote the health of people and the biosphere must surely become our most important goal. At the heart of such an endeavor lies the need, in our view, to replace neoliberalism with an ethical framework and political ideology more conducive to respecting all human rights, promoting democracy, and valuing social justice.

Resulting new initiatives and policy options could facilitate a shift toward a trajectory with the potential for a sustainable future.

Contemplation of health and how it could be improved within the preceding, broadened perspective requires historical insight into the implications of perpetuating current upstream causal processes that are compromising global/planetary health and destroying the resilience of our natural environment on which all life is crucially dependent. Lessons need to be learned from the collapse of past civilizations that have flourished and declined – not least because of a variety of human behavioral excesses.

The difficulty in achieving this lies in the fact that the 20% of people who consume 80% of world's energy and who enjoy most of its resources are reluctant to overcome complacency about the quality of their lives, modify their ongoing expectations, and admit that current global ecological and health predicaments are to a considerable extent attributable to their endless entitlements and wasteful consumption patterns. This complacency is complicated by the fact that the major impetus to "progress" for the 20% who benefit has arisen from the invisibility of power structures and indeed invisibility of the *belief system in which* power is embedded and that determines the *way we think and* how we *frame* our ideas, values, and actions.

It is unlikely that sufficient progress can be made in the health of whole populations globally without some changes to how the global political economy operates, promotion of more sustainable consumption patterns, new resource distributive mechanisms, and conceptions of power such as cooperative "power with" (instead of coercive "power over") that could enhance mutually beneficial endeavors.

All of this will require a major global shift toward a more uniformly held, ecologically oriented belief system – a prospect that may seem unlikely but is arguably essential. At the very least, such an agenda is deserving of the attention of scholars and concerned citizens of the world. The future international order will be shaped by those who have the power and collective will. The question is whether the world's democracies will (again) rise to that challenge (Kagan, 2009).

References

Albrecht, G. (2016). Exiting the Anthropocene and entering the Symbiocene. *Minding Nature* **9**(2), 12–16. Available at www.humansandnature.org/filebin/pdf/minding_nature/may_2016/Albrecht_May2016.

Alexander, T. (1996). *Unravelling Global Apartheid: An Overview of World Politics*. Cambridge, UK: Polity Press.

Anderson, E. (2015). Liberty, equality, and private government (Tanner Lectures in Human Values). Available at https://tannerlectures.utah.edu/Anderson%20manuscript.pdf.

Astroulakis, N. (2014). An ethical analysis of neoliberal capitalism: alternative perspective from development ethics. *Éthique et économique/Ethics and Economics* 11(2), 94–108. Available at https://papyrus.bib.umontreal.ca/xmlui/handle/1866/10931 (accessed December 4, 2019).

Atkinson, A. (2015). *Inequality: What Can Be Done*. Cambridge, MA: Harvard University Press.

Baudet, J. (ed.) (2000). *Building a Global Community: Globalization and the Common Good*. Copenhagen: Royal Danish Ministry for Foreign Affairs.

Barnosky, A. D., et al. (2012). Approaching a state shift in Earth's biosphere. *Nature* **486**: 52–58.

Benatar, S. R. (2001). The coming catastrophe in international health: an analogy with lung cancer. *International Journal* 56(4), 611–631.

Benatar, S. R. (2005). Moral imagination: the missing component in global health. *Public Library of Science Medicine* 2(12), e400.

Benatar, S. R. (2011). Global leadership, ethics and global health: the search for new paradigms, in Gill, S. (ed.), *The Global Crisis and the Crisis of Global Leadership*. Cambridge, UK: Cambridge University Press, pp. 127–143.

Benatar, S. R. (2016). Politics, power, poverty and global health: systems and frames. *International Journal of Health Policy and Management* 5(10), 599–604.

Benatar, S. R. (2017). A divided world in entropy. *Society* **55**, 200–206.

Benatar, S. R., & Upshur, R. (2013). Virtue in medicine reconsidered: individual health and global health. *Perspectives in Biology and Medicine* **56**(1), 126–147.

Benatar, S. R., Daar, A. S., & Singer, P. A. (2003). Global health ethics: a rationale for mutual caring. *International Affairs* 79, 107–138.

Benatar, S R., Daibes, I., & Tomsons, S. (2016). Inter-philosophies dialogue: creating a paradigm for global health ethics. *Kennedy Institute of Ethics Journal* 26(3), 323–346. doi:10.1353/ken.2016.0027.

Benatar, S. R., Gill, S., & Bakker, I. C. (2011). Global health and the global economic crisis. *American Journal of Public Health* **101**(4), 646–653.

Benatar, S., Upshur, R., & Gill, S. (2018). Understanding the relationship between ethics, neoliberalism and power as a step towards improving the health of people and our planet. *Anthropocene Review* **2018**, 1–22.

Bensimon, C. A., & Benatar, S. R. (2006). Developing sustainability: a new metaphor for progress. *Theoretical Medicine and Bioethics* 27:(1), 59–79.

Birn, A.-E., Pillay, Y., & Holtz, T. (2018). Globalisation, trade, work and health, in *Textbook of Global Health*, 4th ed. New York: Oxford University Press, pp. 377–424.

Brock, G. (2009). *Global Justice: A Cosmopolitan Account*. Oxford, UK: Oxford University Press.

Caplan, G. (2008). *The Betrayal of Africa*. Toronto: Groundwood Books.

Cesaire, A. (2001). *Discourse on Colonialism*. New York: Monthly Review Press.

Chatwood, S., Paulette, F., Baker, R., et al. (2015). Approaching etuaptmumk: introducing a consensus based mixed method for health services research. *International Journal of Circumpolar Health* 4(1), 27438.

Collins, M. (2015). *The Bank Bailout*. Available at www.forbes.com/sites/mikecollins/2015/07/14/thebig-bank-bailout/#13595fd72d83.

Cooper, V., & Whyte, D. (eds.) (2017). *The Violence of Austerity*. London: Pluto Press.

DeGraw, D. (2010a). The economic elite have engineered an extraordinary coup, threatening the very existence of the middle class. Available at www.alternet.org/story/145667 (accessed September 20, 2012).

DeGraw, D. (2010b). The richest 1% have captured America's wealth: what's it going to take to get it back? Available at www.alternet.org/story/145705.

Drayton, R., & Motadel, D. (2018) Discussion: the futures of global history. *Journal of Global History* **13**(1), 1–21.

Emmott, B. (2017). *The Fate of the West: The Battle to Save the World's Most Successful Political Idea*. New York: Public Affairs Press.

Garrett, L. (1994). *The Coming Plague: Newly Emerging Diseases in a World Out of Balance*. New York: Farrar, Straus & Giroux.

Garrido, M. (2003). The free trade charade. *Asia Times*, June 11. Available at www.atimes.com/atimes/Global_Economy/EF11Dj01.html.

Gergen, K. (1985). The social constructivist movement in modern psychology. *American Psychologist* **40**, 266–275.

Gill, S. (1995). Globalisation, market civilisation and disciplinary neoliberalism. *Millennium: Journal of International Studies* 23(3), 399–423.

Gill, S. (2008). *Power and Resistance in the New World Order*. New York: Palgrave Macmillan.

Gill, S. (ed.) (2011). *Global Crises and the Crisis of Global Leadership*. Cambridge, UK: Cambridge University Press.

Gill, S. (2015). At the historical crossroads: radical imaginaries and the crisis of global governance, in Gill, S. (ed.), *Critical Perspectives on the Crisis of Global Governance: Reimagining the Future*. New York: Palgrave Macmillan, pp. 181–196.

Gill, S., & Benatar, S. R. (2016). Global health governance and global power: a critical commentary on The Lancet–University of Oslo Commission Report. *International Journal of Health Services* **46**(2), 346–365.

Gill, S., & Benatar, S. R. (2019). Reflections on the political economy of planetary health. *Review of International Political Economy* **27**(1), 167–190.

Greenwood, M., de Leeuw, S., & Lindsay, N. M. (2018). *Determinants of Indigenous Peoples' Health Beyond the Social*, 2nd ed. Toronto: Canadian Scholars Press.

Grantham, J. (2018). The race of our lives revisited. GMO White Paper. Available at www.gmo.com/docs/default-source/research-and-commentary/strategies/asset-allocation/the-race-of-our-lives-revisited.pdf.

Grice, F. (2016). Towards non-Western histories in international relations textbooks. Carnegie Council for Ethics in International Affairs. Available at www.carnegiecouncil.org/publications/ethics_online/0105 (accessed January 14, 2016).

Hanlon, R. J., & Christie, K. (2016). *Freedom from Fear, Freedom from Want: An Introduction to Human Security*. Toronto: University of Toronto Press.

Harvey, D. (2005). *A Short History of Neoliberalism*. New York: Oxford University Press.

Hayek, F. A. (1944) *The Road to Serfdom*. Chicago: University of Chicago Press.

Jamison, D., Summers, L. H., Alleyne, G., et al. (2013). Global health 2035: a world converging within a generation. *Lancet* **382**(9908), 1898–1955.

Johnstone, D. J. (2017). *Missing the Tide: Global Governments in Retreat*. Montreal: McGill-Queens's University Press.

Kaebnick, G. E. (2013). *Humans in Nature: The World as We Find It and the World as We Create It*. Oxford, UK. Oxford University Press.

Kagan, R. (2009). *The Return of History and the End of Dreams*. New York: Vintage Books.

Katz, J. D. (2011). Who benefited from the bailout? *Minnesota Law Review* **95**, 1568. Available at www.minnesotalawreview.org/wpcontent/uploads/2011/05/Katz_PDF.pdf.

Klein, N. (2008). *The Shock Doctrine: The Rise of Disaster Capitalism*. London. Penguin Books.

Kolbert, E. (2014). *The Sixth Extinction: An Unnatural History*. New York: Henry Holt & Co.

Kopp, R. E., Shwom, R., Wagner, J., et al. (2016). Tipping elements and climate economic shocks: pathways toward integrated assessment. *Earth's Future* **4**, 346–372.

Manuel, A., & Derrikson, R. (2017) *The Reconciliation Manifesto: Recovering the Land, Rebuilding the Economy*. Toronto. James Lorimer and Company.

McMichael, A. J. (2013). Globalization, climate change, and human health. *New England Journal of Medicine* **368**, 1335–1343.

Mishra, P. (2017). *The Age of Anger*. New York: Farrar, Straus & Giroux.

Monbiot, G. (2004). *The Age of Consent: A Manifesto for a New World Order*. London: Harper Perennial.

Monbiot, G. (2016). *How Did We Get into This Mess?* London: Verso.

Nettelford, R. (1995). *Inward Stretch, Outward Reach: A Voice from the Caribbean*. London: Caribbean Diaspora Press.

Oreskes, N., & Conway, E. M. (2013). The collapse of Western civilization: a view from the future. *Daedalus* **142**(1), 40–58.

Pinker, S. (2017). *Enlightenment Now: The Case for Reason, Science, Humanism, and Progress*. New York: Viking Press.

Piketty, T. (2013). *Capital in the Twenty-First Century*. Cambridge, MA: Harvard University Press.

Porter, E., & Barry, J. (2016). *Planning for Coexistence: Recognizing Indigenous Rights Through Land-Use Planning in Canada and Australia*. London: Routledge.

Potter, V. R. (1971). *Bioethics: Bridge to the Future*. Englewood Cliffs, NJ: Prentice-Hall.

Pradella, L., & Marois, T. (eds.) (2015). *Polarizing Development: Alternatives to Neoliberalism and the Crisis*. Chicago: University of Chicago Press.

Ralston Saul, J. (2014). *The Comeback*. Toronto: Viking Press.

Rockstrom, J., & Foley, S. W. (2009). A safe operating space for humanity. *Nature* **461**, 472–475.

Rowden, R. (2009). *The Deadly Ideas of Neoliberalism: How the IMF Has Undermined Public Health and the Fight Against AIDS*. London: Zed Books.

Schlossberg, T. (2017). Era of "biological annihilation" is underway, scientists warn. *New York Times*, July 11. Available at www.nytimes.com/2017/07/11/climate/mass-extinction-animal-species.html.

Shiffman, J. (2014). Knowledge, moral claims and the exercise of power in global health. *International Journal of Health Policy Management* **2014**(3), 297–299.

Singer, P. A., Benatar, S. R., Bernstein, P., et al. (2003). Ethics and SARS: lessons from Toronto. *British Medical Journal* **327**, 1342–1344.

Standing, G. (2014). *The Precariat: The New Dangerous Class*. London: Bloomsbury Academic.

Stiglitz, J. E. (2015). *The Great Divide*. New York: W.W. Norton and Company.

Talaga, T. (2018). *All Our Relations: Finding the Way Forward*. Toronto: House of Anansi Press.

Tarnas, R. (2006). *Cosmos and Psyche: Intimations of a New World View.* New York: Penguin Books.

Tomsons, S., & Meyer, L. (eds.) (20034). *Philosophy and Aboriginal Rights: Critical Dialogues.* Oxford, UK: Oxford University Press.

Tooze, A. (2017). Tempestuous Seasons (Review of *In the Long Run We Are All Dead,* by Geoff Mann). *London Review of Books*, September 13, pp. 19–21.

Wagamese, R. (2008). *One Story, One Song.* Toronto: Douglas & McIntyre.

Wallerstein, I. (1992). America and the world: today, yesterday and tomorrow. *Theory Society* **21**, 1–28.

Waters, C., Zalasiewicz, J., Summerhayes, C., et al. (2016). The Anthropocene is functionally and stratigraphically distinct from the Holocene. *Science* **35**(2689), 137. Available at http://science.sciencemag.org/content/351/6269/aad2622.

Welsh, J. (2016). *The Return of History: Conflict, Migration and Geopolitics in the 21st Century* (2016 Massey Lectures). Toronto: House of Anansi Press.

Westley, F., Olsson, P., Folke, C., et al. (2011). Tipping toward sustainability: emerging pathways of transformation. *Ambio: A Journal of the Human Environment* **40**(7), 762–780.

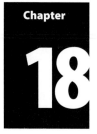

Morbid Symptoms, Organic Crises, and Enclosures of the Commons
Global Health Since the 2008 World Economic Crisis

Stephen Gill, Isabella Bakker, and Dillon Wamsley

The crisis consists precisely in the fact that the old is dying and the new cannot be born; in this interregnum a great variety of morbid symptoms appear.
(Antonio Gramsci, 1971: 276)

Introduction

We have previously argued that the 2008 global financial and economic crisis was a clear manifestation of an unstable and contradictory world characterized by a disjunction between (1) massive economic growth and unprecedented advances in science, technology, and medical care and (2) the widening of disparities in wealth and health within and between nations. We also argued that the global financial crisis was much more than a crisis of capitalist accumulation or a necessary self-correction aided by macroeconomic intervention and bailouts. The crisis also reflected a process of enclosure of the social commons and the contradictions of what we call "market civilization" – an individualistic, consumerist, privatized, energy-intensive, and ecologically myopic pattern of lifestyle and culture that is currently dominant in world development (Gill, 1995, 2008).

Indeed, in our *Power, Production, and Social Reproduction: Human in/Security in the Global Political Economy*, we hypothesized that we are in a period of global contradiction where, on the one hand, we see the intensified power of capital through neoliberal political and constitutional reforms and, on the other hand, a weakening of the conditions for stable and sustainable social reproduction (Bakker & Gill, 2003). This contradiction goes well beyond the global financial and economic crisis of 2008 and its aftermath.

Rather than simply constituting an economic or financial crisis, we argued that the meltdown could best be characterized as part of a *global organic* crisis – one that is simultaneously an economic crisis, a social crisis, and a crisis in the relationship between human

beings, their forms of livelihood, and nature. These concurrent crises have numerous social connections with global health and are framed by what we referred to as new enclosures that undermine public provisioning and access to healthcare.

Whereas the unfolding of the world financial and economic crisis had serious implications for global health financing, the decade since then has seen a continuation of intensifying inequality, tepid economic recovery, and widespread global austerity. Although varying widely by country, after a brief period of fiscal stimulus in the immediate aftermath of the financial crisis, as private debt became socialized, austerity packages were implemented across Europe throughout the Eurozone countries, some of which were mimicked across the Global South, with a new range of structural adjustment programs introduced by the International Monetary Fund (IMF) in the post-2008 period (Kentikelenis, Stubbs, & King, 2016; Ruckert & Labonte, 2017). In the United States, the government, by contrast, sought to stimulate the economy by lowering interest rates; extending government support for banks, corporations, pension funds, and asset holders; and expanding government debt and liabilities to help keep US capitalism afloat. In the European Union, persistent austerity has continued to put pressure on public-sector spending, affecting social services and social safety nets, all of which have exacerbated social, economic, and health inequalities across a range of countries.

The deep crisis of global capitalism from 2007 to 2009 and the decade of virtual nonrecovery and continuing austerity since then have undermined some of the basic conditions of existence for the majority of the world's population, thus endangering their human security and posing severe threats to global health, understood as the health of the global population as a whole. This compounds the desperate issues of malnutrition and climate change discussed at length in this chapter, dramatized by a global food crisis involving over a billion people who are either food insecure or actually starving and threats to the collective future of the planet posed by global warming, pollution, and more general ecological degradation. It is a crisis of the dominant development model that we call *market civilization* – on a world scale. In short, the global organic crisis is posing fundamental threats to the survival and well-being of billions of people who command very few economic resources and little ownership, in contrast to the very small numbers of superwealthy billionaire plutocrats who have gained control over the lion's share of global assets and who have been the primary beneficiaries of government bailout packages and subsequent austerity measures since 2008.[1]

Many of these issues and problems can be connected to the basic logic of the dominant pattern of accumulation in the global political economy – which we call *disciplinary neoliberalism* – and, in turn, to the form of unequal and unjust social development that it fosters. This pattern of social development is also ecologically unsustainable. It is premised on energy-intensive, consumerist, and ecologically myopic patterns of economic activity – a market civilization that by definition is exclusive and can only be available to a minority of the population of the planet but that is nevertheless serving to consume the vast bulk of global resources.

In this chapter, we outline a number of key concepts and hypotheses to help make sense of some of the characteristics of the global organic crisis. We link them to a reading of some of the patterns of social development and social distribution associated with what we call a *global enclosure movement*. We then analyze such developments in terms of their implications for global health, now and in the future.

We conclude with some reflections on public finance, at both the local and global levels, because

a significant reorientation of taxation and expenditure policies might better address fundamental human needs and provide for a healthier, more just, and more sustainable global society. These issues are taken up further in Chapter 38.

Some Key Concepts and Hypotheses

To advance our analysis, we now introduce a number of foundational political economy concepts that correspond to some of the dominant historical structures (understood as the patterned or institutionalized forms of human agency) of globalized capitalism. We think that these concepts help explain some of the transformations and contradictions to which we have just referred. Three of these key structures can be conceptualized as *new constitutionalism*, *disciplinary neoliberalism*, and *exploitative social reproduction*. These concepts are intimately connected to the projects of neoliberal reform that have increasingly shaped global society and economy over the past 30 years. We reflect on some of the effects of these reforms on the structures of everyday life associated with communities and caring institutions.

Disciplinary Neoliberalism

Disciplinary neoliberalism is the dominant discourse of political economy that has shaped our times. It is often associated with the so-called Washington Consensus of Wall Street, the IMF, the World Bank, and the US Treasury on economic policy. It refers to the liberal ideas, institutions, political forces, and policies that are intended to deepen the power of capital and shape patterns of global economic and social development, partly by extending market values and economic and financial disciplines ever further into politics and society and into the ways that human beings relate to nature and the basic issues of livelihood. Its wider context is the advocacy of a free-enterprise economic system dominated globally by the giant firms that control most large industries (e.g., in food, pharmaceuticals, and software).

Disciplinary neoliberalism is politically shaped by (and is intended to be consistent with and support) the interests of big corporate capital (especially financial capital) and the state in not only the G8, especially the United States, but also in so-called large emerging nations such as China and India. Disciplinary neoliberalism, whether in the form of the Washington consensus or World Bank structural adjustment and

---

[1] Oxfam's recent report estimates that the world's wealthiest 26 people now own as much wealth as the poorest half of humanity, or 3.8 billion people (Oxfam, 2019). Credit Suisse's 2018 report similarly notes how the lower half of the world's population owns less than 1% of global wealth, whereas the richest 10% own 85%. If these trends continue, by 2030, the richest 1% is on course to hold 64% of the world's wealth (Michael Savage, Richest 1% on target to own two-thirds of all wealth by 2030, *The Guardian*, April 7, 2018).

IMF stabilization, or in terms of strictures of the European Union, tends to emphasize the need for free enterprise, privatization, and liberalization of trade and investment flows. It has become central to defining programs of political and economic reform – as well as shaping responses to the economic crises of ever-increasing severity since the late 1970s, originating in the orthodox economic measures that were mandated to deal with the third-world debt crises of the 1980s.

Indeed, one of the political characteristics of the present deep crisis is the way that most of the debate about the appropriate responses has been dominated by disciplinary neoliberal forces – by contrast, in the 1930s, there were a variety of significant political alternatives to capitalism in the form of Soviet communism and a variety of forms of Nazism and fascism. Today, political forces opposed to disciplinary neoliberalism, such as socialism and communism, seem to be relatively weak. Indeed, organized political opposition to the status quo is often fragmented and divided. At the same time, there has also been a convergence of political forces toward neoliberalism, in which social democratic, socialist, and some left-wing political forces have increasingly adopted the pro-market economic policies and platforms of neoliberalism. These transformations have drastically narrowed the political avenues to advance viable alternatives to neoliberalism in much of the world. The dominance of neoliberal concepts and associated market forces thus has shaped and channeled political debates concerning the limits, possibilities, and alternatives for change in the twenty-first century.

New Constitutionalism

New constitutionalism is a political-juridical counterpart to disciplinary neoliberalism, which, in the terminology of the World Bank, is intended to "lock in" liberalization of, for example, formerly closed or socialized economies and sectors so that they are exposed to market disciplines. The goal is to allow market forces to govern more and more areas of social, political, and economic life, assuming that these are profitable. This is achieved through a variety of legal and constitutional mechanisms. Some of these mechanisms are entirely new liberal constitutions (as in the former communist states as they are transformed into capitalist states) or else are supported by means of treaties that codify new rights and freedoms for investors and firms – for example,

the huge number of bilateral trade and investment agreements, multilateral agreements under the World Trade Organization (WTO), or regionally by the former North American Free Trade Agreement that has been recently renegotiated by the Trump administration in the United States (now renamed the United States–Mexico–Canada Agreement [USMCA]). Other key new constitutional mechanisms are internal laws mandating balanced budgets and statutes creating independent central banks to give a hybrid of public and private control to monetary policy, one of the most vital and fundamental economic policies that any government could practice. This means that in practice, central banks are "independent" of democratic pressures, a situation often justified by the argument that they need to concentrate on their mandates of fighting inflation without "political" interference. Much of the authority in central banks lies mainly in the hands of private financial interests who tend to have a majority on the governing boards. Such "independence" was crucial in the way that central banks were able to commit gigantic amounts of public funds to bail out the global financial system after 2008 (and again in 2020 in response to the COVID-19 pandemic and economic emergency) and the ways in which "quantitative easing" policies (as they are called in Europe) has supplied cheap money into the hands of financiers in ways that have led to artificially inflating the price of financial assets.

Thus, whereas much of contemporary capitalist development can be very short term in outlook, and concerned with speeding up the turnover time of transactions so as to increase profits (e.g., in the global financial markets or speed-up in the factories), a key characteristic of new constitutionalism is that it is longer term and intended to create a legal platform that minimizes uncertainty for investment calculations and, in the case of central banks, serve as a lender of last resort and as an ultimate guarantor of financial capitalism. New constitutionalism is manifested therefore in laws, rules, and regulations that are very difficult to change. These structures serve to legally reinforce and, to a degree, legitimate the rules of the political economy that tend to favor private power holders such as giant corporations and wealthy investors. A good example of new constitutionalism is the way that the jurisdiction over intellectual property (IP) rights at the global level has shifted to the WTO and how such IP rights are now principally considered as commodities that can be privately owned and therefore bought, sold, licensed, and protected over the long term by patents, copyrights, and trademarks.

In the sphere of health, this has very significant implications not only for access to affordable medicines and medical equipment but also for the already highly skewed processes of research and development in the provision of new medicines and treatments, a process that tends to focus on cures and palliatives for the maladies of the richer parts of the world at the expense of those afflicting poorer people, especially those in developing countries.

Exploitative Social Reproduction

Social reproduction can be defined as the social processes, human relations, and social institutions associated with the creation and maintenance of human beings, communities, and social institutions – on which all production and exchange and the global political economy must ultimately rest.[2] Social reproduction in the postwar "mixed" capitalist economies involved not only state provisions associated with health and welfare and the socialization of risk (e.g., pensions, unemployment insurance, social safety nets, and kinship networks) but also structures associated with the long-term reproduction of the socioeconomic system such as education. These processes, institutions, and ideas shaped the way that individuals, families, and communities viewed the social, political, material, and indeed moral order. More generally, no economic system (perhaps with the exception of slavery) can sustain itself without an appropriate set of social, cultural, and economic values and practices. As we argue, such elements vary across societies and change across time and jurisdictional and geographic space. Following transitions away from the more socialized models of capitalism that emerged after post-1945 reconstruction, in many parts of the world they are increasingly shaped by disciplinary neoliberalism and new constitutionalism so that provisions for social reproduction are increasingly subject to market forces. Under these historical structures, they tend to be more individualized and privatized and lead to the desocialization of risk so that it becomes more market based. Such

shifts are often premised on the ideology of the *self-help society*. Under this ideology and its associated governmental practices, people are deemed to be individually and wholly responsible for their own situations. People are expected to fend for themselves. They are forced to rely more on the capitalist market for their social reproduction, where provisions are provided for profit. We therefore refer to the structures of social reproduction associated with marketized, often subordinated patterns of development as *exploitative*. They involve greater levels of exploitation of labor, social processes, and nature by capitalist accumulation processes, for example, private healthcare, private schools, and public–private hybrids that administer welfare or workfare programs.

Such concepts can be used to help generate a number of secondary hypotheses that connect to our central hypothesis of an emerging contradiction between the extended power of capital (and its protection by the state) and the possibility for attaining more progressive and socially just forms of social reproduction in ways that result in increased human security for a majority of the world's population.

Thus, one of our secondary hypotheses – which relates directly to health provisioning – is that the trend toward disciplinary neoliberalism and market forces, and in some contexts, the reprivatization of the governance of social and caring institutions (e.g., the shift toward more privatized medical and health systems) has tended to contribute to the deterioration in health and healthcare provisioning for a majority of people. This hypothesis is further connected to an increase in the range, scope, and depth of socioeconomic exploitation in global capitalism amid wider conditions of *primitive accumulation* – as well as increased exploitation of nature or the biosphere in ways that may not be sustainable.

By primitive (or original) accumulation, we refer to a term that was advanced by Marx to explain a process by which large segments of the population are violently divorced from their traditional means of self-sufficiency and livelihood, for example, peasants who are forced off their land as it becomes privately owned and fenced in to create larger land holdings. As peasants are forced off the land, they become "free laborers" who have no choice but to sell their labor power to the private owners of the basic means of production in order to survive. Thus, food, which they may have previously produced for themselves, is now obtained in markets mediated by the ability to pay the "market price." As we argued in our earlier

---

[2] Social reproduction has three principal components: (1) biological reproduction of the human species, (2) reproduction of the labor force, and (3) reproduction of provisioning and caring needs.

work, primitive accumulation is an *ongoing* tendency of globalizing capitalism and not a one-off moment in its history. It includes not only the recent privatization of state assets but also the privatization of previously socialized institutions connected with social provisioning (Bakker & Gill, 2003: 19). Both of these trends have strengthened the relative power of capital while also undermining forms of social provisioning.

Perspectives on Capitalism and Crisis

In the first edition of this book, we illustrated how there are at least three distinct perspectives to interpret the 2008 financial and economic crisis, each of which has different implications for understanding the wider depth of the current global organic crisis of social reproduction (Gill & Bakker, 2011). These three perspectives can broadly be conceived of as those of (1) "pure" neoliberals, (2) "compensatory" neoliberals, and (3) radical and heterodox perspectives that offer alternatives to pure and compensatory neoliberals. Pure neoliberals can be understood as an amalgamation of politicians, corporate leaders, governmental technocrats, and Chicago School economists espousing the creed of capitalism as a self-regulating, efficiency-maximizing system optimized to meet the needs of consumers through market mechanisms of exchange. Compensatory neoliberals, including mainstream and some Keynesian economists and intellectuals, as well as politicians and businesspeople, conceptualize capitalism as an unstable yet manageable system that can be governed institutionally through macroeconomic stabilization and government regulation. Radical and heterodox thinkers associated with left-wing forces, by contrast, understand capitalism as a power-based system that is incapable of meeting the social needs of populations and is prone to continual contradictions and crises. The radical view of capitalism is that it does not involve the accumulation of goods for livelihood and social well-being but rather the accumulation of monetary values, which, in turn, allows for control over society and the labor of others. In short, capital relentlessly pursues profits and seeks to further its power over society and social reproduction partly by enclosing the social commons. Thus heterodoxy may involve alternative visions to govern the political economy (e.g., socialism).

We previously argued that the crisis of 2008 was deeply connected to transformations in global finance since the 1970s (Gill & Bakker, 2011). This included the proliferation of risky patterns of highly leveraged borrowing and financial securitization. This occurred alongside the decades-long stagnation of real incomes for many workers and the consequent need to finance social reproduction through increased consumer borrowing. Cheap borrowing policies were launched, most importantly, by the US Federal Reserve. Originating in the US subprime housing market, the global financial crisis morphed into a Eurozone sovereign debt crisis that extended throughout the global economy to other lower- and middle-income countries. The aftermath of the crisis was characterized by massive government bailout packages for private banks and firms alongside enormous quantitative easing borrowing policies by the world's central banks, which, as we have noted, indirectly channeled wealth to financiers and those who own the majority of financial assets – in an attempt to reinject money into the economy.

The *Financial Times* noted in 2017 that the United States has technically recovered more than the total cost of the bailouts since 2007. Other countries, such as Ireland and Greece, in which the impact of the bailouts reached almost 30% as a percentage of gross domestic product (GDP), have not recovered, continuing to bear the costs with higher public debt. What is also at issue, however, is the effectiveness of the bailout strategies and the distribution of resources absorbed since the crisis. Indeed, such bailout policies not only have failed to generate a significant economic recovery but also have indirectly contributed to an unprecedented redistribution of wealth to the world's billionaire class. As a recent report indicates, the decade since 2008 has seen the number of billionaires around the world double (Oxfam, 2019).

We also previously noted that financial crises produce far more significant declines in overall economic activity than those characterized by shortfalls in aggregate demand (theorized by the heterodoxy as crises of overproduction and underconsumption). The last decade of economic activity seems to illustrate this principle. It has been marked by continued economic stagnation and austerity (what the liberal perspectives define as slower growth of GNP) across much of the global economy. Moreover, this period has also seen steeply unequal distributions of national incomes and wealth, continued wage stagnation for the poor, both nationally and globally, and marginal recovery based primarily on a large and unsustainable accumulation of debt. Policy choices have prioritized bailouts and been coupled with decisions to socialize many of the losses of banks, financial houses, and corporations. Many countries in the European Union have therefore continued to feel the aftermath of the economic crisis in the form of sovereign indebtedness, continued austerity, high unemployment, and steep cuts to public expenditures and services. This has directly undermined the public means of social reproduction for a majority in these countries.

Greece in particular has experienced continued austerity enforced by the IMF and other international financial institutions. A recent downturn saw nearly a third of the population living in poverty as of 2018, while Italy recently slid into its fourth recession since 2008. Countries such as the United States, the United Kingdom, and Canada have experienced low-growth stagnation, characterized by a large accumulation of unsustainable consumer debt, increased market volatility, persistent austerity, an increase in part-time, precarious employment, and deepening social inequalities. Even larger economies such as China have also experienced unsustainable debt in areas such as its shadow-banking sector, in addition to its sharp and growing internal inequalities. These economic conditions, as well as continued global political volatility, have prompted the IMF to warn of another impending financial crisis.

Many countries across the Global South, although not hit as hard by the financial crisis as Eurozone countries, have experienced similar economic stagnation, particularly following the global commodity collapse of 2014. Across the Global South – from Haiti to Afghanistan, Jamaica, and elsewhere – countries have been compelled to implement austerity programs to finance government debt in a new round of structural adjustments similar to those of the 1990s and early 2000s. Budget cuts have had significant effects on public-sector spending, on social services, and on community population health. As Kentikelenis, Stubbs, & King (2016: 554) conclude after surveying the landscape of IMF policies from 1985 to 2014, "[t]he most recent data reveal a rising trend for the burden of conditionality since 2008," indicating that structural adjustments across the Global South have increased in the aftermath of the 2008 crisis, with severe implications for public-sector spending and health.

The decade since the global financial crisis has seen prioritization of debt repayment and consequent austerity, which has had significant negative effects on global health and health inequalities. Moreover, the trajectory of the post-2008 world for the affluent members of the world population has largely been connected to restoring, albeit with some effort to use resources more efficiently, much of the very energy-intensive kind of consumerist growth associated with market civilization. By contrast, the poor often go hungry.

Morbid Symptoms 1: Hunger, the Global Food Crisis, and New Constitutionalism in Mexico

Sufficient nutritious food is a fundamental component of health. Lack of nutritious food therefore has very serious consequences for global health outcomes. In the aftermath of the global financial crisis, more than 1 billion people were eating less, switching to cheaper and lower-quality food, or forgoing spending on healthcare and education simply in order to eat (Gill & Bakker, 2011). Poor nutrition is known to impair mental development, particularly for the young, and it weakens the immune system and the ability to ward off disease. Hunger involves inequalities of class, race, and gender: 70% of those living in absolute poverty globally are women, more than 60% of those suffering malnutrition are women, and most of them live in the developing world. Recent UN reports show that in *every* region in the world, women are more likely to be food insecure than men.

Although mainstream indices from the United Nations and the World Bank typically portray a world of declining poverty and hunger, as Jason Hickel (2016) has convincingly argued, these narratives have been constructed by a process of "shifting the goal posts" of development measures and goals. Indeed, Hickel (2016: 761) has illustrated how through the Millennium Development Goals and UN antipoverty programs, "the UN has misrepresented the true extent of poverty and hunger in the world" by shifting the metrics by which hunger and poverty are measured. If more realistic measures are used to measure poverty and the basic nutritional and dietary needs of global populations, in reality, as of 2016, he argues, between 1.5 billion and 2.5 billion people did not have access to adequate food, whereas between 3.5 billion and 4.3 billion were in poverty.

In the post-2008 period, in the absence of a clear break from the developmental patterns of disciplinary neoliberalism, austerity and persistent inequalities have continued to exacerbate the global food crisis. According to a UN report on global nutrition, out of the world's 7.6 billion people, roughly 2 billion or more suffer from micronutrient malnutrition, and another 800 million suffer from caloric deficiency. Out of the world's adults, perhaps 2 billion are overweight or obese. Indeed, our world is one where close to 50% of the population suffers from malnutrition – however, 25% of those who are malnourished are in fact overfed, overweight, and obese; the other 25% – those just referred to – are underfed or starving. As a 2017 report by the UN indicates, childhood obesity is increasing in most regions of the world, with more than 41 million children under the age of five seen as overweight. At the epicenter of market civilization, more than two-thirds of Americans are overweight, mainly eating unhealthy processed foods that contain many chemicals, hormones, and other additives, with their diets based on consumption of too much meat, sugar, and salt. This phenomenon is not simply associated with wealthy countries like the United States and the United Kingdom; Mexico is second only to the United States in obesity rates and, perhaps not surprisingly, in per capita consumption of soft drinks. This overconsumption of unhealthy foods has been linked to diseases and chronic conditions such as diabetes that exact their toll on hard-pressed public health systems (Albritton, 2009: 106–107).

Malnutrition is exacerbated in situations of economic crisis. One reason is that wealthy donor governments tend to cut social expenditures and foreign aid to the poor countries because these revenue lines do not necessarily have strong domestic political constituencies supporting them. All of these factors are intimately connected to questions of human security, global health, and basic humanity.

Much of the global food crisis has contributed to ongoing poverty and undernourishment across the Global South. Some of the world's most affluent countries have also not been immune to poverty, hunger, and suffering in the decade of austerity that has followed the 2008 crisis. Indeed, Professor Phillip Alston, Special Rapporteur to the United Nations in 2018, reported on the stark conditions of rising poverty and declining living standards in the United Kingdom in the aftermath of the Conservative government's austerity measures implemented since 2010. He illustrates that in the world's fifth largest economy of 67 million people, more than one-fifth of the population and almost one in two children live

in poverty. More than 1.5 million people are considered destitute, unable to afford the basic material essentials of livelihood. Noting the precipitous decline in living standards in the United Kingdom since 2010 and the effects of the universal credit system – which represents an amalgamation of six benefits programs and with it the decline of the social safety net in the United Kingdom – Alston (2018: 1) concludes that "Britain is not just a disgrace, but a social calamity and an economic disaster, all rolled into one." Austerity, particularly since 2008, has worsened social and economic inequalities, poverty, and misery even in the richest nations, particularly in Eurozone countries.

Countries across the Global South continue to be uniquely affected by the volatility of market prices of food. In the aftermath of the 2008 economic crisis, rich countries drastically reduced funds given to the UN World Food Program, so global food aid reached its lowest level in 20 years, with all the major donors reducing their contributions. This occurred despite the fact that food prices, already at record high levels in 2008, were in many parts of the world even higher in 2009, contributing to increased global hunger in the context of rising unemployment and poverty (Gill & Bakker, 2011).

While global food aid has been restored to its 2008 levels in recent years, this has occurred within a global context in which economic growth has contracted for many countries since the global financial crisis and government expenditures have declined, particularly in low-income countries. After 2007–2008, world food prices surged once again from 2011 to 2014, dropping moderately after the 2014 global commodity price collapse. Overall the UN Food and Agriculture Organization's global food price index rose from 80 in 2000 to 210 in 2008, before it dropped back to 140 in 2009. From 2011 to 2014, the food price index similarly surged to well over 200. The consequences of soaring food prices have been disastrous for the several billion people living on less than US$2 a day. The world market has become the arbiter of a situation of mass global starvation.

The 2009 food crisis originated with sharp increases in the price of major food grain prices, which the United Nations estimated as being responsible for pushing more than 100 million people back into poverty (Gill & Bakker, 2011). Contrary to the explanations of these crises offered by orthodox views, as we have previously illustrated, the deeper answer is more complex and involves recent trends toward centralization of ownership and control and greater enclosure of global food supplies by large corporations. Food prices also rose as a result of government and corporate strategies.

In effect, the structure of the current world market in food dates back to changes in US policies some 40 years ago, and it relates to the changing ways in which developing countries have become integrated into the capitalist world market for food. Of course, this was done forcibly into an imperial world market during the colonial era. After World War II, however, linked to the ideology and practice of self-determination, there was a trend in the developing world toward relative self-sufficiency in agriculture and food sovereignty.

Important changes occurred in the 1970s with a shift in US agricultural policies focused on giving subsidies to farmers for increasing yields to improve the US balance of trade. This had powerful consequences, including rapid concentration of control and the undermining of agricultural systems in developing countries, and was part of a general shift toward an oil- and pesticide-dependent food production system.[3] Food also became a geopolitical as well as an economic issue at that time, particularly because food prices rose rapidly as a result of massive Soviet grain purchases from the United States – a process overseen by the US Department of Agriculture and huge agribusinesses such as Cargill. Since then, the market has been dominated by a small number of corporations (oligopolies) – such as the large agricultural conglomerates Cargill and Archer Daniels Midland. Nevertheless, until the turn of the twenty-first century, this has largely meant an era of stable food prices.[4]

One reason for this was the growth in global production. Partly as a result of bad harvests and rising prices in the 1970s, agricultural producers in the developing world were encouraged to use new seed hybrids and other new technologies associated with the so-called green revolution and to gradually move toward a more export-oriented agriculture. These developments were further encouraged by global organizations such as the World Bank. The result was a shift toward cash crops and a general reorientation of agriculture toward the world market. This shift also included, as noted, more pesticide-intensive and other industrial methods to increase the turnover time of crop and livestock yields linked to sales for the world market.

Thus an era of cheaper food emerged with the result that at some point during the early 1990s, the prevailing discourse concerning "food security" came to be redefined as access to food by relying on an "efficient" global market. This seemed to make sense with respect to grains, because abundant American production of heavily subsidized products flooded the world market, and thus prices were kept low. However, because the global market was now dominated by American production, itself controlled by a small number of giant corporations, this had the side effect of wiping out many small producers not only in the United States but also in the developing world, concentrating capital in agriculture, further undermining local self-sufficiency, and promoting a general shift toward crop monocultures and larger farms. Production by independent and small farmers both in the United States and throughout the world became more integrated into the global corporate system, with crops often based on the use of so-called terminator seeds that are disease resistant and produce higher yields. However, these seeds need to be obtained on an annual basis from the seed companies (the corporations) because they cannot be used in future crops. The seeds therefore need to be repurchased annually; the seeds are the IP of the corporations that own them rather than the farmers who may actually grow the crops.

The Case of Mexico

Mexico in the 1990s illustrates how this process of centralization, control, and enclosure is also intimately connected to both new constitutionalism and subsequent fluctuations in the world market prices for food. Mexico entered into the new constitutional North American Free Trade Agreement (NAFTA) in 1994, which guaranteed the right of US producers to sell their grain in Mexico, and vice versa. However, because market prices in the United States were much lower than the cost of production not only in the

---

[3] The release of greenhouses gases from nitrogen-based fertilizer use is, according to Albritton (2009: 151), roughly 296 times more potent than carbon dioxide.

[4] The concentration of power in this market rests on a close and strategic relationship between the big agribusinesses and the US and EU governments. In most of the rest of the world, particularly in poor nations, however, firms are much smaller and tend to be less subsidized – emerging large food exporters such as Brazil are partial exceptions to this rule. Thus there is oligopolistic domination of global food production.

United States but also in Mexico owing to large US production subsidies, this had obvious consequences in terms of the competitiveness of Mexican production on the local market, production that, by contrast, was not subsidized. Indeed, once Mexico had signed NAFTA, it was legally obliged to continue with this arrangement despite the fact that since the Revolutionary Constitution of 1917 it had maintained its own constitutional protections for small farmers (*ejidos*) and their right to livelihood on the land. Mexico made at least 30 constitutional amendments in order to legally comply with the strictures of NAFTA. Some of these amendments abolished these rights to livelihood, with the result that more than 1 million Mexican farmers were displaced from agriculture following trade liberalization: they simply could not compete with cheap grains from the United States. Now Mexico, like many other countries, is increasingly dependent on world market prices for its food, and in addition, its prevailing diets have shifted toward the relatively unhealthy US model.

Thus one of the many consequences of the intersection between higher food prices and global poverty is the destruction of livelihoods and the creation of new enclosures – the *ejidos* of Mexico have lost their means of livelihood. This is precisely why the Zapatista rebellion was announced on January 1, 1994, to coincide with the official starting date of NAFTA. In much of Africa, even in locations where harvests have been good, because prices of food subsequently rose, many very poor people have been selling off their livestock, such as goats, which are used for milk, to livestock dealers in order to pay for food or seeds, to the point where they have nothing left to sell. Another example is in West Africa, where the governments of poorer countries have sold off their industrial fishing licenses to European industrial fishing fleets in order to be able to provide funds to the public revenues – for example, in Mauritania, 30% of its budget comes from such licenses. However, the result is not only long-term depletion in regional fishing stocks but also the exclusion of local fishermen from what were previously common fishing grounds – a classic example of primitive accumulation, or accumulation by dispossession. The best fish is exported to the markets of North America, Western Europe, and Japan; local people who used to eat very good fish are now simply excluded or priced out of the market.

Not surprisingly, in a world where one in seven people is severely malnourished or starving, as prices rose in 2007 and 2008, food riots broke out throughout the world – at least 37 nations were experiencing intense food crises. And understandably, people throughout the world questioned the wisdom of defining food security in terms of access to the world market. Indeed, throughout the world, grassroots movements associated with different conceptions of production, consumption, and distribution have been strengthening over the past decade. Important examples include the international organization of farmers Via Campesina, as well as the Landless Workers' Movement (Movimento dos Trabalhadores Rurais Sem Terra [MST]) in Brazil, which has taken advantage of clauses that remain in the Brazilian constitution that allow the landless access to the use of land that is not being productively deployed by its owners (large landowners control the vast majority of the land in Brazil, and much of it is not used for farming or for pasture).

These and other grassroots peoples' organizations continue to press for *food sovereignty*, a concept of self-sufficiency in food based on more organic production and on more diverse crop varieties and that involves production relations that are based on more egalitarian social organization and distribution. These approaches draw on hybrids of traditional and modern concepts of environmental stewardship and sustainability. Some of the pressure from the grassroots movements has been significant in the developing world. For example, in April 2009, 58 governments from the Global South agreed to engage in programs that would seek to redirect agriculture to support small-scale farmers, especially poor women, and to support local knowledge and to do so in ways that would counter global warming.

So it would appear that the trend toward relatively autonomous and self-sufficient agricultural production may be gaining some momentum, and this, one would hope, will not only alleviate hunger but also produce more environmentally and socially sustainable patterns of agriculture, creating a nutritional base for the populations.

At least some of leading figures in the G8 countries have become aware of the fact that the ethical (if not the political) debate is slipping away from them. Indeed, the food crisis has posed enormous issues of legitimacy for global capitalism. Some political leaders in both the G8 and G20 were concerned at being accused of being responsible for (or doing nothing to alleviate) a global humanitarian disaster. Moreover, wealthy private interests such as reflected in the Bill and Melinda Gates Foundation and the Clinton Global Initiative have decided to prioritize the world food crisis in their agendas for action. Nevertheless, it needs to be pointed out that the mechanisms they support for doing so still seek to preserve the world market as the principal means of "food security"; they assume that the market and business innovation can find ways to deliver food more efficiently and in so doing alleviate hunger.

New Enclosures of the Social Commons

Here we outline in more detail the concept of new enclosures that was raised in previous subsections in relation to land and food. The concept of the social commons also enables us to show that access to health systems is coming to be defined by the ability to pay in a much more commodified system in the era of disciplinary neoliberalism and global capitalism.

Marx and more recent critical scholars have noted that key capitalist accumulation processes were made possible through active strategies of the enclosure of the commons (Bakker & Gill, 2003). These strategies were designed, in turn, to increase people's dependence on capitalist markets for their social reproduction and livelihoods (DeAngelis, 2007: 133). Marx's concept of so-called primitive or original accumulation has been subject to debate within the critical literature. For some, it refers to the original historical processes or moments that gave rise to the development of capitalism as a mode of production following feudalism. For others, it is a condition for a fundamental aspect of capitalism: the separation of workers from the ownership of the conditions of the realization of their labor, a process that still continues today (Marx, 1976: 874; DeAngelis, 2007: 136). In this sense, primitive accumulation is both a historical and ongoing process of divorcing producers from the means of production and livelihood, particularly the communal access to common lands and facilities.

Enclosure of "the commons" is a concept that originates from medieval England, where the commons describes parcels of land that were used "in common" by peasant farmers. Their lives depended on access to and use of shared land to pasture livestock and obtain water from streams, ponds, and wells and wood and fuel from forests. Landowners had ownership of these lands, but the importance of the commons to the survival of populations was legally recognized. Strict rules required landowners to ensure access to the commons by peasants. However, landowners began to bar the use of these lands coupled with the idea of physically removing commoners and their traditional settlements, enabling the landowners to use the land solely for themselves, building fences that subsequently prevented further access by commoners. These "enclosures" were eventually sanctioned by the British Parliament, which passed the Enclosure Acts stripping commoners of their customary property rights so that by 1795, about 0.5% of the population of England and Wales owned almost 99% of the land (Bocking, 2003: 26). Deprived of their access to livelihoods, peasants were forced to move to the cities. Some became laborers in the factories of the industrial revolution; others were forced into vagrancy, prostitution, and destitution.

Rather than this being a moment in the development of capitalism, we suggest that enclosures are a continuous characteristic of capital logic that makes the world through commodification and enclosure, thereby fragmenting and destroying "commons" that represent social spheres of life that provide various protections from the forces of the capitalist market. The term *social commons* relates to the community-based and collectivist alternatives to the capitalist enclosures or appropriation of social spending, taxation, and other entitlements associated with privatization or sale of such public provisions and revenues by the state (Bakker & Gill, 2003; DeAngelis, 2007: 135, 148).

Thus, as DeAngelis (2007: 144) notes, all strategies and types of enclosure share the common characteristic of forcibly separating people from whatever access to social wealth they have, thus leaving them only with access to livelihoods mediated by capitalist markets and money as capital. We would agree that the enclosing force we have described is not simply an outcome of neoliberalism but represents an immanent drive of capital that is common to different historical periods. This drive may be part of a conscious strategy such as the English enclosures or, more recently, privatization of public services and healthcare systems and the liberalization of trade and investment regimes (Gill & Bakker, 2006).

One of the most notable developments in the new enclosure movements is the way in which legal and juridical guarantees of private property rights and IP rights in particular have enabled increasing corporate ownership over many aspects of social and cultural life, as well as over life forms, in ways that have significantly shaped the trajectory of ecological systems and healthcare. Under conditions of increasing corporate concentration, for example, in pharmaceuticals and agribusiness, IP rights for corporations have expanded into ownership over foods, plants, and seeds; medicines; bodily organs; and blood supplies – monopoly rights that are guaranteed legally and often constitutionally by international and bilateral trade agreements (Gill & Benatar, 2019). Consequently, many elements of public health and the means by which communities reproduce themselves – aspects of the social commons – have been turned into commodities by large corporations and removed from the social and ecological needs of those communities.

Thus the neoliberal realignment of social institutions over the past 40 years, including those of the care sector (e.g., health and education), involves a shift away from public and authoritative regulation that was previously coupled with some socialized provisioning for the broader population in the "health for all" initiatives that encompassed much of the capitalist, socialist, communist, and developing worlds after World War II.

There has been a retreat from the idea of extended health provisioning as a public good in both rich and poor countries. In healthcare, there has been a shift toward a pay-as-you-go system involving user fees and other forms of self-provisioning. These changes have sometimes produced public–private hybrids but more generally have narrowed the framework of access and entitlements according to level of income and ability to pay. These changes have disproportionately impacted poorer countries in the Global South, which continue to rely on external funding for their healthcare systems – under very difficult and challenging conditions where their countries carry the preponderance of the global disease burden.

Such developments tend to reinforce our argument set out earlier that the new enclosures of the social commons represent wider shifts to private provisioning (privatization) and the growing imposition of hyper-commercial norms on the state. The effect of all this is to remove more and more of the population from access to collective social wealth, in this case to healthcare services. And at the same time, a combination of IP rights and the pricing strategies of many pharmaceutical firms means that it is not possible for the poor to gain access to vital medicines at reasonable prices, that is, prices that should be judged in terms of the prices very poor people could actually afford.

Morbid Symptoms 2: Global Health Financing

In this context, there continue to be numerous problems within the structure of global health financing relating to lower economic growth, fiscal restraints imposed by IMF conditionality, and continued reliance on external sources for health financing. Since the global financial crisis, although average global health spending has steadily increased, particularly in high-income countries, health inequalities have grown throughout much of the world. The increased expenditures in wealthier countries reflect both increasing demand for healthcare services and the need for fiscal stimulus, partly to offset the effects of austerity. Nonetheless, even in wealthier countries, aggregate spending measures tend to mask persistent health inequalities. This unequal pattern is also replicated both within and between the majority of countries, and these trends have continued since 2008. More globally, even though only 20% of the world's population lives in high-income countries, these countries account for more than 80% of global spending on health, a trend that has remained unchanged since 2000 (Xu et al., 2018).

We have previously illustrated how the immediate effects of the 2008 global financial crisis led to a sharp reduction in global economic output, posing additional difficulties for developing-world governments because of a loss of tax and other revenues owing to the decline in aggregate demand and the collapse of trade finance (Gill & Bakker, 2011). Whereas some countries of the Global South have experienced larger growth than high-income countries since the financial crisis, generally speaking, global economic growth has been tepid since 2008. Austerity packages in many countries have been accompanied by a generalized contraction of economic output. In the Global South, the effects of this are manifested in a loss of export revenues *and* lost revenue from remittances, which can often account for more than twice the total of official development assistance.

IMF loan packages for countries in financial distress have continued to come with conditions that limit governments' ability to spend on health. Recent research indicates that in the postcrisis period, increases in "high-conditionality programs" from the IMF have been implemented in countries such as Afghanistan, Bangladesh, Bosnia, Ghana, Greece, Haiti, Jamaica, and elsewhere (Kentikelenis et al.,

2016: 553). As the authors indicate, there has been an "emphatic return of conditionality in recent years," indicating that not much has changed within the IMF's policy apparatus. As we have argued, such structural reforms and conditionalities have a long and documented record of delaying long-term infrastructural spending and limiting spending on social services and protections, both of which can significantly affect health service provisioning, service delivery, and the general health and well-being of populations.

Recent trends also indicate that domestic health expenditures in lower-income countries have in fact been falling, with government spending on health as a share of total government spending declining from 7.9% in 2000 to 6.8% in 2016 (Xu et al., 2018: 22). While middle-income countries have increased domestic spending on health, transitioning away from reliance on external funding for healthcare, government spending on health as a proportion of total expenditures has declined since 2000 in low-income countries, whereas reliance on external funding has increased since 2008 (Xu et al., 2018). Moreover, and as noted earlier, while varying considerably between countries, many low-income countries continue to rely on external and private sources for the majority of their funding for primary care, preventative care, and immunization, a trend that has continued since 2008 (Xu et al., 2018). The knock-on effects of crisis are known to be particularly harsh for women and young children, who are the first to be affected by a deteriorating financial situation and food availability.

Public Finance and the Fiscal Squeeze of the Social Commons

We argued earlier that enclosures of common social property are an ongoing process. However, such enclosures are also continuously being contested. Many of the public institutions related to social provisioning, such as health and education, for example, are the products and a legacy of such resistances. These public institutions, structures, and social relations represent the fruits of a historic and ongoing organized struggle concerning the limits and uses of democratic control over economic life. Such struggles are now taking place in the current context of the pressures to liberalize cross-border investments and transactions in money, goods, services, people, and

information. They are also taking place under conditions of a "fiscal squeeze" (Grunberg, 1998) for state finances that has arisen and created increasing pressure to sell off state assets to investors in order to service bailouts and public debt in ways that allow for further enclosures of the social commons through selling off assets and services via privatization. We call the selling of state assets to achieve a fiscal balance the *fiscal squeeze of the social commons*.

These pressures highlight the importance of focusing on ways of reversing privatizing trends so that we can consider how to strengthen progressive state financing of the social commons so as to counter new enclosures that curtail entitlements and limit or reduce social spending. However, it is also important to identify some of the obstacles to realizing change. These obstacles, we argue, are more long term and diverse than the financial crisis and represent the ongoing legacy of the strategies of disciplinary neoliberalism and new constitutionalism we have outlined in our earlier discussion of global organic crisis (some of these strategies are discussed in more length in our later contribution, Chapter 38).

The most fundamental forces driving the fiscal squeeze relate to both the pressures on governments that stand from a legacy of accumulated debts owed to creditors ("fiscal crisis") and the need to refinance government activities with new loans in order to be able to pay for current government expenditures. What seems to be a common pattern in this process, however, is that conditionality is associated with these loans – especially from the IMF but also indirectly or directly from private creditors – so that operations are disciplined by neoliberal principles. The terms of such loans are often codified in international agreements and constitutional arrangements of the type that we have discussed under the rubric of new constitutionalism. These agreements protect the property rights of investors and underpin the expansion of the concept of IP rights that are increasingly treated as if they are commodities in the world of trade and investment. Under new constitutionalism and disciplinary neoliberalism, these are deemed to be inviolable and not subject to interference by governments (except for situations of extreme emergency) so that, for example, pharmaceutical patents cannot be revoked. This often prevents governments from manufacturing cheaper generics to make them available at much lower prices to their populations.

Thus IP rights are not considered part of the common knowledge pool of humankind but have come to be redefined as a salable commodity that can be legally owned by private individuals or corporations in ways that are also codified in treaties and trade agreements such as those covered by the WTO. This concept and practice contrast with technical and scientific knowledge being treated as part of the global commons, derived as it necessarily is from the broad intellectual and scientific heritage of humankind. Although there is clearly a case to be made for the protection of innovations and works of art, music, and literature by copyrights and patents, the already expansive range of IP rights as commodities is widening rapidly. In this process, forms of social and scientific knowledge – indeed, innovations produced in public institutions – are becoming privately owned by corporations and protected by such private IP rights. In short, a widening range of knowledge forms and intellectual products become not part of the public domain of culture and civilization but legally deemed to be commodities that can be privately owned, bought, and sold in the capitalist marketplace. These trends suggest that an accelerated form of enclosure of the "knowledge commons" is taking place.

This process affects knowledge systems more generally as the thrust of privatization increasingly enters into the world's education systems and as more and more universities and schools turn to private sources for funding. Of course, private funding for research often comes with a price. In this way the conception of education as a public good to be made universally accessible to all comes under pressure. Inequalities develop between institutions on the basis of their ability to raise private funds and not simply their capacity to attract the best brains in the world (as well as the offspring of the wealthy and powerful). Harvard University has a private endowment that is bigger than the GDP of many countries, much of it invested on the stock and bond markets.

There are a number of more specific mechanisms that are connected to the problem of protecting and financing the global commons, not least of which is the prevailing trend toward increasing liberalization of trade and finance, which allows for many corporations and wealthy investors to avoid taxes and thus their contribution to financing the commons, and thus undermine the tax base of governments.

This is why the French call tax havens *les paradis fiscaux*, because they allow for tax evasion on a truly monumental scale. Transnational corporations also have a long history of evading taxes through complex accounting measures such as transfer pricing that locate the losses and profits of their activities in the most favorable jurisdictions where taxes are lowest. At the same time, there has been intense tax competition between different jurisdictions as capital has become more mobile. To attract such capital companies must provide a favorable investment climate, which inevitably means lower corporate tax rates as well as enormous subsidies and tax holidays for new investments. As a means of broadening the tax base under these circumstances, many governments throughout the world have shifted to indirect taxes, such as value-added taxes, which are "regressive" insofar as they exact the same amount of tax per transaction on each consumer irrespective of that person's income level, whether that person is a low-income worker or a billionaire. These taxes are particularly regressive because poorer people spend a greater proportion of their income on everyday necessities such as food, fuel, and housing. A hamburger plus tax amounts to the same price to a billionaire as it does to a pauper.

Grunberg (1998: 595–596) links many global trends and tax-related developments back to the United States. She notes that the 1986 US Tax Reform Act influenced all Organisation for Economic Co-operation and Development (OECD) countries in a number of significant ways: (1) the tax base was broadened in ways that simultaneously removed many tax privileges and exemptions but also included low-income families in the tax base, (2) the very top direct tax rates were reduced dramatically, and (3) fewer tax brackets were created, with the result that the income tax structure overall became much less progressive. Recently, the United States enacted the highly regressive Tax Cuts and Jobs Act of 2017 that gave a massive tax cut and windfall to the wealthy and to corporations. This will likely put pressure on other nations to respond in kind or risk losing business and competitiveness.

Despite needed public finance requirements to pay for restructuring, retraining workers, social safety nets, and healthcare, the fiscal situation of many developing-world countries is desperate. As we noted long ago, in addition to tax losses owing to falling remittances, transfer pricing, capital flight to tax havens, and declining tax revenues resulting from trade liberalization, many developing-world countries (as well as many wealthy ones) lose billions of dollars of potential income each year because of: (1) ineffective domestic tax systems that do not reach landowners, foreign corporations, and wealthy individuals and (2) regressive tax cuts and tax exemptions for foreign investors (e.g., there are currently more than 3,000 export-processing zones, which have similar effects to offshore financial centers insofar as they allow for lower taxes or indeed tax evasion; Gill & Law, 1988: 191–223). Finally, one of the characteristics of our era has been the rampant growth of the so-called covert or informal economy, which is a nationally and globally widespread means of avoiding and evading taxes. Estimates of tax evasion vary but are on the rise. According to the *OECD Observer*, "No-one knows exactly how much public money is lost illicitly to tax havens after all; if it could be measured, it would already be taxed." We discuss taxes and related issues in Chapter 38 in relation to the need for new paradigms – or a new "common sense" – to address some of the challenges for global health.

References

Albritton, R. (2009). *Let Them Eat Junk: How Capitalism Creates Hunger and Obesity*. London: Pluto Press.

Alderman, L. (2019). "The middle class shrinks in Europe," *New York Times*.

Alston, P (2018). Statement on Visit to the United Kingdom, by Professor Philip Alston, UN Special Rapporteur on extreme poverty and human rights. United Nations Office of the High Commission for Human Rights, February 16. Available at www.ohchr.org/EN/NewsEvents/Pages/DisplayNews.aspx?NewsID=23881&LangID=E (accessed March 25, 2019).

Bakker, I., & Gill, S. (2003). *Power, Production, and Social Reproduction: Human In/Security in the Global Political Economy*. Basingstoke, UK: Palgrave Macmillan.

Benatar, S. R., Gill, S., & Bakker, I. (2009). Making progress in global health: the need for new paradigms. *International Affairs* **85**(2), 347–372.

Bocking, R. (2003). Corporatism, privatization drive enclosure of the commons. *Canadian Centre for Policy Alternatives Monitor* October, 26–28.

Davies, J. B. (2006). *The World Distribution of Household Wealth*. Helsinki: United Nations University – WIDER.

De Angelis, M. (2007). *The Beginning of History: Value Struggles and Global Capital*. London: Pluto Press.

Faiola, A. (2008). Where every meal is a sacrifice. *Washington Post*, April 28.

Gill, S. (1995). Globalisation, market civilisation, and disciplinary neoliberalism. *Millennium* **23**(3), 399–423.

Gill, S. (1997). Finance, production and panopticism: inequality, risk and resistance in an era of disciplinary neo-liberalism, in Gill, S. (ed.), *Globalization, Democratization and Multilateralism*. New York: Macmillan, pp. 51–76.

Gill, S. (2008). *Power and Resistance in the New World Order*. Basingstoke, UK: Palgrave Macmillan.

Gill, S., & Bakker, I. (2006). New constitutionalism and the social reproduction of caring institutions. *Journal of Theoretical Medicine* **6**(4), 1–23.

Gill, S., & Bakker, I. (2011). The global crisis and global health, in Benatar, S. R., & Brock, G. (eds.), *Global Health and Global Health Ethics*. Cambridge, UK: Cambridge University Press, pp. 221–238.

Gill, S., & Benatar, S. R. (2019). Reflections on the political economy of planetary health. *Review of International Political Economy* **26**(6).

Gill, S., & Law, D. (1988). *The Global Political Economy: Perspectives, Problems and Policies*. Baltimore: Johns Hopkins University Press.

Gramsci, A. (1971). *Selections from the Prison Notebooks of Antonio Gramsci*. New York: International Publishers.

Grunberg, I. (1998). Double jeopardy: globalization, liberalization and the fiscal squeeze. *World Development* **26** (4), 591–605.

Hickel, J. (2016). The true extent of global poverty and hunger: questioning the good news narrative of the Millennium Development Goals, *Third World Quarterly* **37** (5), 749–767.

Inman, P. (2018). World economy at risk of another financial crash, says IMF. *The Guardian*, October 3.

Kentikelenis, A., Stubbs, T., & King, L. (2016). IMF conditionality and development policy space, 1985–2014. *Review of International Political Economy* **23**(4), 543–582.

Marx, K. (1976). *Capital: A Critique of Political Economy*, Vol. **1**. New York: Penguin Books.

Oxfam (2019). *Public Good or Private Wealth?* Oxford, UK: Oxfam UK.

Ruckert, A., & Labonte, R. (2017). Health inequities in the age of austerity: the need for social protection policies. *Social Science and Medicine* **187**, 306–311.

Sen, G. (2009). SRHR and global finance: crisis or opportunity? *DAWN Informs* **October**, 5–6.

Smith, A., & Foley, S. (2017). Bailout costs will be a burden for years. *Financial Times*, August 8.

Stuckler, D., King, L., & McKee, M. (2009). Mass privatisation and the post-communist mortality crisis: a cross-national analysis. *Lancet* **374**(9686), 315–323.

World Health Organization (WHO) (2009). *The Financial Crisis and Global Health: Report of a High-level Consultation*. Geneva: WHO, pp. 1–34.

Xu, K., Soucat, A., Kutzin, J., et al. (2018). *Public Spending on Health: A Closer Look at Global Trends*. Geneva: WHO.

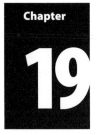

Chapter

19

Challenging the Global Extractive Order
A Global Health Justice Imperative

Ted Schrecker, Anne-Emanuelle Birn, and Mariajosé Aguilera

Introduction: The Global Economy, Global Extractive Order, and Health

Contemporary economic activity depends on massive throughputs of extracted material and energy, which typically cross multiple national borders in commodity, supply, or value chains – the terminology varies with the discipline – dominated by transnational corporations (TNCs). For instance, Apple's iconic iPhone is assembled in China from components manufactured in a variety of countries, mainly in Asia, but approximately half the world's supply of a critical ingredient – the cobalt used in lithium-ion batteries – is mined, often on an artisanal basis,[1] in the Democratic Republic of the Congo (DRC) under horrific conditions that have nothing in common with the life worlds of Apple's shareholders and executives or of most iPhone users (Amnesty International, 2016; Clarke & Boersma, 2017). Amnesty International (2016) and Sovacool (2019) have documented child labor and extremely hazardous working conditions, along with severe environmental damage linked to cobalt and columbite–tantalites (i.e., coltan) mining in the DRC. In another example, much of the world's palm oil – used in everyday household products and ultraprocessed foods – is produced from plantations in Indonesia and Malaysia (Kadandale, Marten, & Smith, 2019). These have expanded rapidly at the cost of devastating environmental impact, including forest clearing, burning, and destruction, with associated loss of livelihood and extensive air pollution (Varkkey, Tyson, & Choiruzzad, 2018; Rulli et al., 2019), and have exploited "thousands of child laborers and workers who face dangerous and abusive conditions" (Skinner, 2013).

Nothing is new about large-scale extraction of resources from territories and populations that occupy a subaltern position in the world system; think of the trade of enslaved persons that was central to the economy of parts of the United States until the middle of the nineteenth century and the daily horrors and millions of deaths that accompanied extraction of value from rubber plantations in what was then the Belgian Congo (Hochschild, 1998). These illustrations also foreground the point that although extractive industries are conventionally defined with reference to mining and oil and gas extraction, it is useful to consider situations in which other resource-based economic activities – such as large-scale agribusiness and associated land and water grabs – are similarly organized around what sociologist Saskia Sassen (2010: 25) calls "logics of extraction." Central to our analysis of extractive industries and global (health) justice is the concept of a *global extractive order* that is fundamentally intertwined with issues of health injustice. Most aspects of extraction have substantial (mainly negative) health implications that are asymmetrically experienced by those whose lands and labor are extracted compared with those who own, profit from, and enjoy the end use of extracted materials.

In the next section of this chapter, we summarize the case for considering the extractive order's impact on health as a matter of global justice. Following this, we take a skeptical view of the argument that extraction can be managed to benefit health through expansion of resources available for social provision and poverty reduction. We then examine land and water grabs – a relatively new form of cross-border resource appropriation with potentially far-reaching effects on health. The final section sets out, in a necessarily abstract way, some prerequisites and challenges for transforming the extractive order to meet the requirements of global justice.

---

[1] Estimates of the proportion of cobalt exported from the DRC that is of artisanal origin range from 20%–60% (Zeuner, 2018: 2).

Extraction and Health: Pathways to Impact

Iconoclastic US epidemiologist Nancy Krieger has argued that "analysis of causes of disease distribution requires attention to the political and economic structures, processes and power relationships that *produce* societal patterns of health, disease, and wellbeing via shaping the conditions in which people live and work" (Krieger, 2011: 168, emphasis in original; see also Birn, Pillay, & Holtz, 2017: 92–95, 285–333). Production of health and illness is not a metaphor but a literal description of how conditions of life and work enable healthy lives or, conversely, sicken, disable, and kill. The political economy of health perspective is thus organized around identifying micro–macro connections between health outcomes and the economic and political context within which inequalities in the conditions of life and work are situated.

The evidence base is fragmented: domestic research capacity is often limited, it can be difficult to conduct research in jurisdictions where extractive industries dominate the economy (Baumüller et al., 2011: 17), and official data may be incomplete or compromised (see, e.g., Reed, 2009: 13). A review of research on the health impact of the mining, oil, and gas industries (Brisbois et al., 2019) emphasized these limitations and found that available research tends to focus on proximal workplace or environmental exposures rather than longer-term systemic effects, such as losses of livelihood, increases in food and water insecurity, and the material and psychosocial effects of social powerlessness. Even more than in other situations involving complex causal pathways from macro-scale processes to health outcomes, assessing health impacts of the global extractive order must rely on multistage mappings of causal pathways using the best available evidence from comparable settings (Schrecker, Birn, & Aguilera, 2018).

It is possible to identify at least five generic pathways from macro-scale information about the operation of extractive activity to health outcomes: (1) environmental degradation, (2) workplace exposures, (3) dispossession, loss of livelihood, and exposure to violence, (4) loss of food and water security, and (5) effects, both positive and negative, on poverty (a key social determinant of ill health) and social provision (Schrecker, Birn, & Aguilera, 2018). The environmental damage associated with mining, especially in the poorly regulated context of

many low- and middle-income countries (LMICs), is axiomatic but also occurs in higher-income countries, as shown by the case of mountaintop mining in the Appalachian United States (Bernhardt et al., 2012; Purdy, 2016). Mining generates air pollution and contaminates and depletes soil and water in nearby communities, notably through acid drainage and metal leaching. Mining also denudes mountaintops and slopes of vegetation, provokes erosion and sinkholes, and leads to deforestation and biodiversity loss (Eisler & Wiemeyer, 2004; Bambas Nolen et al., 2014; Hendryx, 2015; London & Kisting, 2016; Birn et al., 2017: 432–433). Such mine tailings must be managed long after operations have ceased. Moreover, fatal tailings dam collapses are disturbingly frequent (Birn et al., 2017: 432–33; Roche, Thygesen, & Baker, 2017), generating worldwide attention after a Brazilian collapse in 2019 that killed hundreds of people (Phillips & Brasileiro, 2019). Beyond direct health damage, environmental degradation jeopardizes farming, fisheries, and Indigenous livelihoods and lands. In the Andes region, for example, contamination and depletion of water have negatively affected agricultural and livestock raising (Brain, 2017); in North America, Indigenous populations similarly deal with the deadly effects of past uranium mining (Cartwright, 2016: 423; Sarkar, 2019).

Oil and gas extraction presents equally serious hazards, including not only spills but also air pollution from flaring (burning off natural gas at the wellhead), which is increasing in some countries (Environmental Rights Action/Friends of the Earth Nigeria, 2005; Birn et al., 2017: 434; Global Gas Flaring Reduction Partnership, 2019). In 2006, an expert group estimated that in the preceding 50 years, the volume of oil spilled in the Niger Delta was equivalent to one *Exxon Valdez* spill *every year* (Federal Ministry of Environment et al., 2006). In 2011, the UN Environment Programme (UNEP) documented hazardous exposures to hydrocarbons in air pollution as well as widespread contamination of surface water and groundwater and made numerous recommendations for urgent action (UNEP, 2011). Five years later, of 27 recommendations, "only three [had] been partially implemented" as a result of government nonchalance and resistance from the Shell Petroleum Development Company – the major private-sector operator in the region (Yakubu, 2017: 2).

Many of extraction's environmental hazards are experienced at higher levels of exposure by those who work in the relevant industries, compounded by workplace accidents. Mining remains "one of the most dangerous occupations in the world, and it is one that often highlights the effects of class and lives lived in situations of structural and physical violence" (Cartwright, 2016: 419; see also Elgstrand et al., 2017). Artisanal mining, typically even less regulated than industrial mining, is extremely dangerous and a desperate last resort for the economically marginalized, who may be permitted to work only on sites that are not viable for large-scale commercial production. In the case of large-scale agribusiness, which operates on an extractive model, a particular hazard is worker exposure to pesticides; many pesticides are banned or severely restricted in high-income countries (HICs) and exported to jurisdictions (especially LMICs) where they are permitted (see, e.g., Hertz-Picciotto et al., 2018). In its first 100 days in office, Brazil's business-friendly Bolsonaro government approved 152 new pesticides for use despite a reported 100,000 poisoning cases annually (Branford & Borges, 2019).

Extractive activity often requires, or is facilitated by, the coerced movement of people off the land. Because most extraction takes place in rural areas where many Indigenous populations live, the latter are disproportionately affected by the dispossession that is central to extractive industry activity (see, e.g., Gordon & Webber, 2008: 67–69; Munarriz, 2008; Holden, Nadeau, & Jacobson, 2011). In the Andes, (forced) displacement of farmers by mining companies onto smaller plots or into towns has shrunk communal grazing lands and threatened land-based livelihoods (Helwege, 2015; Brain, 2017). Importantly, the World Bank – the world's most influential development finance institution – is implicated in many such cases. A 2015 journalistic investigation found that World Bank–financed projects between 2004 and 2013 displaced more than 3 million people through forced resettlement, acquisition of their land, or destruction of their livelihoods, including more than 1.3 million displaced by energy, mining, and agroforestry projects (International Consortium of Investigative Journalists, 2015). Environmental damage can function as a driver of dispossession. A Brazilian team identified 570 environmental conflicts in the country in 2018, most involving agribusiness and mining. The cases predominantly affected family farmers, Indigenous people, Afro-Brazilians (heavily discriminated against in multiple settings), and small-scale fishers. The researchers found that "[i]n 43% of the cases, the disruption of the traditional forms of subsistence led to food insecurity," and "at least 50% of the evaluated cases involved some form of violence … directly or indirectly linked with state, corporate, or other economic agents" (da Rocha et al., 2018: 714–715).

Violence is, in fact, a close companion to extraction. Dispossession of land and livelihoods linked to extractive development has long been enabled by government, paramilitary, and private security firm suppression of activist opposition (Middeldorp, Morales, & van der Haar, 2016; Imai, Gardner, & Weinberger, 2017), with diplomatic officials of investor countries tacitly or even actively supporting this violence (Gordon & Webber, 2016). Mines in Tanzania and Papua New Guinea controlled by Canadian-based Barrick Gold, for example, have been the focus of repeated complaints about violence by both private security forces and policing agencies, which have been brought before a United Nations (UN) human rights working group (Coumans, 2019b; Watts, 2019b). The civil society organization Global Witness found that in 2017, more than 200 people opposing environmentally destructive projects were killed, with agribusiness and mining and extractives the most dangerous sectors for opponents (Global Witness, 2019). In one context alone – opposition to illegal but lucrative sand mining in India, which has resulted in widespread water degradation – an activist has observed that "[m]urders, threats and acts of intimidation … probably number in the hundreds" (quoted in Tweedie, 2018). Journalists reporting on such opposition face similar dangers (Schapiro, 2019; Watts, 2019a).

Yet a further dimension of the nexus linking violence and the global extractive order involves situations in which control over resources either triggers or finances warfare – a situation exemplified by the two Congo wars between 1996 and 2003, in which millions of people died. In an unusually forthright report, a UN panel (Panel of Experts, 2003) detailed that the commercial activities of over 100 transnational mining companies contributed to and benefited from the DRC wars, but host country governments initially declined to investigate the role of these corporations in the conflict (Kneen, 2009). Evidence on the effectiveness of subsequent responses, specifically the US Dodd-Frank legislation of 2010, is equivocal. A later UN report concluded that "the implementation of mineral traceability … has considerably reduced instances of armed groups directly benefiting from the exploitation and trade of tin, tantalum and tungsten" (Group of Experts, 2017: 2), but another analysis found not only that Dodd-Frank requirements enabled the DRC government to help industrial mining companies displace artisanal miners but also that battles, looting, riots, and violence against civilians in gold-mining areas increased after the requirements were put in place (Stoop, Verpoorten, & van der Windt, 2018). There is thus a web of interconnections in need of further detailed investigation between outcomes (including violence) on the ground and the ownership structures that connect extractive industries in LMICs to investors in HICs, the policies of their governments, and alliances with local economic and political elites (see, e.g., Fitzgibbon, Hamilton, & Schilis-Gallego, 2015; Imai, Gardner, & Weinberger, 2017).

Development, the Resource Curse, and the Supposed Absence of Alternatives

It is superficially plausible to argue that economic growth associated with the expansion of extractive industries can raise incomes, create jobs, and/or increase government revenues, thereby reducing poverty and enabling increased investment in health systems. In the context of advocacy for the UN Sustainable Development Goals' (SDGs) universal health coverage (UHC) target, a Chatham House study of financing options identified increasing natural resource revenues through more favorable tax and royalty regimes or state ownership as one of the revenue sources that LMICs should consider; it also underscored the need to address various corporate tax avoidance strategies (Meheus & McIntyre, 2017; see also Ridde, Campbell, & Martel, 2015) that deprive national treasuries of needed revenues.

Interesting parallels exist between the argument about the benefits of resource extraction and the claim that trade and investment liberalization "is good for your health, mostly" because of the benefits in terms of poverty reduction (Feachem, 2001: 504). As in that case (Banerjee et al., 2006: 53; Kawachi & Wamala, 2007: 129–132), the evidence is weak and, under many circumstances, the contribution of extractive industries to equitable development is nonexistent or limited. The development studies literature is rich in discussions of the so-called resource curse in which

resource-rich economies are observed to underperform relative to others on growth and, especially, social indicators (for nontechnical overviews, see Karl, 1999; Gary & Karl, 2003: 21–24). A recent authoritative review of the resource curse literature concludes: "[T]here is strong evidence that one type of resource wealth – petroleum – has at least three important effects: It tends to make authoritarian regimes more durable; it leads to heightened corruption; and it helps trigger violent conflict in low- and middle-income countries, particularly when it is located in the territory of marginalized ethnic groups" (Ross, 2015: 240).

Prime illustrations are Nigeria and Angola – Africa's dominant oil exporters. Nigerian official figures show a consistent increase in poverty over more than three decades (United Nations Development Programme, 2015), whereas oil wealth remains extremely concentrated (Wallis, 2014). On some rankings, Luanda, the capital of Angola, ranks as the world's most expensive city (Ngugi, 2017), and although Angola is a middle-income country based on World Bank criteria, 30% of the population lived below the World Bank's unrealistically low extreme poverty threshold in 2008, *before* the oil price decline that led to an economic implosion, a collapse of public services, and an associated outbreak of yellow fever (PriceWaterhouse Coopers, 2016; World Health Organization, 2016). Sovacool (2019: 2) points out that "[d]espite having vast natural resources, more than half (63%) of Congolese citizens live below the national poverty line of less than $1 per day." Where does the money go?

A review of studies of the effects of mining and oil and gas extraction on poverty identified six potential pathways to reduced poverty and seven to increased poverty (Gamu, Le Billon, & Spiegel, 2015), revealing that industrial mining is more frequently associated with worsening poverty than reducing it. For the Sub-Saharan context, "Extractive industries are especially ill-suited to generate technology and skill diffusion, and have limited potential for poverty reduction" (Sundaram & von Arnim, 2012: 499). Similar observations have been made by the Economic Commission for Latin America and the Caribbean (2016: 87–133) about the limited contribution of the mining industry in Latin America to direct employment or industrial development through either backward or forward linkages. The Economic Commission for Latin America and the Caribbean does note the increased contribution to government revenues during the commodity price boom of this century's first decade but emphasizes the cyclical and uncertain nature of that contribution, as demonstrated (as in many other cases) when the boom collapsed. Resource revenues arguably created fiscal space for such measures as Brazil's expanded public healthcare provision (Castro et al., 2019) and the Bolsa Família cash-transfer program, but these are now under attack for reasons both global (the decline in commodity prices) and domestic (the ascent of a far-right government) (Alston et al., 2018; Lima, 2018).

Meanwhile, the activities of transnational mining firms in the region have been associated with a variety of direct and indirect negative health consequences (Birn, Shipton, & Schrecker, 2018). Tellingly, the 2019 tailings dam collapse that killed hundreds of Brazilians occurred at a mine owned by a Brazilian transnational, Vale, that has expanded into the high-income world through such ventures as acquisition of much of Canada's nickel-mining capacity.[2] It was also just one in a long series of such fatal disasters in Brazil, drawing attention to the generic weakness of regulatory capacity in states heavily dependent on resource industries, regardless of their ownership.

Still, for some researchers, an equitably managed extractive sector that is adequately regulated with regard to health and environmental effects is not a priori implausible. Ridde et al. (2015: 915) argue that "[a] well-managed mining sector in the mineral-rich countries of Africa and more specifically in the Sahelian countries is possible" despite past failures; even nominally progressive Latin American governments have embraced "neoextractivism" given the limited alternative development options available in the current global economic order (Cáceres, 2015; North & Grinspun, 2016). However, a long history of corporate intransigence shows that the affected industries actively resist efforts to increase governments' share of revenues and to reduce negative environmental, health, and social effects. Instead, these extractive TNCs divert attention to alleged weaknesses in host-country "governance" when the real issues are rather domestic and cross-border power imbalances, exemplified by the active promotion of highly destructive corporate activity by home-country governments, such as Canada's (Birn et al., 2018; Coumans, 2019a).

Inevitably, the opportunity for financial gains associated with control over natural resources creates multiple opportunities for corruption and therefore incentivizes resistance to improved management (Le Billon, 2011). Returning to the question of where the money goes, massive amounts of revenue are lost through corporate bribes and kickbacks, simple theft by political leaders (as in the case of some African petrostates), capital flight to tax havens, transfer mispricing to minimize corporate tax liabilities, and other tax avoidance strategies that the "international community" and HICs have made only limited efforts to control (Brock, 2009: 125–130; Zucman, 2014; Ridde et al., 2015: 913–914; High Level Panel, 2015). In the context of global justice, the focus on governance in the Global South undoubtedly diverts attention from incentives for predation created by a global financial system that welcomes ill-gotten gains with open arms.

A Case Example: The Neglected Health Consequences of Land Grabs

Prices of many food commodities on international markets rose rapidly in 2007–2008, in parallel with the price of oil – a key input for agricultural production and transportation. The effect was to undo much recent progress in reducing undernutrition and food insecurity (Dawe & Drechsler, 2010; Prain, 2010; Ruel et al., 2010; Mason et al., 2011; Ortiz, Chai, & Cummins, 2011). Importantly, food commodity prices did not consistently follow oil prices downward thereafter, suggesting that other characteristics of the world food system, such as its increasing financialization (Clapp & Isakson, 2018), were also involved. Supply concerns on the part of food-importing countries combined with identification of agricultural land as an investment in the context of the financial crisis and growing demand for biofuels accelerated large-scale transnational acquisitions of arable land (*Economist*, 2009; Dell'Angelo, D'Odorico, & Rulli, 2017; Dell'Angelo, Rulli, & D'Odorico, 2018).

On the most reliable estimate, between 2000 and 2019, approximately 47.2 million hectares of land – roughly three times the agricultural land area of the United Kingdom – had been acquired by foreign investors and the governments of food-importing countries[3] (Land Matrix, 2019). In one of the more

---

[2] In another example, an Indian corporation has received approval to open a major coal mine in Australia, the first of several such proposed projects (*Economist*, 2019).

[3] This figure covers acquisitions for multiple purposes, although agriculture was the dominant intended use. Notably, forestry and mining are also intended uses in many transactions.

extreme examples, approximately 30% of cultivated land in Mozambique, with one of the world's highest rates of malnourishment, has been the target of land grabs; this process has been found to aggravate the feminization of poverty (Porsani, Caretta, & Lehtilä, 2019), and most of that land remains out of production (Rulli et al., 2018), both phenomena exacerbating ill health. This lends support to the characterization of land grabs as "wide-ranging global 'land reform' – in this case, a regressive land reform where governments take land from the poor and give (or sell or lease) it to the rich" (White et al., 2012: 620). Africa is the most targeted continent for land grabs despite what has been described as a "looming crisis" of arable land availability on the continent (Gettleman, 2017) and the fact that Sub-Saharan Africa is the world's poorest region in terms of income per capita.

It is conceivable, although disputed, that some such acquisitions improve food supply and security by improving the productivity of agriculture for domestic markets. However, there is little evidence that this is happening; more evidence supports the argument that such acquisitions are part of a larger agenda, backed by such actors as the World Economic Forum, of increasing corporate control of the global agrifood system (see, e.g., McKeon, 2014), which, in turn, threatens not only food security but also food sovereignty. On one estimate, *circa* 2014, land grabs had cut off local access to land that could otherwise produce food for 190 million to 235 million people, even without substantial investment in raising productivity (Rulli & D'Odorico, 2014).

As in the case of industrial mining, the input-intensive agricultural practices associated with "grabbed" land tend to create few employment opportunities that generate local income (Borras & Franco, 2013; Aguilar-Støen, 2016). Conversely, among the more immediate local consequences is loss of livelihood as existing users of the land become dispossessed (Nolte, Chamberlain, & Giger, 2016). For instance, Ethiopia's government nationalized large tracts of land only to resell them to private interests, simultaneously forcing local farmers and pastoralists onto unproductive land (Human Rights Watch, 2012; Moreda & Spoor, 2015). A study of 56 cases of coerced dispossession from agricultural land by the world's leading research team on the topic, *circa* 2019, found that "[a]cquisitions are generally characterized by imbalanced power relations" and "most of the cases of conflict (including violent and non-violent conflict) emerged when the land was acquired through

government lease" (Dell'Angelo, et al., 2017: 8). The health effects of losing agricultural and other related livelihoods – an impact that is disproportionately concentrated among the most economically vulnerable (Davis, D'Odorico, & Rulli, 2014) – may be compounded by reduced food sovereignty as domestic resources are appropriated for export production. To this loss of livelihood must be added the health effects of social dislocation because loss of "control over destiny" generates negative health outcomes across multiple scales, including at the macro level through "traumatic social transitions" (Whitehead et al., 2016: 58).

A further important consideration with regard to land grabs is that when crops are exported, so is, necessarily, the water required to grow them – comprising a "virtual water trade" that has grown dramatically since the mid-1980s (D'Odorico et al., 2018: 37). Chen et al. (2018: 938, 941) have mapped the extent to which both land and water are "exported" in global trade, finding that 37% of agricultural land and 29% of agricultural water "are embodied in interregional trade" and identifying "significant net transfers of these two resources … from resource-rich and less-developed economies to resource-poor and more developed economies." Among the top net "exporters" of agricultural land (in the sense that the products of the land are exported) are Mongolia, Argentina, Madagascar, and Ethiopia; among the top net exporters of fresh water are Pakistan, India, Egypt, Myanmar, and Chile, currently and potentially generating large-scale water insecurity and its associated negative health consequences. Not all these exports are attributable to land grabs, of course, but land grabs are likely substantial contributors in many of the countries in question. Such a pattern of exports of land products and water raises the prospect of an escalating global bidding war for resources that are prerequisites for health in which the poor lose out, often with the active participation of their political leaders, much as city dwellers of limited means have lost out worldwide in the course of metropolitan gentrification (United Nations Human Settlements Programme, 2003; Lees, Shin, & López-Morales, 2015).

Land grabs instantiate an element of complexity in global health politics that is likely to become more important with the southward and eastward shift of the world's center of economic gravity (Dobbs et al., 2012). Mapping land grabs shows many countries outside the north as "grabbers" (Rulli, Saviori, & D'Odorico, 2013; O'Brien et al., 2017) and some countries, notably Brazil, being both targets and acquirers (Rulli et al., 2013; Wolford & Nehring, 2015). Chinese and Saudi actors have acquired substantial land and water rights in the United States (O'Brien et al., 2017; Markham, 2019). As with other elements of the global extractive order, such observations are only the starting point for what should be a serious inquiry into the distribution of health hazards and benefits *within* both acquiring and target countries – informed by detailed knowledge of the contexts involved, as well as the trajectory of future health implications.

Possibilities for a Health-Equitable Global Extractive Order

The multiple "power asymmetries" identified by the Lancet–University of Oslo Commission on Global Governance for Health (Ottersen et al., 2014) are very much in evidence in the global extractive order. The most immediately obvious asymmetry is that between large, usually transnational corporations and those who bear the health consequences of their activities. However, it must be emphasized that the asymmetries in question do not all involve North–South relations. Many corporate actors and economic elites based in what is now conventionally referred to as the Global South are actively involved in and profiting from the exploitative dynamics of the global extractive order. Many governments undertake systematic predation against their own populations. Returning to our example of Congolese cobalt mining, it should not be assumed that conditions in industrial mines run by domestic corporations or state-owned Gécamines are less dangerous than transnational corporation–owned mines, given the limited evidence base.

A minimal condition for a just extractive order is accountability. At present, international law allows a national government to control and dispose of resources within its borders on whatever terms and conditions it chooses and without regard for the domestic human consequences – the "resource privilege" (Brock, 2009: 25–26, 122–125; Schuppert, 2014). The resource privilege in fact connects the asymmetries just identified: "Because foreigners benefit so greatly from the international resource privilege, they have an incentive to refrain from challenging the situation or, worse, to support or finance

oppressive governments" (Brock, 2009: 25). Wenar (2013: 299) has used a dramatic hypothetical to contrast this situation with what holds within the borders of at least those countries characterized by a legally robust system of property rights: "Imagine New York declared that whoever can seize any property in New Jersey will thereby gain the legal right to sell that property to New Yorkers … so long as the New Jersey vendor had physical control over the goods at the time of sale." This, he argues, approximates the situation codified by the resource privilege. Thus, for him, "[t]he most salient reform of international commerce must be to remove the 'might makes right' rule that vests the right to sell resources in whoever can control a population by force" or via a variety of autocratic and unaccountable institutions (Wenar, 2008: 15).

Such reform would, to say the least, constitute a remarkable departure from the current international order and confront formidable political obstacles. But it would not be enough. A quick canvass of the current global extractive order suggests several experiences where, within functioning institutions of formal democracy, a political plurality: accepts demagogues' choices about distribution of resource revenues and risks or supports extractive activities that disproportionately impose health (and economic) dangers on subaltern or marginalized populations (Indigenous peoples; racialized, linguistic, or religious groups; disfavored regions); fails to satisfy minimal criteria of gender justice; or accepts selective impoverishment for a perceived greater good. It is therefore necessary to apply additional frameworks above and beyond political accountability to make the global extractive order even minimally just.

Schuppert (2014: 72) rather optimistically states that "[b]oth in practice and in normative theory sovereignty is understood to be limited by the demands of people's universal human rights," but if taken seriously, human rights – in particular the economic and social rights codified in the International Covenant on Economic, Social and Cultural Rights – would constitute such a framework. He advances an intriguing proposal for an International Court of the Environment, which would not directly challenge the resource privilege but rather create a framework that limits how states can exercise it based on such normative principles as "no harm, precaution, equitable use, sustainable development, and intergenerational equity," perhaps also including the "polluter pays" principle. Most of these norms are already embedded to some degree in international "soft law."

The problem with such mechanisms, as we know from the experience of, *inter alia*, the International Criminal Court and global climate governance, is that those states whose actions most clearly demand such restraints are least likely to agree to be bound by them. Nevertheless, human rights norms are the most widely recognized limitation (at least at the level of rhetoric) on what governments may permissibly do to those over whom they rule. In this context, it is worth noting that the United Nations' independent human rights experts, now known as "Special Procedures" (United Nations, 2019), have generated incisive critiques of the health impacts of globalization (Schrecker et al., 2010: supplementary online material) and domestic austerity programs (Alston et al., 2018); they have also scrutinized the food security implications of land grabs (De Schutter, 2009). The mandate holders have no power beyond "naming and shaming," but it is nevertheless worth advocating the establishment of a thematic mandate that would ask hard questions about the global extractive order using the conceptual lens we have provided here and examining both specific national case studies – because nation-states are the principal duty bearers under international human rights law, although not the only ones – and the operation of international institutions and norms of international law.

Yet a further set of issues, suggested by the imagery of bidding wars and the empirics of land grabs, is between the users of extracted resources and those who bear the health consequences of their extraction while often receiving minimal or no economic benefit or redress for harms. The UNEP has estimated, based on a formula that converts various forms of resource consumption to a common metric and adjusts domestic resource use to account for resources imported and exported in either raw or processed form, that the countries that rank highest on the UN Development Programme's Human Development Index (HDI) consume roughly twice the mass of resources per person as the next group of countries ("high HDI" rather than "very high HDI"). The pattern exists despite the fact that the very high HDI economies are actually less materials intensive, per unit of gross domestic product (GDP), and the minimum material throughput required for a very high HDI has been declining over the past few decades (Schandl et al., 2016: chapter 4).

Despite recent slight decreases in the material intensity of some very high HDI economies, the information economy that some envision as a route to dematerialization is in fact highly materials and energy intensive because of such factors as the electrical and water demands associated with cloud servers and semiconductor fabrication facilities (Ensmenger, 2018). And the assumption that technological innovation will radically mitigate climate change and extraction harms remains misguided, as per the current vogue for electric cars, which have important environmental and health implications, *inter alia*, because of the material requirements for lithium batteries that are, as of this writing, the preferred energy storage medium and due to the deleterious environmental effects of lithium mining (Katwala, 2018; Lombrana, 2019).

If we take seriously (as we should) the aspirations of all of humanity for global health equity and justice, what are the resource implications? Even if we disregard considerations of sustainability that do not involve health, is there any prospect even of approximating this egalitarian objective while avoiding negative health impacts from extraction and the extractive order? Space does not permit considering this question here, beyond suggesting that global health justice and equitable well-being may require far more radical approaches to (de-)growth and dematerialization than are currently anticipated.

Acknowledgments

Much of the research for this chapter was carried out as part of the work of the University of Oslo Independent Panel on Global Governance for Health, with partial financial support from the University of Oslo, and presented to the Panel as a paper by Mariajosé Aguilera, Anne-Emanuelle Birn and Ted Schrecker in October 2017. However, the views expressed are exclusively those of the named authors. The valuable research assistance of Leah Shipton is gratefully acknowledged.

References

Aguilar-Støen, M. (2016). Beyond transnational corporations, food and biofuels: the role of extractivism and agribusiness in land grabbing in Central America. *Forum for Development Studies* 43, 155–175.

Alston, P., Bohoslavsky, J. P., Boly Barry, K., et al. (2018). Information received concerning the negative impacts of budget cuts, structural adjustment and austerity measures implemented since 2014, on several human rights, notably the rights to health, education, social security, food, as well as on gender equality, and in particular the negative impacts linked to the Constitutional Amendment No 95, also known as "Expenditure Ceiling", in force for over 16 months. Office of the High Commissioner for Human Rights, Geneva. Available at https://spcommreports.ohchr.org/TMResultsBase/DownLoadPublicCommunicationFile?gId=23789.

Amnesty International (2016). *"This Is What We Die For": Human Rights Abuses in the Democratic Republic of Congo Power the Global Trade in Cobalt.* London: Amnesty International. Available at www.amnesty.org/en/documents/afr62/3183/2016/en/.

Bambas Nolen, L., Birn, A.-E., Cairncross, E., et al. (2014). *Case Study on Extractive Industries Prepared for the Lancet Commission on Global Governance.* Oslo: University of Oslo. Available at www.med.uio.no/helsam/english/research/global-governance-health/background-papers/extrac-indus.pdf.

Banerjee, A., Deaton, A., Lustig, N., et al. (2006). *An Evaluation of World Bank Research, 1998–2005.* Washington, DC: World Bank. Available at http://siteresources.worldbank.org/DEC/Resources/84797-1109362238001/726454-1164121166494/RESEARCH-EVALUATION-2006-Main-Report.pdf.

Baumüller, H., Donnelly, E., Vines, A., & Weimer, M. (2011). *The Effects of Oil Companies' Activities on the Environment, Health and Development in Sub-Saharan Africa* (EXPO/B/DEVE/FWC/2009–01/Lot5/11). Brussels: Policy Department, Directorate-General for External Policies of the Union, European Parliament. Available at www.europarl.europa.eu/RegData/etudes/etudes/join/2011/433768/EXPO-DEVE_ET(2011)433768_EN.pdf.

Bernhardt, E. S., Lutz, B. D., King, R. S., et al. (2012). How many mountains can we mine? Assessing the regional degradation of central Appalachian rivers by surface coal mining. *Environmental Science & Technology* **46**, 8115–8122.

Birn, A.-E., Pillay, Y., & Holtz, T. (2017). *Textbook of Global Health*, 4th ed. New York: Oxford University Press.

Birn, A.-E., Shipton, L., & Schrecker, T. (2018). Canadian mining and ill health in Latin America: a call to action. *Canadian Journal of Public Health* **109**, 786–790.

Borras, S. M., & Franco, J. C. (2013). Global land grabbing and political reactions "from below.". *Third World Quarterly* **34**, 1723–1747.

Brain, K. A. (2017). The impacts of mining on livelihoods in the Andes: a critical overview. *Extractive Industries and Society* **4**, 410–418.

Branford, S., & Borges, T. (2019). Bolsonaro administration authorizes 150+ pesticides in first 100 days. Mongabay (online). Available at https://news.mongabay.com/2019/05/bolsonaro-administration-authorizes-150-pesticides-in-first-100-days/.

Brisbois, B. W., Reschny, J., Fyfe, T. M., et al. (2019). Mapping research on resource extraction and health: a scoping review. *Extractive Industries and Society* **6**, 250–259.

Brock, G. (2009). *Global Justice: A Cosmopolitan Account.* Oxford, UK: Oxford University Press.

Cáceres, D. M. (2015). Accumulation by dispossession and socio-environmental conflicts caused by the expansion of agribusiness in Argentina. *Journal of Agrarian Change* **15**, 116–147.

Cartwright, E. (2016). Mining and its health consequences: from Matewan to fracking, in Singer, M. (ed.), *A Companion to the Anthropology of Environmental Health*. Chichester, UK: John Wiley & Sons, pp. 417–434.

Castro, M. C., Massuda, A., Almeida, G., et al. (2019). Brazil's unified health system: the first 30 years and prospects for the future. *Lancet* **394**, 345–356.

Chen, B., Han, M. Y., Peng, K., et al. (2018). Global land-water nexus: agricultural land and freshwater use embodied in worldwide supply chains. *Science of the Total Environment* **613–614**, 931–943.

Clapp, J., & Isakson, S. R. (2018). *Speculative Harvests: Financialization, Food, and Agriculture.* Halifax: Practical Action Publishing and Fernwood Publishing.

Clarke, T., & Boersma, M. (2017). The governance of global value chains: unresolved human rights, environmental and ethical dilemmas in the Apple supply chain. *Journal of Business Ethics* **143**, 111–131.

Coumans, C. (2019a). Minding the "governance gaps": re-thinking conceptualizations of host state "weak governance" and re-focussing on home state governance to prevent and remedy harm by multinational mining companies and their subsidiaries. *Extractive Industries and Society* **6**, 675–687.

Coumans, C. (2019b). Submission to the United Nations Working Group on the Use of Mercenaries: in regard to the relationship between private military and security companies and extractive industry companies from a human rights perspective in law and practice. MiningWatch Canada, Ottawa. Available at https://miningwatch.us4.list-manage.com/track/click?u=c89185f430617e4dc1a02762e&id=bbbec74b10&e=9e15bb0108.

D'Odorico, P., Davis, K. F., Rosa, L., et al. (2018). The global food-energy-water nexus. *Reviews of Geophysics* **56**, 456–531.

da Rocha, D. F., Porto, M. F., Pacheco, T., & Leroy, J. P. (2018). The map of conflicts related to environmental injustice and health in Brazil. *Sustainability Science* **13**, 709–719.

Davis, K. F., D'Odorico, P., & Rulli, M. C. (2014). Land grabbing: a preliminary quantification of economic impacts on rural livelihoods. *Population and Environment* **36**, 180–192.

Dawe, D., & Drechsler, D. (2010). Hunger on the rise: number of hungry people tops one billion. *Finance and Development* **March**, 40–41.

De Schutter, O. (2009). Report of the Special Rapporteur on the right to food – Addendum: Large-scale land acquisitions and leases: a set of minimum principles and measures to address the human rights challenge (No. A/HRC/13/33/Add.2). United Nations, New York. Available at http://dacess-dds-ny.un.org/doc/UNDOC/GEN/G09/177/97/PDF/G0917797.pdf?OpenElement.

Dell'Angelo, J., D'Odorico, P., & Rulli, M. C. (2017). Threats to sustainable development posed by land and water grabbing. *Current Opinion in Environmental Sustainability* **26–27**, 120–128.

Dell'Angelo, J., Rulli, M. C., & D'Odorico, P. (2018). The global water grabbing syndrome. *Ecological Economics* **143**, 276–285.

Dell'Angelo, J., D'Odorico, P., Rulli, M. C., & Marchand, P. (2017). The tragedy of the grabbed commons: coercion and dispossession in the global land rush. *World Development* **92**, 1–12.

Dobbs, R., Remes, J., Manyika, J., et al. (2012). *Urban World: Cities and the Rise of the Consuming Class*. Washington, DC: McKinsey Global Institute. Available at www.mckinsey.com/~/media/McKinsey/dotcom/Insights%20and%20pubs/MGI/Research/Urbanization/Urban%20world%20-%20Rise%20of%20the%20consuming%20class/MGI-Urban-world_Full%20Report_June%202012.ashx.

Economic Commission for Latin America and the Caribbean (2016). *Foreign Direct Investment in Latin America and the Caribbean 2016*. Santiago: ECLAC. Available at https://repositorio.cepal.org/bitstream/handle/11362/40214/S1600662_en.pdf?sequence=6&isAllowed=y.

Economist (2009). Buying farmland abroad: outsourcing's third wave. *Economist*, May 21.

Economist (2019). Black in business. *Economist*, June 29, pp. 54–55.

Eisler, R., & Wiemeyer, S. N. (2004). Cyanide hazards to plants and animals from gold mining and related water issues. *Reviews of Environmental Contamination and Toxicology* **183**, 21–54.

Elgstrand, K., Sherson, D. L., Jørs, E., et al. (2017). Safety and health in mining, part 1. *Occupational Health Southern Africa* **23**, 10–20.

Ensmenger, N. (2018). The environmental history of computing. *Technology and Culture* **59**, S7–S33.

Environmental Rights Action/Friends of the Earth Nigeria (2005). *Gas Flaring in Nigeria: A Human Rights, Environmental and Economic Monstrosity*. Amsterdam: Climate Justice Programme, Friends of the Earth International. Available at www.foe.co.uk/sites/default/files/downloads/gas_flaring_nigeria.pdf.

Feachem, R. G. A. (2001). Globalisation is good for your health, mostly. *British Medical Journal* **323**, 504–506.

Federal Ministry of Environment, Nigeria Conservation Foundation, WWF UK, & CEESP-IUCN Commission on Environmental, Economic and Social Policy (2006). *Niger Delta Natural Resource Damage Assessment and Restoration Project*. Gland, Switzerland: International Union for the Conservation of Nature. Available at https://cmsdata.iucn.org/downloads/niger_delta_natural_resource_damage_assessment_and_restoration_project_recommendation.doc.

Fitzgibbon, W., Hamilton, M. M., & Schilis-Gallego, C. Ã. (2015). Australian mining companies digging a deadly footprint in Africa. International Consortium of Investigative Journalists (online). Available at www.icij.org/project/fatal-extraction/australian-mining-companies-digging-deadly-footprint-africa.

Gamu, J., Le Billon, P., & Spiegel, S. (2015). Extractive industries and poverty: a review of recent findings and linkage mechanisms. *Extractive Industries and Society* **2**, 162–176.

Gary, I., & Karl, T. L. (2003). *Bottom of the Barrel: Africa's Oil Boom and the Poor*. Baltimore: Catholic Relief Services. Available at www.justiceinitiative.org/db/resource2/fs/?file_id=15674.

Gettleman, J. (2017). Vanishing land fuels "looming crisis" across Africa. *New York Times*, July 29. Available at www.nytimes.com/2017/07/29/world/africa/africa-climate-change-kenya-land-disputes.html?hp&action=click&pgtype=Homepage&clickSource=story-heading&module=second-column-region&region=top-news&WT.nav=top-news.

Global Gas Flaring Reduction Partnership (2019). The new ranking: top 30 flaring countries (2014–2018). World Bank (online). Available at http://pubdocs.worldbank.org/en/645771560185594790/pdf/New-ranking-Top-30-flaring-countries-2014-2018.pdf.

Global Witness (2019). *At What Cost? Irresponsible Business and the Murder of Land and Environmental Defenders in 2017* (updated January 2019). London: Global Witness. Available at www.globalwitness.org/documents/19595/Defenders_report_layout_AW4_update_disclaimer.pdf.

Gordon, T., & Webber, J. R. (2008). Imperialism and resistance: Canadian mining companies in Latin America. *Third World Quarterly* **29**, 63–87.

Gordon, T., & Webber, J. R. (2016). *Blood of Extraction: Canadian Imperialism in Latin America*. Winnipeg: Fernwood.

Group of Experts on the Democratic Republic of the Congo (2017). Letter dated 8 August 2017 from the Group of Experts on the Democratic Republic of the Congo extended pursuant to Security Council Resolution 2293 (2016) addressed to the President of the Security Council (S/2017/672/Rev.1). United Nations Security Council, New York. Available at www.securitycouncilreport.org/atf/cf/%7B65B

FCF9B-6D27-4E9C-8CD3-CF6E4FF96FF9%7D/s_2017-67 2_rev_1.pdf.

Helwege, A. (2015). Challenges with resolving mining conflicts in Latin America. *Extractive Industries and Society* **2**, 73–84.

Hendryx, M. (2015). The public health impacts of surface coal mining. *Extractive Industries and Society* **2**, 820–826.

Hertz-Picciotto, I., Sass, J. B., Engel, S., et al. (2018). Organophosphate exposures during pregnancy and child neurodevelopment: recommendations for essential policy reforms. *PLoS Medicine* **15**, e1002671.

High Level Panel on Illicit Financial Flows from Africa (2015). Track it, stop it, get it! Illicit financial flows, in *AU/ECA Conference of Ministers of Finance, Planning and Economic Development*. Addis Ababa. Available at www .uneca.org/sites/default/files/PublicationFiles/iff_main_re port_26feb_en.pdf.

Hochschild, A. (1998). *King Leopold's Ghost*. Boston: Houghton Mifflin.

Holden, W., Nadeau, K., & Jacobson, R. D. (2011). Exemplifying accumulation by dispossession: mining and indigenous peoples in the Philippines. *Geografiska Annaler: Series B, Human Geography* **93**, 141–161.

Human Rights Watch (2012). *"Waiting Here for Death": Forced Displacement and "Villagization" in Ethiopia's Gambella Region*. New York: Human Rights Watch. Available at www.hrw.org/sites/default/files/reports/ethio pia0112webwcover_0.pdf.

Imai, S., Gardner, L., & Weinberger, S. (2017). *The "Canada Brand": Violence and Canadian Mining Companies in Latin America* (Legal Studies Research Paper Series No. 17). Toronto: Osgoode Hall Law School, York University. Available at https://dx.doi.org/10.2139/ssrn.2886584.

International Consortium of Investigative Journalists (2015). Evicted and abandoned: the World Bank's broken promise to the poor. International Consortium of Investigative Journalists (online). Available at www.icij.org /project/world-bank.

Kadandale, S., Marten, R., & Smith, R. (2019). The palm oil industry and noncommunicable diseases. *Bulletin of the World Health Organization* **97**, 128.

Karl, T. L. (1999). The perils of the petro-state: reflections on the paradox of plenty. *Journal of International Affairs* **53**, 31–48.

Katwala, A. (2018). The spiralling environmental cost of our lithium battery addiction. *Wired* (online). Available at www .wired.co.uk/article/lithium-batteries-environment-impact.

Kawachi, I., & Wamala, S. (2007). Poverty and inequality in a globalizing world, in Kawachi, I., & Wamala, S. (eds.), *Globalisation and Health*. Oxford, UK: Oxford University Press, pp. 122–137.

Kneen, J. (2009). Mining in the Democratic Republic of Congo. MiningWatch Canada (online). Available at https://

miningwatch.ca/blog/2009/5/6/mining-democratic-republic-congo.

Krieger, N. (2011). *Epidemiology and the People's Health: Theory and Context*. Oxford, UK: Oxford University Press.

Land Matrix (2019). Online public database on land deals. Available at http://landmatrix.org/en/ (accessed July 4, 2019).

Le Billon, P. (2011). *Extractive Sectors and Illicit Financial Flows: What Role for Revenue Governance Initiatives?* (U4 Issue No. 13). Bergen: Chr. Michelsen Institute. Available at http://hdl.handle.net/11250/2474929.

Lees, L., Shin, H. B., & López-Morales, E. (eds.) (2015). *Global Gentrifications: Uneven Development and Displacement*. Bristol, UK: Policy Press.

Lima, R. (2018). Austerity and the future of the Brazilian Unified Health System (SUS): health in perspective. *Health Promotion International* **34**, i20–i27.

Lombrana, L. M. (2019). Saving the planet with electric cars means strangling this desert. Bloomberg Hyperdrive (online). Available at www.bloomberg.com/news/features/ 2019-06-11/saving-the-planet-with-electric-cars-means-strangling-this-desert.

London, L., & Kisting, S. (2016). The extractive industries: can we find new solutions to seemingly intractable problems? *New Solutions: A Journal of Environmental and Occupational Health Policy* **25**, 421–430.

Markham, L. (2019). Who keeps buying California's scarce water? Saudi Arabia. *Guardian*, March 25. Available at www .theguardian.com/us-news/2019/mar/25/california-water-drought-scarce-saudi-arabia.

Mason, N. M., Jayne, T. S., Chapoto, A., & Donovan, C. (2011). Putting the 2007–2008 global food crisis in longer-term perspective: trends in staple food affordability in urban Zambia and Kenya. *Food Policy* **36**, 350–367.

McKeon, N. (2014). The new alliance for food security and nutrition: a coup for corporate capital. TNI Agrarian Justice Programme policy paper. Transnational Institute, Amsterdam. Available at www.tni.org/files/download/the_ new_alliance.pdf.

Meheus, F., & McIntyre, D. (2017). Fiscal space for domestic funding of health and other social services. *Health Economics, Policy and Law* **12**, 159–177.

Middeldorp, N., Morales, C., & van der Haar, G. (2016). Social mobilisation and violence at the mining frontier: the case of Honduras. *Extractive Industries and Society* **3**, 930–938.

Moreda, T., & Spoor, M. (2015). The politics of large-scale land acquisitions in Ethiopia: state and corporate elites and subaltern villagers. *Canadian Journal of Development Studies* **36**, 224–240.

Munarriz, G. (2008). Rhetoric and reality: the World Bank development policies, mining corporations, and Indigenous communities in Latin America. *International Community Law Review* 10, 431–443.

Ngugi, F. (2017). What makes Luanda most expensive city in the world? Face2Face Africa (online). Available at https://face2faceafrica.com/article/luanda-expensive-2.

Nolte, K., Chamberlain, W., & Giger, M. (2016). *International Land Deals for Agriculture: Fresh Insights from the Land Matrix. Analytical Report II.* Bern: Centre for Development and Environment, University of Bern. Available at www.landmatrix.org/media/filer_public/ab/c8/abc8b563-9d74-4a47-9548-cb59e4809b4e/land_matrix_2016_analytical_report_draft_ii.pdf.

North, L. L., & Grinspun, R. (2016). Neo-extractivism and the new Latin American developmentalism: the missing piece of rural transformation. *Third World Quarterly* 37, 1483–1504.

O'Brien, E., Nhamire, B., Niu, S., et al. (2017). China spins a global food web from Mozambique to Missouri. *Bloomberg News*, May 22 (online). Available at www.bloomberg.com/news/features/2017-05-22/china-spins-a-global-food-web-from-mozambique-to-missouri.

Ortiz, I., Chai, J., & Cummins, M. (2011). Escalating food prices: the threat to poor households and policies to safeguard a recovery for all. Social and Economic Policy Working Paper. UNICEF, New York. Available at www.unicef.org/socialpolicy/files/Escalating_Food_Prices.pdf.

Ottersen, O. P., Dasgupta, J., Blouin, C., et al. (2014). The political origins of health inequity: prospects for change. *Lancet* 383, 630–667.

Panel of Experts on the Illegal Exploitation of Natural Resources and Other Forms of Wealth of the Democratic Republic of the Congo (2003). Final Report to the Secretary-General (S/2003/1027). United Nations, New York. Available at https://miningwatch.ca/sites/default/files/N0356736.pdf.

Phillips, D., & Brasileiro, D. (2019). Brazil dam disaster: firm knew of potential impact months in advance. *Guardian*, March 1. Available at www.theguardian.com/world/2018/feb/28/brazil-dam-collapse-samarco-fundao-mining.

Porsani, J., Caretta, M. A., & Lehtilä, K. (2019). Large-scale land acquisitions aggravate the feminization of poverty: findings from a case study in Mozambique. *Geojournal* 84, 215–236.

Prain, G. (2010). *Effects of the Global Financial Crisis on the Food Security of Poor Urban Households: Synthesis Report on Five City Case Studies.* Leusden: Resource Centres on Urban Agriculture and Food Security Foundation. Available at www.ruaf.org/sites/default/files/Synthesis%20report%20final.pdf.

PriceWaterhouse Coopers (2016). *The Choice to Change: Africa Oil and Gas Review.* PwC in South Africa. Available at www.pwc.co.za/en/assets/pdf/africa-oil-and-gas-review-2016.pdf.

Purdy, J. (2016). The violent remaking of Appalachia. *The Atlantic* (online). Available at www.theatlantic.com/technology/archive/2016/03/the-violent-remaking-of-appalachia/474603/.

Reed, K. (2009). *Crude Existence: Environment and the Politics of Oil in Northern Angola.* Berkeley: University of California Press.

Ridde, V., Campbell, B., & Martel, A. (2015). Mining revenue and access to health care in Africa: could the revenue drawn from well-managed mining sectors finance exemption from payment for health? *Development in Practice* 25, 909–918.

Roche, C., Thygesen, K., & Baker, E. (eds.) (2017). *Mine Tailings Storage: Safety Is No Accident.* Nairobi: United Nations Environment Programme. Available at https://gridarendal-website.s3.amazonaws.com/production/documents/:s_document/371/original/RRA_MineTailings_lores.pdf?1510660693.

Ross, M. L. (2015). What have we learned about the resource curse? *Annual Review of Political Science* 18, 239–259.

Ruel, M. T., Garrett, J. L., Hawkes, C., & Cohen, M. J. (2010). The food, fuel, and financial crises affect the urban and rural poor disproportionately: a review of the evidence. *Journal of Nutrition* 140, 170S–176S.

Rulli, M. C., Casirati, S., Dell'Angelo, J., et al. (2019). Interdependencies and telecoupling of oil palm expansion at the expense of Indonesian rainforest. *Renewable and Sustainable Energy Reviews* 105, 499–512.

Rulli, M. C., & D'Odorico, P. (2014). Food appropriation through large scale land acquisitions. *Environmental Research Letters* 9(064030), 1–9.

Rulli, M. C., Passera, C., Chiarelli, D. D., & D'Odorico, P. (2018). Socio-environmental effects of large-scale land acquisition in Mozambique, in Petrillo, A., & Bellaviti, P. (eds.), *Sustainable Urban Development and Globalization: New Strategies for New Challenges – With a Focus on the Global South.* Cham: Springer International Publishing, pp. 377–389.

Rulli, M. C., Saviori, A., & D'Odorico, P. (2013). Global land and water grabbing. *Proceedings of the National Academy of Sciences USA* 110, 892–897.

Sarkar, A. (2019). Environmental impact assessment of uranium mining on Indigenous land in Labrador (Canada): biases and manipulations. *Environmental Justice* 12, 61–68.

Sassen, S. (2010). A savage sorting of winners and losers: contemporary versions of primitive accumulation. *Globalizations* 7, 23–50.

Schandl, H., Fischer-Kowalski, M., West, J., et al. (2016). *Global Material Flows and Resource Productivity: Assessment Report for the UNEP International Resource Panel.* Nairobi: United Nations Environment Programme. Available at http://hdl.handle.net/20.500.11822/21557.

Schapiro, M. (2019). What happens to environment journalists is chilling: they get killed for their work. *Guardian*, June 18. Available at www.theguardian.com/commentisfree/2019/jun/18/environment-journalists-killed.

Schrecker, T., Birn, A. E., & Aguilera, M. (2018). How extractive industries affect health: political economy underpinnings and pathways. *Health & Place* **52**, 135–147.

Schrecker, T., Chapman, A., Labonté, R., & De Vogli, R. (2010). Advancing health equity in the global marketplace: how human rights can help. *Social Science & Medicine* **71**, 1520–1526.

Schuppert, F. (2014). Beyond the national resource privilege: towards an International Court of the Environment. *International Theory* **6**, 68–97.

Skinner, E. B. (2013). Indonesia's palm oil industry rife with human-rights abuses. *Bloomberg Businessweek* (online), July 18. Available at www.bloomberg.com/news/articles/2013-07-18/indonesias-palm-oil-industry-rife-with-human-rights-abuses.

Sovacool, B. K. (2019). The precarious political economy of cobalt: balancing prosperity, poverty, and brutality in artisanal and industrial mining in the Democratic Republic of the Congo. *Extractive Industries and Society* **6**, 915–939. doi:10.1016/j.exis.2019.05.018.

Stoop, N., Verpoorten, M., & van der Windt, P. (2018). More legislation, more violence? the impact of Dodd-Frank in the DRC. *PLoS ONE* **13**, e0201783.

Sundaram, J. K., & von Arnim, R. (2012). Economic liberalization and constraints to development in Sub-Saharan Africa, in Noman, A., Botchwey, K., Stein, H., et al. (eds.), *Good Growth and Governance in Africa*. Oxford, UK: Oxford University Press, pp. 499–535.

Tweedie, N. (2018). Riddle of the sands: the truth behind stolen beaches and dredged islands. *Observer*, July 1. Available at www.theguardian.com/global/2018/jul/01/riddle-of-the-sands-the-truth-behind-stolen-beaches-and-dredged-islands.

United Nations (2019). Special Procedures of the Human Rights Council. Office of the High Commissioner for Human Rights (online). Available at www.ohchr.org/EN/HRBodies/SP/Pages/Welcomepage.aspx.

United Nations Development Programme (2015). *National Human Development Report, 2015: Human Security and Human Development in Nigeria*. New York: UNDP. Available at http://hdr.undp.org/sites/default/files/2016_national_human_development_report_for_nigeria.pdf.

United Nations Environment Programme (UNEP) (2011). *Environmental Assessment of Ogoniland*. Nairobi: UNEP. Available at https://postconflict.unep.ch/publications/OEA/UNEP_OEA.pdf.

United Nations Human Settlements Programme (2003). *The Challenge of Slums*. London: Earthscan. Available at www.unhabitat.org/pmss/getPage.asp?page=bookView&book=1156.

Varkkey, H., Tyson, A., & Choiruzzad, S. A. B. (2018). Palm oil intensification and expansion in Indonesia and Malaysia: environmental and socio-political factors influencing policy. *Forest Policy and Economics* **92**, 148–159.

Wallis, W. (2014). Nigeria's super elite laps up luxury as 60% live in severe poverty. *Financial Times* (online). Available at www.ft.com/cms/s/0/54a6d688-bb14-11e3-948c-00144feabdc0.html#axzz3L1QwcUwU.

Watts, J. (2019a). Jagendra Singh: the Indian journalist burned to death. *Guardian*, June 17. Available at www.theguardian.com/environment/2019/jun/17/writing-truth-weighing-heavily-on-my-life-murder-jagendra-singh.

Watts, J. (2019b). Murder, rape, and claims of contamination at a Tanzanian goldmine. *Guardian*, June 18. Available at www.theguardian.com/environment/2019/jun/18/murder-rape-claims-of-contamination-tanzanian-goldmine.

Wenar, L. (2008). Property rights and the resource curse. *Philosophy and Public Affairs* **36**(1), 2–32.

Wenar, L. (2013). Fighting the resource curse. *Global Policy* **4**, 298–304.

White, B., Borras, S., Hall, R., et al. (2012). The new enclosures: critical perspectives on corporate land deals. *Journal of Peasant Studies* **39**, 619–647.

Whitehead, M., Pennington, A., Orton, L., et al. (2016). How could differences in "control over destiny" lead to socio-economic inequalities in health? A synthesis of theories and pathways in the living environment. *Health & Place* **39**, 51–61.

Wolford, W., & Nehring, R. (2015). Constructing parallels: Brazilian expertise and the commodification of land, labour and money in Mozambique. *Canadian Journal of Development Studies* **36**, 208–223.

World Health Organization (WHO) (2016). Angola grapples with worst yellow fever outbreak in 30 years. World Health Organization (online). Available at www.who.int/features/2016/angola-worst-yellow-fever/en/.

Yakubu, O. H. (2017). Addressing environmental health problems in Ogoniland through implementation of United Nations Environment Program recommendations: environmental management strategies. *Environments* **4**, 12–19. doi:10.3390/environments4020028.

Zeuner, B. (2018). An obsolescing bargain in a rentier state: multinationals, artisanal miners, and cobalt in the Democratic Republic of Congo. *Frontiers in Energy Research* **6**, 123.

Zucman, G. (2014). Taxing across borders: tracking personal wealth and corporate profits. *Journal of Economic Perspectives* **28**, 121–148.

The Environment, Ethics, and Health

20

David B. Resnik

Introduction

The relationship between human health and the physical, biological, and social environment raises novel bioethical issues that extend beyond clinical medicine to encompass interactions between human beings and nonhuman species, habitats, ecosystems, the atmosphere, oceans, and the biosphere. These issues may arise at a local, national, or international level and often have implications for public health, global health, social justice, international justice, future generations, economic development, public policy, and human rights. This chapter provides an overview of environmental health ethics and explores some of the issues that arise in this area of study.

Potter's Vision

When bioethics originated as an area of scholarship in the early 1970s, Van Rensselaer Potter articulated a vision of the discipline as environmental and global in scope (Jonsen, 1998; Whitehouse, 2003; ten Have, 2012). Potter argued that bioethics should address not only issues that arise in the clinical setting (such as euthanasia, abortion, informed consent, and organ transplantation) but also those which pertain to humanity's interaction with the environment (such as pollution, animal experimentation, industrial agriculture, and species preservation; Potter, 1971). Social justice concerns in bioethics should include not only those which affect individuals and societies (such as access to healthcare) but also those which impact everyone living on planet Earth (such as population control, deforestation, and energy use). Unfortunately, Potter did not persuade many bioethicists to adopt his vision, and different areas of the discipline began to emerge and diverge. The main division that occurred was between biomedical ethics, which focuses on issues that arise in healthcare and clinical medicine (Beauchamp & Childress, 2008), and environmental ethics, which deals with issues relating

to the environment (Attfield, 2003). There was very little interchange between scholars working in these different areas of inquiry or recognition of overlapping intellectual interests (Resnik, 2012; Lee, 2017).

The division between biomedical and environmental ethics began to break down at the beginning of the twenty-first century because of a growing awareness of the need to address the public and environmental health impacts of clinical decisions (Pierce & Jameton, 2001; Childress et al., 2002) and the realization that many environmental ethics issues have implications for human health and social justice (Dwyer, 2009; Gardiner, 2010). The overuse of antibiotics in medicine and agriculture, for example, can lead to antibiotic resistance, which has dire consequences for the health of human and animal populations around the globe (Selgelid, 2007). Waste management impacts public health and the environment and has implications for human rights and social justice (Shrader-Frechette, 2002; Cranor, 2011). Climate change as a result of human activity has had adverse impacts on public health, species survival, ecosystem stability, and biodiversity (Macpherson, 2013). Scholars began to recognize that to adequately address these and other ethical and policy issues, it was necessary to consider the relationship between human health and the environment more closely (Childress et al., 2002; Jameton, 2010; Resnik, 2012; Lee, 2017; Buse et al., 2018).

Health and the Environment

The environment impacts human health in numerous ways. At the most basic level, the environment provides and supports the necessities of life, such as water, air, food, clothing, shelter, energy, and raw materials. The environment is where we live, raise children, work, travel, and recreate. Although we depend on the environment for our existence and livelihood, human activities can impact the environment in ways that threaten our health by increasing the risk of cancer, birth defects, diabetes, and cardiovascular, respiratory, and neurologic diseases. Many of these adverse health impacts come from substances that enter the environment because of human activities, such as air and water pollution; household, commercial, and hazardous wastes; pesticides; and industrial chemicals. Other adverse health impacts come from changes we make to the environment through processes such as deforestation, urban development, and energy production (Frumkin, 2010). One might conclude that promoting human health and protecting the environment go hand in hand: to promote human health, we should always safeguard the environment.

The relationship between human health and the environment is not that simple, however, because some activities that promote human health can adversely impact the environment. For example, hospitals play a key role in healthcare, but they also produce a tremendous amount of waste and pollution and use considerable energy (Pierce & Jameton, 2010). Using dichlorodiphenyltrichloroethane (DDT) to control populations of mosquitoes that carry malaria can have adverse impacts on some types of birds and aquatic life forms, and spraying pesticides on crops to kill insects that feed on them can threaten other species of insects, such as some types of bees and butterflies (Resnik, 2012). Dams can promote human health by providing clean water for growing human populations but can also destroy habitats and ecosystems and threaten animal and plant species.

Environmental Health Ethics

Because the relationship between human health and the environment raises moral concerns related to nonhuman species, habitats, ecosystems, and the biosphere, environmental health ethics must take into account both human-centered and environmental values. Most of the articles and books on biomedical ethics focus on human-centered values (Jonsen, 1998; Gert et al., 2006; Arras et al., 2015; Moskop, 2016). In their highly influential book *Principles of Biomedical Ethics,* Beauchamp and Childress (2008) articulate four principles for making ethical decisions in medicine and healthcare: autonomy (respecting the choices and actions of morally autonomous persons), nonmaleficence (avoiding harming other people), beneficence (doing good for others), and justice (treating people fairly). Beauchamp and Childress argue that

one must balance and prioritize these different principles when making ethical decisions. For example, in deciding whether adults with highly infectious, dangerous diseases, such as tuberculosis, should receive mandatory treatment, one must consider whether a concern for protecting public health (beneficence) overrides their right to refuse treatment (autonomy). Facts relevant to the decision, such as the communicability of the disease and its health impacts and the availability of treatment, can make a difference in how one prioritizes competing principles (Beauchamp & Childress, 2008). Although bioethicists have developed methods of ethical decision making that differ from Beauchamp and Childress's approach, such as virtue ethics, the ethics of care, and case-based reasoning (or casuistry), most tend to focus on the human values at stake in medicine and healthcare (Moskop, 2016).

Most of the literature in environmental ethics, by contrast, tends to focus on philosophical issues concerning conflicts between human interests and the environment while paying scant attention to the relationship between human health and the environment per se (Norton, 1987; Attfield, 2003; ten Have, 2006; Brennan, 2015). One of the key questions in environmental ethics is whether nonhuman entities, such as other species, habitats, ecosystems, and the biosphere, have intrinsic moral value that is independent of human interests or whether these things are valuable only extrinsically, that is, because they promote human interests (Attfield, 2003). According to anthropocentric approaches to environmental ethics, the environment is valuable only as a means for promoting human interests. Anthropocentric approaches recognize that it is important to protect the environment because it provides food, water, air, energy, and other things that promote human interests. However, when human interests conflict with protecting the environment, human interests should take priority. For example, in deciding whether to build a dam, we should prioritize human interests (such as providing clean water and energy for the human population) over environmental concerns (such as protecting nonhuman species, habitats, or ecosystems). According to nonanthropocentric approaches, the environment has moral value that is independent of humanity and can take precedence over human interests (Brennan, 2015). For example, one might oppose building a dam on the grounds that this would threaten nonhuman species, habitats, or ecosystems.

Whereas the debate between anthropocentrism and nonanthropocentrism is an important issue in environmental ethics, it tends to gloss over differences among the human values at stake, such as health, food production, energy procurement, economic development, and so on. For example, one might defend construction of a dam as a means of providing clean water necessary for human health but not as a means of stimulating local economic development. It matters, from a moral point of view, which types of human interests are at stake when they conflict with environmental concerns (Resnik, 2012).

Because most approaches to biomedical and environmental ethics do not have the conceptual tools needed to deal with the range of ethical questions and problems related to interactions between human health and the environment, to address these issues effectively, it is necessary to develop an approach to decision making that combines theories, ideas, and principles from biomedical and environmental ethics, that is, environmental health ethics (Resnik, 2009, 2012). As an area of study, environmental health ethics addresses ethical, social, legal, and policy issues related to interactions between human health and the environment. It incorporates insights from humanistic disciplines, such as philosophy, law, ethics, and public policy, as well scientific ones, such as toxicology, ecology, public health, occupational health, medicine, economics, genetics, epidemiology, and exposure biology (Resnik, 2012). Environmental health ethics is a new and underappreciated discipline, but it is likely to increase in importance and prominence in the decades ahead as citizens, policymakers, and researchers grapple with the complex issues related to health and the environment, such as climate change, genetically modified organisms, waste management, and chemical regulation (Lee, 2017).

Principles of Environmental Health Ethics

Numerous authors (e.g., Beauchamp & Childress, 2008; Gert et al., 2006; Shamoo & Resnik, 2015) argue that ethical decision making involves the application of general principles or rules to specific cases. The principles are based on our commonsense intuitions of right and wrong and are supported by diverse moral theories, for example, Kantianism, utilitarianism, virtue ethics, and so on. For example, most people would agree that it is wrong to harm others,

and virtually all moral theories would support this axiom. Although the principles provide useful guidance for action in most cases, situations may arise in which they conflict, and one must decide which one should have the highest priority. For example, suppose that a woman is working at a factory job that exposes her to dangerous chemicals. The woman becomes pregnant, and her employer decides to transfer her to a different job to protect her fetus from harm. The woman protests this reassignment because she likes her old job better than the new one. This case involves a conflict between respecting the woman's right to make decisions concerning her own body and protecting her fetus from harm. To decide what should be done in this case, one must determine which principle should have priority. Very often, attending to the relevant facts pertaining to an ethical dilemma can help us to set priorities. For example, the degree of risk to the fetus posed by the factory job is a relevant fact that we should consider in this case. Another relevant fact would be the availability and effectiveness of techniques (such as protective clothing or masks) to reduce exposure risk. One might argue that if the job would expose the woman's fetus to a significant risk of birth defects or long-term health problems that cannot easily be minimized, then a transfer would be warranted.

Because environmental health ethics addresses issues related to human interests and protection of the environment, ethical principles should include human-centered and environmentally oriented rules. What follows is a brief summary of some ethical principles and metaprinciples, that is, decision-making strategies.

Human-Centered Principles

Autonomy: Do Not Interfere with the Choices of Moral Agents

The basic idea behind this principle is that we should allow moral agents to make their own decisions and act on them. Moral agents are people who have the ability to understand and follow moral rules and make responsible, well-informed decisions. The principle of autonomy implies various rights, such as rights to life, liberty, property, and the pursuit of happiness. Moral agents should have freedom of movement, thought, expression, religion, and socialization. They should be able to control their own bodies and choose their own endeavors and occupations. However, autonomy can be restricted to prevent moral agents from harming other people (see "Nonmaleficence" below).

Nonmaleficence: Do Not Harm Other People or Place Them at Unreasonable Risk of Harm

To harm someone is to negatively impact their interests. Harms may include physical harms (such as murder, assault, or rape), psychological harms (such as emotional abuse), and property harms (such as theft or vandalism). Unreasonable risks are risks that are not justified in terms of their social benefits. For example, driving an automobile is reasonable risk because driving has many benefits for society in that it is a means of gaining and keeping employment, attending school, visiting friends, and so on. Driving while intoxicated is an unreasonable risk because it places other people at a high risk of serious harm but does not provide any significant social benefits.

Beneficence: Promote Good Consequences for Other People

The basic idea here is that we should do things that benefit others, such as consoling despondent friends or family members, feeding people who are hungry, and conducting scientific research that leads to treatments for disease. Benefits may accrue to individuals, groups, or society as a whole. Benefits may be personal, social, medical, or economic in nature. The principle of utility, which instructs us to maximize benefits/harms for all people, can be understood as a combination of beneficence and nonmaleficence.

Justice: Treat People Fairly

Justice is a complex concept that includes procedural justice (i.e., following fair procedures), distributive justice (i.e., distributing social and economic goods fairly), retributive justice (i.e., administering fair punishments for wrongdoing), restorative justice (i.e., rehabilitation of criminal offenders through reconciliation with victims and the community at large), and corrective justice (i.e., correcting injustices fairly). There are different approaches to distributive justice, including libertarianism (i.e., a distribution of goods is fair if it results from following fair procedures and respects rights to property), egalitarianism (i.e., a distribution is fair if it gives people an equal portion of what they are entitled to, such as equality of opportunity), and utilitarianism (i.e., a distribution is fair if it maximizes benefits/harms). As we shall see later, environmental justice issues may arise at the local, national, or international levels (Dwyer, 2009; Resnik et al., 2018).

Justice is a very important consideration in environmental health (Shrader-Frechette, 2002). The environmental justice movement began in the United States in the 1980s when some low-income minority communities objected to the placement of waste sites near their neighborhoods. Their objections were twofold: (1) they had not been appropriately consulted about the placement of the waste sites, and (2) placement of the waste sites unfairly exposed them to health risks (Resnik, 2012). Since then, justice has become a hot-button issue in environmental health policy. For example, the Environmental Protection Agency (EPA) has adopted a policy that requires fair treatment and meaningful involvement of people affected by its decision making, regardless of race, ethnicity, or income (Resnik, 2012).

Environmentally Oriented Principles

Animal Welfare: Avoid Unnecessarily Harming Sentient Animals

This principle recognizes that we should avoid harming some nonhuman species, that is, sentient animals. A sentient animal is an organism that is capable of suffering or experiencing physical pain or psychological stress. For example, nonhuman primates, dogs, cows, horses, cats, mice, whales, and dolphins would be considered to be sentient animals because we have evidence that they can suffer or experience pain or stress. *Unnecessarily* is a key point of contention in the application of this principle to real cases because one might argue that it is necessary to kill sentient animals for food or use them in scientific experiments that can benefit human beings.

Stewardship: Take Good Care of Environmental Resources

The basic idea behind this principle is that we should be good stewards of environmental resources, such as the air, water, soil, nonhuman species, habitats, ecosystems, and the biosphere as a whole. Human activities, such as air and water pollution, waste disposal, deforestation, urban development, agriculture, and fishing, can damage, deplete, or threaten environmental resources (Frumkin, 2010). Stewardship must be balanced against human-centered principles such as beneficence because many activities that negatively impact environmental resources may also provide important medical, social, or economic benefits to people. An extreme version of the stewardship principle, which is endorsed by some environmentalists, would prohibit human beings from doing anything that damages or threatens the environment. This principle would require a drastic restructuring and downsizing of human civilization (Brennan, 2015; Crist, 2018).

Sustainability: Practice Sustainable Uses of Environmental Resources

Sustainability is closely related to stewardship because sustainability involves good stewardship of resources over time. Sustainability recognizes the important point that future generations will also need to use environmental resources and that we have obligations to ensure that they have sufficient resources to live and prosper (Dwyer, 2009). A use is sustainable if we can continue doing it indefinitely without permanently damaging or depleting environmental resources. For example, cutting down trees for firewood is sustainable if we also replant new ones. In some cases, a practice may be considered sustainable if it substitutes new resources with lower environmental impacts for depleted ones. For example, using a nonrenewable resource such as oil for energy is sustainable if we also are developing alternative sources of energy with lower environmental impacts, such as biofuels, as a replacement.

Metaprinciples

Precaution: Take Reasonable Measures to Prevent, Minimize, or Mitigate Threats to Public Health or the Environment That Are Plausible and Significant Even When We Lack Scientific Certainty That They Will Transpire

Most of the decisions we make – as individuals and as a society – involve taking risks for the sake of obtaining benefits. Sometimes we have enough information to make decisions based on the probabilities of different outcomes related to our choices. For a simple example, suppose that I am considering whether to ride my bike to work today, and I know that the chance of rain is 50%. I can take this information into account when deciding whether the risk of getting wet is worth the benefit of biking to work (e.g., saving gasoline and exercising). Decisions made by regulatory agencies charged with protecting public

health or the environment are usually based on a careful analysis of scientific research related to the probabilities concerning different outcomes. For example, when the Food and Drug Administration (FDA) decides whether to approve a new drug, it carefully reviews the scientific research pertaining to the safety and efficacy of the drug and calculates the likely impacts of approval on public health.

However, sometimes we must make decisions when we lack enough information to estimate the relevant probabilities. For example, a government agency might need to decide whether it should allow beef to be imported from a country where there was an epidemic of mad cow disease a year ago. While it is possible that some of the beef is infected, the agency does not have enough information to estimate the probability that this is case. In the 1980s, scholars and policy analysts developed the *precautionary principle* (PP) as an approach to decision making when we lack enough scientific information to estimate probabilities related to the outcomes of important public policy choices, such as decisions related to climate change, genetically modified organisms (GMOs), or chemical regulation (Resnik, 2012). The basic idea behind the PP is that we should take steps to deal with significant threats to public health or the environment, even when we don't have all the facts or scientific data needed to decide what to do. For example, the government agency mentioned earlier could ban importation of beef from a country where mad cow disease has been detected within the last three years to protect the public from harm.

The PP has generated considerable controversy, largely because of its vagueness (Resnik, 2003; Steel, 2014). Strong formulations of the PP are highly risk-aversive maxims that instruct us to avoid doing anything (such as developing new technologies) that could pose a significant threat to public health or the environment. Others are so weak that they would seem to impose almost no constraints on risk taking (Steel, 2014). To think clearly about the PP, two points need to be considered. First, the threats we face need to be plausible; that is, they should not be fanciful, alarmist scenarios with no solid basis in scientific fact or theory. While the PP is relevant to situations where we face considerable uncertainty, this does not mean that science has no bearing on our risk taking. Second, the measures we take to prevent, minimize, or mitigate these threats should be reasonable; that is, they should reflect a judicious weighing of the possible benefits and harms of different courses of action. Precautionary measures we take to address potential harms often have social and economic costs (Munthe, 2011). If we ban a type of technology because we are concerned about how it may threaten public health or the environment, then we forego the potential benefits of that technology. We must consider the costs of precaution when we apply the PP to actual cases (Munthe, 2011; Steel, 2014).

Community Engagement: Take Appropriate Steps to Consult with and Obtain Approval from the Affected Community before Implementing an Environmental Health Intervention

Fair and effective community engagement is part of environmental justice (see earlier discussion) because it helps to ensure that decisions that impact communities follow fair procedures by including meaningful community input. Community engagement is also important for promoting benefits and avoiding harms at the community level because community members can provide information to public health officials concerning their needs and concerns. Many different environmental health decisions significantly impact communities. Some of these include placement of waste sites, factories, highways, schools, and shopping malls; policies concerning urban development, housing, and air or water quality; and introduction of GMOs into environment (Resnik, 2012).

Environmental Health Ethics Issues

As mentioned previously, environmental health ethics issues arise at the local, national, and international levels and involve conflicts among human-centered and environmentally oriented principles. The remainder of this chapter provides a summary of some of these issues (see Sharp et al. [2008], Jameton [2010], Resnik [2012], and Zölzer & Meskens [2019] for discussion of issues not covered in this chapter).

Waste Management

Human activities generate various forms of waste, including household waste, industrial waste, electronic waste, sewage, and hazardous waste (e.g., radioactive or biological waste). Proper disposal of waste is necessary to protect human beings and nonhuman species from exposure to harmful substances (Frumkin, 2010). Although waste disposal sites are usually designed to contain materials and prevent

them from leeching into the environment, containment is often not completely effective, and people living near waste disposal sites may face higher health risks than those who live further away. Whereas proper waste disposal promotes public health and protects the environment, deciding where to locate waste disposal sites raises ethical issues because it results in differential exposure to health risks. People who live near waste disposal sites may object to noxious odors and health problems (such as cancer or respiratory or gastrointestinal diseases) related to exposure to materials in the sites. Waste disposal therefore raises issues of environmental justice and often involves conflicts between population-level beneficence (or utility) and distributive justice (Shrader-Frechette, 2002; Resnik, 2012). Effective community engagement is therefore paramount when making decisions concerning the location of waste sites. Waste disposal may also raise issues of international justice if one country decides to accept waste from another country to reap economic benefits (such as receipt of fees for waste disposing or access to materials, such as metals, that can be recycled, processed, and sold).

Air and Water Pollution

Human activities generate various pollutants that contaminate the air and water. Air pollutants include ozone, particulate matter, carbon monoxide, carbon dioxide, sulfur dioxide, nitrogen oxides, volatile organic compounds, chlorofluorocarbons, and heavy metals. Water pollutants include sewage, wastewater treatment products, disinfectants, industrial waste, metals, agriculture waste, petroleum and coal hydrocarbons, pesticides, and phosphates, nitrates, and other fertilizers. Air and water pollution adversely impacts public health and the environment in numerous ways. Air pollution increases the risk of asthma, lung cancer, and cardiovascular disease. Water pollution can increase the risk of cholera, *Salmonella* infection, typhoid, diarrhea, gastritis, and cancer (Frumkin, 2010). While access to clean air and water is essential for promoting public health and protecting the environment, policies designed to control pollution raise ethical issues because they may restrict beneficial human activities, such as agriculture, industry, transportation, and urban development. Most developed nations have agencies that establish standards for acceptable levels of air and water pollution. Ethical conflicts between public health and environmental protection, on the one hand, and social and economic development, on the other, may arise when agencies deliberate about air and water quality standards (Resnik, 2012). Air and water pollution may also raise issues of environmental justice because some vulnerable groups, such as children, the elderly, and asthmatics, may be more susceptible to the effects of pollution than others. Societies may need to decide whether air and water quality standards should be aimed at providing an acceptable level of protection for average members of the population or should be tailored to meet the health needs of vulnerable populations (Resnik et al., 2018).

Chemical Regulation

Human activities produce many types of chemical compounds that can pose risks to public health and the environment. Chemicals are used in consumer products, industry, medicine, manufacturing, building construction, transportation, agriculture, and many other applications. Some of these chemicals can produce severe toxicity and even death at high, short-term exposure levels. Others, such as asbestos, polychlorinated biphenyls (PCBs), formaldehyde, benzene, and various flame retardants, can increase the risk of cancer at low exposure levels over longer periods of time (Frumkin, 2010). Many types of pesticides, including neonicotinoids, organophosphates, dichlorodiphenyltrichloroethane (DDT), and glyphosate (the active ingredient in the herbicide Roundup), can have adverse impacts on nonhuman species such as insects, birds, aquatic organisms, and plants. Some chemicals used in plastics, such as bisphenol A, can interfere with the body's endocrine system and increase the risk of developmental problems in infants and children and cancer in adults. Various drugs can have adverse side effects, ranging from nausea and dizziness to kidney or liver toxicity, even when used as directed (Resnik, 2012).

The central ethical dilemma concerning chemical use is deciding on the appropriate level of regulation, if any (Resnik & Elliott, 2015). The degree of regulation for a chemical tends to be proportional to the degree of public health or environmental risk posed by exposure to the chemical. Pesticides are highly regulated because they are known to pose significant risks to humans and nonhuman species. Pesticides must undergo extensive animal testing before receiving approval by the EPA for use in the United States.

The EPA also imposes significant restrictions on the use of pesticides that have been approved for marketing. Drugs are also highly regulated because they can pose significant risks to human health, especially if not used appropriately. Drugs must undergo extensive animal and human testing prior to receiving approval by the Food and Drug Administration (FDA) for use in the United States. Once a drug has been approved, it may be available only under a physician's prescription. In many countries, including the United States, premarket regulatory approval is not required for thousands of chemicals produced by industry and in consumer products because they are presumed to be safe at typical exposure levels, an assumption that is often mistaken (Cranor, 2011).

Various ethical principles come into play when making decisions concerning chemical regulation. On the one hand, chemicals often have significant benefits for human health (e.g., drugs), agriculture (e.g., pesticides), housing (e.g., flame retardants, wood products), and the economy (e.g., consumer products). On the other hand, chemicals can pose risks to human health and the environment. Regulatory decision making involves judicious balancing of these benefits and risks. Because we often have little knowledge about the impacts of various chemicals on public health and the environment, a precautionary approach often may be warranted (Resnik & Elliott, 2015). In the United States and most developed nations, regulatory agencies such as the EPA have the authority to ban or restrict chemical compounds when they have convincing evidence that these products pose significant risks to human health or the environment. Because evidence accumulates over time, a dangerous chemical could be on the market for many years before an agency regulates it. For example, asbestos was used in insulation and as a fire retardant for decades until evidence emerged linking it to lung cancer and other health problems. The EPA began taking steps to restrict the use of asbestos in the 1970s (EPA, 2018).

A key question related to precaution is whether chemicals should undergo any safety testing prior to marketing (Cranor, 2011). As noted earlier, pesticides and drugs must undergo safety testing prior to marketing, but many chemicals used by industry and in consumer products do not need to meet this requirement because they are presumed to be safe at typical exposure levels. Mandating premarket testing for these chemicals could put many companies out of business and significantly raise prices for consumers. One might argue that such a policy would be an overreaction to the risks posed by these chemicals but that a more reasonable approach would be to require companies to provide some basic information about their chemicals to regulatory authorities prior to marketing. Regulatory authorities could use this information to decide whether additional oversight, research, or monitoring is needed.

Agricultural Practices

Agriculture supplies human beings with food, which is necessary for life. Although agriculture has existed since the dawn of civilization, it has become highly industrialized since the 1850s. Industrial farming is highly mechanized and scientific and takes advantage of economies of scale. Although small farms have not vanished, many crops are produced on large farms owned or operated by corporations. In the twentieth century, farmers began using chemical pesticides and fertilizers to increase crop yields, and in the 1990s, they started planting and harvesting genetically modified (GM) crops, such as corn, soybeans, and tomatoes, to increase yields and reduce reliance on pesticides. In the near future, industrial farms could include GM poultry, livestock, and fish. Many farmers supplement animal feed with antibiotics to prevent disease and increase weight (Resnik, 2012). Agriculture also uses a significant amount of land, water, and energy. Whereas the practices associated with industrial agriculture can produce many important benefits for human societies, they also can impose significant risks to human health and the environment. For example:

- As mentioned earlier, pesticides can be toxic to human beings at high doses. Low-dose exposure to pesticides may also carry some health risks. Pesticides can also adversely impact nonhuman species and ecosystems. Overuse of pesticides can lead to pesticide resistance.
- Agricultural waste, such as animal feces and chemical fertilizers, can contaminate the water supply.
- The use of antibiotics in agriculture can increase antibiotic resistance, which is a significant public health problem.
- Using water in agriculture can deplete the supply of drinkable water needed to sustain the human population.

- Clearing of land for agriculture can lead to deforestation, which is a key factor in climate change (see discussion later).
- The use of fossil fuels in agriculture contributes to climate change.
- Long-term ingestion of some types of GM crops may pose health risks that are not well understood at this time.
- People who live near some types of agricultural facilities, such as hog farms, may be exposed to greater health risks than those living further away.
- GM animals and plants that are not well contained may adversely impact native species and disrupt habitats and ecosystems.
- Excessive fishing and hunting for food can threaten species and disrupt ecosystems.
- Eating meat (especially beef) is a highly inefficient use of land, water, energy, and feed grain that contributes to climate change.

Deciding how to manage these hazards involves a careful assessment of the impacts of agriculture and strategies for risk minimization and mitigation. It may be possible, in many cases, to reach compromise solutions that balance competing principles and provide reasonable solutions to complex problems. As noted earlier, government agencies restrict the use of pesticides to minimize adverse impacts on public health and the environment. Additionally, farmers could administer antibiotics to animals orally or intravenously to treat or prevent disease but not add antibiotics to their food to increase weight, nations could reach agreements to prevent overfishing, farmers could use recycled (i.e., gray) water to minimize their use of drinking water, and human populations could reduce the percentage of beef in their diet.

The Built Environment

The built environment consists of the structures human beings create to support various activities and includes houses, schools, factories, roads, sidewalks, bridges, airports, hospitals, dams, sewage treatment plants, farms, electric power lines, shopping malls, and cities, among other structures (Frumkin, 2010). Because the structures we build impact public health and the economy as well as other species, habitats, and ecosystems, decisions we make concerning the built environment raise ethical issues, such as

- Clearing away land for structures that benefit human beings can threaten species (via habitat loss), disrupt ecosystems, and reduce biodiversity. Additionally, because trees remove carbon from the atmosphere, deforestation is a significant factor in climate change (discussed later).

- Draining of wetlands to create spaces for human structures or control mosquito populations can threaten species, destroy habitats, disrupt ecosystems, and reduce biodiversity. Also, wetlands play an important role in removing toxins from the water, and coastal wetlands can prevent saltwater from contaminating freshwater and serve as a barrier against storm surges.

- Dams (mentioned earlier) can provide human beings with drinking water and hydroelectric power but can threaten habitats and species, disrupt ecosystems, and reduce biodiversity.

- Safe housing is important for promoting public health, but it costs money. Housing standards therefore often involve tradeoffs between public health/safety (i.e., beneficence, utility) and affordability/access (i.e., distributive justice).

- Safe work environments are important for promoting public health, but they also cost money. Occupational health standards therefore often involve tradeoffs between public health and business interests/economic development.

- The design of urban areas can impact health in various ways. Uncontrolled development around the edge of a city, otherwise known as *urban sprawl*, increases automobile traffic and decreases walking and biking as forms of transportation. Urban sprawl therefore contributes to air pollution, obesity, diabetes, and heart disease. Policies designed to combat urban sprawl and promote healthier urban areas may restrict property rights and interfere with economic development.

- People who live near factories, electric power plants, oil pipelines, oil wells, natural gas wells, freeways, and other structures may face greater health risks than those living further away. Decisions concerning construction and placements of these structures therefore raise issues of procedural and distributive justice.

Climate Change

There is considerable scientific evidence that global surface temperatures have been rising in the last hundred years and that human activities, such as greenhouse gas production and deforestation, are largely responsible for this recent change in the Earth's climate (Intergovernmental Panel on Climate Change, 2013). Although estimates from different climate models vary, mean global surface temperatures are likely to continue rising at least 1.5°C in the twenty-first century (relative to the period from 1850 to 1900) unless we drastically cut back on the activities that contribute to climate change. Chief sources of greenhouse gases (e.g., carbon dioxide and methane) include the combustion of oil, natural gas, coal, and biomass for transportation, industry, and heating; cement production; and industrial meat production. Global warming is likely to have numerous adverse impacts on public health and the environment, such as rising sea levels; increased severe weather, flooding, droughts, forest fires, heat-related deaths, and infectious and respiratory diseases; habitat loss; and decreased drinkable water, agricultural productivity, and biodiversity (Intergovernmental Panel on Climate Change, 2014). The two basic responses to climate change include mitigation, which involves taking steps to minimize or mitigate expected changes in global temperatures, and adaptation, which involves taking steps to adapt to climate change. International treaties pertaining to climate change, such as the Kyoto Protocol and the Paris Agreement, address these responses (Resnik, 2012).

Because global warming chiefly results from diverse human activities taking place all over the planet, the ethical issues raised by climate change are complex, multidimensional, and wide ranging in scope (Dwyer, 2009; Gardiner, 2010; Macpherson, 2013). Some of these include

- **Public health and environmental protection versus economic development.** Two of the most discussed policy options for mitigating climate change are (1) imposing an additional tax based on the carbon content of fossil fuels (i.e., a carbon tax) to reduce consumption and (2) implementing a cap and trade system for large producers of greenhouse gases (such as electric power companies) to limit their production of greenhouse gases. However, increased taxes on fossil fuels could impair economic development because most economic activities are highly dependent on fuel, and increases in fuel costs will lead to increased costs and decreased productivity and efficiency. Cap and trade systems could also have negative economic impacts by driving up the cost of electricity, which is also essential to the economy. The United States has refused to participate in climate change treaties, in part because of concerns about the economic impacts of policies that reduce greenhouse gases emissions (Resnik, 2012).

- **International justice.** Climate change is likely to affect different countries differently. For example, small island nations are likely to suffer greater impacts from rising sea levels than land-locked nations. Developing nations are more likely to have difficulty adapting to the impacts of climate change than developed ones because they have fewer resources to draw on (Macpherson, 2013). Furthermore, different countries differ with respect to their roles in causing climate change. Developed nations produce more greenhouse gases per capita than developing ones (Intergovernmental Panel on Climate Change, 2013). A key issue is whether developed countries should be allowed to continue with the pattern of resource use that has spurred their economic development or should radically reduce their use and thus expect lower rates of economic growth. Climate change mitigation policies may also affect different countries differently. For example, developing nations may suffer more severe economic consequences from policies designed to reduce greenhouse gas emissions than developed ones because their economies are less developed. These differences concerning the causes and consequences of climate change raise issues of international justice and have led to some disputes related to climate change treaties. For example, developing nations have argued that developed nations should compensate them for the impacts of climate change by providing them with funds to adapt to rising global temperatures (Resnik, 2012). While few people disagree with some form of compensation for developing nations, there are disagreements about how much compensation should be given or what form it should take (e.g., money, climate change treaty concessions, etc.). Developing nations have also argued that they should not be required to adopt policies that increase fossil fuel or electricity costs until their economies become more developed (Resnik, 2012). Also, some countries, such as the United States, refuse to participate in climate change treaties unless countries that produce a large amount of greenhouse gases, such

as China and India, also participate (Resnik, 2012). Although the United States produces a higher amount of greenhouse gases per capita than these countries, one might argue that total production matters when negotiating international treaties because countries expect cosigners to abide by the same rules.

- **Geoengineering.** Some scientists and engineers have argued that we should develop and implement methods designed to alter the climate at a global scale, known as *geoengineering*. Although this is essentially a technological solution to a social problem, some scientists and engineers favor this solution because they doubt that countries will be able to cooperate to mitigate climate change. Some geoengineering methods include removing carbon from the atmosphere and sequestering it; fertilizing the oceans with iron to stimulate the growth of algae, which remove carbon from the air; and spraying aerosols (such as sulfur dioxide) into the atmosphere to block sunlight (Resnik & Vallero, 2011). Environmentalists have objected to geoengineering on the grounds that some of these strategies, such as fertilizing the oceans and blocking sunlight, may have adverse environmental impacts that are difficult to predict or control and that pursuing geoengineering as a policy option will undermine political support for other, more effective climate mitigation policies, such as fossil fuel taxes or cap and trade systems (Gardiner, 2010). Scientists and engineers have responded to these objections by asserting that all reasonable options should be on the table when it comes to dealing with a serious problem like climate change and that the risks of geoengineering can be managed by beginning with small-scale projects before pursuing global ones (Resnik & Vallero, 2011).

- **Population control.** The growth of the human population increases greenhouse gas emissions and deforestation and contributes to pollution, waste production, overfishing, and other activities that negatively impact the environment (Crist, 2018). The current global population of 7.6 billion is likely to grow to 8.6 billion in 2030, 9.8 billion in 2050, and 11.2 billion by 2100 (United Nations, 2017). As long as the population continues to grow at its current pace, aggregate greenhouse emissions will continue to rise even if per capita emissions decline significantly (Lutz, 2017). Policies to control population growth by imposing restrictions on the number of children are ethically and politically controversial, however. First, some religious traditions hold that we have a moral duty to reproduce. Second, policies that restrict the number of children that one may have interfere with procreative liberty, which is widely regarded as a basic human right, although some would argue that it can be limited for worthwhile social goals (Resnik, 2012).

Conclusion

To conclude, the relationship between human health and the environment raises a variety of ethical issues that have implications for public health, global health, social justice, international justice, future generations, public policy, economic development, and human rights. Some of these issues, such as waste disposal, are mostly local in scope; others, such as chemical regulation, are largely national in scope; and still others, such as climate change, are global in nature. These issues merit further discussion among philosophers, theologians, lawyers, natural scientists, social scientists, policymakers, and others who can contribute to our understanding of the ethics of environmental health.

Acknowledgments

This research was supported by the Intramural Program of the National Institute of Environmental Health Sciences (NIEHS), National Institutes of Health (NIH). It does not represent the views of the NIEHS, NIH, or the US government.

References

Arras, J. D., Fenton, E., & Kukla, R. (2015). *The Routledge Companion to Bioethics*. New York: Routledge.

Attfield, R. (2003). *Environmental Ethics*. Cambridge, UK: Polity Press.

Beauchamp, T., & Childress, J. (2008). *Principles of Biomedical Ethics*, 6th ed. New York: Oxford University Press.

Brennan, A. (2015). Environmental ethics, in *Stanford Encyclopedia of Philosophy*. Available at https://plato.stanford.edu/entries/ethics-environmental/ (accessed November 26, 2018).

Buse, C. G., Smith, M., & Silva, D. S. (2018). Attending to scalar ethical issues in emerging approaches to environmental health research and practice. *Monash Bioethics Review*, June 4.

Childress, J. E., Faden, R. R., Gaare, R. D., et al. (2002). Public health ethics: mapping the terrain. *Journal of Law, Medicine, and Ethics* **30**(2), 170–178.

Cranor, C. (2011). *Legally Poisoned: How the Law Puts Us at Risk from Toxicants*. Cambridge, MA: Harvard University Press.

Crist, E. (2018). Reimagining the human. *Science* **362**(6420), 1242–1244.

Dwyer, J. (2009). How to connect bioethics and environmental ethics: health, sustainability, and justice. *Bioethics* **23**(9), 497–502.

Elliott, K. C. (2011). *Is a Little Pollution Good for You? Incorporating Societal Values in Environmental Research*. New York: Oxford University Press.

Environmental Protection Agency (EPA) (2018). Federal Bans on Asbestos. Available at www.epa.gov/asbestos/us-federal-bans-asbestos (accessed December 11, 2018).

Frumkin, H. (ed.) (2010). *Environmental Health: From Global to Local*, 2nd ed. New York: John Wiley & Sons.

Gardiner, S. (2010). Is "arming the future" with geoengineering really the lesser evil? Some doubts about the ethics of intentionally manipulating the climate system, in Gardiner, S., Caney, S., Jamieson, D., et al. (eds.), *Climate Ethics: Essential Readings*. New York: Oxford University Press, pp. 284–312.

Gert, B., Culver, C. M., & Clouser, D. K. (2006). *Bioethics: A Systemic Approach*, 2nd ed. New York: Oxford University Press.

Intergovernmental Panel on Climate Change (2013). *Climate Change 2013: The Physical Science Basis*. Available at www.ipcc.ch/report/ar5/wg1/ (accessed December 9, 2018).

Intergovernmental Panel on Climate Change (2014). *Climate Change 2014: Impacts, Adaptation and Vulnerability*. Available at www.ipcc.ch/report/ar5/wg2/ (accessed December 9, 2018).

Jameton, A. (2010). Environmental health ethics, in Frumkin, H. (ed.), *Environmental Health: From Global to Local*, 2nd ed. New York: John Wiley & Sons, pp. 195–226.

Jonsen, A. R. (1998). *The Birth of Bioethics*. New York: Oxford University Press.

Lee, L. M. (2017). A bridge back to the future: public health ethics, bioethics, and environmental ethics. *American Journal of Bioethics* **17**(9), 5–12.

Lutz, W. (2017). How population growth relates to climate change. *Proceedings of the National Academy of Sciences USA* **114**(46), 12103–12105.

Macpherson, C. C. (2013). Climate change is a bioethics problem. *Bioethics* **27**(6), 305–308.

Moskop, J. C. (2016). *Ethics and Health Care: An Introduction*. Cambridge, UK: Cambridge University Press.

Norton, B. G. (1987). *Why Preserve Natural Variety?* Princeton, NJ: Princeton University Press.

Munthe, C. (2011). *The Price of Precaution and the Ethics of Risk*. Dordrecht, Netherlands: Springer.

Pierce, J., & Jameton, A. (2001). *Environmentally Responsible Healthcare*. New York: Oxford University Press.

Potter, V. R. (1971). *Bioethics: Bridge to the Future*. Englewood Cliffs, NJ: Prentice-Hall.

Resnik, D. B. (2003). Is the precautionary principle unscientific? *Studies in the History and Philosophy of Biology and the Biomedical Sciences* 34(2), 329–344.

Resnik, D. B. (2009). Human health and the environment: in harmony or in conflict? *Health Care Analysis* 17(3), 261–276.

Resnik, D. B. (2012). *Environmental Health Ethics*. Cambridge, UK: Cambridge University Press.

Resnik, D. B. (2014). Ethical issues in field trials of genetically modified disease-resistant mosquitoes. *Developing World Bioethics* 14(1), 37–46.

Resnik D. B. (2018). Ethics of community engagement in field trials of genetically modified mosquitoes. *Developing World Bioethics* 18(2), 135–143.

Resnik, D. B., & Elliott, K. C. (2015). Bisphenol A and risk management ethics. *Bioethics* 29(3), 182–189.

Resnik, D. B., & Vallero, D. A. (2011). Geoengineering: an idea whose time has come? *Journal of Earth Science and Climate Change* S1, 1.

Resnik, D. B., MacDougall, D. R., & Smith, E. M. (2018). Ethical dilemmas in protecting susceptible subpopulations from environmental health risks: liberty, utility, fairness, and accountability for reasonableness. *American Journal of Bioethics* 18(3), 29–41.

Richie, C. (2015). What would an environmentally sustainable reproductive technology industry look like? *Journal of Medical Ethics* 41(5), 383–387.

Selgelid, M. (2007). Ethics and drug resistance. *Bioethics* 21(4), 218–229.

Shamoo, A. E., & Resnik, D. B. (2015). *Responsible Conduct of Research*, 3rd ed. New York: Oxford University Press.

Sharp, R. R., Marchant, G. E., & Grodsky, J. A. (eds.) (2008). *Genomics and Environmental Regulation*. Baltimore: Johns Hopkins University Press.

Shrader-Frechette, K. S. (2002). *Environmental Justice: Creating Equity, Reclaiming Democracy*. New York: Oxford University Press.

Steel, D. (2014). *Philosophy and the Precautionary Principle*. Cambridge, UK: Cambridge University Press.

ten Have, H. A., (ed.) (2006). *Environmental Ethics and International Policy*. Paris: UNESCO Publishing.

ten Have, H. A. (2012). Potter's notion of bioethics. *Kennedy Institute of Ethics Journal* 22(1), 59–82.

United Nations (2017). *World Population Prospects: The 2017 Revisions*. Available at www.un.org/development/des a/publications/world-population-prospects-the-2017-revision.html (accessed December 9, 2018).

Whitehouse, P. J. (2003). The rebirth of bioethics: extending the original formulations of Van Rensselaer Potter. *American Journal of Bioethics* 3(4), W26–W31.

Zölzer, F., & Meskens, G. (eds.) (2019). *Environmental Health Risks: Ethical Aspects*. New York: Routledge.

Chapter 21

Ecological Ethics, Planetary Sustainability, and Global Health

Colin D. Butler

Introduction: The Scope of This Chapter

This chapter links ethics, sustainability, and global health. It proposes that a deep reason for our peril, as a quasi-global civilization, is inequality. But inequality itself has deep, self-reinforcing causal roots. There is no "first" cause, and there is no easy solution.

Human population now approaches 8 billion. Despite the fancies of some visionaries, Earth is the only planet on which human life has existed and (apart from orbiting spacecraft and perhaps some missions to the moon and Mars) will be our only home for decades, if not millennia, to come. The conditions for life on our planet were once completely due to nonhuman factors – to natural laws such as physics and evolution, to our proximity to the sun, and to our progression through the great glacial and interglacial cycles, now mostly thought to be determined by orbital factors or changes in Earth's geometry, such as distance from the sun and slight, but recurring, variations in Earth's tilt and wobble.

As with all of science and thought, these theories rely on the work of many people but are particularly associated with the ideas and research of the Serbian Milutin Milankovitch. According to a website provided by the US National Aeronautics and Space Administration (NASA), the life work of Milankovitch, born within three months of Albert Einstein, was largely overlooked for about half a century. However, it may be fairer to consider that a better appreciation of his genius was enabled by research undertaken after his death that was not possible in his life.

We can only know the world through our observations, our memory, and our glimpses into the historical record and similarly constrained exploration of the work and ideas of others, conveyed in literature (including scientific literature), in media, and in discussions. Important scientific advances, including in medicine, are not always sequential and have sometimes been long delayed by prejudice and inertia. Today's dogma may be tomorrow's fallacy. It is thus prudent to practice self-reflection and humility. Even in our era, increasingly called the *Anthropocene*, neither science nor think tanks (whether conservative, liberal, or in between) are omniscient.

Despite these caveats, this chapter presents arguments and discusses data in support of the idea that civilization, and therefore population health, is in great peril. This conclusion will not seem plausible to all readers. Written in 2019, some ideas may not be testable, or able to be confirmed, for decades. But their lack of imminent verification is not sufficient ground to dismiss them in 2019 and probably not even in 2029.

Although scientific knowledge today may one day seem primitive, there is much about the near future (e.g., the next two centuries) that we can already forecast. These predictions are not confined to cosmic events such as eclipses or the timing of the next ice age, now thought to be deferred, by unwitting human action, for tens of millennia, far beyond that which would have seemed likely to an Earth scientist, were there one, at the start of the Holocene, the current interglacial (warm) period.

Nor are predictions restricted to the observations that human society, if it is to survive, will require supplies of energy, food, water, and mineral resources in quantities that greatly exceed that of the recent past. It is also likely to require a persisting balance between the three great competing nuclear powers, China, the United States, and Russia. Upsetting this balance is conceivable but may be associated with enormous disruption, including, possibly, nuclear war.

Natural science, especially relating to the Earth system (the linked fields of science that consider our planet as an integrated unit), is now rich in forecasting the evolution of the planetary climate, especially for the remainder of this century. This includes predictions for phenomena such as average and extreme temperatures (regional and global), storms and other extreme weather events (including droughts), and regional and global sea-level rise. Ecologists increasingly warn of the *sixth great extinction*, presenting evidence from the demise of megafauna to the loss of many insect populations. The Institute for Health Metrics and Evaluation, based in Seattle, Washington, produces a stream of reports analyzing recent and future trends in global and regional life expectancy. The United Nations Population Division provided detailed estimates of global and regional human population size under a range of scenarios until 2100.

However, integration of the data and trends analyzed in producing these forecasts is more scarce, with important exceptions including the limits to growth modelers and polymaths such as Paul and Anne Ehrlich and Martin Rees, a former president of the Royal Society. Even the authors of the "Planetary Boundaries" studies couch their concerns for the human prospect vaguely (Steffen et al., 2015), perhaps demonstrating a phenomenon Hansen called *scientific reticence.*

There are an increasing number of other exceptions. Perhaps the most distinguished living political critic, Noam Chomsky, is now focusing on the threat to human well-being from the global environmental crisis. Chomsky recently stated that "every single journal should have a shrieking headline every day saying we are heading to total catastrophe. In a couple of generations, organized human society may not survive" (Hackett, 2019: 2).

Following a lecture given at the University of Cambridge in late 2018 (Read, 2018), eco-philosopher Rupert Read stated that if humans were to prevent an overwhelming environmental crisis, then "green" governments would have had to have been elected at least a generation ago. Read understands the lags and feedbacks involved. He suggested that the chaos in Yemen and the Democratic Republic of the Congo may be foretastes of our common future in processes that the late epidemiologist Tony McMichael called *planetary overload.*

In support of the claim that we have lost much time, Wallace-Wells, author of *The Uninhabitable Earth: Life After Warming*, refers to claims that if the world had started global decarbonization in 2000, greenhouse gas emissions would only have needed to have been reduced by 2% per year to have a 66%

chance of remaining in the *carbon budget* (Wallace-Wells, 2019). This task now is much more daunting, as some scientists have long warned.

Michael Mann, who shared the 2019 Tyler Prize for Environmental Achievement for his work on climate change science, recently stated that

the science that we are doing is a threat to the world's most powerful and wealthiest special interests. The most powerful and wealthiest special interest that has ever existed: the fossil fuel industry. They have used their immense resources to create fake scandals and to fund a global disinformation campaign aimed at vilifying the scientists, discrediting the science, and misleading the public and policymakers. Arguably, it is the most villainous act in the history of human civilization, because it is about the short-term interests of a small number of plutocrats over the long-term welfare of this planet and the people who live on it. (Page & Mann, 2019: 5)

This might sound overstated, yet, despite the unprecedented scientific capacity to understand the Earth system, there is enormous disrespect for science, even dismissed as fake news not only by US President Donald Trump but by part of the media. Some of the reasons for this are intimately connected to inequality, particularly in developed countries.

From Life-Support Mechanisms to the Determinants of Civilization

Appreciation that human well-being at the planetary scale is underpinned by ecological *support systems* widened (albeit probably from a very small base) among health workers in the 1960s, at a time of rising awareness of the links between environment and health, led by writers including Rachel Carson, René Dubos, and Frederick Sargent. Planetary consciousness was strongly accelerating because of the space program, including the first photographs of the whole Earth, taken by astronauts orbiting the moon, a dazzling image called "Earthrise."

In 1972, Sargent wrote, in *The American Journal of Public Health*, that "interventions in and manipulations of the processes of the planetary life-support system (ecosystem) have produced a set of complex problems, problems that constitute the essence of human ecology" (Sargent, 1972: 629). McMichael, who led the first Intergovernmental Panel on Climate Change (IPCC) chapter on health, frequently wrote and spoke of eroding *life-support mechanisms.*

Certainly, users of this term, seek to convey a profound risk to human well-being and health. However, although many life forms are in danger, even including through reduced oxygen in the ocean (Breitburg et al., 2018), our species remains overwhelmingly anthropocentric. Might the phrase *civilization-support system* help to motivate us to more effective action to save ourselves, in a way that *life-support system* so far has not?

Many authors from fields outside health have warned of the fragility of modern civilization. However, apart from groups such as the International Physicians for the Prevention of Nuclear War (IPPNW), comparatively few writers with a health background have contributed to these warnings (Benatar, 1998; Butler, 2000, 2016; Hancock, 2011).

If global civilization decays, then so, too, will global health. Despite the lack of official recognition, not only might average life expectancy decline this century, but even the size of the human population may fall, as warned by the simulations of the "Limits to Growth" pioneers (under the "business as usual" scenario) and many authors since, a few of them health based (Butler, 2017).

The Interaction of Environmental Change and Social Responses

Like Albert Schweitzer, the most recent health-related Nobel Peace Laureate, the International Campaign to Abolish Nuclear Weapons (ICAN), has recognized that civilization is in peril. In 1992, the Union of Concerned Scientists coordinated the "World Scientist's Warning to Humanity," signed by more than 1,700 leading scientists (but no public health workers). This warning was repeated in 2017, with far more signatories (including many health workers). In 2018, the *Bulletin of the Atomic Scientists* moved its Doomsday Clock forward to 11.58 pm, reflecting the highest level of concern since 1953.

Climate change is an important constituent of the ecosocial factors that threaten human civilization and thus global health, but it is part of an even bigger syndrome of threats (see Table 21.1). Humans have always been exposed to environmental risk, whether from predatory mammals, floods, or droughts. As humans spread from Africa, they were also exposed to severe cold. Past environmental change has led, via a series of cascades, to the collapse of many empires,

from Sumeria to the Mayans. The collapse of the Western Roman Empire is now thought to have been precipitated, in part, by immense volcanic eruptions in the fifth century depressing crop yields. But such collapses (with rare exceptions, such as the Roman town of Pompeii, buried by volcanic ash) have never been solely the result of the loss of environmental "goods"; social factors are also at play.

In the presence of temporary and moderate resource scarcity, societies may successfully adapt, such as by greater sharing. However, beyond thresholds of scarcity, such cooperation is inevitably stretched and can break down, contributing, for example, to famine and conflict. Today, it is our quasi-global civilization that is at risk not only because of ecological change (a subset of environmental change) but also because of social responses to it (see Table 21.1). Such responses include the chance of a persistent currency crisis that will greatly diminish trade and economic confidence and, even more disturbingly, nuclear war.

In 1987, "Our Common Future" (the Brundtland Report) popularized the term *sustainable development*. Perhaps reflecting good intentions, the term *ecologically* (or *environmentally*) *sustainable development* consequently became popularized in some places. But either descriptor erroneously implies that sustainable development is chiefly an environmental issue. In fact, the Brundtland Report tried to unite the issues of global equity and human development. It pointed out how the poor and disadvantaged need economic opportunity, but without irreparable harm to natural capital, such as from global warming. The framers of the Brundtland Report understood that humans need abundant natural resources to flourish.

Climate Change as an Existential Threat

Human-induced climate change is increasingly recognized as a global crisis, akin to the dangers of the cold war. Although it will have its greatest, and generally earliest, impact on the poorest and most disadvantaged of the world's people, high-income populations are already affected. Examples of the latter include the people in the small Californian city of Paradise (population approximately 30,000), which was largely destroyed by wildfire in 2018, and the deaths, by drowning and starvation, of over 500,000 head of cattle because of an extreme weather event in

Table 21.1 Some of the Main Forms of Harm and Risk to the Global Ecosocial System

Major form of loss or harm	Examples (causes)
Biodiversity	Insects, wild animals, large fish, microbiome, soil erosion, wetland clearance, corals, (population increase, rising affluence, habitat loss, climate change, overfishing)
Pollution	Particulate matter (in air), plastics (ocean and land), "novel entities" (e.g., endocrine disruptors), heavy metals, arsenic and fecal contamination of groundwater and other sources of freshwater, coastal dead zones, marine hypoxia
Climate change (global warming)	Heat waves, stalled weather patterns, waviness of the jet stream, stronger storm winds and surges, droughts, fires, impaired agricultural yields, rising sea levels, coastal retreat, island abandonment, some infectious disease changes, coral loss (fossil fuel use, forest clearing, methane emissions from ruminants)
Resource depletion	Fossil fuel, phosphate, copper, rare earths, aquifers, soil (population increase, rising affluence, technologies)
Adverse social responses, beyond thresholds	Public health and health system breakdown, mass migration and population displacement, conflict, undernutrition, anxiety, famine

Note: The growth in human numbers, ingenuity, and affluence is an underlying cause for all of these forms.

Queensland, Australia, in 2019. In Finnish Lapland, the reindeer that used to keep the Saami alive in winter are now kept alive by the Saami because climate change has reduced access to nutritious lichen (Jaakkola et al., 2018).

"Dangerous" climate change, once suggested as 2 or even 3°C above 1990 levels, now seems more likely to occur at or before 1.5°C above preindustrial levels,[1] a level of heating that the signers of the 2015 Paris Agreement pledged to try to avoid (Hawkins et al., 2017). An increasing number of writers (Knutti et al., 2016; Xu et al., 2018) argue that that level is too risky,

and yet we may reach it by 2030 (Tollefson, 2018).[2] The recent IPCC report on the difference between 1.5 and 2°C of average warming attracted enormous publicity (which is encouraging), but emissions of greenhouse gases continue at a record level. These emissions are still subsidized in many countries; according to researchers at the International Monetary Fund (IMF), global subsidies for fossil fuels exceed 6% of global gross domestic product (GDP; Coady et al., 2017).

If it were to be more widely accepted that climate change has already contributed to the Syrian war (Gleick, 2017), to the rise in global food prices that accompanied the 2010 drought and heat wave in Russia (Wegren, 2011), and the 2018 wildfire season, then the threshold of danger might already be widely seen as having long been exceeded.

However, recognition of the existential risk of climate change among health workers is limited, apart from the period 1989–1993, when the majority of published papers warned of at least one large-scale, potentially devastating consequence such as conflict, famine, or mass migration (Butler, 2018a). In subsequent years, most of the climate and health literature focused on a particular aspect, usually heat, an infectious disease, or another indirect effect, such as allergies.

However, in 2009, a highly cited paper warned that climate change could be the biggest threat to global health in the twenty-first century (Costello et al., 2009). Following its publication, more integrative papers appeared, but they were outnumbered by a large increase in reductionist papers. For the period 2014–2017, the literature was more conservative than in the previous five years, based on a random sample of 5% of the relevant papers identified as published in that period. This reticence cannot be because of evidence suggesting a reduced risk from climate change (there isn't any) but instead suggests a disconnect between the level of risk and its declining appreciation by funders, researchers, reviewers, and most journals (Butler, 2018a).

Climate Change and Global Health

In his inaugural address to staff, Tedros Ghebreyesus, director of the World Health Organization (WHO), identified climate change as one of the top four threats to human health, continuing WHO's long-standing

---

[1] The issue of baseline temperature is inconsistent and confusing.

[2] According to Tollefson (2018), the 2014 IPCC assessment estimated that the world would breach 1.5°C by the early 2020s, if the current rate of emissions continues.

recognition of this issue. The most obvious ways by which climate change will harm health (*primary* effects) are through heat stress, extreme weather events (not only from heat waves but also from stronger storms and intensified droughts, floods, and rainstorms), and changes in the distribution of vectors (e.g., mosquitoes and ticks) and other effects on infectious disease epidemiology (Butler, 2018a; Haines & Ebi, 2019). Other indirect (*secondary* effects) include reduced food diversity, diminished micronutrient concentrations in crops (owing to higher carbon dioxide levels), allergies, and cardiorespiratory and neurologic effects, such as from worsened tropospheric air pollution, or from climate change–aggravated fires and effects on some chronic diseases, such as cardiac failure and diabetes.

However, as long recognized by a minority of health workers, climate change threatens to act as a *risk multiplier* for *tertiary* impacts, which can affect millions or even hundreds of millions of people simultaneously (Haines et al., 1993). Such effects include rising food prices, famine, conflict, and mass migration (Butler, 2018a). In turn, enough of these tertiary effects may contribute to the collapse of civilization.

Heat and Climate Change

For decades, there has been appreciation that excessive heat, especially in humid settings, where the capacity of sweating to reduce heat loss is lowered, can cause fatal heat stroke. This is, for example, well recognized in military settings, where otherwise fit young men sometimes die suddenly while engaged in strenuous weight-bearing training exercises. Excess heat exposure has many other dangers, especially for the poor, the elderly, and those with chronic diseases. In hot settings, such as India, laborers face a stark choice between income and health (Sett & Sahu, 2014). Kidney stones and renal impairment are common in some hot work settings, aggravated by limited water access. The sudden death of construction workers in the Middle East has been linked to excess heat and insufficient water (Acharya et al., 2018). A lack of toilets, especially for women, may lead to deliberately reduced fluid intake in hot weather, contributing to renal disease, urinary infections, and perhaps hypertension (Venugopal et al., 2016). A raised body temperature slows nerve conduction and worsens the symptoms of multiple sclerosis and perhaps other neurologic diseases (Dutta et al., 2015). Excessive heat may impair cognition (Wallace et al.,

2016) and thus learning, adding another causal layer to the perpetuation of poverty in many developing countries. Finally, excessive heat exposure interferes with sleep and exacerbates chronic diseases such as cardiac failure (Tait et al., 2018).

Infectious Diseases and Climate Change

Many infectious diseases are sensitive to climatic conditions. In warmer conditions, bacteria in food and nutrient-loaded water multiply. Studies in the United Kingdom, Australia, and Canada have shown a clear relationship between short-term higher temperature and the rate of occurrence of *Salmonella* food poisoning. Changes in rainfall patterns affect river flows, flooding, sanitary conditions, and the spread of diarrheal diseases, including cholera. Many vector-borne infections, transmitted by mosquitoes, other insects, or rodents, are sensitive to temperature, rainfall, humidity, and wind. As temperature rises, infectious agents within mosquitoes (e.g., the protozoan parasite *Plasmodium falciparum* and dengue virus) mature more quickly, whereas mosquitoes reproduce more efficiently and must feed (blood meal) more often. Surface water patterns influence mosquito breeding, and humidity affects mosquito survival. Many zoonotic infectious diseases that spill over into human populations from animal sources are influenced by eco-climate-related changes affecting the density and movement of *reservoir* animal species and, sometimes, the chance of human contact (see Table 21.2).

Health Effects of Social and Cultural Disruption

Around one-fifth of the world's population lives in coastal areas affected by rising seas and natural disasters – especially those living in major river deltas (e.g., Bangladesh, Egypt), parts of Central America, eastern China and India, and many small island states. Populations in the Maldives, Tuvalu, Kiribati, and parts of the Caribbean face the risk of whole-nation displacement.

The World Bank has recently increased its projection of displaced people from climate change (without dramatic action) to affect over 100 million by 2050 (Rigaud et al., 2018). The mental health consequences of these social and cultural disruptions, and of associated perceptions of future threats, pose an increasingly important risk to health. This may apply

Table 21.2 Important Characteristics of Significant Zoonotic[a] and Vector-Borne Diseases

Pathogen/ disease	Animal host/ vector (postulated ecosocial cofactor)	Regions affected
Dengue	Humans, *Aedes* mosquitoes	Widespread tropical
Ebola	Nonhuman primates[b]/bats[b] (palm oil plantations[?], conflict)	Central and West Africa
Malaria	Humans[c]/ *Anopheles* mosquitoes	Widespread, with highland expansion (e.g., Ethiopia, Colombia)
Ross River virus	Kangaroos/*Culex mosquitoes*	Australia
Tick-borne encephalitis	Rodents, deer/ ticks[d]	Northern Europe
West Nile fever	Birds/*Culex* mosquitoes	North America, Europe, Africa
Yellow fever	Primates/*Aedes* mosquitoes[d]	Africa, South America, not Asia
Zika	Primates/*Aedes*	Widespread in tropics

[a]Definitions of zoonoses vary in the literature. The only animal reservoir for dengue and most forms of malaria is human; these are generally called anthroponoses.

[b]Putative.

[c]Only human reservoir for most kinds.

[d]Proven human vaccine.

particularly to children. Long-standing expectations, at least in higher-income countries, of continued material gains and ever-improving conditions of life should now be superseded by an understanding that the environmental and social consequences of climate change associated with endless consumption cannot be ignored.

Intergenerational Inequity

Climate change also raises stark issues of intergenerational injustice. Some deleterious health effects of past industrialization are being experienced today (e.g., environmental lead and asbestos exposures). Greenhouse gases (GHGs) started to rise at the start of industrialization, but even though their theoretical effect on the climate was suggested in the nineteenth century, widespread understanding of the scale and risk of GHG-related climate change is more recent. The impacts of past and continuing climate change will be increasingly felt in the future. Because of their immature organ systems, neurobiology, and dependence on caregivers, children are particularly susceptible to heat stress, gastroenteritis, and natural disasters, as well as to family stresses linked to droughts, loss of livelihood, and familial dislocation – and these will have long-term health consequences for many children (Strazdins et al., 2011).

Complacency on the Upper Decks of the Human *Titanic* – and Its Reasons

Despite the evidence, humanity remains largely calm. It is as if most of us are enjoying dinner on the "human *Titanic*," not yet conscious of the consternation on the face of the lookout. A goal of this chapter is to convince uncertain readers to act in ways that might nudge our home vessel away from the iceberg. Although millions of people now sense our collective danger, our number is still too small to persuade those who control civilization's course to alter it. But the number is growing, including school children. If there really is a *noosphere*, a form of planetary consciousness, then one would expect children to be at its vanguard. But, while one such schoolchild, 16-year-old Greta Thunberg, spoke at the World Economic Summit in Davos, Switzerland, in January 2019, we do not yet know if those with real economic power paid attention. If they didn't, it could be because they have already abandoned ship, in their minds.

I first published the idea of the *Titanic* as an analogy to civilization in 2000 (Butler, 2000), arguing that the inequality evident on the White Star liner and the "gilded age" to which some of its most illustrious passengers belonged has lessons for today. When the *Titanic* sank, survival of children in steerage (the lowest deck) was far lower than that from its upper decks.

There are many reasons for the failure of most of humanity to act to solve climate change and its allied environmental ills. To start, almost 1 billion people are counted as undernourished in macronutrient terms (i.e., protein and/or calories). Up to an additional 2 billion people are chronically deficient in micronutrients, especially iron and zinc. The cognitive capacity of undernourished people is generally harmed, meaning that even if they are aware that climate change is occurring, they are very unlikely to have access to effective methods to reduce it. This population (the third and fourth global *clastes*; Butler, 2000) is also the most vulnerable to climate change and its associated threats.

Another reason that has been advanced is that few humans, even if adequately nourished, are scientifically literate, and thus they fail to understand (focusing on climate change) how increased concentrations of trace molecules in the atmosphere can trap heat. However, few humans understand the laws of flight or how electricity works; this lack of comprehension does not prevent millions of people, every day (mostly from the first and second clastes), from switching on a reading light at an altitude of 30,000 feet. Nonetheless, the concept that humans are now akin to a great natural force, able to even defer the next glacial period or trigger a new geologic era (the Anthropocene), may be too subtle for many people to grasp, even if they are well nourished and literate (Butler et al., 2014). After all, humanity had trouble accepting heliocentrism and evolution. Today, most people in the world follow one of the great faiths. Although (for example) His Holiness Pope Francis has called for humans to contribute to planetary stewardship, it must be cognitively difficult for most people of faith, who literally believe in an afterlife, to act in this life in ways that reduce their level of consumption of climate-harming goods and services, although some steps, such as reduced meat eating, are feasible and have definite health benefits.

Unlike many scientific insights, climate change (and some other aspects of limits to growth) has been, for decades, the subject of sophisticated and well-funded propaganda campaigns designed to vilify and discredit climate scientists and to confuse the public, raising doubt and delaying effective action. Five years after the release of the Brundtland Report, the US government, led by President George W. Bush, actively worked to undermine the effectiveness of the Earth Summit held in Rio de Janeiro, Brazil. Bush, for example, stated: "The American way of life is not up for negotiations. Period." Reflecting on this summit, Sir Geoffrey Palmer, a former New Zealand minister for the environment and prime minister, noted:

> Twenty years after Stockholm, we are deeper in the mire and no closer to getting out. The biggest diplomatic gathering in the history of the world, which more world leaders attended than any international conference before, did not summon up the collective political resolve necessary to deal with the global environmental challenge. Progress was, simply, insufficient, due to a general failure of political will. Rio produced too little, too late. … We have had plenty of rhetoric-the time for rhetoric is past. The time for binding international instruments that actually produce change has arrived.*(Palmer, 1992: 1028)*

It is now 27 years since the Rio summit and 22 years since the Kyoto Protocol was signed, the first international treaty intended to curb global heating and climate disruption. In 1987, the year of the Brundtland Report, the atmospheric level of the main GHG, carbon dioxide (CO_2), averaged 349 parts per million (ppm), having risen from approximately 280 ppm in the preceding two centuries as a result of the burning of fossil fuels (coal, oil, and gas), the clearing of forests, and the expansion of animal farming, especially of cattle. In 2018, CO_2 provisionally averaged 409 ppm, more than 2.25 ppm higher than 12 months earlier. The anthropogenic increment to the level of average global CO_2 has more than doubled since the Brundtland Report, and its rate of increase is rising still.

CO_2 is not the only important GHG; levels of methane (CH_4) and nitrous oxide (N_2O) are also rising. There is increasing evidence of adverse feedback effects, by which global heating triggers additional GHG release, such as methane or through forest or peat fires, potentially leading to runaway warming and a "hothouse" Earth (Steffen et al., 2018). Most excess heat is stored in the ocean, reducing (so far) the severity of heat waves, but a warmer ocean changes the climate on land in many ways, including through more intense rainfall and expanded oceanic volume. The polar ice is melting, and sea levels rising at accelerating rates. The strength of the carbon sink in the ocean is also weakening. If this effect intensifies, it is likely to accelerate warming of the atmosphere, ocean, and land.

Reasons for Our Danger, Including Global Inequality

A major reason for the campaigns of misinformation that impede effective climate change action is that the erosion of environmental goods (*natural capital*) has helped to make possible the enjoyment of living standards, for many, that were recently undreamed of, even by emperors. Humans have been seduced by the sight and taste of impending cornucopia, the horn of plenty, an ancient image in Greek mythology. Humans, part of the animal kingdom, aspire to be God-like. This longing for abundance is perhaps encoded in our DNA, but it now threatens our collective existence. It is very seductive for most of those with a high environmental footprint (including a high carbon footprint) to underestimate the harm that our everyday actions impose, both cumulatively and collectively. Our cognitive dissonance and denial allow us to continue our daily tasks, perhaps with slight adjustments, but mostly with a clear conscience.

The aviation industry is a major contributor to global warming, not only through fossil fuel combustion but also via contrails and land-use changes for airports. Climate scientists and climate policymakers make a disproportionate contribution to global warming; with few exceptions, they, too, seem to rationalize this behavior. Aviation tycoon Richard Branson is well aware of climate change. In 2017, Necker Island, his 30-hectare Caribbean haven, was in the path of Hurricane Irma, which devastated it. Branson has invested in biofuels as a way to keep flying without harming the climate; however, the *net energy* of biofuels (the usable energy available after their production) approximates the energy used to create them. In other words, without extraordinary technological breakthroughs, biofueled planes will not slow global warming.

However, no one died on Necker Island, unlike on the American protectorate of Puerto Rico, which soon after was ravaged by Hurricane Maria, which crippled its already fragile and damaged infrastructure (especially its electrical power), ultimately leading to about 4,000 excess deaths over the next few months (Kishore et al., 2018). Most of the houses and wineries that were burned in the 2017 Napa Valley fire in California are likely to have been insured, but the poor living in nearby trailer homes are less likely to have been. As climate change deepens, however, insurance companies are likely to become increasingly resistant to insuring for climate change–related disasters, such as from fires, flooding, and storm surges.

Many right-wing think tanks completely dismiss the risks of climate change. Notoriously, US President Donald Trump claims climate change as a Chinese hoax. Brazilian President Bolsonaro wants to accelerate the clearing of the Amazon rain forest, a major regulator of climate change, as well as

a reservoir of biodiversity and home for Indigenous people.

Yet the problem is not confined to right-wing politicians and their advisors. Scientists display *scientific reticence*, hiding the worst consequences (or even the worst fraction of consequences) from themselves and from their audience. "Crying wolf" is viewed as unscientific and discouraged, even though worst-case scenarios are commonly used as tools for leverage by agents of the powerful, such as to justify bank bailouts, increase military spending, or launch invasions. Funding for the military-industrial complex rarely challenges the income, status, or influence of those with the greatest wealth.

Although the IPCC is often accused of being alarmist, many of the models it relies on are conservative (optimistic). For example, panel members ignore the possibility of GHG accelerating feedbacks such as from melting tundra or burning peat. The melting of sea-level ice, from both Antarctica and Greenland, is far faster than IPCC reports have anticipated. The Gulf stream is weakening as the North Atlantic freshens. This weakness, if it persists, places much of Western Europe at risk of paradoxical cooling. This possibility is also absent from IPCC models.

William Nordhaus and Ecological Economics

William Nordhaus, a corecipient of the 2018 Nobel Prize in Economics, has long accepted the reality of climate change and was probably the first prominent nonecological economist to publish prolifically on this subject. In his early career, Nordhaus was dismissive of the "Limits to Growth" study, using arguments convincingly refuted by Ugo Bardi, who showed that Nordhaus then had a poor understanding of complex systems (Bardi, 2018). But Nordhaus has been extremely influential, even being credited as key in delaying the *precautionary principle*, allegedly because he argued that economic growth will offset considerable harm from climate change (Cho, 2018). In the early 1990s, a time when serious action to slow climate change may have bought humanity valuable breathing space (which would be greatly appreciated today), Nordhaus reportedly claimed that 3°C of warming was an acceptable tradeoff, leaving climate change as technologically manageable (Cho, 2018).

In researching this chapter, I read a paper Nordhaus published in 1993 (Nordhaus, 1993).

Although it is technologically optimistic, even then, Nordhaus was well aware of the potential for catastrophic surprise arising from climate change. He wrote:

> Scientists raise the specter of shifting currents turning Europe into Alaska, of mid-continental drying transforming grain belts into deserts, of great rivers drying up as snow packs disappear, of severe storms wiping out whole populations of low-lying regions, of surging ice sheets raising ocean levels by 20 to 50 feet, of northward migration of old or new tropical pests and diseases decimating the temperature regions, of environmentally induced migration overrunning borders in search of livable land. Given the potential for catastrophic surprises, perhaps we should conclude that the major concern lies in the uncertainties and imponderable impacts of climate change rather than in the smooth changes foreseen by the global models.   *(Nordhaus, 1993: 23)*

At least in this paper, Nordhaus does not state a view that 3°C of warming is acceptable, though he does report a survey in which "experts" were asked to estimate lost income for scenarios of both 3 and 6°C warming, an exercise in hubris, at least with hindsight. His paper ends philosophically, devolving the responsibility of what is acceptable to leaders, presumably including President Bush, whose opposition to meaningful action to protect Earth was already then clear.

While it is tempting to single out Nordhaus as the culprit for slowing action on climate change, it may be more accurate to ascribe his prominence as arising because he seemed a considered voice, aware of the risks of climate change, technologically optimistic, but one whose research could be used, at the highest level, to justify inaction. Had Nordhaus been more strident in sounding a warning, he would probably have been ignored, the fate of the Club of Rome (which commissioned the "Limits to Growth") and the discipline of ecological economics (economics as if the Earth matters).

Ecological economics, to which Nordhaus was (and may still be) opposed, was well established by the time of the Earth Summit, pioneered by figures such as Kenneth Boulding, E. F. Schumacher, and Herman Daly. Unlike Nordhaus, its recommendations did threaten vested interests and were thus ignored by most governments, although they had some influence in the 1960s and 1970s, including on assassinated US presidential candidate Bobby Kennedy and (still-living) US President Jimmy Carter. To date, no ecological economist has been recognized by the Royal Swedish Academy.

The Most Recent Rise of Inequality

I was born within a decade of World War II, in a period sometimes called the "great compression" (Goldin & Margo, 1992: 1). In this time, in most Western countries, the wages of the working and middle class increased, including as a proportion. Substantial inheritance taxes were expected, and even bankers and executives practiced self-restraint (Krugman, 2002). In the United States, the world's richest country, unrestrained capitalism was kept partly in check by the still raw, recent memory of the Great Depression (Butler, 2000). It was also a time when the great project of the United Nations was taken seriously, at least by three Western nuclear states, France, the United Kingdom, and the United States. It was also a time of decolonization and a pledge, made in 1969 at a conference chaired by Canadian Prime Minister and Nobel Peace Laureate Lester Pearson, by developed countries to provide 0.7% of their GDP as aid.

For people of my age, living in the West, it thus once seemed normal, even sensible, to perceive social justice and health for all as plausible aspirations. But the declaration of "Health for All" in 1978 can now be seen as a transient crest in the long struggle for an enduring global civilization. Since then, the trajectory has been downhill, now steeply.

Today, in countries from Mexico to Russia, hundreds of billionaires exist, many taking advantage of new rules that have made wealth accumulation easier. In supposedly democratic countries, inequality has been facilitated by the "wealth dynasty defense industry," accountants and lawyers who seek to evade the spirit of tax laws. Partly as a result, as few as eight people (six of them American) now own the same wealth as half the world's population (Oxfam, 2017).

Rigging the System

Billionaires and their agents have systematically lobbied for rules to facilitate increased inequality. For years, Citigroup and other players in the financial services industry fought for the reversal of legislation introduced by former US President Franklin Roosevelt restricting the capacity of US banks to speculate in order to lessen the chance of another Great Depression. Then newly elected US President Clinton acceded to this pressure, overseeing passage of the Glass-Steagall Act (1993), further fueling inequality and a key step in incubating the 2008 global financial crisis. In 2017, the government of US President Trump enabled legislation to exempt the first US$22.4 million gifted from parents to children from the estate tax.

This pattern of the wealthy rigging the system to promote inequality has many names, including the *law of increasing returns*, the *Matthew effect*, and *he who has, gets*. The perpetuation and deepening of inequality have many social cofactors and many subtle elements, from the effective theft of cognitive potential from the poor through means such as undernutrition, disease, and inadequate schooling to epigenetic factors associated with poverty and many forms of environmental pollution.

Branko Milanovic, a leading inequality analyst, argues that global inequality has declined slightly in recent years, even as domestic inequality has increased in some countries (Milanovic, 2013). This is plausible because an increasing fraction of the population in the Global South has escaped the most abject poverty, especially in China. But even this analysis concedes that global income inequality is more extreme than in any single nation. That is, the majority of the global population has almost no political or economic power.

Increasing domestic inequality in many high-income countries, especially in the United States, has also contributed to delayed action on climate policy. For example, in the United States, where inequality has been rising for decades, a poorly educated, socially excluded working class can easily succumb to allegations that climate change is "fake news," in turn, supporting the climate views of President Trump.

The nexus between inequality and climate change operates in many ways (see Figure 21.1). When inequality becomes excessive, corrective measures occur, such as revolutions and, perhaps, catastrophes. Occasionally, societies may voluntarily reduce extreme inequality; examples include Roosevelt's New Deal (which triggered the start of the "Great Compression") and the British response to the French Revolution. One way that global inequality could be reduced is via the failure of civilization, fueled, in part, by climate change, by human-driven global warming.

Conclusion

Adverse global environmental change is the stepchild of inequality and human ingenuity. Humans are an animal species engaged in competition not only with other species but also with fellow humans. At the close of World War II, statesmanship generated the United

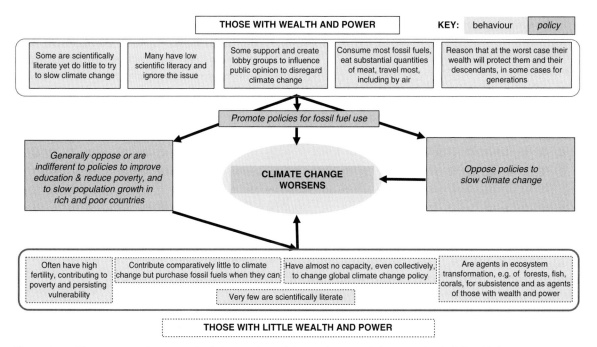

Figure 21.1. There are many dimensions that link inequality and climate change, including via policy, belief, and behavior.

Nations, the WHO, and the Universal Declaration of Human Rights at a time when civilization seemed young again. But we are forgetting that collective wisdom. Too many of the generation in power seem indifferent to the lessons that the postwar leaders learned through the suffering of their populations. Instead of collective good, too many seek national gain. Humans, the product of evolution, now have the capacity to provide unprecedented levels of abundance for billions of people. However, collectively, we are unable to slow the assault on nature; it is as if we are severing the limb of the tree on which we sit. Very few human groups voluntarily cede power or resources to another human group. Although humans cooperate in large groups, including multinational military alliances, "fear of the other" continually inhibits the cooperation that is needed for us to live within planetary limits (Butler, 2018b; Butler et al., 2019).

Most scientists, grant makers, and policymakers remain blind to the severity and intractability of the risks described in this chapter. Excessive faith is placed in technological solutions, such as vaccines, biomass energy, and carbon capture and storage (Butler, 2019). Yet, when seemingly miraculous technologies do appear, such as photovoltaic cells, their rollout is slowed in too many places by the lingering power of the fossil fuel industry, allied with the inertia of too many old men who do not conceive that they, or even their grandchildren, may inherit an unlivable, desolate, hothouse.

It is customary, when writing of these issues, to give hope. There is some. The most industrialized country in Europe, Germany, announced in 2019 its decision to eliminate coal-fired electricity by 2038. Los Angeles wants to reach this goal by 2025. The school strike started by Thunberg has reached many wealthy countries. "Extinction Rebellion" demonstrations slow traffic in British cities. The next generation is acting to try to save itself in ways that my generation failed. These steps are encouraging. At best, sufficient advanced knowledge will survive to enable our descendants to rebuild a wiser, fairer, and more sustainable civilization.

References

Acharya, P., Boggess, B., & Zhang, K. (2018). Assessing heat stress and health among construction workers in a changing climate: a review. *International Journal of Environmental Research and Public Health* **15**, 247.

Bardi, U. (2018). Why economists can't understand complex systems: not even the Nobel Prize, William

Nordhaus. Cassandra's Legacy. Available at https://cassandralegacy.blogspot.com/2018/10/why-economists-cant-understand-complex.html (accessed February 28, 2019).

Benatar, S. R. (1998). Global disparities in health and human rights: a critical commentary. *American Journal of Public Health* **88**, 295–300.

Breitburg, D., Levin, L. A., Oschlies, A., et al. (2018). Declining oxygen in the global ocean and coastal waters. *Science* **359**, eaam7240.

Butler, C. D. (2000). Inequality, global change and the sustainability of civilisation. *Global Change and Human Health* **1**, 156–172.

Butler, C. D. (2016). Sounding the alarm: health in the Anthropocene. *International Journal of Environmental Research and Public Health* **13**, 665.

Butler, C. D. (2017). Limits to growth, planetary boundaries, and planetary health. *Current Opinion in Environmental Sustainability* **25**, 59–65.

Butler, C. D. (2018a). Climate change, health and existential risks to civilization: a comprehensive review (1989–2013). *International Journal of Environmental Research and Public Health* **15**, 2266.

Butler, C. D. (2018b). Planetary epidemiology: towards first principles *Current Environmental Reports* **5** 418–429.

Butler, C. D. (2019). Philanthrocapitalism: promoting global health but failing planetary health. *Challenges* **10**, 24.

Butler, C. D., Bowles, D. C., McIver, L., et al. (2014). Mental health, cognition and the challenge of climate change, in Butler, C. D. (ed.), *Climate Change and Global Health*. Wallingford, UK: CABI, pp. 251–259.

Butler, C. D., Higgs, K., & McFarlane, R. A. (2019). Environmental health, planetary boundaries and Limits to Growth, in Nriagu, J. (ed.), *Encyclopedia of Environmental Health*. Amsterdam: Elsevier, pp. 533–543.

Cho, A. (2018). Nobel Prize for the economics of innovation and climate change stirs controversy. *Science* **10**, 986 . Available at www.sciencemag.org/news/2018/10/roles-ideas-and-climate-growth-earn-duo-economics-nobel-prize?r3f_986=https://www.google.com/ (accessed February 28, 2019).

Coady, D., Parry, A., Sears, L., et al. (2017). How large are global fossil fuel subsidies? *World Development* **91**, 11–27.

Costello, A., Abbas, M., Allen, A., et al. (2009). Managing the health effects of climate change. *Lancet* **373**, 1693–1733.

Dutta, P., Rajiva, A., Andhare, D., et al. (2015). Perceived heat stress and health effects on construction workers. *Indian Journal of Occupational and Environmental Medicine* **19**, 151–158.

Gleick, P. H. (2017). Climate, water, and conflict: commentary on Selby et al. 2017. *Political Geography* **60**, 248–250.

Goldin, C., & Margo, R. A. (1992). The Great Compression: the wage structure in the United States at mid-century. *Quarterly Journal of Economics* **107**, 1–34.

Hackett, R. (2019). Noam Chomsky: "In a couple of generations, organized human society may not survive." *National Observer (Canada)*, February 12. Available at www.nationalobserver.com/2019/02/12/features/noam-chomsky-couple-generations-organized-human-society-may-not-survive-has-be (accessed February 28, 2019).

Haines, A., & Ebi, K. (2019). The imperative for climate action to protect health. *New England Journal of Medicine* **380**, 263–273.

Haines, A., Epstein, P. R., & McMichael, A. J. (1993). Global health watch: monitoring impacts of environmental change. *Lancet* **342**, 1464–1469.

Hancock, T. (2011). It's the environment, stupid! Declining ecosystem health is THE threat to health in the 21st century. *Health Promotion International* **26**(S2), 168–172.

Hawkins, E., Ortega, P., Suckling, E., et al. (2017). Estimating changes in global temperature since the pre-industrial period. *Bulletin of the American Meteorological Society* **September**, 1841–1856.

Jaakkola, J. J. K., Juntunen, S., & Näkkäläjärvi, K. (2018). The holistic effects of climate change on the culture, well-being, and health of the Saami, the only Indigenous people in the European Union. *Current Environmental Health Reports* **5**, 401–417.

Kishore, N., Marqués, D., Mahmud, A., et al. (2018). Mortality in Puerto Rico after Hurricane Maria. *New England Journal of Medicine* **379**, 162–170.

Knutti, R., Rogelj, J., Sedláček, J., et al. (2016). A scientific critique of the two-degree climate change target. *Nature Geoscience* **9**, 13–18.

Krugman, P. (2002). For Richer. *New York Times*, October 20. Available at www.nytimes.com/2002/10/20/magazine/20INEQUALITY.html?ex=1036790476&ei=1&en=6ea98b6c61d57124 (accessed February 28, 2019).

Milanovic, B. (2013). Global Income Inequality in numbers: in history and now. *Global Policy* **4**, 198–208.

Nordhaus, W. D. (1993). Reflections on the economics of climate change. *Journal of Economic Perspectives* **7**, 11–25.

Oxfam (2017). Just 8 men own same wealth as half the world. Available at www.oxfam.org/en/pressroom/pressreleases/2017-01-16/just-8-men-own-same-wealth-half-world (accessed February 28, 2019).

Page, S., & Mann, M. E. (2019). The most villainous act in the history of human civilisation. *Cosmos*. Available at https://cosmosmagazine.com/climate/the-most-villainous-act-in-the-history-of-human-civilisation-tyler-prize-winner-michael-e-mann-speaks-out (accessed February 28, 2019).

Palmer, G. (1992). Earth Summit: what went wrong at Rio. *Washington University Law Quarterly* **70**, 1005–1028.

Read, R. (2018). This civilisation is finished: so what is to be done? (IFLAS Occasional Paper 3). Available at www.youtube.com/watch?v=uzCxFPzdO0Y (accessed February 28, 2019).

Rigaud, K. K., de Sherbinin, A., Jones, B., et al. (2018). *Groundswell: Preparing for Internal Climate Migration.* Washington, DC: World Bank.

Sargent, F. (1972). Man–environment: problems for public health. *American Journal of Public Health* **62**, 628–633.

Sett, M., & Sahu, S. (2014). Effects of occupational heat exposure on female brick workers in West Bengal, India. *Global Health Action* **7**, 219–223.

Steffen, W., Richardson, K., Rockström, J., et al. (2015). Planetary boundaries: guiding human development on a changing planet. *Science* **347**, 736–746.

Steffen, W., Rockström, J., Richardson, K., et al. (2018). Trajectories of the Earth system in the Anthropocene. *Proceedings of the National Academy of Sciences USA* **115**, 8252–8259.

Strazdins, L., Friel, S., McMichael, A. J., et al. (2011). Climate change and children's health: likely futures, new inequities? *International Public Health Journal* **2**, 493–500.

Tait, P. W., Allan, S., & Katelaris, A. L. (2018). Preventing heat-related disease in general practice. *Australian Journal of General Practice* **47**, 835–840.

Tollefson, J. (2018). IPCC says limiting global warming to 1.5°C will require drastic action. *Nature* **562**, 172–173.

Venugopal, V., Rekha, S., Manikandan, K., et al. (2016). Heat stress and inadequate sanitary facilities at workplaces: an occupational health concern for women? *Global Health Action* **9**, 31945.

Wallace, P. J., Mckinlay, B. J., Coletta, N. A., et al. (2016). Effects of motivational self-talk on endurance and cognitive performance in the heat. *Medicine & Science in Sports & Exercise* **48**, 191–199.

Wallace-Wells, D. (2019). Time to panic. *New York Times*, February 16. Available at www.nytimes.com/2019/02/16/opinion/sunday/fear-panic-climate-change-warming.html (accessed February 28, 2019).

Wegren, S. K. (2011). Food security and Russia's 2010 drought. *Eurasian Geography and Economics* **52**, 140–156.

Xu, Y., Ramanathan, V., & Victor, D. G. (2018). Global warming will happen faster than we think. *Nature* **564**, 30–32.

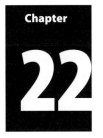

Chapter 22

Mass Migration and Health in the Anthropocene Epoch

Christine Straehle

Introduction

In a piece published in *The Atlantic* in December 1994, the authors discuss Jean Raspail's novel *The Camp of the Saints*, published in 1973. The novel depicts a dystopian future in which migrants from poor countries arrive on the shore of rich Europe:

> Now, stretching over that empty sea, aground some fifty yards out, [lay] the incredible fleet from the other side of the globe, the rusty, creaking fleet that the old professor had been eyeing since morning . . . . He pressed his eye to the glass, and the first things he saw were arms . . . . Then he started to count. Calm and unhurried. But it was like trying to count all the trees in the forest, those arms raised high in the air, waving and shaking together, all outstretched toward the nearby shore. Scraggy branches, brown and black, quickened by a breath of hope. All bare, those flesh-less Gandhi-arms . . . thirty thousand creatures on a single ship![1]

The protagonist in the novel observes the black name-less mass on the horizon waiting to come ashore. In the 1994 piece, the authors warned that unless the causes for migration were taken seriously as a *global* challenge, the dystopia would become true. Twenty-five years later, the figures speak for themselves: 272 million people were estimated to be migrants in 2019, up from 258 million in 2017, up from 248 million in 2015, 220 million in 2010, 191 million in 2005, and 173 million in 2000.[2] Migration is one of the most pressing issues of our times. Arguably the second most pressing issue is climate change. And, indeed, the two are connected.

In this vein, consider the 2016 United Nations Global Compact for Refugees, which departs from the standard definition of refugees as those who face persecution for reasons of ethnic, religious, or national persecution. Instead, the authors of the compact acknowledge that "while not in themselves causes of refugee movements, climate, environmental degradation and natural disasters increasingly interact with the drivers of refugee movements" (United Nations High Commissioner for Refugees [UNHCR], 2016: 2). Similar mention of climate-induced migration can be found in the 2015 UN Paris Agreement, where the authors mention climate and migration in the preamble and in the goal to protect people and foster resilient communities. This should be taken as a clear signal that the Anthropocene epoch is no longer simply a description of a historical epoch or one that causes environmental concerns; instead, the Anthropocene is now accepted as the background that defines specific ethical challenges and a context that adds to the specific challenges that migration poses for the international order of nation-states.

Definitions of what we mean by the Anthropocene vary. For instance, the *Oxford English Dictionary* defines the term rather neutrally as "[t]he epoch of geological time during which human activity is considered to be the dominant influence on the environment, climate, and ecology of the earth, a formal chrono-stratigraphic unit with a base which has been tentatively defined as the mid-twentieth century."

Among many geoscientists and natural scientists, however, the time of the Anthropocene is now strongly linked to changes in weather and climate that may make human life in some parts of the world difficult or impossible (for an overview, see Revkin [2011] and *The Economist* [2011]). What concerns me here is that some of the developments brought about by human activity are billed as responsible for driving many people, especially in agricultural areas, from their land toward unregulated slums

---

[1] www.theatlantic.com/past/politics/immigrat/kennf.htm.
[2] Figures from https://migrationdataportal.org/sites/default/files/2019-10/key-global-migration-figures.pdf; www.un.org.

growing in urban centers. As I will explain below, this raises moral as well as practical concerns. Morally, the question is what is owed to those who are forced to leave their homelands behind. Practically, we need to think about how to deal with the specific challenge of unregulated climate-induced migration nationally and internationally. In this instance, the Anthropocene epoch is associated with "(1) an increase in the intensity and frequency of extreme weather events and climate-related disasters; (2) loss of arable and habitable land, such as people who lose island habitats or coastal or riverine terrestrial land due to sea-level rise; and (3) adverse impacts on eco-systems that are important sources of amenity and livelihood, including land degradation, declining abundance of fish, erosion of river banks and beaches, declining freshwater availability, and coral degrad-ation" (McMichael, 2015: 548).

In what follows, I will refer to such developments when employing the term *Anthropocene*. I will join those who use it as shorthand to describe the slowly deteriorating living conditions for many inhabitants of the Earth.

At the same time as individuals flee degraded and unlivable conditions in their homelands, the govern-ments in safer countries have fine-tuned their legal instruments to enforce the protection of their bor-ders. Australia, Canada, the United States, and the European Union have made it clear that they intend to screen those who arrive to their territories to claim asylum. Many states have adopted policies of deterrence and *nonentrée* to prevent entry, that is, policies and measures that prevent individuals from entering the territory of signatory states in the first place. Hence, we can witness the Italian coastguard patrolling the Mediterranean, supplying nongovern-mental organization (NGO)–run boats in the same waters, only to ensure that their passengers do not set foot on Italian soil (see *The Guardian*, February 14, 2019). Similarly, the European Union has entered into agreements with Libya and Turkey for the latter to protect the land borders of the European Union, at times in blatant disregard for the demands of human rights.

Once in the territory of asylum states or in the care of an international organization with which they can lodge their request for asylum, individual asylum seekers are protected against being sent straight back to their country of origin by the Geneva Convention and the principle of *nonrefoulement* therein enshrined.

According to Article 33(1) of the 1951 Convention, "No Contracting State shall expel or return (*refouler*) a refugee in any manner whatsoever to the frontiers of the territories where his life or freedom would be threatened on account of his race, religion, nationality, membership of a particular social group or political opinion."

Instead of being sent back, asylum seekers should be provided with basic healthcare: they are checked for communicable diseases and provided with medi-cation and emergency care to address urgent health needs, if necessary. The UNHCR states in its *Global Strategy for Public Health Report* (UNHCR, 2014b: 4) the vision that "all refugees are able to fulfill their rights in accessing life-saving and essential health care, HIV prevention, protection and treatment, reproductive health services, food security and nutri-tion, and water, sanitation and hygiene services."

Amid the current discussion of migration, and against the background of policies of *nonentrée* that make it almost impossible to reach the shores of rich states, more and more voices demand that the needs of those displaced by the effects of climate change should be considered on par with traditional asylum seekers who fall under the protection of the Geneva Convention. Therein, a refugee is identified as a person who "owing to a well-founded fear of being persecuted for reasons of race, religion, nationality, membership of a particular social group or political opinion, is outside the country of his nationality and is unable or, owing to such fear, is unwilling to avail himself of the protection of that country; or who, not having a nationality and being outside the country of his former habitual residence, is unable or, owing to such fear, is unwilling to return to it" (Geneva Convention, 1951, Article 1(A)II).

Philosophers, in calling for environmental migrants to be considered in need of asylum and refuge, argue that they resemble politically and religiously persecuted individuals who have lost access to the protection of their original state because the state of origin either cannot or will not protect them (Nine, 2010; see also Kolers, 2012; Risse, 2009). Others have established the normative framework that justifies taking the effects of the Anthropocene as a valid reason for protection (Lister, 2014). Should the international community expand the traditional definition of a refugee?

In this chapter, I tackle this question through the lens of health. In particular, I argue that all migrants should be able to access vitally necessary health resources. This is simply a demand of the protection guaranteed in the context of human rights. In earlier work, I argued that a prudential approach to public health warrants extensive access to health, even for irregular migrants, to stem possible public health emergencies that arise when migrants fall through the cracks of the health provision system (Straehle, 2019). Here I want to focus on the human rights aspect of health provision (see also Klingler et al,, 2018). But what should count as the vitally necessary health resources I just demanded? A growing number of health justice theorists have discussed different measures to define what kind of health resources are needed in a justice context, whether this should include specialized and potentially expensive treatments such as renal analysis and heart surgery, or whether the threshold of vital necessity should be set lower. I won't take a position in this debate here, but suffice to say that climate-induced migrants should be protected at least against the health risks that are due to the specific threat of climate change and the risks that are associated with climate-induced migration. I discuss four different sets of risks in the latter category below.

In this vein, climate change should be accepted as a sufficient reason to extend special protective measures toward those displaced by the consequences of the Anthropocene. In line with other groups who fall outside the traditional refugee regime, and for whom *complementary protection* may be warranted (Lister, 2014), climate migrants should also benefit from such protective measures. However, the anticipated numbers of climate-induced migrants to come are staggering. Simply looking at the worst affected areas, Africa and Asia, and their populations, 1.2 billion and 4.5 billion, respectively, suggests that it won't be possible to apply the standard measures known so far to protect the anticipated number of climate-induced migrants. The volume of displaced individuals will simply be too high. Moreover, the known strategies fail to address the specific needs of climate-induced migrants. For instance, supplementary protection – a status conferred to rejected asylum seekers who are "tolerated" in a safe third country because it would endanger their life if they were sent back to their country of origin – would not be helpful to address the plight of those who can't return home. When "home" is gone, the idea

of territorial return becomes incoherent. Instead, the specific needs of those displaced by climate change require a specific social and global policy response that has yet to be developed.[3]

However, it would be a mistake to think of the necessary kind of protection as "asylum." What unites asylum seekers and climate migrants, one could say, is the moral obligation that flight from religious and political persecution and flight from climate disasters generates. Both call for protections necessary to secure basic needs. Second, both kinds of migration are a last resort, a last answer to an emergency. Put otherwise, neither traditional asylum seekers nor climate refugees opt for migration of their own volition; instead, both groups are coerced to adapt to changed conditions in their home state. Yet their needs are different and should be addressed differently.

I will first provide some background to my discussion, starting with a short review of the link between the Anthropocene and its effects on health, before turning to the focus of this chapter – the nexus between climate change, migration, and health. In the second part of this chapter, I will provide my own take on the moral obligations that arise in the face of mass migration due to climate change. I will suggest that the moral obligation arises not because of causal responsibility for climate change but because of remedial responsibility to ensure that the basic needs of all human beings are met. This is notwithstanding the fact that the basic needs of many go unmet today, even before increased mass migration occurs. My argument here is a normative one: I use basic needs as a reference point to define what form remedial responsibility should take. If people have to move because of climate change, they should at least have their basic needs protected. These include access to health resources. For many, this requires provisions in their state of origin, in other parts of their country of origin, or in neighboring countries. Not many may want to resettle elsewhere, as I illustrate later on. However, actively barring entry through policies of *nonentrée* to those who want to resettle and who migrate toward rich countries without protecting the human right to health otherwise neglects international moral obligations in two fundamental ways. The populations of rich developed countries are the countries that may be able to weather climate change most easily, either through adaptation or through protection (Shue, 2014). They are also very often

---

[3] For a very encompassing proposal that also applies basic human needs as a measure of policy development, see Gough (2017).

among the biggest polluters contributing to climate change and those who benefit most from past pollution to advance their economies. Policies of *nonentrée* thus constitute a moral failure because they represent a failure to protect and enable human rights (Caney, 2009). Second, they represent a failure to accept the responsibility that especially wealthy countries have for climate change (Shue, 2014).

Effects of the Anthropocene Epoch on Health

When thinking about health in the context of the Anthropocene, I distinguish several different aspects. First, researchers have pointed to the specific health risks that climate change *in itself* has on affected populations. "Epidemiological studies have identified health risks associated with, for example, differences and extremes in temperature, climate-related natural disasters, altered food yield and water supply, and changing infectious disease patterns" (McMichael, 2015: 549).

It is because of such effects that climate change figures prominently on the agenda of international and national health agencies. For instance, the recently published research agenda of the World Health Organization (WHO) is now in line with the findings of the Intergovernmental Panel on Climate Change, aiming to heighten awareness of the effects of climate change on health. In particular, the authors argue that climate change has negative effects on health because of negative effects on the social and environmental determinants of health. Climate change undermines conditions for clean air, safe drinking water, secure food supply, and the possibility for many to find shelter (WHO, 2017). Lacking these conditions of health is worrisome enough. Access to these goods, moreover, is promised to all human beings in the United Nations Declaration of Human Rights.[4] Therein, Article 25 stipulates that everyone has the right to a standard of living adequate for the health and well-being of himself or herself and of his or her family, including food, clothing, housing, and medical care and necessary social services and the right to security in the event of unemployment, sickness, disability, widowhood, old age, or other lack of livelihood in circumstances beyond his or her control.

The nexus between climate change and possible violations of human rights to bodily security and safety leads some international law specialists to argue that climate migrants should be given the same *legal* status in international law as traditional refugees (Höing & Razzaque, 2012). I will return later to the question of needs and rights and the moral obligations that arise when needs are unmet.

Climate change affects individual health not only through its effects on social determinants of health; it also affects individuals directly. The WHO estimates that "between 2030 and 2050, climate change is expected to cause approximately 250, 000 additional deaths per year, from malnutrition, malaria, diarrhea and heat stress" (WHO, 2017). Add to this an increase in respiratory diseases that other researchers have signaled (D'Amato et al., 2014).

A third detrimental effect of climate change on individuals is the nefarious consequences to people's health resulting from migration *driven by* climate change, as I explain now.

Mass Migration and Health in the Anthropocene

A note on terminology: I will refer to those whose reasons to migrate include reasons of environmental degradation as *climate migrants, climate-induced migrants,* or *environmental migrants.* I follow here the definition of the International Organization for Migration (IOM) in its definition of environmental migrants as "persons or groups of persons who, predominantly for reasons of sudden or progressive changes in the environment that adversely affect their lives or living conditions, are obliged to leave their habitual homes, or choose to do so, either temporarily or permanently, and who move within their country or abroad" (IOM, 2018: 13).[5]

This is not to suggest that changes in the environment are the sole reason for decisions to migrate, because the reasons most obviously derive from changes in the capacity to earn a livelihood and

---

[4] Again, I take the UNDHR as a reference point of what ought to be done rather than an account of the status quo. This is to say that it is sadly true that for many, even the most basic human rights are not protected, such as access to food and water and safe sanitation.

[5] The term *environmental refugee* was originally coined by Essam El-Hinnawi working for the United Nations Environment Programme in 1985. El-Hinnawi identified three categories of environmentally displaced peoples: (1) those temporarily displaced due to natural hazards, (2) those permanently displaced because of a marked environmental disruption (natural and/or triggered by people), and (3) those who migrate permanently or temporarily because of ecological changes in their environment and cannot afford to mitigate the changes.

make a home. Climate migrants are those who can no longer gain a secure livelihood in their homelands because of drought, soil erosion, desertification, deforestation, and other environmental problems. This does not deny that other push factors such as high levels of existing poverty are prevalent. Instead, referring to some as climate migrants acknowledges that it is increasingly difficult to separate environmental from economic factors, especially in agriculturally based societies (Myers, 2002). As I noted earlier, following the language of the UN compact for refugees, it seems uncontroversial to say that climate interacts and possibly intensifies other drivers of migration.

The literature examining the connection between climate change, migration, and health is only emerging (but see McMyers and Schwerdtle), yet the need for an integrated analysis is proven by the latest figures on climate migration. For instance, the International Displacement Monitoring Center (IDMC) reports that "[t]he risk to humans of being displaced through sudden natural disasters is 60 percent higher today than it was forty years ago. Today, an average of 24.4 million people are displaced every year as a consequence of natural disasters" (Greenpeace, 2017: 6). To put these figures into context, in 2018, the UNHCR registered 70.8 million forcibly displaced people overall (UNHCR, 2018). This is to say that nearly a third of all displaced people worldwide are considered displaced for environmental reasons.

More specifically, researchers distinguish between displacement for reasons of natural disasters and displacement due to weather-related and geophysical disasters. Looking at the figures for 2015, countries worst affected by the former are predominantly in Eastern Asia and the Pacific, Southern Asia, Latin America and the Caribbean, and Sub-Saharan Africa. More than 19 million people in these regions are estimated to have been displaced. Displacement as a result of weather-related and geophysical disasters such as floods, storms, earthquakes, forest and bush fires, and extreme temperatures affect an estimated 203 million people globally (Greenpeace, 2017: 13).

Climate migration is largely a phenomenon of the Global South. The IDMC data cited earlier show a concentration of environmental displacements in Asia, with 82% of total displacement there between 2008 and 2014 (cited in Ionescu, Mokhnacheva, & Gemenne, 2017). Asia is the continent with the biggest proportion of countries affected by displacement (11 of 20). Contrast this with displacement in Europe and Oceania, which together account for only 0.5 percent of the overall figures of displaced (Ionescu, Mokhnacheva, & Gemenne, 2017: 16). Many migrants move internally, adding to the growing number of internally displaced people who fall through the statistical cracks. Moreover, data for their destination countries are limited, so it is unclear where those who are displaced settle. Yet "[i]t is widely agreed . . . that most displaced people remain within the same countries. In many situations, people stay close to their original homes; and though some may cross international borders, global data on such situations are also lacking" (Ionescu, Mokhnacheva, & Gemenne, 2017: 16).

According to most commentators, mass migration for climate reasons poses specific health risks to individual migrants and to host societies. These can be separated into four different categories, each of which is expanded on below (see also Schwerdtle, Bowen, & McMichael, 2018):

Risk through migration into urban slums

Risk of exposure to environmental hazards in unknown territory

Risk of long-term effects of ill-health due to neglect or the fact of being trapped

Risk of communicable diseases in country of migration

Risks of Migration into Urban Slums

Displacement for environmental reasons raises specific health-related concerns because of the largely unregulated nature of the movement, which is reflected in the lack of data mentioned earlier. Cities are considered safer than the countryside and seem to offer better opportunities to find a new livelihood. Especially in largely agricultural societies, migration into cities is often the only option under conditions of climate degradation that make agriculture not profitable enough to provide a livelihood. Moreover, most agriculture-based economies don't dispose of vacant land that migrants might take over, hence limiting the possibilities of pursuing agriculture for those driven from their plots individually. The situation is different in government-led resettlement projects, in which governments relocate entire villages and population groups. I will discuss these adaptation strategies later on.

However, many migrants arrive in bigger cities only to find themselves living in urban slums. Rather than alleviating their suffering, moving into the city thus bears new dangers for environmental refugees through the unregulated nature of most urban slums. Exposure to violence and diseases that come from lack of sanitation present increased health risks (Greenpeace, 2017: 21).

Risk of Exposure to Environmental Hazards in Unknown Territory

This risk also often stems from the choice of migration destination into large cities. The locations of the slums in low-lying outskirts of the cities are often threatened by further environmental hazards, such as flooding and landslides, that pose new and unexpected challenges to those unfamiliar with the local territory. "In Southeast Asia . . . observers have noted that migrant groups were less able to protect themselves against heavy storms than local inhabitants because they could not assess dangers and were not familiar with protective measures" (Greenpeace, 2017: 90).

Risk of Long-Term Effects of Ill-Health Due to Neglect or the Fact of Being Trapped

One of the most worrying trends is the fact that many who migrate for climate reasons disappear in the statistics. Not recognized officially as refugees, and often internally or regionally displaced, those settling in urban slums or neglected rural areas add to the growing population of the global poor. Their health needs, because of their undocumented nature, are not addressed or even diagnosed in the first place.

Risk of Communicable Diseases in Place of Migration

Migrants are often considered possible bearers of problems in health settings (see University College London–Lancet Commission on Migration and Health, 2016). First, migrants may be carriers for communicable diseases to which the local population has not been exposed.[6] Prior health status of a population, including immunity, plays a major role when assessing negative health outcomes in migration settings. The level of immunization of migrants varies depending on their country of origin, and those migrating from health-sector-poor countries are more likely to lack immunizations and to carry pathogens.[7] Second, migrants may themselves be prone to disease, especially if they have been weakened by their migration or have suffered food insecurity and other deprivations in their country of origin and during their migration. Malaria, for instance, is a constant threat to those on the move (Schwerdle et al., 2018).

Climate Migration and Adaptation

Earlier I suggested that climate migrants and traditional asylum seekers have different needs, which makes it questionable whether designating climate migrants as *climate refugees* is helpful, conceptually and practically. From a health perspective, providing access to necessary care, providing immunizations, and preventing downward migration into urban slums may be a first basic step to address the specific risks to individual health triggered by climate migration. Addressing health needs in a neighboring country or within the country of origin may be better suited to address the moral wrong that climate change inflicts than resettlement in a new home. The needs of climate migrants, in other words, are different from the needs of those requesting asylum for reasons of religious and political persecution who request surrogate membership and the protection of their religious and political rights in another state than their original one (Price, 2009).

Climate migrants may indeed wish to stay closer to home regardless of the fact that migration or resettlement elsewhere could have positive effects on the social determinants of health: migration may enable access to more secure food sources than in the country of origin, or it may lead to settlement in a country with less extreme weather patterns, such as floods or exposure to heat. Thus, from a health perspective, one could argue that planned and organized relocation can have benefits for those relocated (Schwerdle et al., 2018). This was the motivation of the authors

---

[6] "Infectious disease risk is affected by migration. International and internal migration increases chances for illness as migrating people are exposed to infection in new locations, service as carriers of infection during transit and to their new sites of residence, or reintroduce infectious agents during return migration" (McMichael, 2015: 556).

[7] "International and internal migration alters the distribution and incidence of infectious disease as migrating people are exposed to infection in new locations, serve as carriers of infection during transit and to their new sites of residence, or reintroduce infectious agents during return migration" (McMichael, 2015: 549).

of the Cancun Framework to include specific recommendations for relocation as an adaptive measure to climate change (see IOM, 2018; UNHCR, 2014). And indeed, several governments around the world have begun to relocate threatened population groups. Proactive governments in Vietnam, Papua New Guinea, and the Maldives but also the Netherlands and the United States have begun planning relocation measures that climate change has made necessary (for an overview, see Ionescu, Mokhnacheva, & Gemenne, 2017: 26ff).

Yet case studies show that even well-thought-out and planned relocation is not easily accepted and adopted by populations under threat from climate change. To give an example, take the case of the Carteret Island population in Papua New Guinea.

> In 2007, the Council of Elders of the Carteret Islands formed an NGO called Tulele Peisa (Sailing the Waves on Our Own). Tulele Peisa developed the Carteret Integrated Relocation Project, a community-led relocation model, to coordinate the voluntary relocation of Carteret Islanders to Bougainville Island, 100 km to the north-east. The location of the relocation site was critical to ensure sufficient land for the Carteret families to be economically self-sufficient. The relocation also prioritised food security by ensuring access to traditional fishing grounds, which was important for nutritional and cultural reasons. . . . Nevertheless, despite the apparent opportunity for livelihoods, food security and access to health services, the future through relocation was seen as uncertain and few wished to relocate to the new site.
>
> *(Schwerdtle et al., 2018: 3)*

How should governments react in the face of resistance to relocation? Because of such resistance, relocation is potentially contentious and needs to be carefully guided. One possible framework to guide relocation measures is the measure of individual basic needs in the context of human rights.

What precisely categorizes needs as morally relevant and duty grounding is subject to debate (see Brock, 1998). Suffice to say that most commentators accept that the "notion of need can play a valuable role in political discourse" (Wringe, 2005: 187; see also Doyal & Gough, 1991). This is particularly obvious if basic needs are taken to ground the core of individual rights that liberal democratic states are called on to protect and implement. In this respect, a link between basic needs and access to a set of rights is often stipulated to justify a conception of generally accepted

human rights (Shue, 1980; Miller, 2014). Moreover, access to a set of *equal* rights also expresses the equal moral status that all human beings are promised. The equal moral status all individuals should enjoy is most commonly expressed in the form of equal protection through rights. The most relevant category of rights to be considered are human rights, especially the human right to health.

One way to interpret official relocation efforts would be to say that governments aim to protect the human rights of their citizens – something they ought to do – but that the only viable way to secure access and protection to the human right to health stipulated in Article 25(1) of the UNHDR would be to relocate those parts of the population that are under threat through climate change. To put this differently, governments may refer to the "right to a standard of living adequate for the health and well-being" to justify their relocation efforts. Similarly, other governments, such as those of the European Union and North America, could suggest that they are eager to contribute to relocation efforts in order to help protect the human right to health. In this vein, international agreements such as the Cancun framework mentioned earlier go to the core of the question of responsibilities and moral obligations in the face of climate change.

However, these obligations have to be weighed in relation to other obligations liberal-democratic governments have toward their citizens, most prominently the one to protect the bases of individual autonomy and the capacity to be self-determining. In medical ethics, a patient's consent has to be granted before any health intervention can be justified, and we can assume that individuals should have a say in being subjected to relocation efforts by governments, even if these aim to improve the social and environmental determinants of health.

Moral Obligations and Responsibilities in the Anthropocene

I want to distinguish between the obligations of state governments in the face of climate change and the obligations of the international community. Within the first group, it is important to distinguish further: first, there are governments that are willing to act to protect the human rights and, in particular, the right to health of their citizens. Examples in this category include countries that engage in relocation efforts, such as Vietnam and Papua New Guinea. As the example of the Cateret Island relocation proposal suggests, however, the cases of governments eager to act but that encounter resistance from the population will be the most difficult to assess morally. On the face of things, one would be hard pressed to fault these governments for their efforts, even if the health outcomes are uncertain in the face of resistance. In other words, it seems fair to say that relocation under these circumstances comes close to satisfying the moral obligations that arise in the context of climate change and access to health, in particular in the context of the social determinants of health. The tragedy lies in the fact that the best-intentioned governments may still have to act against the wishes of at least some of their citizens to promote the best possible outcomes in these circumstances (see Blake [2019] on tragedy in politics).

As I said at the outset, what unites traditional asylum seekers with climate migrants is the need to act in the face of coercion. And while the coercion in the context of climate change is less tangible than that arising from persecution on religious or political grounds, lacking an alternative to relocating in order to ensure their survival still counts as coercion. The coercion takes the shape of climate change negatively affecting and changing the range of options individuals have to lead the kind of life they hope to lead (Anderson, 2008).

Climate-induced migrants are coerced in several ways. In the first instance, they are coerced to leave because of erosion of their fields, farms, or land, more generally. In addition, and if their government wants to relocate them, they may be coerced by their government if they resist relocation. Moreover, although relocation may address individual needs such as access to secure forms of livelihood and employment and may improve social determinants of health, there may be collective needs such as the one to protect cultural goods that may require access to traditional lands and subsistence practices. In this light, the concern for protecting human rights and basic needs has to be weighed against the concern for individual autonomy and self-determination and the demands of self-determination of cultural communities. Especially this last concern supports my critique of the equivalence strategy to address the needs of climate-induced migrants through the lens of asylum: in contrast to individual asylum seekers and their families, climate-induced migration is often a collective

phenomenon. As the example of the Cateret Islands illustrates, for some environmentally displaced people, the concern of climate change is not only missing livelihoods and protection of human rights, it may also be a concern for cultural survival.

Second, we can identify governments that could act but are not willing to act in the face of climate change and environmental disaster – either because of a denial of climate change or because of a lack of political will. One example discussed in this category is the United States in the face of Hurricane Katrina, which devastated parts of New Orleans and in the face of which the US government was slow to respond in addressing the needs of those affected (Ionescu, Mokhnacheva, & Gemenne, 2017). The moral assessment here seems much easier as it seems obvious that the US government should have acted more promptly than it did and with more urgency.

Both sets of governments have in common that their responsibility in question is remedial. This is to say that governments are responsible not because they brought about climate change or deteriorating conditions for their citizens but because they have to protect those of their citizens who need help (Miller, 2007: 81ff).

Finally, we need to differentiate those state governments who are willing to act and accept remedial responsibility but who are unable to do so because they lack the resources. In some cases, there is no territory to which to relocate. This is the case for Pacific Island states such as Tuvalu, which hase appealed for international help because the possibilities to remedy the worsening situation for its citizens are limited.

It is at least at this point that obligations of the international community have to be considered. The debate how to address climate change internationally has long been mired in deadlock between those who propose redistributive accounts of climate justice (e.g., Caney, 2009; Shue 2014) and those who don't aim for redistribution. What concerns me here is the applied question of how to deal with the displacement of people for reasons of climate change and environmental disaster and the violation of their human right to access health resources, including, most minimally, safe housing, clean drinking water, and food security. As I explained earlier, the statistics of climate-induced displacement indicate that Europe and Oceania are relatively unaffected continents, with only 0.5% of all climate displacement recorded there, whereas 82% of climate-related displacement occurs in Asia. I also explained that rich countries in the North have historically benefited most from CO_2 emissions that are taken to worsen climate change compared with the relatively poorer countries in the Global South.

This suggests a remedial responsibility to assist those governments, whose resources assisting their own citizens are limited, should be uncontroversial. Rich countries such as those in Europe and Oceania should come to the help of Tuvalu to find solutions and remedies to escape climate disaster. The measures that could be taken should be based on the needs of climate migrants. As I have assumed so far, and following the UNDHR, all humans need access to clean drinking water, safe food supplies, and basic healthcare. The satisfaction of these needs in the face of climate change should set the policy agenda.

How to satisfy obligations and responsibilities arising from climate change may be open to debate. Most minimally, it should again be uncontroversial that all governments should implement climate-related policies that are necessary to achieve international climate targets and to keep global warming below 2°C. Moreover, though, governments should accept specific targeted responsibilities that are tied to the challenge of realizing the human right to health.

Let me return at this point to the question with which I began. In light of my argument so far, would it thus not be better to accept the proposals by those who call for the equivalence between climate migrants and traditional asylum seekers? Should we not accept the category of climate refugees? Originally, I suggested that this equivalence strategy neglects the different needs of climate migrants, who may not wish to relocate elsewhere, or at least not very far, but whose needs, including their health needs, should be satisfied closer to home. As my discussion of the specific risks of climate-induced migration has indicated, unless migration takes the form of planned and government-led relocation, climate migration so far seems to worsen health outcomes for many rather than improve them. Climate migration leads to downward integration into the unregulated and unsanitary urban slums.

In this vein, the remedial responsibility of rich developed states should not only address climate change in their own countries but also include measures to help governments who are less well positioned to cope with climate disaster. Finally, though, let's think about Tuvalians, say, and all the others who may have to leave their state of origin behind simply because there is no more "there" there. Some climate migrants may have to start anew elsewhere. In light of this individual adaptation strategy, which is what migration obviously is, policies of *nonentrée* are a moral failure, in particular when implemented by relatively climate-secure states. Put differently, the plight of some who aim to migrate to safer shores so that they can live lives in which their human rights are protected may render these policies into a moral hazard causing more suffering. Governments such as Italy that prevent entry of people from African countries under threat of desertification, say, neglect individual needs further, thus adding to the moral wrong that climate change inflicts.

Conclusion

It is clear that climate change will lead to further migration of those who lose their livelihoods. Climate-induced migration will potentially dwarf the numbers of all migrants the world has witnessed so far. Yet climate-induced migration poses challenges that cannot be addressed with the known instruments of asylum and refuge. Especially when thinking about basic needs, and in particular health needs of climate migrants, providing for asylum in a country elsewhere doesn't obviously address the problem. For one, much of the migration is internal, thus falling through the cracks of statistical data. To be sure, this may change with increasing population pressure in poor countries hit by climate change. However, the idea described by Raspail, that people aim for Europe as the Promised Land is true only insofar as Europe seems largely immune yet to climate catastrophe. Left to their own devices, most people would prefer to lead a decent life back home. This should be one of the guiding principles informing policies dealing with climate-induced migration. When analyzing health needs of climate migrants, it seems clear that assistance should be provided in the country of origin through relocation within the country. Relocation, though, may be resisted by individual migrants and their collectives. In such instances, those framing global health policy have to weigh individual health needs with the demands of individual autonomy and collective self-determination. The one certainty to be had is that rich countries have an obligation to reduce emissions so as not to further contribute to degrading conditions in climate-change-affected countries. They also have an obligation to allow immigration by those few climate migrants who wish to settle somewhere safe.

References

Anderson, S. (2008). Of theories of coercion: two axes and the importance of the coercer. *Journal of Moral Philosophy* **5**(3), 394–422.

Blake, M. (2019). Asylum, speech and tragedy, in Miller, D., & Straehle, C. (ed.), *The Political Philosophy of Refuge*. Cambridge, UK: Cambridge University Press.

Brock, G. (1998). Morally important needs. *Philosophia* **26**(1), 165–178.

Caney, S. (2009). Climate change human rights and moral thresholds, in Humphreys, S. (ed.), *Human Rights and Climate Change*. Cambridge, UK: Cambridge University Press, pp. 69–90.

Connelly, M., & Kennedy, P. (1994). Must it be the rest against the West? *The Atlantic*. December. Available at www.theatlantic.com/past/politics/immigrat/kennf.htm.

D'Amato, G., Cecchi, L., D'Amato, M., & Annesi-Maesano, I. (2014). Climate change and respiratory disease. *European Respiratory Review* **23**, 161–169. DOI:10.1183/09059180.00001714.

Doyal, L., & Gough, I. (1991). *A Theory of Human Need*. New York: Gilford Press.

The Economist (2011). Available at www.economist.com/leaders/2011/05/26/welcome-to-the-anthropocene. May 26, 2011

Greenpeace (2017). *Climate Change, Migration and Displacement: The Underestimated Disaster*. Available at www.greenpeace.de/sites/www.greenpeace.de/files/20170524-greenpeace-studie-climate-change-migration-displacement-engl.pdf.

Gough, I. (2017). *Heat, Greed and Climate Change*. London: Elgar.

Höing, N., & Razzaque, J. (2012). Unacknowledged and unwanted? Environmental refugees in search of legal status. *Journal of Global Ethics* **8**(1), 19–40.

International Organization for Migration (IOM) (2018). *Mapping Human Mobility (Migration, Displacement and Planned Relocation) and Climate Change in International Processes, Policies and Legal Frameworks*. Available at https://unfccc.int/sites/default/files/resource/WIM%20TFD%20II.2%20Output.pdf.

Ionesco, D., Mokhnacheva, D., & Gemenne, F. (2017). *The Atlas of Environmental Migration*. New York: Routledge.

Klingler, C., Odukoya, D., & Kuehlmeyer, K. (2018). Migration, health, and ethics. *Bioethics* **32**, 330–333. https://doi.org/10.1111/bioe.12473.

Kolers, A. (2012). Floating provisos and sinking islands. *Journal of Applied Philosophy* **29**, 333–343.

Lister, M. (2014). Climate change refugees. *Critical Review of Social and Political Philosophy* **17**(5), 618–634.

McMichael, C. (2015). Climate change-related migration and infectious disease. *Virulence* **6**(6), 548–553.

Miller, D. (2007). *National Responsibility and Global Justice*. Oxford, UK: Oxford University Press.

Miller, D. (2014). Personhood versus human needs as grounds for human rights, in Crisp, R. (ed.), *Griffin on Human Rights*. Oxford, UK: Oxford University Press, pp. 152–169.

Myers, N. (2002). Environmental refugees: a growing phenomenon of the 21st century. *Philosophical Transactions: Biological Sciences* **357**(1420), 609–613.

Nine, C. (2010). Ecological refugees, states borders, and the Lockean proviso. *Journal of Applied Philosophy* **27**, 359–375.

Price, M. E. (2009). *Rethinking Asylum: History, Purpose, and Limits*. Cambridge, UK: Cambridge University Press.

Risse, M. (2009). The right to relocation: disappearing island nations and common ownership of the earth. *Ethics & International Affairs* **23**(3), 281–300.

Revkin, A. (2011). Confronting the Anthropocene. *New York Times*, May 11. Available at https://dotearth.blogs.nytimes.com/2011/05/11/confronting-the-anthropocene/.

Schwerdtle, P., Bowen, K., McMichael, C., et al. (2018). The health impacts of climate-related migration. *BMC Medicine* **16**, 1. https://doi.org/10.1186/s12916-017-0981-7.

Shue, H. (1980). *Basic Rights: Subsistence, Affluence, and US Foreign Policy*. Princeton, NJ: Princeton University Press.

Shue, H. (2014). Human rights, climate change and the Triliionth ton, in Denis, G. (ed.), *Climate Ethics*. Oxford, UK: Oxford University Press, pp. 293–314.

Straehle, C. (2019). Asylum, refuge and justice in health. *Hastings Center Report* **49**(2), 1–5.

Türk, V. (2016). Prospects for responsibility sharing in the refugee context, *Journal on Migration and Human Security* **4**(3) 45–59.

United Nations High Commissioner for Refugees (UNHCR) (2014). *Planned Relocation as an Adaptation Strategy*. Geneva: UNHCR. Available at www.unhcr.org/543e78a89.pdf.

United Nations High Commissioner for Refugees (UNHCR) (2014b). *Global Strategy for Public Health 2014–2018*. Geneva: UNHCR. Available at www.unhcr.org/protection/health/530f12d26/global-strategy-public-health-unhcr-strategy-2014-2018-public-health-hiv.html.

United Nations High Commissioner for Refugees (UNHCR) (2018). *Global Trends: Forced Displacement in 2018*. Geneva, UNHCR. Available at www.unhcr.org/dach/wp-content/uploads/sites/27/2019/06/2019-06-07-Global-Trends-2018.pdf.

University College London–Lancet Commission on Migration and Health (2016). *Lancet* 388. https://doi.org/10.1016/S0140-6736(18)32114-7.

World Health Organization (WHO) (2017). *Climate Change and Health*. New York, WHO. Available at www.who.int/news-room/fact-sheets/detail/climate-change-and-health.

Wringe, B. (2005). Needs, rights, and collective obligations. *Royal Institute of Philosophy Supplement* **80** (57), 187–208.

Animals, the Environment, and Global Health

David Benatar

Introduction

When people talk about global health and the ethics thereof, they almost invariably mean global *human* health. This is not because it is impossible to have more expansive notions of global health that include other species. Instead, it is because most people who are concerned about global health, like most of those who are concerned about local health, are either not concerned at all or are much less concerned with the health of other species. Thus, global health ethics, although expanding the reach of health ethics geographically, has not extended moral concern to other species within that global space.

This is unfortunate for at least two reasons. First, there is good reason to think that not only humans but also some other animals, the sentient ones, are worthy of moral consideration. That is to say, they are the sorts of beings to which we have moral duties. I shall not argue for this conclusion here, in part, because it has been defended extensively elsewhere (e.g., Regan, 1983; Singer, 1990; DeGrazia, 1996) but also because overlooking animal welfare in the way that people generally do poses a considerable threat to global human health. Thus, even those who fail to recognize the moral standing of nonhuman animals but do recognize the moral standing of humans should be more attentive to animal well-being on account of its instrumental value for human health.

There are those who think that not only nonhuman animals but also the natural environment itself – plants, as well as local ecosystems and the global aggregation of these – is worthy of moral consideration.[1] I do not share this view. However, one need not go as far as attributing moral standing to the environment to think that we have duties to preserve it. Although we may have no (direct) duties

to the environment, we could still have (indirect) duties *concerning* the environment. The latter duties could be grounded in the interests that sentient beings, either human or nonhuman or both, have in an environment that is conducive to their own health and general well-being. Global human (and animal) health can be affected by the state of the global environment.

There is now considerable awareness of the impact of the environment on human health and thus of the need to act in environmentally responsible ways. This is so even if most people do not do enough in response to this awareness. Matters are quite different, however, when it comes to the connection between animal and human interests. Indeed, arguably the most common view on this matter is that advancing or protecting human interests regularly requires overriding animal interests. Humans, it is thought, want to eat animals, need to experiment on them to advance medical science, and must cull them when they present a nuisance or a threat. In all these cases, animal and human interests are thought to conflict rather than coincide – a disputable view that I shall not evaluate here.

Although people realize that humans pay a price for environmental damage, they often do not realize the human costs of much maltreatment of animals. I propose to rectify this by noting the ways in which human and animal interests coincide. I shall also make reference to the manner in which environmental degradation threatens global human health. Once these facts have been described, albeit briefly, I shall raise and respond to various arguments for the view that we nonetheless have no duty, based on human interests alone, to preserve the environment or to improve our treatment of animals.

Animal Interests and Global Human Health

Animal interests and human health intersect in a variety of ways, but not all of these ways are equally

---

[1] On this view, *global health* takes on an additional meaning. It refers also to the health of the globe, of planet Earth.

relevant for *global* human health. For example, vegetarian diets advance animal interests in not being killed. The humans who benefit most directly from vegetarian diets are the vegetarians themselves. They benefit from not consuming animal flesh. Although these advantages could aggregate to have an impact on global health, the contribution to global health is merely the sum of benefits to individuals.[2] This is unlike other factors impacting human health, where the harms or benefits to some spill over into affecting others and that are thus more likely to impact global health.

Consider infectious diseases, for example. They contribute significantly to the global burden of disease. By their nature, they are also the diseases that carry the greatest threat of suddenly spreading and thus, at least for a period, affecting and killing many more people than they usually do. For this reason, their capacity to cause fear in addition to illness and death is considerable.

Some have suggested that "[a]ll human viral infections were initially zoonotic in origin" (Weber & Alcorn, 2000: 6), although the precise animal source and route of transmission to humans are often a matter of some dispute.[3] Whether or not it is true that *all* human viral infections have animal origins, it certainly seems that *many* do. Consider some examples. Severe acute respiratory syndrome (SARS) arose in the live-animal (i.e., "wet") markets of China (Guan et al., 2003).[4] Variant Creutzfeldt-Jakob disease probably arose from bovine spongiform encephalopathy (BSE; Will et al., 1996; Scott et al., 1999). And the source of the human immunodeficiency virus (HIV), which causes AIDS, is widely thought to be the simian immunodeficiency virus that is found in nonhuman primates (Gao et al., 1999; Sharp et al., 2001). The animal origins of avian and swine influenzas are reflected in their colloquial names.

Although these latter two diseases have not as yet killed as many people as was feared, the fears are not without some justification. Influenza epidemics arise periodically. Although not all are equally dangerous, the fears of dangerous epidemics and pandemics are grounded both in historical experience of such lethality and in the knowledge that the ongoing process of mutation could yield more deadly strains. The relevant questions, therefore, are not whether a new epidemic will arise, but rather *when* it will arise and *how bad* it will be (Osterholm, 2005).

It transpires that we did not need to wait long for the first of those questions to be answered. A novel coronavirus emerged in Wuhan, China, in late 2019 and became pandemic in early 2020. At the time of inserting this update, we already know that the implications for global human health and well-being are very severe, although the full extent of that severity remains to be seen. Now that we know that the COVID-19 pandemic was the next to arise, the obvious next question is, When will the *next* epidemic emerge? Again, it is not a question of *whether*, but rather *when*?

Although some zoonoses are probably unavoidable, much human suffering resulting from zoonotic diseases could probably have been avoided had humans treated animals better. Consider, for example, the wet markets from which an influenza or SARS epidemic could be launched and from which the novel coronavirus of 2019 may have emerged (Zhang, 2020). The other likely source for the latter is one of the many mixed wildlife-livestock farms in China (Gorman, 2020). In these markets, live animals of diverse kinds are kept in large numbers and cruelly close quarters ready for sale and fresh slaughter. The concentration of animals, their overlapping sojourns in the markets (allowing disease to spread through vast numbers of animals), and their interactions with humans (facilitating human infection) make these markets ripe for zoonoses (Webster, 2004). Once an epidemic starts among animals, it can also spread to animals reared in less cruel conditions.[5]

If humans did not eat wet-market animals, there would be fewer of them (because fewer would be bred), the animals would not suffer from being housed in close quarters, and they would not be slaughtered. Consequently, the risk of zoonoses would be greatly

---

[2] To clarify, vegetarianism does have *indirect* global health benefits, to which I shall turn soon. For now, I am only showing that not all human benefits from vegetarianism impact as markedly on *global* health.

[3] This sentence is from David Benatar (2007). The chickens come home to roost. *American Journal of Public Health* **97**(9), 1545–1546. Reprinted, with permission of the copyright holder, the American Public Health Association.

[4] This sentence and the next two are from David Benatar (2007). The chickens come home to roost. *American Journal of Public Health* **97**(9), 1545–1546. Reprinted, with permission of the copyright holder, the American Public Health Association.

[5] This paragraph and the next are from David Benatar (2007). The chickens come home to roost. *American Journal of Public Health* **97**(9), 1545–1546. Reprinted, with permission of the copyright holder, the American Public Health Association.

diminished. In the case of variant Creutzfeldt-Jakob disease, humans would not have become infected had some humans not killed and eaten cows infected with BSE. Moreover, BSE would not spread among cattle if humans did not process offal, including neural matter from BSE-infected cattle, to produce feed for other cattle, a practice that was prompted by the volume of cattle that humans eat. If the plausible hypothesis that HIV resulted from simian immunodeficiency virus is indeed true, then the most likely causal route of transmission was through infected simian blood during the butchering of these animals. The butchering itself was most likely for the purposes of providing nonhuman primate meat (*bushmeat*) for human consumption, a practice that continues today.

Now it might be suggested that there is no use closing the barn door once the virus has bolted across the species barrier to humans. This, however, is a myopic view. It sees only the damage that has already been done and ignores the likelihood that unless we close the door on treating animals in the ways they have been treated in the past, new diseases (or new strains of diseases) will still emerge.

Nor are the relevant diseases only viral or prion diseases. Millions of pounds of antibiotics are added to animal feed in so-called factory farms. The antibiotics have a dual purpose – to prevent the spread of bacterial disease between animals in intensive confinement and also to promote growth (Boyd, 2001: 647). This volume of antibiotic use would be unnecessary if animals were not treated as commodities to be fattened as quickly as possible and to be produced in the greatest number possible. The maltreatment necessitates the use of antibiotics, but the widespread use of antibiotics, in turn, poses a longer-term threat to humans because it can be expected to breed resistant strains of the organisms currently targeted by the antibiotics (Boyd, 2001: 650).

The Environment and Global Human Health

The impact, both actual and potential, of the environment on global human health is much more widely recognized than is the connection between animal welfare and human health. Nevertheless, the main themes are worthy of mention.

Whereas for most of human history environmental degradation had only local effects, today things are very different. Many of the effects of environmental damage are now global. There are two broad interrelated reasons for the greater impact humans are having on the environment. First, there are many more humans than there used to be. For most of human history, there were no more than a few tens of thousands of humans and for long periods considerably fewer than this. However, the human population began to increase exponentially just a few hundred years ago. There were about half a billion humans by the middle of the seventeenth century. This increased to 1 billion by 1804, 2 billion by 1927, 3 billion by 1960, 4 billion by 1974, 5 billion by 1987, and 6 billion by 1999 (McMichael, 2001: 188). At the time of writing, there are in excess of 7.6 billion human beings (and the number continues to grow).

The second reason why humans are having a much greater impact on the environment now than they did for much of their history is that the per capita consumption of the Earth's resources has also burgeoned, attributable in large part to technological developments since the industrial revolution. Nonrenewable resources (such as fossil fuels) and slowly renewable resources (such as groundwater, fertile soil, and forestation) are being depleted. Current levels of usage are thus not sustainable. Moreover, it is not merely that these resources are being depleted but that their use, particularly at massively increased rates, has effects on the environment. For example, burning fossil fuels increases atmospheric levels of carbon dioxide, one of the major greenhouse gases (GHGs) responsible for global warming. The increase in carbon dioxide is exacerbated by the depletion of forests (Houghton, Jenkins, & Ephraums, 1990: xv) because plants remove carbon dioxide from the atmosphere. Concentrations of another GHG, methane, have also increased significantly. Among the causes of this are biomass burning, coal mining, and massive increases in the number of cattle being reared for human use (Houghton, Jenkins, & Ephraums, 1990: xv). Chlorofluorocarbons, which were only invented in the 1930s and which were widely used in subsequent decades, are destructive of the ozone layer and were thereby another major contributor to global warming (Houghton, Jenkins, & Ephraums, 1990: xv) until they began to be phased out under the Montreal Protocol.

Global warming can be expected to have further environmental effects. For example, sea levels will rise as polar ice melts (Houghton, Jenkins, & Ephraums, 1990: 275). This will have devastating effects for low-lying islands and coastal areas (McMichael, 2001: 305–306) and the large proportion of humanity living there. It can also be expected to affect weather patterns and food production, both of which will have an impact on health. Pathogens that thrive in warmer temperatures could cause outbreaks and the geographic spread of various infectious diseases (McMichael, 2001: 300–303).

Global warming is not the only environmental change likely to have an impact on global health. Deforestation, in addition to contributing to global warming, also leads to increased flooding. Ozone depletion, while contributing to global warming, also threatens higher levels of skin cancer and adverse effects on vision and possibly also on the immune system (McMichael, 1993: 183–194). Irresponsible use of land can lead to desertification, with a resulting impact on food production and access to potable water.

The dislocation of people caused by rising sea levels, combined with shortages of water and arable land, likely will result in conflicts over scarce resources (McMichael, 2001: 300).

Humans tend to think of themselves as a highly successful, adaptable species, but they often forget that adaptability is *to an environment* and thus is heavily constrained by the environment. In other words, although humans can adapt to some changes in environment, they cannot adapt to most possible changes. Humans can currently survive in only a very small part of one universe, and it is only relatively recently in the history of our small planet that conditions became conducive to the emergence of humans.[6] Given both how recent the human species is and how many millions of other species have become extinct, any evidence of the resilience of our species is extremely limited.[7]

Responding to Arguments That Humans Have No Duty to Treat Animals and the Environment Better

So far I have shown that some maltreatment of animals and the environment can have an adverse impact on global human health. Accordingly, even those who are not concerned about animals or the environment have anthropocentric reasons to avoid the relevant maltreatment. Those who would prefer not to alter their treatment of animals and the environment may nonetheless want to resist the conclusion that we have a duty to make these changes. Sometimes they do this by denying the factual claims I have made. They deny, for example, that humans are contributing to global warming or otherwise damaging the environment in ways that will cause human suffering. This is not the place and I am not the person to evaluate that challenge. The overwhelming majority of the relevant scientific community accepts the factual claims I have made, and thus, whereas I cannot exclude the possibility that the majority of relevant scientists are mistaken, the dominant scientific view is not an unreasonable starting point. On the assumption that the factual claims are true, I shall, in the following sections, consider and reject three philosophical arguments for the view that humans have no duty to change the way they treat animals and the environment.

The Argument from Insignificant Difference

One commonly advanced argument is that any individual's actions make no noticeable contribution to the unfortunate effects described. For example, even if rearing many animals in cramped conditions makes the emergence of new zoonotic diseases more likely, no individual's purchase of meat makes a discernible difference to the likelihood of the unfortunate outcome.[8] Similarly, even if humans are collectively causing global warming, any individual's actions make no significant contribution to that trend (Sinnott-Armstrong, 2005). Thus, many are inclined to assume that they are not harming anybody in purchasing their meat or driving their petrol-guzzling cars.

It is tempting to see this as an instance of what Derek Parfit (1984: 75ff) has termed a "mistake of moral mathematics." As others have also noted, there is a difference between making an imperceptible difference to an outcome and making no difference at all. If each person performing an action, such as purchasing meat, causes zero harm, then the sum of all meat purchases must also cause no harm because the sum of any number of zeros is zero. However, we know that

---

[6] A. J. McMichael (1993: 1) notes that "*Homo sapiens* has existed for less than one ten-thousandth of Earth's lifespan – and, indeed, for less than one-thousandth of the time since animal life ventured from the oceans onto the dry land."

[7] Unlike most, I do not find the prospect of human extinction regrettable in itself (see Benatar, 2006). However, there are better and worse ways for humans to become extinct, and the suffering of masses of people inhabiting an increasingly inhospitable environment is among the worse ways.

---

[8] This sort of argument, although in a version discussing animal rather than human interests, is advanced by Shafer-Landau (1994).

the sum of all meat purchases certainly does cause harm because without those purchases, there would be no demand for meat, and without the demand, billions of animals would not be treated cruelly and killed. Thus, if the sum of all meat purchases causes a vast amount of harm, individual purchases cannot make no difference, even though they may make only an imperceptible difference. Jonathan Glover (1975: 174) recommends what he calls the "Principle of Divisibility" – "that the harm done in such cases should be assessed as a fraction of a discriminable unit, rather than as zero." He provides an engaging and helpful example to illustrate the problem that results from rejecting the principle of divisibility:

> Suppose a village contains 100 unarmed tribesmen eating their lunch. 100 hungry armed bandits descend on the village and each bandit at gunpoint takes one tribesman's lunch and eats it. The bandits then go off, each one having done a discriminable amount of harm to a single tribesman. Next week, the bandits are tempted to do the same thing again, but are troubled by new-found doubts about the morality of such a raid. Their doubts are put to rest by one of their number who does not believe in the principle of divisibility. They then raid the village, tie up the tribesmen, and look at their lunch. As expected, each bowl of food contains 100 baked beans. The pleasure derived from one baked bean is below the discriminable threshold. Instead of each bandit eating a single plateful as last week, each takes one bean from each plate. They leave after eating all the beans, pleased to have done no harm.
>
> *(Glover, 1975: 174–175)*

Rejecting the principle of divisibility, he suggests, entails that it makes a moral difference whether each bandit takes one plate of food from one tribesman or each takes one bean from each tribesman. However, because there is actually no moral difference between these alternatives, we should accept rather than reject the principle of divisibility.

The problem is that the analogy of the bandits does not seem applicable to the sorts of harms I have described. Most important, the contribution that each person makes to these harms is not part of a linear, cumulative process as it arguably is in the case of the bandits.[9] Given the complexity of the causal chain linking individual actions to the harms caused to animals and the harms caused via environmental damage, many individual actions will make not an imperceptible difference but rather no difference at all to the amount of harm.

For example, while the number of animals maltreated and killed is somewhat responsive to the demand for meat and animal products, it is not so sensitive to demand that every single purchase of meat, let alone every meat meal, will result in further harm being caused to an animal. Instead, there are (unknown) thresholds that, if met, will trigger substantial harm. Matters are even more complicated in the case of environmental damage, given the interplay between one's actions and multiple complex systems. Nor do all emissions cause harm. For example, some particular emitted carbon dioxide molecules will be taken in by plants and used during photosynthesis, and a very small proportion of the carbon dioxide that enters the ocean is eventually stored in carbonate rocks, thereby causing no damage at all.

Given these facts, the principle of divisibility may not be the best solution to the problem of insignificant difference, at least as it arises in the case of animals and the environment. It has thus been suggested (Matheny, 2002) that we should instead respond to the problem of insignificant difference by calculating the *expected utility* of our actions. The expected utility of an action is the product of the utility resulting from the action and the probability of that utility occurring. In the sorts of cases we are considering, the probability of a bad outcome is low, but this is offset by the severity of the badness when it does occur.

For example, imagine that meat production is sensitive to every hundred purchases (the precise number does not matter). Whereas only one in a hundred purchases will make a difference to the amount of suffering caused, the difference that the hundredth purchase will make will be all the suffering and death required to generate meat for a hundred purchases. In other words, when it comes to expected utility, the difference is not insignificant. Although the risk of causing harm is small, the amount of harm one does cause in those rare cases is great enough to make the expected utility of each purchase significant.[10]

---

[9] Another way in which the bandits are a poor analogy is that they constitute a coordinated group acting in concert, whereas meat eaters and contributors to environmental damage tend not to be acting in a coordinated manner.

[10] One important reason for employing expected rather than actual utility is that the former but not the latter can be known in advance of acting and is thus a better basis for decision making.

The argument from insignificant difference, which I have now rejected, should not be confused with an overlapping but distinct argument: the egoistic argument that I could lack a *self*-interested reason to desist from actions that aggregated with similar actions of others will cause us all harm. This is the so-called tragedy of the commons. Every individual has a self-interested reason to consume as much as possible of a common resource, even though everybody's doing likewise will deplete the resource, making everybody worse off in the long run. This is because everybody can reason as follows: "If I desist from consuming, I lose out whether or not others are partaking. If they *are* partaking, I lose the advantage of joining them before the resource is depleted, and if others are *not* desisting, I can benefit without the resource being depleted."

The egoistic argument just sketched can acknowledge that my actions aggregated with similar actions of others will cause us all harm, but it can deny that I have a self-interested reason to desist. By contrast, the argument from insignificant difference can acknowledge that I should consider the interests of others, but it denies that the interests of others are negatively affected by the specified actions of an individual.

However, the two arguments do overlap: in both cases, the difference the individual makes to bringing about the tragic outcome is too small to be noticeable. This overlap is instructive because we can apply to the argument from insignificant difference a solution that is regularly applied to the tragedy of the commons. This solution, which involves a shift in focus from the individual to the aggregation of individuals, may appeal even to those who were not persuaded by the expected utility response to the argument from insignificant difference.

The tragedy of the commons can be avoided by establishing an authority over the commons – an authority that regulates its use and, by penalizing violators, provides a self-interested reason to individuals to comply with the regulations that promote the common good. Similarly, a shift in focus, from individual action to public policy, provides a second solution to the argument from insignificant difference. Good public policy will prohibit or at least disincentivize the *kinds* of actions (as distinct from individual actions) that cause harm. The makers of public policy are not interested in your action independently of the actions of everybody else. They are interested in the aggregated actions of individuals. It is quite clear that

the aggregation of certain individual actions causes harm. There is thus good reason to adopt policies that protect global health.

Two Kinds of Discounting Argument

I have described a number of ways in which maltreatment of animals and damage to the environment can adversely affect global human health. Some people who think that we have no duty to prevent these adverse affects do so because these effects are not immediate but rather will be felt only in the future. In this section and the next, I consider arguments of this kind.

First, in this section, I consider two kinds of *discounting* argument – a radical one and a more moderate one. The radical argument concludes that we need not consider the interests of future people at all. The moderate argument concludes that the interests of future people, although worthy of moral consideration, should not weigh as heavily as the interests of present people. Thus, whereas the radical version of the discounting argument "discounts" in the sense of "does not count at all," the more moderate argument "discounts" in the sense of "counts less."

Radical Discounting

Consider, first, the radical discounting argument. It denies that we have *any* duties to some humans. According to this view, morality (or justice) should be understood in terms of reciprocity. Morality, on this view, is a contract between parties who undertake to bear the costs of the contract in exchange for the more substantial benefits that the contract yields. On this view, morality is grounded in rational self-interest: you agree not to stab my back, and I agree not to stab yours.

One of the implications of such a view is that we have no duties, even no negative duties, to future people.[11] We do nothing wrong if we harm them. This is because there can be no reciprocity with future people. First, we cannot enter into agreements with them. When we exist, they do not, and when they exist, we do not. Second, whereas we can affect their lives, they can do nothing to us.[12] Thus,

---

[11] Some people, for reasons that will be implicit in what follows, might wish to restrict this claim to those future people whose lives do not overlap (or do not overlap significantly) with ours.

[12] I leave aside here the things they could do to our remains or the memories or records of us.

we would have no self-interested reason to enter into an agreement with them even if we could. This fact is captured in the famous quip: "Why should I care about posterity? What has posterity ever done for me?" This view is different from the one embodied in another famous (or, more accurately, infamous) quotation, the imagery of which is particularly apt in our context: "*Après moi, le deluge.*"[13] This latter view expresses an indifference to the interests of future people, whereas the *morality as reciprocity* view goes further and claims that this indifference is morally acceptable.

The reciprocity view of morality is deeply flawed. Not only does it exclude future people from moral consideration, but it also excludes some currently existing people. Most obviously, it excludes those who, throughout their lives, are sufficiently severely disabled that we either cannot enter into an agreement with them or have no self-interested reason to do so.

This is a difficult conclusion to swallow, and there seems to be good reason not to swallow it. The reciprocity view seems to misunderstand fundamentally what morality is about. Although we have a duty to do what we have agreed to do, it is far from clear that the only duties we have are those we have agreed to. Moreover, it seems that part of the point of morality is to ensure that we give consideration to people irrespective of their ability to do things for or to us. This is not, as Allen Buchanan (1990: 233) says, "mere prejudice or irrational benevolent impulse." Instead, it is "a stable, theoretically embedded practical belief" (Buchanan, 1990: 233). If we reject this view, we are committed to thinking, among other things, that there is nothing wrong with torturing, for one's own pleasure, a severely disabled person with whom one has no self-interested reason to enter into an agreement.

Moderate Discounting

There is a more moderate and arguably more common discounting argument. It does not treat the interests of future people as intrinsically unimportant. Instead, it claims that the further in the future costs are expected, the less weight they should have in decisions about what we should do. This is the *social discount* view, common in economics. The precise *rate* per annum at which future costs should be discounted is a matter of dispute, but I shall attempt to

bypass that specific question and instead shall ask whether future costs should be discounted at all.

Various reasons might be offered for prioritizing current people over future ones.[14] The first and worst reason is that current people exist earlier. There is nothing to recommend this view. The time at which one exists should not, in and of itself, determine how much one's basic[15] interests count. An analogy between geographically and temporally distant people is apt. Although it might be psychologically easier to harm somebody who is far away than somebody who is close by, it is not morally less bad. People's important interests do not count less merely because those people are geographically distant. Nor do they count less merely because they are temporally distant. Consider Joel Feinberg's helpful example of a person who hides a bomb in a kindergarten, setting it to explode six years later, at which time it kills or maims many five-year-olds (Feinberg, 1984: 97). It is hard to see how this person's act is any less bad than if he[16] had set the bomb to explode five minutes after he had left the building.[17]

The problem with the first reason for discounting the interests of future people is that it is arbitrary. The mere fact that people exist later is irrelevant. Other reasons for discounting the interests of future people, therefore, will need to be nonarbitrary. They will need to explain *why* later costs should be counted less. The most common such reason is that a cost should be discounted to the extent that it is less than certain. There can be various reasons to be unsure that a cost will materialize, but one of them is that if it will occur at all, it will only occur later. All things being equal, the later something is projected to occur, the less sure we can be that it will occur. This is because there are so many possible intervening variables that could

---

[13] "After me, the flood." This is usually attributed to Louis XV, but that attribution may be apocryphal.

[14] Simon Caney discusses these issues in more detail than I am able to here. See Caney (2009).

[15] I add this adjective because Simon Caney is correct that one might draw a distinction between more and less important interests with regard to discounting. See Caney (2009: p. 167).

[16] For an argument as to why using the male pronoun is not sexist, please see Benatar (2005).

[17] To be fair, the social discount rate is often set very low – significantly less than 1% per annum – in which case defenders of it would be committed to thinking that it is only marginally less bad to set the bomb to explode in six years' time. Those who think this is an adequate defense need only adapt Professor Feinberg's example such that the bomb is set to explode in the significantly further future.

mitigate or eliminate the outcome. For example, a cost that is projected for the distant future might well never be paid because all life will have become extinct for a reason quite independent of the action that generates the projected cost. Thus, if dangerous increases in global temperature were projected to occur only in a million years time, those concerned about human health should worry less because the chances of humans having become extinct for other reasons by that time are much higher than the chances of humans becoming extinct by next year. Temporal discounting is thus but one kind of discounting for diminished probability. It is not futurity per se but the lower probability that explains the discounting.

Although this explanation has a certain plausibility to it, it is an unconvincing justification for denying that the current generation has a duty to change the way it treats animals and the environment. This is because at least some of the quite serious consequences of environmental damage for global human health are projected (with degrees of probability ranging from "virtually certain" to "likely") to occur in the very foreseeable future (later in the twenty-first century; Pachauri & Resinger, 2007: 11–13). As far as I know, similar risk assessments (for humans) resulting from maltreatment of animals have not been conducted.[18] However, given the historical frequency of epidemics and pandemics of zoonotic infectious diseases, we have strong inductive reason to think that the next one is not so far off as to be significantly discountable. The emergence of the COVID-19 pandemic has demonstrated just how warranted this reasoning was.

Thus, even if social discounting is appropriate, the rate at which we can discount at least some of the serious costs is so minimal as to be practically irrelevant. This is particularly the case because these later costs may be averted without incurring serious costs now. Consuming less need not entail a lower quality of life for current people, or at least for the more affluent among them, who are also the biggest consumers per capita. Shifting to alternative, renewal energy sources, for example, would mean that we could use as much energy without consuming nonrenewal resources and polluting the environment. Eating no or less meat need not

lower quality of life. Indeed, it could even raise it by securing the individual health benefits that come from a diet without meat or with less of it.

There is a third kind of reason that might be advanced for discounting future costs – one that is compatible with (but which does not require) thinking that later people *will* bear the costs. This kind of reason suggests, following some or other preferred principle of distributive justice, that it would be fairer for future generations to bear the cost.[19] Whereas it is impossible to consider all possible distributive principles that could plausibly justify discounting future costs, any such principles, would have to assume that later people were better able to bear the costs, perhaps because they would be wealthier or because they would have the technical capacity to reverse or adapt to the environmental damage.

But even such lines of argument seem doomed. First, this discounting rationale may conflict with the previous one – discounting on the basis of uncertainty. After all, we cannot be sure that future generations will be richer than ours. Indeed, it could be that on account of what we do, they are poorer than we are. (Just think what a deadly pandemic, water scarcity, and millions of refugees from rising sea levels and associated conflicts could do to the global economy.) Second,[20] even if future generations are wealthier than ours, it does not follow that all people within those generations will be. Because the poorest of future people are most likely to suffer the consequences of our actions, any principle based on ability to pay would assign the costs of our actions to us rather than them. Third, even if all future people were richer or technologically more advanced than we are, they might be insufficiently wealthier or technologically advanced to warrant discounting. The costs may increase at a greater rate than the wealth and technical capacity. It may thus be sufficiently cheaper and easier, all things considered, to prevent the problems than to fix them later.

A policy of prevention has the added advantage of avoiding those harms that will creep up on humans, perhaps springing suddenly, and will thus be felt before they are prevented or mitigated. A zoonotic pandemic is just such a possibility. People keep engaging in the risky behavior. Once the lethal pandemic arrives, it will be too late to prevent many

---

[18] This is indicative of the point, made earlier, that there is much greater awareness of the connection between the environment and global human health than there is between animal and human well-being.

[19] Simon Caney raises this possibility in order to reject it. See Caney (2009, pp. 170–175).

[20] The following responses are either drawn or adapted from Simon Caney. See Caney (2009, pp. 170–175).

deaths. Damage control will be the only option. This has been borne out by the COVID-19 experience. Similarly, scientists now fear various climate change "tipping points." These are possible major changes that are irreversible (within human rather than cosmic time frames). They could cause quite considerable human suffering that may be immune to financial and even technical solutions. In other words, a policy of prevention could avoid a situation in which a problem arises that cannot be fixed.

The Nonidentity Argument

The discounting arguments, I noted earlier, take it to be relevant that the effects on humans of our damage to the environment and our maltreatment of animals will be felt in the future. The next argument does the same, but in a different way. Instead of arguing that future people should count less or not at all, it allows that future people *could* count equally. However, it questions whether future people really are harmed by our current actions. This might sound to some like an empirical argument, one that denies that our current actions will lead to epidemics or will damage the environment in the way most scientists think. However, the argument at hand is instead a philosophical one, embodying metaphysical, conceptual, and ethical features.

The metaphysical component pertains to "personal identity in different possible histories of the world" (Parfit, 1984: 351) or, in other words, to the necessary conditions for a particular person's coming into existence. Each one of us emerged from a combination of particular sex cells (a particular ovum and a particular spermatozoon).[21] Thus, for example, had a different spermatozoon (whether of the same man or a different one) fertilized the ovum from which one developed, one would not have come into existence. Somebody else would have existed instead.

Derek Parfit (1984) has famously argued that when we are choosing between a policy of conservation and a policy of depletion, the identity of which people will exist in the future will likely be affected. This, he thinks, is because following such different policies will affect which people meet and procreate, or at least when they will procreate. Because the identity of future people is contingent on the conjunction of two specific gametes, choosing between two very different policies could readily affect who comes into existence.

Consider, next, the conceptual component of the argument. Here *harm* is understood as "making somebody worse off than he or she would otherwise have been." For somebody to be worse off in some state, it is then suggested, one must be able to compare that state to the alternative state in which he or she would have been. However, if that person would *not otherwise have been*, one cannot compare the state in which he or she exists with the alternative.

The problem, then, is that following a policy of depletion instead of a policy of conservation might harm nobody. Nobody who exists at some later time is worse off than they would otherwise have been because if the alternative policy of conservation had been adopted, then different people would have existed. Although the quality of life of those people who exist as a result of a policy of depletion will be worse than the quality of life of those people who would exist as a result of a policy of conservation, it will not be worse than the quality of *their own* lives would have been.

Consider next the ethical component of the argument I am now considering. If the foregoing is correct, then we cannot morally require conservation and prohibit depletion on the grounds that the latter *harms* future generations. This poses a problem for those ethical approaches – so-called person-affecting approaches – that seek to evaluate actions on the basis of whether they affect people.

Thus, it is said, if we are to claim that conservation is preferable to depletion, we must instead appeal to an alternative moral framework, often known as an *impersonal* approach. Impersonal approaches are not concerned with whether an action makes people worse off. Instead, they are concerned with whether one outcome (impersonally considered) is better than the alternative, even if it is not better *for* anybody. Impersonal views can say why we should opt for conservation rather than depletion: the outcome of the former will be better than the outcome of the latter.

Although impersonal views can explain why we should opt for conservation over depletion, such views lead to repugnant and absurd conclusions that call into question whether an impersonal approach is a suitable refuge for those wishing to explain the wrongfulness of depletion policies or practices. In brief, the problems include the following: impersonal views that are interested in producing the greatest *total* good must allow, when choosing between two possible outcomes, that an outcome in which the people have a lower quality of life is preferable if

---

[21] A similar story could be told, *mutatis mutandis*, for clones.

there are sufficient additional people that the total happiness is greater than in the alternative outcome. This means that these impersonal total views must prefer a world in which there are billions of people leading lives that are barely worth living to a world in which there are only a hundred thousand people with very good quality of life, as long as there is more happiness in total in the more populous world. Derek Parfit (1984: 381–390) rightly calls this conclusion repugnant.

The more populous world just described might contain more happiness in total than the more sparsely inhabited one, but it nonetheless contains less happiness *on average* – that is, the total good divided by the number of people. This might lead some impersonal theorists to seek the outcome with the greatest amount of good on average (rather than in total). But this, too, is problematic. Consider the following: You are contemplating whether to have a child. On the impersonal average view, you are permitted to have the child if its existence would raise the average quality of life of all people. This means, to use Derek Parfit's memorable example, that the quality of life of the ancient Egyptians can be relevant to whether or not you may have a child. Yet it seems clear that "research in Egyptology cannot be relevant to our decisions whether to have children" (Parfit, 1984: 420).

If person-affecting views as well as impersonal ones are problematic, then it is unclear what the grounds are for saying that we should avoid actions that will lead future people to suffer. This is clearly a problem, even if it is not clear how the problem can be solved.

Various solutions have been proposed, although it is unsurprising that they have proved contentious. If we focus on the person-affecting approach, one could deny that all changes to our behavior would affect the identities of future people. While abstaining from driving might lead to one's meeting and mating with somebody closer to home and thereby affecting the identity of future people, a change from a vehicle that consumes lots of petrol to a more fuel-efficient one or, in time, to a car powered exclusively by renewable energy sources need not have that effect. Nor is it clear why the choice between rearing animals intensively or not should affect the identity of (many) future people.

Even if we assume that all such changes would alter the identity of future people, we might take issue with the notion that to harm somebody is to make that person worse off (Benatar, 2006: 21). And even if we think that harming somebody is to make him worse off, we might deny that this must involve a comparison between two states of the person (Feinberg, 1992).

However, given how contested these solutions are, I propose to show how we can *bypass* the problem even if we cannot *solve* it. In other words, let us assume, for the sake of argument, that we cannot explain why it is wrong to engage in actions that cause later generations to suffer. I contend that we ought still to desist, for purely anthropocentric global health reasons, from damaging the environment and maltreating animals. This is because the evidence suggests that not changing our actions will later harm people who *already* exist. Some of the youngest people on the planet can expect to be around for up to another 80 or 90 years, a time span within which significant effects of our actions are likely to be felt (Pauchauri & Reisinger, 2007: 11–13). Our current actions also threaten older people and those disadvantaged young people whose life expectancy is not as long as more advantaged children. The intensive rearing of animals poses an ongoing threat of a deadly zoonotic pathogen emerging and becoming pandemic. The very young and the very old are especially vulnerable, but in the case of very virulent pathogens, people in the prime of their lives are also at serious risk. All this, too, has been borne out by the COVID-19 experience. It is thus simply a mistake to think that our actions will have an impact only on the quality of life of future humans – those who have not yet come into existence. Our actions will impact them, and even if these impacts will be more serious than earlier ones, sufficient damage could be done to existing people to warrant our desisting from the actions in question.

"The End [of This Chapter] Is Nigh"

There have been those, throughout human history, who have predicted "doom soon" – an impending catastrophe and sometimes even the "end of the world."[22] Whereas such doomsayers are *sometimes* (or will someday be) correct, most of them make the mistake of telescoping the future of humanity or some component thereof. Telescopes make things look closer than they really are. A far more common error is either to look through the wrong

---

[22] That is the *human* world, because the Earth itself will survive the fulfillment of many such predictions.

end of the telescope, making the consequences of our actions look further away, or not looking at the future but rather focusing myopically on the present. This is one reason why humans act the way they do. Just as smokers pay more attention to their immediate gratification than to the long-term costs to themselves, so do many people maltreat animals and contribute to the destruction of the environment for their immediate gratification without thinking of the longer-term consequences of their actions for themselves and others.

This shortsightedness and attention to more immediate gratification is, of course, but one of many reasons why humans are not doing more to curb their excesses. Another, related problem is the mistaken perception or assumption of the invulnerability of the human species. This connects with the previous point in that the sense of invulnerability is fed by taking a more immediate view rather than a longer view. But it is also attributable to a widespread faith in the human capacity to adapt. There is a tendency to think that we can find a solution to any problem. Indeed, all too often, the focus is on cures rather than on prevention. This explains, for example, why so little attention has been given to preventing new pandemics by avoiding exploitative treatment of animals and why so much attention has been given to responding to pandemic threats when they do occur. This attitude increases animal suffering. Having bred them in intensive conditions or otherwise mistreated them, thereby generating the pandemic threat, humans then cull animals in their millions when the threat begins to materialize, or they experiment on them in order to produce vaccines or cures. These reactive instead of proactive inclinations also harm humans. Trying to nip a pandemic in the bud or, worse still, attempting to curb it once it is in full vigor is generally less effective than preventing it upstream.

The world is laden with suffering – both human and animal. It will remain that way as long as there is sentient life on the planet. However, there are things we can do to influence just how much suffering there is. I have shown how current human practices damage the environment and bring suffering to animals in ways that can be expected also to cause human suffering. I have rejected various arguments that we need not desist from these practices. In so doing, I have suggested that instead of "killing two birds with one stone," we, in one go, could and should be sparing two kinds of beings – human and nonhuman animals – from suffering.

References

Benatar, D. (2005). Sexist language: alternatives to the alternatives. *Public Affairs Quarterly* **19**, 1–9.

Benatar, D. (2006). *Better Never to Have Been: The Harm of Coming Into Existence*. Oxford, UK: Oxford University Press.

Benatar, D. (2007). The chickens come home to roost. *American Journal of Public Health* **97**, 1545–1546.

Boyd, W. (2001). Making meat: science, technology and American poultry production. *Technology and Culture* **42**, 631–664.

Buchanan, A. (1990). Justice as reciprocity versus subject-centered justice. *Philosophy and Public Affairs* **19**, 227–252.

Caney, S. (2009). Climate change and the future: discounting for time, wealth and risk. *Journal of Social Philosophy* **40**, 163–186.

DeGrazia, D. (1996). *Taking Animals Seriously*. Cambridge, UK: Cambridge University Press.

Feinberg, J. (1984). *Harm to Others*. New York, Oxford University Press.

Feinberg, J. (1992). Wrongful life and the counterfactual element in harming, in *Freedom and Fulfilment*. Princeton, NJ: Princeton University Press, pp. 3–36.

Gao, F., Bailes, E., Robertson, D. L., et al. (1999). Origin of HIV-1 in the chimpanzee *Pan troglodytes troglodytes*. *Nature* **397**, 436–441.

Glover, J. (1975). It makes no difference whether or not I do it. *Proceedings of the Aristotelian Society, Supplementary Volume* **XLIX**, 171–190.

Gorman, J. (2020). Significance of pangolin viruses in human pandemic remains murky. *New York Times*, March 30. Available at www.nytimes.com/2020/03/26/science/pangolin-coronavirus.html (accessed April 22, 2020).

Guan, Y., Zheng, B. J., He, Y. Q., et al. (2003). Isolation and characterization of viruses related to the SARS coronavirus from animals in Southern China. *Science* **302**, 276–278.

Houghton, J. T., Jenkins, G. J, & Ephraums, J. J. (eds.) (1990). *Climate Change: The IPCC Scientific Assessment*. Cambridge, UK: Cambridge University Press.

Matheny, G. (2002). Expected utility, contributory causation, and vegetarianism. *Journal of Applied Philosophy* **19**, 293–297.

McMichael, A. J. (1993). *Planetary Overload: Global Environmental Change and the Health of the Human Species*. Cambridge, UK: Cambridge University Press.

McMichael, A. (2001). *Human Frontiers, Environments and Disease*. Cambridge, UK: Cambridge University Press.

Osterholm, M. T. (2005). Preparing for the next pandemic. *New England Journal of Medicine* **352**, 1839–1852.

Pachauri, R. K., & Reisinger, A. (eds.) (2007). Summary for policymakers, in *Climate Change 2007: Synthesis Report. A Report of the Intergovernmental Panel on Climate Change.* Geneva: IPCC, pp. 1–22.

Parfit, D. (1984). *Reasons and Persons*. Oxford, UK: Oxford University Press.

Regan, T. (1983). *The Case for Animal Rights*. Berkeley: University of California Press.

Scott, M. R., Will, R. G., Ironside, J., et al. (1999). Compelling transgenetic evidence for transmission of bovine spongiform encephalopathy prions to humans. *Proceedings of the National Academy of Science USA* **96**, 15137–15142.

Shafer-Landau, R. (1994). Vegetarianism, causation and ethical theory. *Public Affairs Quarterly* **8**, 85–100.

Sharp, P., Bailes, E., Chaudhuri, R. R., et al. (2001). The origins of acquired immune deficiency syndrome viruses: where and when? *Philosophical Transactions of the Royal Society of London B* **356**, 867–876.

Singer, P. (1990). *Animal Liberation*, 2nd ed. New York: Avon Books.

Sinnott-Amstrong, W. (2005). It's not *my* fault: global warming and individual moral obligations, in Sinnott-Armstrong, W., & Howarth, R. B. (eds.), *Perspectives on Climate Change: Science, Economics, Politics and Ethics, Advances in the Economics of Environmental Resources*, vol. 5. Amsterdam: Elsevier, pp. 285–307.

Weber, J., & Alcorn, K. (2000). Origins of HIV and the AIDS epidemic. *Medscape General Medicine* **2**, 1–6.

Webster, R. G. (2004). Wet markets: a continuing source of severe acute respiratory syndrome and influenza. *Lancet* **365**, 234–236.

Will, R. G., Ironside, J. W., Zeidler, M., et al. (1996). A new variant of Creutzfeldt-Jakob disease in the UK. *Lancet* **347**, 921–925.

Zhang, L., Shen, F-M., & Lin, Z. (2020). Origin and evolution of 2019 novel coronavirus. *Clinical Infectious Diseases* **71**, 882–883.

Justice and Global Health: Planetary Considerations

Henk ten Have

Introduction

When I started to work in Pittsburgh, a journalist called with a request for an explanation about infant mortality. Recent surveys had shown that infant mortality in some neighborhoods of Pittsburgh was higher than in developing countries such as Nicaragua and the Philippines. These findings caused an uproar on social media. How was this possible? In 42 countries, infant mortality rates are lower than in the United States. For every 1,000 American babies born, an average of 5.82 will die before their first birthday. In Pennsylvania, the average infant mortality rate is 5.9. In Pittsburgh, the average is 6.65, but in some areas it is up to 22, especially among African-American populations. Americans, unaccustomed to not being in a leadership role, cannot imagine why such disparities occur (Smith, 2017). Visiting such neighborhoods reveals the deterioration and desolation associated with high unemployment, no health insurance, no decent housing, irregular waste removal, no schools, and no shops. If children are ill, they simply have no resources for medical care or medication. My question to the journalist therefore was, "Have you ever visited one of these neighborhoods?" Of course, she hadn't. Most people only know them from movies or online videos.

This story illustrates the effects of globalization, vulnerability, and the role of social media. First, it shows that the adverse effects of the globalization of problems are ubiquitous. For a long time, access to medication was restricted to people living in developing countries. Today, the prices of essential medications are so high that even citizens in wealthy countries have increasing difficulty securing the drugs they need. Problems with fake medication that tend to pervade countries such as Bangladesh are now common in Europe and the United States. Infectious diseases such as malaria and yellow fever, once almost controlled in developed countries, are back as public

health threats in most countries. Globalization, characterized by mobility, not only disregards borders but is also a two-way interaction. It is not possible to displace health problems comfortably to distant areas of the globe. Localized dangers have become global.

The second dimension of this story is the significance of vulnerability. This is an ambiguous notion for contemporary bioethics because it has emerged in a specific context of globalization (Ten Have, 2016a). Globalization has created an asymmetry of power with vulnerability as one of the major symptoms. Vulnerability, especially of women in developing countries, is growing. Failing states are blamed for increasing vulnerability because of the persistence of poverty and hunger. The discourse of vulnerability has particularly emerged and expanded in the context of global phenomena such as natural disasters and the pandemic of HIV/AIDS or COVID-19. Vulnerability is not a coincidence but the deliberate outcome of the political and economic logic that drives processes of globalization. Policies have shifted away from maximization of public welfare to the promotion of enterprise, innovation, and profitability. This logic has changed the nature of state regulation, prioritizing the well-being of market actors over the well-being of citizens. Rules and regulations protecting society and the environment are weakened in order to promote global market expansion. A new social hierarchy has emerged worldwide with the integrated at the top (those who are essential to the maintenance of the economic system), the precarious in the middle (those who are not essential to the system and thus disposable), and the excluded at the bottom (the permanently unemployed). According to such analyses, vulnerability is the result of the damaging impact of economic global logic. It is also a symptom of social disintegration. As a consequence of this type of globalization, threats to human well-being are increasing, and coping mechanisms are being eroded. Vulnerability has become the hallmark of globalization; it is everywhere and affects everybody. It is not simply that threats and challenges have multiplied and do not respect borders but rather that people and communities have diminishing abilities to cope with them. Vulnerability is not an individual concern but is produced by social, economic, and political changes associated with globalization. It demonstrates that societies have become subservient to the needs of the economic system (Garrafa et al., 2010).

This story furthermore illustrates the power of social media. Findings about infant mortality and health in general interest people; they comment, share their views and experiences, and search for explanations. In 2017 in the United Kingdom, the parents of Charly Gard launched a social movement with several hundred thousand supporters across the world. They contested decisions of medical doctors and courts concerning their severely handicapped child. In a short time, they raised $1.67 million for possible treatment. Through mobilizing support for their case with the use of social media and the internet, the parents created a global controversy.

Bioethics witnessed another outbreak of moral outrage at the end of November 2018 when Jiankui He, a Chinese researcher, announced that he had produced two genetically edited babies. He had used the gene-editing technology known as CRISPR to alter the genome and make the twin babies resistant to future HIV infection. The scientific community was shocked. There was a global outcry of anger and outrage not only about what he has done but also about how he had done it. These events demonstrate that, in general, and in bioethics in particular, debate and protest are motivated by anger and outrage.

Anger seems to play a more prominent role now in contemporary societies. More than 68% of Americans are angry at least once a day. White middle-class women are the angriest. They are especially angry toward politicians because they enact policies that favor the interests of the rich. Healthcare professionals are also confronted with angry patients, whose anger is directed both at them and at the profession with its paternalism.

It is argued that social media have transformed the expression of moral outrage. It is rare to encounter norm violations in person; only 5% of people report that in daily experiences they witness immoral acts (Crockett, 2017). The internet, however, exposes people to a vast range of misdeeds, corruption,

trafficking, dishonesty, and fraud. Nowadays, most people learn about immoral acts online. This online content is also widely shared. There is evidence that immoral acts encountered online incite stronger moral outrage than immoral acts faced in person or via traditional media. Digital media seem to alter the subjective experience of outrage. Because there is continuous experience of immoral conduct, there can be possible outrage fatigue. But it is also easier to express outrage because the threshold for expressing is lower. Because there is not much chance of encountering the wrongdoer, there is little risk of physical retaliation. The costs of shaming are lower, although people's lives can be made difficult with online retaliations. Anger and moral outrage can be destructive; they can elicit a desire for revenge. They can lead to the perception that offenders are less than human ("monsters") and that they lack core human qualities (Bastian, Denson, & Haslam, 2013).

Moral Outrage

Although the language of moral outrage is common in bioethical debates, it is often not taken seriously. It employs conceptions such as revulsion and repugnance and lack of decency, dignity, respect, and humanity rather than anger. The focus is on injustices such as lack of access to essential medicine, exploitation of vulnerable populations, and public services that provide polluted water. Moral outrage is anger because a moral standard is violated or injustices are witnessed. It is a powerful moral emotion and a source of motivation to engage in action to reaffirm or reestablish the moral standard. Anger and outrage also have a positive meaning. They signal moral quality to others. They clarify that some injustices are not acceptable.

This more positive view is endorsed in a recent publication from Charles Duhigg. He argues that anger has always been an important emotion for human beings. The main question is how to deal with anger and indignation. Anger can make bad situations better because people are listening, speak more honestly, and are more accommodating to complaints and grievances. Moral indignation can be a force for good. It transforms practical and economic complaints into emotional and moral issues. The protests of the "yellow vests" in France, for example, or the *indignados* in Spain are not simply about higher taxes but also about justice and equality. People do not merely want higher wages or better working conditions;

their angry movement also demands rectification of injustices. Moral indignation therefore locates their protest and discontent within a broader fight about rights and wrongs; it reframes complaints into moral offences. Duhigg concludes that we "need moral outrage that motivates citizens to push for a more just society" (Duhigg, 2019: 75).

Nowadays, there is a growing rejection of the idea that the world is a global community. Globalization is regarded as exploitation of trust by an elite minority that reaps most of the benefits. Inequality is growing between and within countries. The driving force of all policies seems to be the maximization of profits. Politicians brag that it is smart to evade taxes and not contribute to the common good. Public policies no longer reflect the interests of average citizens. Social media are an important tool to mobilize people denouncing the concentration of wealth and the growth of inequality at the expense of the majority of the population. They also criticize a practice of democracy that is not really representative. More important, the shared indignation motivates collective action that transforms into connective action – not focused on formal organization but on the use of digital media and sharing of personalized content through social media networks. This kind of action is more fluent and less stable. Activists and self-organizing networks are more autonomous than traditional vehicles of social change.

Destruction of the Environment

One of the major challenges for healthcare and thus bioethics today and a source of injustice and thus moral outrage is environmental degradation (Ten Have, 2019). Potter, who conceived the notion of bioethics in the 1970s, included environmental ethics in the new discipline. But its subsequent development focused on biomedical issues and ignored environmental concerns. Nowadays, bioethical analysis and debate can no longer ignore environmental issues. Climate change, toxic waste, air pollution, ozone depletion, extreme weather events, and loss of biodiversity have significant impacts on health and healthcare. Deforestation and destruction of habitat are associated with the emergence of new virus diseases such as Ebola, Zika, or COVID-19. Focusing on care, treatment, or vaccination of individual patients therefore cannot be disconnected from the wider environmental context in the management of epidemics. A broader concept of bioethics is needed, as

advocated by Potter. Biomedical and environmental ethics should be reconnected in an encompassing ethical approach. One reason is that health and environment are clearly interconnected.

This is not a new idea. It has been a crucial element in social medicine, occupational healthcare, and public health. But its significance has changed recently, transforming the environment from an additional consideration as one of the determinants of health into a crucial global condition for the pursuit of health. This transformation will require the development of "green bioethics" – a broader ethical perspective acknowledging that human beings and nature are deeply connected (Resnik, 2012).

Another reason is that biomedical ethics and environmental ethics as currently conceived have a reductive approach that is too narrow for today's ethical problems. For example, in natural disasters, medicine and public health cannot be separated from environmental challenges (Moreno, 2005). Threats to health arise in a global context of social injustice and environmental damage. Biomedical solutions are therefore often inadequate, and the social, economic, environmental, and political determinants of health are not addressed. Bioethics discourse should do more than focus on individual problems; it should develop a collective, global vision of how human existence can be improved (Benatar, Daar, & Singer, 2003; Sherwin, 2011).

Justice

One of the major ethical principles in the global approach to bioethics is justice. There are several reasons why justice has become a dominant concern. Globalization is associated with increasing inequality and inequity. It has not led to one world that is flat for everybody. It is benefiting a minority that often controls the economic and political decision making. Most people, however, live in other worlds pervaded by hunger, austerity, unemployment, growing insecurity, and vulnerability. Another reason is that the consumption of natural resources is not equal. Total consumption of all resources produces an ecological deficit. We consume more than the Earth can sustain. But the "we" in this case are living in a limited number of countries. People in most other countries do not have a just share of the planet's resources. They suffer from disparities in health and disease, food and water.

Furthermore, biodiversity is not equally distributed. Biodiversity-rich countries are generally poor and not powerful within the global system. Their resources are often exploited by developed countries. Destruction of biodiversity, in contrast, is often the result of lifestyles and policies in developed countries, whereas the negative impact affects people in developing countries.

Policies to protect biodiversity can have unjust consequences. Establishment of protected areas and national parks leads to displacement, especially of Indigenous peoples who provided stewardship for those areas for centuries. Another reason for the emphasis on justice is concern with future generations. Biodiversity emphasizes that contemporary and future living beings are interconnected. They all need a healthy biodiversity to survive. But whose interests will prevail; how do we weigh intragenerational and intergenerational justice?

Finally, the bioeconomic paradigm that prevails in environmentalism, since the adoption of the Convention on Biological Diversity, is another reason for considering issues of justice. In practical policies, biodiversity is regarded as a global resource that generates benefits. Nature is an economic asset. But this paradigm results in appropriation, lack of access, and exclusion, thus raising questions of justice and injustice.

The principle of justice is an important normative tool in the implementation of global bioethics discourse. It transcends the usual emphasis on the autonomous individual and focuses critical attention on the underlying structures and power constellations that determine the social, economic, and environmental conditions in which people live. It not merely criticizes the inequalities produced by neoliberal policies and practices but most of all argues that the benefits of globalization should accrue to everybody. In regard to the environment, justice as an abstract principle has been translated into social movements and activism across the world calling attention for health justice, environmental justice, food justice, and water justice.

Health Justice

New infectious diseases are emerging mostly from world regions with deteriorating biodiversity. They also strike countries that are the least able to defend themselves. Pandemics such as COVID-19 bring havoc to countries with inadequate health infrastructures and an insufficient number of health professionals. Similar disparities occur for many other diseases (Sparke & Anguelov, 2012). A harrowing example of unequal care is tuberculosis. Over 95% of the 1.8 million people who died from this disease (in 2015) lived in low- and middle-income countries. Health justice scholars and activists argue that these health disparities are the result of an unfair system of global governance that gives priority to security rather than health. The current dominance of biosecurity focuses on the dangers of contagion and invasion. When a mortal infection is raging in developing countries, the first concern of other countries is not assistance but protection; they send military, not health professionals. They regard themselves as vulnerable, not the people in affected countries. The discourse of biosecurity has only increased vulnerability, further articulating structural violence, suffering, and dispossession and producing more anxiety and fear. At the same time, the discourse has shifted the blame and responsibility toward the most vulnerable people; they should be resilient, manage their own risks, and learn how to cope, adapt, and recover. However, for them, the most significant biothreat is not terrorism but everyday violence, the terrors of daily human survival (Chen & Sharp, 2014).

Health justice is also important for another dimension of global governance: the intellectual property (IP) rights regime. Patent activity is concentrated in a relatively small number of companies in the Global North. This is especially clear in biotechnology: 90% of all patents on life forms are held by northern companies (Beall, Blanchet, & Attaran, 2017). The global IP regime is not only reinforcing inequalities but also itself the result of an unfair global institutional order (as argued by Pogge, 2013). The establishment of the World Trade Organization (WTO) and the Agreement on Trade-Related Aspects of Intellectual Property Rights (TRIPS) were the outcome of coordinated pressures of Western countries and international businesses as the owners of property rights on developing countries. There was no fair representation of countries involved, no sharing of full information, no democratic bargaining, but a mixture of political and economic threats and coercion. Public involvement was also absent; all negotiations were behind closed doors. But it is not only the process that is unfair. The globalization of IP has primarily benefited the Western countries. The international legal context has been created by owners of IP and in their primary interest. The IP rights regime is an illustration that the global context of health and healthcare itself is unfair.

Environmental Justice

Since the 1970s, the environmental justice movement has criticized the unjust distribution of environmental benefits and harms. Toxic waste used to be dumped and processed close to vulnerable populations, specifically poor neighborhoods. Local and grassroots movements denounced the connections between poverty, ethnicity, and environmental hazards. Instead of the usual emphasis in environmentalism on wilderness and nature, they focused attention on the circumstances in which people are living. Activists criticized the context of oppression, disrespect, and dehumanization that exposed them disproportionally to risks (Scholsberg, 2007). The success of this movement in the United States was followed by increased outsourcing of toxic waste. Dumping in poor and developing countries has generated similar environmental justice movements around the globe. The sense of injustice at the global level is deepening. The dumping sites are usually countries that are not responsible for toxic waste and that generally do not benefit from the lifestyle and consumption patterns associated with waste production (Timmons Roberts, 2007).

Food Justice

As an essential determinant of human life and health, food should be available to everybody. Nonetheless, people are hungry not because there is a lack of food but because global distribution is unequal. People die of starvation in countries that are exporting food. Intensive agriculture has replaced traditional ways of growing food. Numerous small farms in rural areas have been eliminated and their farmers driven into slums and poverty. Powerful agrobusinesses control the production, transport, processing, and marketing of food. Their interest primarily is in trade, less in health and environmental sustainability.

Food justice movements have emerged all over the world (e.g., fair trade, slow food, local food) influencing the global food regime. They attack the power and shortsightedness of corporations and international organizations that transform food into commodities and that are not concerned with biodiversity and global health. They develop alternative approaches to the dominant agricultural model. Social movements such as La Via Campesina claim back sovereignty over food production. Consumer movements nowadays make critical choices. Food is a basic and daily concern for everybody. Many people also care about health and biodiversity. They prefer food that is healthy and green. Because food is not merely a commercial commodity, issues of justice go beyond questions of distribution, scarcity, and access. They also concern respect for diversity and recognition of cultural identity, reducing inequalities in power and control over food production and consumption and participation of people in decision-making processes, not as consumers but as citizens (Alkon & Agyeman, 2011).

Water Justice

Most people regard water as a prime example of the global commons. It is a good that should benefit all: everybody should have equal access, and its management should be a shared responsibility. Nonetheless, continuous efforts are undertaken to enclose these commons and privatize water resources and services. When governments and the United Nations were reluctant to go this way, the same drivers of the IP rights regime as in the fields of drugs and food started to promote the idea that water is a commodity. The World Bank joined with private water companies to establish nongovernmental organizations (NGOs) such as the World Water Council. They constructed a "water crisis," arguing that there is growing scarcity of drinking water and that the only remedy is a market approach of privatization. These neoliberal policies generated vigorous responses and resistance focusing specifically on injustices. The idea of scarcity is contested. The main ethical problem is lack of access to water. Privatization will only increase inequalities in the availability and affordability of water. A blatant example of injustice occurred in Flint, Michigan, one of the poorest and most dangerous cities in the United States. In 2014, drinking water was contaminated with lead following the decision of authorities to change the water source because it was cheaper.

Water justice movements argue that water requires democratic governance (because it is a common good) and should not be controlled by powerful global corporations and agencies. They emphasized that the water crisis can only be solved by common action. Individual water-saving activities will have limited impact. Fresh water is a collective challenge (Peppard, 2014). These movements have been successful in turning back the drive toward privatization of water resources.

Injustices

Justice is an abstract notion. Different theories of justice are not easy to apply. In practice, the emphasis is often on injustices, for example, a tuberculosis patient who can be cured but does not receive treatment because it is too expensive, a child may be hungry because food is not available in his or her region because it is being exported, and a village runs out of water resources because a bottled water company is massively extracting the water. These are concrete examples that ask for responses. They can also be cases for theoretical debate over justice and various theories.

But focusing on injustices is not a theoretical exercise. Injustices have many faces. They direct attention to human responsibility; they are not misfortunes but the result of human activities. Human beings have created and are supporting systems, structures, and regimes that are unfair. These systems do not benefit everyone; they are often imposed and can be violent; and they victimize vulnerable groups and populations.

Judith Shklar (1990) has argued that civilizations advance when what is commonly perceived as misfortune becomes considered injustice. She explains how we might address injustices. Actively unjust agents violate the rules of justice and therefore produce injustices. Of course, these violations should be examined, prosecuted, and punished. Perhaps even more important is passive injustice. This occurs when people do not prevent or oppose wrongs when they are able to do so. They remain indifferent. According to Shklar, this is a failure of citizenship, a civic vice. The sense of injustice should motivate citizens to raise their voices, to protest, and to resist. This is what many are doing when confronted with increasing loss of biodiversity and threats to health, drugs, food, and water.

Justice Is More than Sharing

To address the inequalities of biodiversity, most frequently a concept of justice is used that emphasizes fair exchange between two parties. The Convention on Biological Diversity has defined equitable sharing as one of its goals. Justice is regarded as equitable distribution of benefits and harms. The concept of distributive justice acknowledges that parties usually are in unequal positions. It defines the criteria to establish a fair distribution of goods and services.

The question, however, is whether this concept of justice is sufficient to address the global context and practices of injustice. The emphasis on distribution accommodates very well to the neoliberal ideology and neoliberal regimes. It proceeds with a similar interpretation of biodiversity as a collection of resources that can be used for human needs. These resources can be owned by private agents and agencies.

The main concern is that benefits and harms are shared. However, the question of whether it is fair to privatize such common resources in the first place is not posed. Traditional knowledge is not recognized and protected. Indigenous populations are not respected, and their rights are ignored. In decisions about distribution of benefits, weaker parties such as the poor, minorities, women, and Indigenous people are usually not involved. Neoliberal policies and regimes that promote the concept of distributive justice to address the problem of global injustices are in fact applying the same approach that created the problem as its solution. With this notion of justice, the underlying causes of maldistribution do not need to be taken into consideration. Yet the focus on distribution cannot disregard how inequalities and inequities are produced and sustained (Williams, 2005).

That injustice is more than maldistribution is particularly clear in environmental justice movements. They articulate other dimensions of justice: recognition, participation, and capabilities for human functioning and flourishing not only for individuals but also for communities. They protest against dumping of toxic waste in their neighborhoods because it does not respect them as citizens. People of color and poor populations feel undignified and abused because their health and well-being are disregarded like those of the citizens of Flint. They are subjected to power that ignores their interests and denies their rights. They are also denied any participation in decision-making processes about their own environment. Usually, they are marginalized and excluded. Respect and dignity as preconditions for distributive justice refer to a context of dominion and oppression that first must be addressed if one talks about justice.

This is the message of the critical discourse of biopiracy, for example. Biopiracy is not simply theft of biodiversity resources that can be compensated by fair distribution and benefit-sharing arrangements. Basically, it is a phenomenon of inequalities of power and not so much of distribution of resources.

It is not a market failure that can be addressed by reallocating resources. In the first place, it is a consequence of an ideology that does not recognize differences and identities, that excludes many people from political participation, and that undermines capabilities of individuals and groups. Stories of injustice are motivating movements in environmental justice as well as health, food, and water justice that are based on a plurality of notions of justice (Schlosberg, 2007).

The Role of Imagination

More and more bioethicists nowadays argue that bioethical discourse needs to change. It should rethink its agenda that is focused on "sexy" topics arising in wealthy countries while common global issues are not addressed. Bioethics should develop into a critical discipline that examines the social processes that determine bioethical problems. It is too distanced from the values of ordinary people and too far from the social context in which problems arise. The environment of injustice and inequality frequently denies the fruits of science and medicine to many people (Farmer & Campos, 2004; Benatar, Daar, & Singer, 2005). A helpful suggestion for remedies is offered by Solomon Benatar: what is necessary is a greater moral imagination, enabling us to alter our outlook and actions (Benatar, 2005).

Metaphors and imaginary visions are cognitive ways for thinking about the world and acting on the world. Imaginary visions are not just rhetorical devices. Many metaphors today are mechanistic: the organism as a machine and genes as building blocks. Metaphors do not provide explanations but furnish ways of thinking, give structure to ideas. The concept of solidarity, for example, may broaden the moral imagination of bioethics by shaping sensibility to go beyond particular acts and individual agents (Jennings & Dawson, 2015).

Another example is the notion of vulnerability. Rather than imagining vulnerable people as victims, or as weak and miserable, they can be imagined as dignified persons, as human beings with potential, because they struggle to overcome negative forces and circumstances. Imaginary visions can reflect negative as well as positive experiences: deception and trust, horror and fascination, hope and despair, disgust and admiration, and compassion and self-interest.

In her final book, Mary Midgley focuses on patterns, world pictures and frameworks, ways of thinking to explore the constantly changing world. She argues that there are always different perspectives available. In her view, imaginative visions of how the world is "are the necessary background of all our living. They are likely to be much more important to us, much more influential than our factual knowledge" (Midgley, 2018: 73). There is a close relation between how we think and how we live. We should be looking at life as a whole and thus considering different perspectives. For example, there are always two aspects of human health: the physical aspect appropriate for medicine and science and the imaginative or sympathetic social aspect, reflecting the point of view of the patient and the subject. Philosophy suggests new ways of thinking that call for different ways of living.

It is important to emphasize that bioethics is not a homogeneous discourse. It comprises various discursive practices. It moves from cases and specific situations to more elaborate and abstract arguments. This can be done in multiple ways. Imaginary processes play a role in this movement so that a richer and broader conceptual and analytical apparatus may emerge, giving voice to discourses that are easily silenced. Moral imagination, as a creative faculty of the mind, is not phantasy. It activates value systems that are not dominant and provides alternative styles of thinking that can create other norms and can resist the imposition of current norms.

That ideas can be powerful and have the potential to change norms is illustrated in field of *disease diplomacy*. States have been redefining their interests and responsibilities in regard to emerging infectious diseases. Now that local outbreaks of diseases quickly develop into global threats, national approaches and the traditional norms of containment (quarantine and border control) are no longer sufficient. The need for collective action, sharing information, and transparency to secure global health has changed the normative behavior of states. A new set of expectations concerning responsibilities of states, a new set of norms, has been created, based on a greater sense of global solidarity (Davies, Kamradt-Scott, & Rushton, 2015).

These possibilities for change through broader normative discourse problematize the usual stance of bioethics as a rational and objective discourse. Bioethics identifies itself as an academic discipline that is neutral. It assumes that there are clear boundaries between academic analysis and political engagement. Bioethics provides a "detached authority" that overrides the responses of patients, parents, families, and communities that are often emotional and not well informed, as demonstrated in the Charlie Gard case. Ethical activism in this view will compromise the credibility of bioethics (Ashby & Morrell, 2018). Angus Dawson et al. (2018) have argued that this neutrality is a myth. They are right. Mainstream bioethics is not a neutral discourse. It endorses the ideologies of neoliberalism and scientism, neglects issues of vulnerability and solidarity, and treats justice merely as the distribution of resources. Confronted with human rights violation, for example the inhuman treatment of asylum seekers in Australia and elsewhere, bioethicists should criticize policies that directly harm the most vulnerable people and seriously affect their health.

Finally, bioethics is not only crucial for democracy, as argued by Solomon and Jennings (2017), but it is also essential for civilization. Moral imagination locates us within the stories of "undesirables," "disposables," and "victims." It interrogates our relationships to other people and how they are affected by scientism and neoliberalism. It questions the rules of civilization and standards of appropriateness. The inhumane treatment of other persons threatens "society's conception of civilized life" (Kekes, 1992: 443). Concepts such as respect, recognition, and dignity will then be reconfigured from a moral perspective that primarily applies to individuals into a perspective that is fundamental for society. Human dignity, for example, has motivated the search for shared humanity and therefore human rights (Horton, 2004). It is the basis for mutual respect in decent societies. Bioethics learns that to understand patient cases and medical problems, interpretation of moral experiences is unavoidable. Imagination is important to facilitate interpretation; it generates and produces worldviews, ideals, and values to guide moral perception. Imagination is reshaping and reconstructing our experiences. Philosopher John Dewey has argued that we all have the capacity to imagine (Dewey, 1934; Adams et al., 2015). It is the creative ability to make the absent become present. Imagination projects ideals and values, offers possibilities for thinking and acting, helps us to bring new realities into existence, and conceives alternatives to problematic situations. It also makes use of past experiences because they suggest alternative possibilities. Imagination is therefore a crucial activity for ethics.

Expanding the Circle of Moral Concern

Moral imagination is not merely an inventive power that gives us different ways of seeing the world. It is also especially important for global bioethics. First of all, it provides the capability to empathize with others. It helps us to experience the situation of other human beings, to recognize situations like ours, and to notice the moral demands that others make on us. Second, moral imagination identifies various possibilities for acting. It encourages us to envision how action might help or hurt, to anticipate possible consequences of action, and to project possibilities into the future (Wright, 2003).

The first capability was described by Edmund Husserl, the founder of phenomenology. He argued that imagination brings us beyond the limitations of empirical experience. Imagination is the ability to make the absent become present. It brings new realities into existence. His disciple Edith Stein elaborated the role of imagination in our ability to empathize with others (MacIntyre, 2007). We can imagine ourselves as the other because we recognize what we share, what is essential for all human beings, and what are invariable human goods. Imagination makes us aware of values beyond the limits of our own experience. This characteristic of imagination was furthermore developed by John Dewey (1922). Imagination brings us together as human beings. It is the extension of experience beyond our limited and familiar realm of everyday life. It fosters sympathy and dialogue because it involves taking the perspective of others. Without imagination we cannot see situations from the viewpoint of other persons and cannot understand the experiences of others. It is the capacity to understand the experiences of other.

Processes of globalization have contributed to an emerging global consciousness. More people than ever regard themselves as citizens of the world, living on a common planet and sharing similar fundamental challenges. Global bioethics is developing on the basis of this idea of common humanity (Ten Have, 2016b). It is argued that over time, the circle of moral concern has expanded; our moral horizon has enlarged so that the perspectives of other persons have been taken into account. Siep Stuurman (2017), who extensively studied this historical process, concludes that it is the result of cross-cultural encounters and exchanges producing a dialectic between particularism and universalism. The language of common humanity emerged in critical reflection on prevailing notions of otherness and inequality. The urge to adopt a globally inclusive concept of equality mainly came from Asian, African, and Latin American states. The discourses of otherness and inequality were ceding ground to notions of common humanity. The empathic circle gradually widened, creating a global language of universal equality and respect for human rights and dignity.

The second capability of moral imagination is its creative power. Dewey (1922) describes several roles of the imagination in the process of inquiry. It is conceiving alternatives to problematic situations, it suggests means to reach specific ends, and it evaluates these means through considering possible consequences. The imagination not only enables us to bring to mind future possibilities but also enables us to make use of past experiences (Chambliss, 1991; English, 2016). Social imaginaries, for example, present a conception of the moral order of society. They articulate principles of sociality. How people are living together is expressed in images and stories. This shared understanding of social existence makes common practices possible (Taylor, 2004).

Conclusion

Moral injustices are experienced as violations of intuitive notions of justice. They often imply that there is no respect for dignity, integrity, or honor. People are denied social recognition. The normative assumptions of social interaction are violated. In many cases, people will react with anger, outrage, and indignation. In the context of global bioethics, the principle of justice plays an important role. It locates the discussion of ethical issues outside the usual space of individual autonomy, directing attention to the social, economic, and political conditions in which people live and focusing on the common good.

Globalization, as argued in this chapter, is associated with generalization of local threats and challenges as well as with growing vulnerability. It has also encouraged the use of social media that have become an important outlet for moral outrage and anger concerning injustices. One of the major sources of injustice today is environmental degradation. Rather than stimulating theoretical discourse, it has been an inspiration for social movements and global activism in

specific areas of health justice, environmental justice, food justice, and water justice. The emphasis in these movements is on injustices, that is, on violations of rights, disrespect for dignity, denial of recognition, and exclusion from participation.

This chapter argues that a different and broader concept of bioethics is necessary to face these global challenges – a concept that can be generated and cultivated through moral imagination. Imagining is a creative way of knowing as well as seeing things differently. It recognizes the complexity of human experience. It corrects the analytical and mechanical approach to the world, providing resistance against dehumanizing tendencies. Moral imagination helps to overcome experiences of disrespect and humiliation. But it also helps to overcome social pathologies such as the economic order that has led to moral impoverishment of the social lifeworld or the process of rationalization that is transforming all phenomena into commodities, that is, objects of economic possession (Honneth, 2007). Moral imagination in this perspective is a remedy against moral injuries that are the result of experiences of injustice and that occur because recognition is refused or withdrawn. Particularly because human beings are not primarily autonomous entities, and because human life is intersubjective, humans are vulnerable, so moral injuries are possible. Fortunately, though, human beings have the capability of moral imagination.

References

Smith, A. (2017). Infant mortality in Pittsburgh and beyond. National Health Corps. Available at www.nationalhealthcorps.org/pittsburgh/blog/infant-mortality-pittsburgh-and-beyond.

Adams, S., Blokker, P., Doyle, N., et al. (2015). Social imaginaries in debate. *Social Imaginaries* 1, 15–52.

Alkon, A., & Agyeman, J. (eds.) (2011). *Cultivating Food Justice: Race, Class, and Sustainability*. Cambridge, MA: MIT Press.

Ashby, M., & Morrell, B. (2018). To the barricades or the blackboard: bioethics activism and the "stance of neutrality." *Journal of Bioethical Inquiry* 15, 479.

Beall, R., Blanchet, R., & Attaran, A. (2017). In which developing countries are patents on essential medicines being filed? *Globalization and Health* 13, 38.

Benatar, S., Daar, A., & Singer, P. (2003). Global health ethics: the rationale for mutual caring. *International Affairs* 79(1), 107–138.

Benatar, Daar, A., & Singer, P. (2005). Global health challenges: the need for an expanded discourse on bioethics.

PLoS Medicine **2**(7)), e143. doi:10.1371/journal.pmed.0020143.

Benatar, S. (2005). Moral imagination: the missing component in global health. *PLoS Medicine* **2**(12), e400. doi.org/10.1371/journal.pmed.0020400.

Bastian, B., Denson, T., & Haslam, N. (2013). The roles of dehumanization and moral outrage in retributive justice. *PLoS One* **8**(4), e61841. doi:10.1371/journal.pone.0061842.

Chambliss, J. (1991). John Dewey's idea of imagination in philosophy and education. *Journal of Aesthetic Education* **25**, 43–49.

Chen, N., & Sharp, L. (eds.) (2014). *Bioinsecurity and Vulnerability*. Santa Fe, NM: School for Advanced Research Press.

Crockett, M. (2017). Moral outrage in the digital age. *Nature Human Behavior* **1**, 769–771.

Davies, S., Kamradt-Scott, A., & Rushton, S. (2015). *Disease Diplomacy: International Norms and Global Health Security*. Baltimore: Johns Hopkins University Press.

Dawson, A., Jordens, C., Macneill, P., & Zion, D. (2018). Bioethics and the myth of neutrality. *Journal of Bioethical Inquiry* **15**, 483–486.

Dewey, J. (1922). *Human Nature and Conduct*. New York: Henry Holt & Company.

Dewey, J. (1934). *A Common Faith*. New Haven, CT: Yale University Press.

Duhigg, C. (2019). Why are we so angry? The untold story of how all got so mad at one another. *The Atlantic*, January–February, 63-75.

English, A. (2016). John Dewey and the role of the teacher in a globalized world: imagination, empathy, and 'third voice'. *Educational Philosophy and Theory* **48**, 1046–1064.

Farmer, P., & Campos, N. (2004). Rethinking medical ethics: a view from below. *Developing World Bioethics* **4**, 17–41.

Garrafa, V., Solbakk, J., Vidal, S., & Lorenzo, C. (2010). Between the needy and the greedy: the quest for a just and fair ethics of clinical research. *Journal of Medical Ethics* **36**, 500–504.

Honneth, A. (2007). *Disrespect: The Normative Foundations of Critical Theory*. Cambridge, UK: Polity Press.

Horton, R. (2004). Rediscovering human dignity. *Lancet* **364**, 1081–1085.

Jennings, B., & Dawson, A. (2015). Solidarity in the moral imagination of bioethics. *Hastings Center Report* **45**, 31–38.

Kekes, J. (1992). Disgust and moral taboos. *Philosophy* **67**, 443–447.

MacIntyre, A. (2007). *Edith Stein: A Philosophical Prologue, 1931–1922*. Lanham, UK: Rowman & Littlefield.

Midgley, M. (2018). *What Is Philosophy For?* London: Bloomsbury Academic.

Moreno, J. (2005). In the wake of Katrina, has "bioethics" failed? *American Journal of Bioethics* **5**, W18–W19.

Peppard, C. (2014). *Just Water: Theology, Ethics, and the Global Water Crisis*. Maryknoll, NY: Orbis Books.

Pogge, T. (2013). *World Poverty and Human Rights: Cosmopolitan Responsibilities and Reforms*. Cambridge, UK: Polity Press.

Resnik, D. (2012). *Environmental Health Ethics*. New York: Cambridge University Press.

Schlosberg, D. (2007). *Defining Environmental Justice: Theories, Movements, and Nature*. Oxford, UK: Oxford University Press, pp. 45ff.

Sherwin, S. (2011). Looking backwards, looking forward: hope for bioethics' next twenty-five years. *Bioethics* **25**, 75–82.

Shklar, J. (1990). *The Faces of Injustice*. New Haven, CT: Yale University Press.

Solomon, M., & Jennings, B. (2017). Bioethics and populism: how should our field respond? *Hastings Center Report* **47**, 11–16.

Sparke, M., & Anguelov, D. (2012). H1N1, globalization and the epidemiology of inequality. *Health & Place* **18**, 726–736.

Stuurman, S. (2017). *The Invention of Humanity: Equality and Cultural Difference in World History*. Cambridge, MA: Harvard University Press.

Taylor, C. (2004). *Modern Social Imaginaries*. Durham, NC: Duke University Press.

Ten Have. H. (2016a) *Vulnerability: Challenging Bioethics*. London: Routledge.

Ten Have, H. (2016b). *Global Bioethics: An Introduction*. London: Routledge.

Ten Have, H. (2019). *Wounded Planet: How Declining Biodiversity Endangers Health and How Bioethics Can Help*. Baltimore: Johns Hopkins University Press.

Timmons Roberts, J. (2007). Globalizing environmental justice, in Sandler, R., & Pezzulo, P. (eds.), *Environmental Justice and Environmentalism: The Social Justice Challenge to the Environmental Movement*. Cambridge, MA: MIT Press, pp. 285–307.

Williams, T. (2005). Beyond distributive justice. *Logos: A Journal of Catholic Thought and Culture* **8**, 90–101.

Wright, T. (2003). Phenomenology and the moral imagination. *Logos: A Journal of Catholic Thought and Culture* **6**, 104–121.

Chapter

25

Global Health and Ethical Transculturalism
A Methodology Connecting the East and the West, the Local and the Universal[*]

Jing-Bao Nie and Ruth P. Fitzgerald

Introduction

Contemporary bioethical issues are inherently cross-cultural and global in their nature. This is not surprising because bioethical matters touch everyone in many and different ways. Moral quandaries in healthcare, life sciences, and biotechnology arise ubiquitously across natural and human boundaries, the boundaries between and within nation-states, ethnicities, cultures, communities, and social groups. In addition, the simultaneously large-scale and intimate interactions between and within different cultures and civilizations and the rapid pace at which they change are phenomena that distinguish our times from previous eras. Bioethics – as a particular domain of public discourse and an academic discipline – has thus been rapidly evolving not only in the United States and other Western countries but also on a global scale over the past 50 years. (The field of medical ethics, of course, extends back for several hundred years in modern European and North American traditions and for two to three millennia in India, China, and the West through ancient Greece.)

As a result, an essential prerequisite for contemporary bioethical inquiry to continue to retain its relevance in such times of high interpersonal and institutional mobilities lies in the development of a transcultural and international bioethics, a subfield facing numerous practical and theoretical challenges. How can bioethics help relieve the social suffering, injustice, and inequality that are such a permanent feature of our world and that so frequently transcend local and international borders while simultaneously being created from the legal technicalities that such

borders create? Whereas cultural differences in understanding issues in bioethics are obvious, what are the intellectual and moral implications of these differences, and how should they be dealt with in practical terms? Are cultural and national differences really so radical that the only option open to us is a hoary relativism that holds that "the local is king" or adopting a postmodernist belief about the inevitable clash of cultures and local worlds? Are there universal bioethical values that can transcend widely differing cultural norms and social practices and overcome the coercive power of realpolitik? What would ethical healthcare and medical research look like on a global scale, or are the local variations in biomedicine (despite the strong influence of Western medicine over so many other medical traditions) too great to consider it a global practice? Is there such a thing as global justice, as the newly emerged area of transitional justice would argue? Do human rights matter for a global bioethics, and can the moral vision and language of human rights make any difference and help reform the real sources of various forms of oppression? Can bioethics move beyond its heavy shadow of Western colonialism and imperialism? How can moral traditions of different cultures contribute to the emerging discourse of global bioethics? These are just a few important questions plucked from a long list.

This chapter focuses on the question of how cultural differences in bioethics should be perceived, characterized, and addressed – thus our focus is specifically methodological. While a nascent methodological consciousness is evident in bioethics (e.g., Sugarman & Sulmasy, 2010; McMillan, 2018), the methodological foundations of a transcultural and global bioethics are yet to be placed on its agenda despite the longer-established recognition from several quarters of the *need* for such a study (e.g., Campbell, 1999; Andoh, 2011). Despite growing

---

[*] This chapter is a significantly shortened and revised version of an earlier article: Nie, J.-B., & Fitzgerald, R. (2016). Connecting the East and the West, the local and the universal: the methodological elements of a transcultural approach to bioethics. *Kennedy Institute of Ethics Journal* **26**(3), 219–247.

rapidly, the subfield of transcultural and global bioethics is still dominated by a series of highly problematic methodological modes.

This chapter presents a *transcultural* approach to bioethics and cultural studies. It takes seriously the challenges offered by social sciences and anthropology in particular toward the development of new methodologies for comparative and global bioethics. By the term *transcultural*, we do not mean an international bioethics hemmed in from within particular national borders but transcultural in a sense that allows for the cultural plurality both within and across such borders. The key methodological elements of *ethical transculturalism* include acknowledging the great internal plurality within every culture, highlighting the complexity of cultural differences, upholding the primacy of morality or ethics, incorporating a reflexive theory of social power, and promoting changes or progress toward shared and sometimes new moral values.

A Pervasive Habit: Radically Dichotomizing the East and West, the Local and the Universal

Despite the obvious hegemony of the West, the meeting of diverse cultures constitutes the most visible characteristic of contemporary bioethics. A seminal anthology (Veatch, 2000) has pointed to the breadth of cultural traditions in medical ethics. In the West itself, in addition to a contemporary mainstream bioethics rooted in moral and political liberalism, the Hippocratic tradition and other modified versions of the professional ethics of medicine, as well as Judeo-Christian traditions of medical ethics, are evident, with African and African-American perspectives also featuring. Outside the West, Islam, Hinduism, Buddhism, Confucianism, and Daoism all have developed their own medical ethics traditions. Although not included in the anthology, the Latin American tradition has many additional perspectives to offer (see, e.g., Pessini et al., 2010). Along with these are the varieties of Indigenous and First Nation moral and cultural traditions, which offer critically important insights for contemporary bioethical issues (see, e.g., Tipene-Matua & Wakefield, 2007; McGrath & Phillips, 2008). The list can go on and on.

Yet significant obstacles, both visible and hidden, still exist to achieving adequate cross-cultural understandings and creating ethically sound and culturally sensitive transglobal discourses. Among them is the deeply rooted and still-popular habit of approaching cultural differences through the radical dichotomizing of the East and the West, the local and the universal.

In comparing Western and non-Western cultures, such as the United States and China, one of the most pervasive approaches to defining and representing cultural differences is to set one's own culture against its presumed opposite – "us" versus "them," the East versus the West. This habit of thought goes back to ancient times. It is seen, for instance, in the comparative characterization of Greeks and non-Greeks (such as the peoples of Egypt and Asia) by Herodotus and Aristotle, civilized Chinese and "barbarians" by ancient Chinese. Dichotomizing the East and the West serves as the intellectual foundation of Orientalism, a discourse that has powerfully shaped modern Occidental attitudes toward the Orient. This habit has been vividly expressed by nineteenth-century British poet Rudyard Kipling in his famous lines from "The Ballad of East and West" (1895): "Oh, East is East and West is West, and never the twain shall meet." Although the twain have long since met (and indeed had already met long before Kipling's times) – both in mutually beneficial encounters and in violent conflict – the mentality behind Kipling's words stubbornly refuses to go away.

Dichotomizing cultures is pervasive in the West and probably even more popular in the East. About the Chinese and Western cultures and bioethics, the myth of a "communitarian or collectivist China" versus the "individualistic West" still enjoys a wide circulation in China and the West alike (Nie, 2011, chapter 1). Defining China and Japan in stark contrast to the West constitutes a fundamental way of categorizing cultures and framing a large number of issues in various academic disciplines in not only the humanities and social sciences but also the biological sciences in the two East Asian countries (Sleeboom, 2004). Sociological analysis shows how such a notion of East Asian or Asian bioethics has served academic and political functions such as networking, developing regional identity, and promoting policy changes (Sleeboom-Faulkner, 2016). There is an extremely prevalent but specious idea of Asian bioethics that characterizes Asian cultures as communitarian, collectivist, and family centered in nature, making them radically different from "individualistic" Western cultures (for critiques, see de Castro, 1999; Nie, 2007).

Furthermore, parallel debates exist in other parts of world, for instance, in Africa and Latin America about the nature of African bioethics (see, e.g., Tangwa, 1996; Ujewe, 2016) or Latin American bioethics (see, e.g., Salles & Bertomeu, 2002; Luna, 2006; Pessini et al., 2010) and how these should be distinguished from so-called Western bioethics, whatever this phrase may mean.

One of the numerous examples of dichotomizing the differences of Eastern and Western cultures and bioethics by Asian scholars is a volume entitled, *Beyond a Western Bioethics*, edited by two Filipino physician-bioethicists (Alora & Lumitao, 2001). Their presentation relies on a thoroughgoing opposition between a Filipino bioethics and a Western bioethics:

> The very character of ethics in the West contrasts with ethics in the Philippines not just in terms of the issues and solutions, as well as the context in which each is embedded, but also in the very language and character of moral concern. The focus of Western bioethics is individual; elsewhere it focuses on social units. Western bioethics often is oriented to principles; Filipino bioethics, on the other hand, is not articulated primarily in principles but in lived moral virtues. Whereas Western bioethics is almost always expressed in discursive terms, Filipino bioethics is part of the phenomenological world of living experience. For the West, bioethics is a framework for thought, a conception system. For the Philippines it is a way of life, an embodied activity of virtue.
>
> (Alora & Lumitao, 2001: 4)

Furthermore, these authors have no hesitation in extending these general statements on Filipino ethics to bioethics in the developing world as a whole.

Corresponding to dichotomizing the East and the West is another dichotomy, that between the local and the universal. The volume edited by Alora and Lumitao is introduced by H. Tristram Engelhard, Jr. Based on his postmodernist vision of bioethics as well as a thoroughly dichotomized characterization of Eastern versus Western moralities, Engelhard (2006) has proclaimed a "collapse of consensus" in global bioethics. For him, contemporary cultural and moral pluralism is so well entrenched that culture wars are inevitable, and there is no possibility of a transcultural and transglobal bioethics.

Whether a transglobal bioethics or universalism is possible and feasible is one of the heated debates in bioethics (see, e.g., Macklin, 1999; Engelhard, 2006).

The notion of "common morality" is presented in recent editions of *The Principles of Biomedical Ethics*, by Tom Beauchamp and James Childress (2012), the influential bioethical textbook. Yet, for anthropologists, the everyday workings of multiethnic, multicultural, multifaith, and pluralistic Western societies seriously undermine, if not categorically falsify, any theory of a common morality (Turner, 2003).

The universal appeal of dichotomization is understandable because it offers neat (if simplified and distorting) characterizations of different cultures, both non-Western and Western alike, and also appears to respect the differences between them. It also reflects a good-faith (if misguided) attempt to understand the peoples, practices, and values of cultures and societies other than one's own. However, this oppositional approach has serious drawbacks in various ways. New and more constructive methodologies are therefore much needed

The pervasive and persistent habit of dichotomization in bioethics and cultural studies fosters empirically problematic overgeneralizations, normatively misleading prescriptions, and politically contentious claims. The intellectual fallacies include what have been termed *assumed homogeneity* (the assumption of a fundamentally homogeneous, single, and unified culture, whether Chinese, Philippine, Asian, or Western, and so on), the *manufactured representative* (where the dominant or official position is deemed to be the only authentic representative of the culture concerned), the *grand belief in a peculiar mentality* (assuming that every culture or society has a unique and pervasive mentality), and the *assumption of incommensurability* (assuming that different cultures are radically different and incompatible with each other). The broadly political perils of dichotomizing cultures include "the rejection of trans-cultural similarities or commonalities in morality," "generating contentious and harmful social policies," and "endorsing the tyranny of a reified cultural practice over ethics" (Nie, 2011: 46–49). Under the influence of dichotomization, the proposed mechanism, the only possible mechanism, for the non-Western societies or developing countries to move beyond contemporary bioethics much dominated by the West would be to become the radical other or opponent of the West and to refuse any universal values in bioethics (see, e.g., Alora & Lumitao, 2001).

Rather than throwing light on the differences between cultural practices and norms, the dichotomizing habit reflects and often merely reinforces a variety of myths or stereotypes – explicit or implicit, good or bad. Rather than promoting the cross-cultural understanding and dialogue it purports to offer, this habit often serves to strengthen the invisible existing "walls" between cultures and to create new ones. The thesis of cultural incommensurability that stems from this has led to the popular prophecy that the clash, especially the violent clash, of the Eastern and Western cultures – or of different civilizations in general, as has repeatedly occurred throughout history – is inevitable. The clash of cultures and civilizations is defined as a matter of destiny rather than human choices. But history has also taught us that where there is a will, genuine dialogue between different cultures – like those that take place between diverse moral traditions and viewpoints *within* every culture – is not only necessary but also possible, however difficult its realization may be in practice.

Ethical Transculturalism and Its Methodological Elements: The Complexity of Cultural Differences and the Primacy of Morality

The world today – a world deeply troubled by conflicts, widening disparities, continuing human rights abuses and negligence, and (one may add) persistent tribalism in the forms of patriotism and the globalizing politics of fear – calls for moral imagination and new paradigms of thinking and action. The same applies to bioethics, especially global health ethics. Many scholars have already put forward and are developing different and better theoretical and methodological approaches to global and cross-cultural bioethics (see, e.g., Barilan, 2012). Benatar, Daibes, and Tomsons (2016: table 1) present an illustrating list of some widely accepted major dichotomized differences of the dominant Western and other worldviews related to bioethics. They do so not to accentuate the polar differences but to suggest that the poles are merely components of broad spectra and that it should be possible to find common ground for dialogue where these spectra overlap. As they have pointed out, to characterize differences entirely in opposed polar terms is problematic precisely because this enables us to overlook the common ground where commonalities could be found and thus reject the possibility of meaningful transworldview dialogue. They have also identified a series of inadequacies in the current dominant Western approach embedded in moral and political liberalism in comparison

with and contrast to non-Western and more traditional philosophies. Through these insights, they have offered an innovative methodological paradigm that they call "inter-philosophies dialogue" to enable constructive debates about complex problems (Benatar et al., 2003, 2009, 2016). For some applications in the global health context, see Benatar (2004) and Benatar and Brock (2011). Such a dialogue should be cultural as well as global because the issues about (in)justice, (in)equality, power imbalance, and the need for ethical deliberations are of concern to human beings universally. Their methodology aims to create a collaborative, interdisciplinary, and power-balanced space able to accommodate different worldviews where the dominant paradigm can be challenged and where the marginalized and suppressed perspectives are adequately recognized as coming from equal moral partners in the grand undertaking of global health ethics.

In search of an alternative mode for cross-cultural and comparative bioethics from Chinese reality and cultural traditions, a theoretical and methodological vision of *ethical transculturalism* has been put forward in such works as *Medical Ethics in China: A Transcultural Interpretation* (Nie, 2011) and a special issue on "Transcultural and Transglobal Bioethics: A Search for New Methodologies" for the *Kennedy Institute of Ethics Journal* (Nie & Fitzgerald, 2016). This approach resulted from the efforts primarily to better understand the nature of medical ethics in the sociocultural context of China in a Chinese–Western comparative prospect (see, e.g., Nie, 2005; Nie & Kleinman, 2018). It is designed to resist and hopefully move beyond the aforementioned strong currents in today's world.

The main methodological features of *ethical transculturalism* are as follows (Nie, 2011: 6–13):

- overcoming stereotypes and stereotyping and appreciating the *complexity* of cultural differences;

- taking seriously the internal *plurality* and diversity found within every culture;

- focusing not only on cross-cultural differences but also on transcultural similarities or *commonalities*;

- promoting genuine and deeper *dialogues* between and within different cultures; and

- resisting the tyranny of cultural practices and upholding the necessity of moral judgment and the primacy of *morality* over culture.

In the next section, we will present two additional features: the inclusion of a reflexive theory of social power and a way to conceive of change or progress toward shared and sometimes new moral values. In this section, we highlight *primacy of morality*, the *internal plurality within every culture*, and the *complexity of cultural differences*.

In the discourse of cross-cultural studies and multiculturalism, and in the course of the well-meaning efforts to preserve and cherish cultural differences, there has been a tendency to reify cultural practices over any practical attempt to negotiate and discuss ethical shared ground. The transcultural approach we advocate opposes this position and stresses the necessity of searching for transglobal moral values over cultural practices. One of the reasons for this is that an uncritical reverence for local cultural norms and practices can actually work against the most fundamental values of a given culture and society. But ethical transculturalism aims to advance a bioethics that transcends cross-cultural differences as well as critically engages with the prevailing social practices, both globally and locally, from ethical standpoints.

To once again use Chinese cultures as an example, Confucianism and Daoism (the two major indigenous Chinese moral and political traditions) both teach that it is not existing cultural practices that should be privileged, but whatever is morally right.

> For Confucianism and Daoism, the most fundamental value is precisely the primacy of ethics and morality over existing social and cultural practices, rather than the other way around.... The basic task and highest calling of ethics, transcultural bioethics included, is, first of all, to identify which sociocultural practices are morally justifiable and which are not; and then to begin the process of constantly reforming existing social and cultural practices, however accepted or privileged they are and however difficult it may be to change them, according to ethical ideals and moral imperatives. *(Nie 2011: 13)*

It is in this sense that every culture, every medical ethics tradition, is always an open system – open to new and creative interpretations of the past, open to incorporating positive elements from other systems, open to innovations whether originating from outside or within; and above all, open to the aspirations of human morality and, to invoke the Confucian and Daoist term, the calling of the great Dao (Way).

Fundamentally different from the dichotomizing habit that often overlooks or downplays uncomfortable divisions and plurality of views within one's own cultural group, the transcultural methodological approach emphasizes the great internal moral diversity or radical disagreements within each and every culture or society. The plural voices and radical disagreements over pressing moral issues such as abortion, euthanasia, distribution of resources, and the concept of the just war have been widely acknowledged as one of the most striking features of the contemporary West. This (accurate) characterization of Western societies often carries the hidden assumptions that the same criteria do not apply to non-Western societies such as China or to cultures and societies in the past. The insistence that moral diversity and plurality constitute the *unique* features of postmodern morality is a characteristically contemporary and Western prejudice or stereotype. Yet, to use China as an example again, as in any other culture – Western or Eastern, southern or northern – a rich and wide-ranging internal plurality has long been an essential condition of Chinese moral and sociopolitical life (Nie, 2011). As a result, taking its internal moral plurality seriously is indispensable intellectually – if we are to understand a given culture – and politically – if we are to to formulate ethically sound social policies.

Truth telling about a terminal illness in the Chinese historical and sociocultural context offers a compelling and fascinating case on the empirical and normative problems associated with the dichotomizing habit and the necessity of a transcultural approach. In sharp contrast to today's standard norm of open and honest disclosure in Western countries, in China (including Hong Kong and Taiwan), medical professionals routinely withhold information about terminal illness from patients and usually inform family members only. It is not uncommon for Chinese medical professionals, along with family members, to lie to patients about the diagnosis and prognosis of terminal illness. These striking disparities appear to support the dichotomization.

However, the cultural differences involved are far more complex and nuanced than anything implied by such a crude dualistic schema. By carefully comparing and contrasting cultural attitudes and drawing on primary historical and sociological studies, a number of rarely acknowledged features can be brought to light. *First*, based on extensive primary historical materials, including the biographies of ancient medical sages and famous physicians from various dynasties, a long (albeit forgotten) Chinese tradition of truth telling about terminal illness – a tradition dating back at least 26 centuries – can be recovered. The traditional practice of those well-known health practitioners in history was to disclose their diagnosis and prognosis of terminal illness truthfully and directly to patients. *Second*, this long Chinese tradition is remarkable in itself. It is especially remarkable when compared with the situation in the West, where, historically, concealing the truth about terminal illness was the cultural norm – clearly stipulated in ancient medical writings and modern professional codes of medicine alike (such as the influential 1847 Code of Ethics of the American Medical Association) – and where direct disclosure did not become the standard procedure until the 1960s and 1970s or even later. *Third,* and equally ironically, in tandem with the establishment of Western biomedicine in China from the late nineteenth century, the development of the contemporary mainstream Chinese practice of nondisclosure might be closely connected with the then-dominant Western norm of concealment. *Fourth,* even if medical truth telling were culturally alien to China, as is usually assumed, there are indigenous ethical imperatives at hand to reform the contemporary mainstream Chinese practice of nondisclosure or indirect disclosure because it is increasingly acknowledged that this practice can cause serious harm to patients and their families. *Fifth*, numerous surveys conducted throughout mainland China, like others in Hong Kong and Taiwan, demonstrate that the great majority of Chinese patients want truthful information about their medical condition, even in terminal cases. When asked to imagine that they were patients, the vast majority of medical professionals and family members stated that they would prefer to know the truth. *Sixth*, the Confucian moral outlook mandates truthfulness as an important ethical principle and social virtue that physicians ought to take as their guiding star. *Lastly*, but not least importantly, a historic shift from current practices toward honest and direct disclosure by physicians is now occurring in China. Culturally, this change is not so much following Western (and thus foreign) ways but a return to a long-neglected indigenous Chinese tradition (for a systematic exploration of these issues, see Nie [2011: chapters 6 and 7]).

The other illustration is on an emerging global mental illness issue, attention deficit hyperactivity disorder (ADHD). The current discussion of cross-cultural issues related to the nature of ADHD has been dominated by *double dichotomies*, with the

West versus the non-West paralleled by nature versus culture (biological destiny versus socially and culturally constructed reality) – assumptions unifying different and even apparently opposing positions. However, taking the protagonist of the classic Chinese novel *The Dream of the Red Chamber* as a case study, one can identify the ways in which dichotomization has oversimplified the complexity of Chinese culture and the vast moral plurality evident in China (i.e., the different and radically opposing normative Chinese positions on ADHD-like behaviors) and has ruled out culture(s) as a potential source of similarities or commonalities. The misleading dichotomy of China versus the West thus should be reformulated or, better, abandoned. A transcultural approach can help us think more clearly about the complex cross-cultural differences and transcultural similarities and, consequently, open up new possibilities for much richer transcultural dialogues on ADHD and bioethics (Pickering & Nie, 2016; see also Benatar et al., 2016).

Ethical transculturalism may appear to argue that all cultures are fundamentally the same and that cultural differences do not matter. But this not our view. Our point is that Chinese and Western cultures, like other cultures, *are* different, but not in the ways suggested by popular stereotypes, not in the sense of their being "radical others" to one another. Cultural differences including Chinese–Western ones are far more complicated, subtle, intriguing – and thus more difficult to grasp and articulate – than simplified overgeneralizations. Actually, a transcultural approach endeavors to discover not only similarities or commonalities in differences but also differences in similarities.

Here the Confucian tradition of universalism is another powerful example (see, e.g., Roetz, 1993; Nie & Jones, 2019). As presented in the preceding section, cultural differences are often treated as hard evidence for relativism and against universalism. Because in Western social, political, and moral imagination, China has been persistently perceived as the radical other, it is thus often asserted that one has to set aside moral universalism and subscribe to cultural and ethical relativism in order to respect Chinese cultural values and traditions. However, the question is, what if Chinese ethical traditions are universalistic in essence? Based on the fundamental Confucian moral norm *ren* ("benevolence, love, humaneness, or humanity"), the age-old Chinese ideal of *yi nai renshu* ("medicine as the art of humanity") demonstrates compellingly the inherent universalistic belief in Confucianism and Chinese medical ethics. According to the teachings of Mengzi (Mencius), common humanity is rooted not in an agreement on a set of general ethical principles but in moral sentiments in human nature, what he calls the "four beginnings": the feelings of commiseration, shame, courtesy, and right and wrong as the beginnings of *ren*, *yi* ("righteousness"), *li* ("decorum"), and *zhi* ("wisdom"). Confucian ethical universalism thus not only endorses a vision for a global bioethics embedded in common humanity so that it can overlap with Western universalistic perspectives. At the same time, it also offers an alternative theoretical foundation for such a global bioethics, one that may significantly differ from the current mainstream principle-oriented universalistic frameworks developed from the notions of common morality and human rights. A transcultural approach calls for further transcultural dialogues to identify what these similarities or commonalities are and where differences lie.

Recasting the Local and the Universal

In this section, we consider the techniques and modes of enquiry for bioethicists who wish to contribute to the task of recasting the local and the universal via ethical transculturalism, drawing inspiration from the strongly empirically based subdiscipline of the anthropology of moralities. As a comparative science, anthropology engages in the study of pluralism in order to develop an etic (or universal) understanding of the local (emic) cultural phenomena being discussed. Bioethics also has an interest in an etic understanding of moral pluralism. In addition, it has been experiencing an "empirical turn," and the use of empirical studies of morality as part of this more globalized scope of bioethics has been advocated by bioethicists for some time (Alvarez, 2001). This earlier empirical work provides ad hoc further information toward an appreciation of moral pluralisms, but it is the *systematic* collection of varied case studies that we argue is now the more pressing requirement for a transcultural bioethics. This is the purpose of our focus on methodology rather than to provide a list of methods. A methodologically sophisticated transglobal bioethics requires coherent research designs that allow for sustained and theoretically informed international comparisons.

The elements of a methodology to guide such empirical work are set out later, drawing, where

possible, on exemplars from contemporary bioethicists working already in this empirical tradition. Early proto-examples of this empirical transglobal bioethics approach can be found in the work of bioethicists grappling with the experience of working within increasingly pluralistic societies. Bowman (2004), for example, suggested that a transglobal bioethics would reevaluate the implicit cultural viewpoints of the moral merit of individualism and stoicism in the autonomy principle. Health professionals in pluralistic communities are another academic (and practice) group that, while having a strong commitment to hegemonic bioethics discourse, also engages with ethnic and ethical pluralism on a daily basis. As a result, these health professionals proffer alternative views toward the components of a globalized discourse of bioethics. Harper (2006), for example, draws on nursing science to argue that a universal set of bioethical principles might be beneficence and a respect for persons and communities in a culturally competent manner. The difficulty in assessing this early work analytically is its polyglot nature. Drawing as it does from pressure points in clinical or bioethical practice, its value lies in demonstrating the necessity for a practice-based discipline to create an etic vision of its intellectual contribution, but each work responds to the "itch" of the practitioner's specific professional dilemma. The works are idiosyncratic in their design, highly selective in their references, and intellectually isolated from each other – more methodologically sophisticated research is needed for a mature field of transcultural ethics to emerge.

Deciding what data to collect in a comparative project on such a global scale is a difficult task if the bioethicist is to avoid replicating his or her own moral agenda onto the research topic. Anthropologist Signem Howell (1997) suggests specific data collection concerning the nature of ethical breaches as well as conformities and a study of "reigning orthodoxies," along with a two-level approach to the study of moralities – the pluralities of values within any particular community and the "conflicts of premises and values" at higher-level groupings, that is, national or ethnic. She sums this up concisely as the need to think very carefully as to where to locate (in her disciplinary language) the "anthropological gaze" in such a study, along with a need to understand morality as a dynamic phenomenon emerging from reflection and practices that swing between the *is* and the *ought* and recreate moral orders in so doing. These insights are equally valid, we suggest, for bioethicists working in the transcultural tradition who will be turning this newly empiricist gaze on their research sites. The challenge for emerging empirically trained bioethicists will be to search beyond the "obvious" sites of bioethics discourse in international declarations on universal ethical principles, government committees, and ethical review boards to include other previously neglected sites of ethical discourse as perhaps "descriptive" or "lay."

One example of the complexity that unfolds when one purposefully shifts the location of the research gaze within the study of a single moral issue is a recent study of the ethical regulation of reproductive decision making for prenatal genetic testing of fetuses in New Zealand (Fitzgerald et al., 2015). This study explores the discursive lines of moral reasoning behind the topic of ethical governance of this issue as manifest by the state and its affiliated medical and bioethical instruments and two popular but politically opposed advocacy groups. These groups were the New Zealand Organization for Rare Disorders (NZORD), which supports greater access to genetic testing and screening, and Saving Downs, which wishes to restrict genetic testing and screening availability. Alongside the institutional focus on deontological ethics and principles such as informed choice, the study revealed that the two community groups, rather than engaging in mere political posturing, were in fact carefully articulating alternative lines of moral reasoning on this topic – often developed over decades of careful self-reflection. The oppositional lines of moral reasoning were based on a virtue ethics approach to the provision of choice from NZORD and a citizen's rights approach for disabled citizens from Saving Downs. Both groups and their lines of moral reasoning proved influential in reshaping the institutional interpretation of informed choice.

This dynamism and the productive interrelationship between multiple moral discourses within one community can also be seen in a study on the same topic in Iceland and another in Finland, although with quite different outcomes. In Iceland, the deontological approach at the government level was responded to at the population level by a demographically uncharacteristic loss of the birth of babies with Down syndrome – citizens' moral reasoning appeared to reject the human status of potential people with Down syndrome (Gottfreðsdóttir & Árnason, 2010). In Finland, the government discourse

created an alternative moral discourse for women in which they used social media and peer discussions to develop a moral discourse newly coined as "personalized bioethics" by Meskus (2012). A transglobal bioethics will need to embrace this degree of empirical complexity in its fieldwork and look far beyond its own internal discourses to find where an etic morality (or moralities) lies. Howell (1997) suggests that such an interest in dynamic moral worlds will need to consider wider ideas of morality, including such things as cultural scripts, a shifting focus from moral dilemmas to uncovering moral reasoning styles or thinking (as in the previously cited example of Fitzgerald et al. [2015]), and examining emotionality as well as reasoning in order to be productive of local views.

Anthropologist and medic Didier Fassin's (2012) work on moral anthropology and its exploration of "moral sentiments, judgments and practices" argues for a reflexive subject position for the researcher when engaging in such studies. This reflexive approach is also relevant to a transglobal bioethics, for conventional bioethics has tended to rely on social science rather than internal criticisms of its disciplinary history, aims, and scope of practice. Teasing out the emic from the etic requires a reflexive disciplinary self-awareness – our preceding section has been discussing such a reflexive approach in understanding the hybridity of cultural knowledges and experiences. However, reflexivity will also be required of transglobal bioethicists in relation to their understanding of their own discipline. Marshall and Koenig (2004), for example, have described conventional bioethics as both an academic discipline and an increasingly globalized set of practices, whereas Gaines and Jeungst (2008: 303) argue that bioethics is in fact "a plurality of distinct enterprises with distinct origins and, hence, justifications." They list the various responses of bioethicists to this plurality of aims as that of service, oversight, advice, advocacy, reconnaissance, and support (Gaines & Jeungst, 2008: 306). Systematic cross-cultural comparisons for a transglobal bioethics will need simultaneously to systematically engage with these several internal communities of bioethical practice in order to ensure consistency of comparisons and to identify the researcher's position within this internal disciplinary plurality.

The most difficult part of this project may be in coming to accept that the connection between moral worlds will not necessarily reflect the vision of a classical Euro-American bioethical scholarly tradition as the preceding section's discussion of the teachings of Mengzi suggests. A possible pathway to mitigating the intellectual discomfort associated with this reimagining of the social order is to first deconstruct the apparent unity of the Euro-American ethical discourse itself. Fracturing what Matsuoka (2007: 61) has termed the "ethno-ethics" of American society has already begun, for example, with Häyry's criticisms of the lack of relevance of the American ideal of autonomy as a primary issue in European ethical arenas and his proposal instead that the principles of dignity, precaution, and solidarity may be more relevant (Häyry, 2003). The earlier work by Dickenson (1999) on the regional difference, within Europe, of the prominence of various bioethical principles is also relevant to this task. Far too much of the existing work toward a transglobal bioethics is based on demonstrable untranslatabilities of Western bioethical concepts without recognizing the lack of unity and conceptual difficulties in even defining what the West might be. In a rare exception, Matsuoka (2007) has explored the middle-class bias in classical philosophical American bioethics, drawing on sociologist Fox's observations of the inattention to class and race contexts in various bioethical issues such as end-of-life decision making over neonates in intensive care. Fox notes that while debating the pros and cons of terminating life support for neonates in intensive care, bioethics in general has ignored as irrelevant the wider context that reveals the preponderance of nonwhite teenagers who are mothers of these children (Fox, 1990). More recently, Holloway (2011) has highlighted the systematic inattention to matters of race in American bioethics – noting the manner in which autonomy and privacy are regularly compromised for African-American and female medical clients in US healthcare.

These examples of variations in race and class across a national bioethical discourse are simply one of several often-intersecting lines of difference within national identities. There are also, for example, the voices of Indigenous bioethicists and populations to consider. Examples from our own location in the world include Durie (2008: 20), who has argued that an Indigenous ethics has three very specific ethical domains – "the ethics of eco-connectedness, the ethics of engagement, and the ethics of empowerment." Similarly, McGrath and Phillips (2008) reflect on the very different assumptions about informed consent in two Australian populations (Indigenous versus mainstream). Macer (2014), in an overview of the 2014 AUSN Conference on Bioethics, Public Health and Peace for Indigenous Peoples, has also portrayed these complex interpretive dimensions for a variety of Indigenous populations from an *Americas* rather than an *American* perspective. How to calculate the relative weightings of these (and more) variously standpointed insights toward a transglobal bioethics will be a challenge.

Appiah (2006) is an author who has written substantively on such a task, his cosmopolitan approach to ethics holding much in sympathy with our own arguments. Appiah has argued that such a shared moral vision in a globalized world could be an understanding of obligations to strangers (not overriding the demands of closer connections) but also unable to be completely ignored. Appiah, however, readily acknowledges that detailing the specifics of these obligations is rather difficult without data and a shared research agenda, adding to the urgency for our call for such a systematic approach. The results of such empirical studies will also require a careful analysis of whose word gets to "count" in defining the new transglobal values (Chattopadhyay & De Vries, 2013). The continued existence of hate speech and acts of terror emphasizes the importance of a discriminating awareness of these matters of inclusion/exclusion. These persistent problems amplify the significance of exploring social power and voice in the practice of transglobal bioethics. Thus we can add a sixth item for carrying out a methodologically sophisticated empirical transglobal and comparative bioethics:

- the inclusion of a reflexive theory of social power as a component of its methodologies

We see this as an inevitable and pragmatic methodological response to the loss of intellectual naiveté subsequent to postcolonial and other postmodernist critiques of knowledge production. A growing awareness of such power dynamics (Benatar, 2016) appears in the reports and reflections of bioethicists working in Africa (Gbadegesin, 1993; Andoh, 2011), Central and Latin America (Salles & Bertomeu, 2002; Luna, 2006; Pessini et al., 2010), and Asia (Rafique, 2015; Ghotbi, 2014).

Finally, if we recall one previous argument that a transglobal bioethics also requires us to engage in "constantly reforming existing social and cultural practices," then this comment highlights an additional methodological element to our list:

- a way to conceive of change or progress toward shared and sometimes new moral values

This conceptual dilemma has also been noted by Wallace (2009); Benatar, Daar, and Singer (2003); and Benatar, Gill, and Bakker (2009) for both the foundational and pragmatic approaches to a common morality. For our specific agenda, if we take on board the necessity of acknowledging social power in moral theorizing, then as Prinz (2007: 289) observes: "There is no view from nowhere. We must always assess progress from the inside. In this sense morality is not different from science … theory revision is like rebuilding a raft while we are at sea. We cannot simply abandon our current raft and start anew; we must replace the planks on the raft we already have." Prinz goes on to argue that moral progress is achieved by judging not the merits and truth values of any particular moral tradition but rather through an assessment of nonmoral values associated with the flourishing of various moral traditions.

Movement toward a transglobal bioethics clearly necessitates that we theorize how to recognize and measure moral change. This solution requires us to adopt a more reflexive approach to knowledge production. In this case, it would require recognizing our own moral world and its inherent value predispositions while simultaneously holding to a holistic vision of a wider moral community and assessing our movement toward that vision by (if we follow Prinz [2007]) reference to outcomes and social attributes of other communities such as social cohesion, increased well-being, consistency in interpretation, and so on. The list needs to be flexible for the times and the moment and emerges from pluralistic debates within societies. A modus vivendi approach to these debates in which communities agree on what they can bear to live with rather than delineating all lines of complete agreement seems the more likely contemporary outcome.

We conclude this section with one example of a well-developed but at times neglected subbranch of bioethics that, we argue, should be included in the project of a transglobal bioethics as a shining example of its capacity to reexamine and critically assess its disciplinary roots – feminist bioethics (see, e.g., Tong, 2001; Tong, Donchin, & Dodds, 2004). All the key components of the path toward a transglobal ethics are already underway in the ongoing work of feminist and disability bioethicists (Duran, 2008; Scully, 2008)

who are working from inside the discipline to unravel these lines of force. If we consider feminist bioethics first, this field of knowledge already demonstrates some of the qualities of the empirical agenda we are discussing – strong critical reflection on the history and spatial arrangement of its own body of knowledge (Shildrick, 1997), recognition of the need to incorporate change in ethical values (Rehman-Sutter, 2010), and a pragmatic understanding of the political quality of ethical appeals for shared humanity. For example, Guerrero (2011) provides a detailed discussion of the contemporary diversity of feminisms and their combined aspiration for global human rights. Her work is particularly germane to the preceding discussion for the manner in which she draws attention to the habit of rich countries such as the United Kingdom and Austria to invoke ideas of "tradition" and "culture" to scuttle moves toward honoring international women's rights in as rapid a movement as is commonly ascribed to certain non-Western nations. In a similar critical vein, Scully's (2008) work on disability ethics demonstrates a rich transdisciplinary reading between the social sciences and bioethics in order to address the importance of considering embodied moralities.

The initial misrecognition that might cause us to overlook the subfield of feminist bioethical studies as a proto-transglobal ethics highlights the reflexive and transformative intellectual work that accompanies a commitment to a transglobal bioethics. This thought exercise in imagining feminist bioethical studies as the strongest existing plank in our raft of a transglobal ethics is just the beginning of the disciplinary self-reflection in which our project calls us to engage.

Conclusion

In this chapter we have critically revealed the pervasiveness of the habit of radically dichotomizing cultural differences as well as its main empirical, normative, and political drawbacks. Constructively, we have presented a transcultural approach or the key methodological features of ethical transculturalism, along with a tentative agenda for creating the systematic comparative analytical program that undergirds its future development.

Ethical transcuturalism aspires to connect the East and the West, the local and the universal, as they are and should be. Even Nietzsche, an ethical nihilist and probably the first postmodernist philosopher, was acutely aware of the connectedness of human existence and ideas. He wrote in 1876, before falling into insanity, that despite their obvious differences, the striking "similarities and affinities" between Kant and the Eleatics, between Schopenhauer and Empedocles, and between Aeschylus and Richard Wagner serve as "an almost intangible reminder of the relative nature of all concepts of time; it almost seems as though some things belong together, and time is only a mist that makes it hard for our eyes to see that they do" (cited in Ewans, 1982: 255). Why should we believe that the *space* between the different cultures in this small global village is unbreakable and never to be bridged? Why should we *not* believe that the space, just like time, is relative, a mist? The transcultural and transglobal approach is proposed so that however thick the mist of time and space may appear to be, we still can see the profound similarities, affinities, and interconnection of different cultures amid significant differences.

References

Alora, A. T., & Lumitao, J. M. (2001). *Beyond a Western Bioethics: Voices from the Developing World*. Washington, DC: Georgetown University Press.

Alvarez, A. A. (2001). How rational should bioethics be? The value of empirical approaches. *Bioethics* 15(5–6), 501–519.

Andoh, C. T. (2011). Bioethics and the challenges to its growth in Africa. *Open Journal of Philosophy* 1(2), 67–75.

Appiah, K. (2006). *Cosmopolitanism: Ethics in a World of Strangers*. New York: W.W. Norton.

Barilan, Y. M. (2012). *Human Dignity, Human Rights, and Responsibility: The New Language of Global Bioethics and Biolaw*, 1st ed. Cambridge, MA: MIT Press.

Beauchamp, T. L., & Childress, J. F. (2012). *The Principles of Biomedical Ethics*. New York: Oxford University Press.

Benatar, S. R. (2004). Towards progress in resolving dilemmas in international research ethics *Journal of Law, Medicine and Ethics* 32(4), 574–582.

Benatar, S. (2016). Politics, power, poverty and global health: systems and frames. *International Journal of Health Policy & Management* 5(10), 599–604.

Benartar, S. R., & Brock, G. (2011). *Global Health and Global Health Ethics*. Cambridge, UK: Cambridge University Press.

Benatar, S. R., Daar, A., & Singer, P. A. (2003). Global health ethics: the rationale for mutual caring. *International Affairs* 79(1), 107–138.

Benatar, S., Daibes, I., & Tomsons, S. (2016). Inter-philosophies dialogues: creating a paradigm for global health ethics. *Kennedy Institute of Ethics Journal* 26(3), 323–346.

Benatar, S. R., Gill, S., & Bakker, I. (2009). Making progress in global health: the need for a new paradigm. *International Affairs* 85(2), 347–371.

Bowman, K. (2004). What are the limits of bioethics in a culturally pluralistic society? *Journal of Law, Medicine & Ethics* 32(4), 664–669.

Campbell, A. V. (1999). Presidential address: Global bioethics: dream or nightmare? *Bioethics* 13(3–4), 193–190.

Chattopadhyay, S., & De Vries, R. (2013). Respect for cultural diversity in bioethics is an ethical imperative. *Medicine, Health Care and Philosophy* 16, 639–645.

de Castro, L. (1999). Is there an Asian bioethics? *Bioethics* 13(3–4), 227–235.

Dickenson, D. L. (1999). Cross-cultural issues in European bioethics. *Bioethics* 13(3–4), 249–255.

Duran, J. (2008). Global bioethics and feminist epistemology. *International Journal of Applied Philosophy* 22(2), 303–310.

Durie, M. (2008). Bioethics in research: the ethics of indigeneity. Presented at the 9th Global Forum on Bioethics in Research, Auckland, New Zealand.

Engelhard, Jr., H. T. (ed.) (2006). *Global Bioethics: The Collapse of Consensus*. Salem, MA: M&M Scrivener Press.

Ewans, M. (1982). *Wagner and Aeschylus: The Ring and the Oresteia*. London: Faber & Faber.

Fassin, D. (ed.) (2012). *A Companion to Moral Anthropology*. Oxford, UK: Wiley Blackwell.

Fassin, D. (2013). On resentment and *ressentiment*: the politics and ethics of moral emotions. *Current Anthropology* 54(3), 249–267.

Fiester, A. (2012). What "patient-centered care" requires in serious cultural conflict. *Academic Medicine* 87(1), 20–24.

Fitzgerald, R. P., Legge, M., & Park, J. (2015). Choice, rights and virtue: prenatal testing and styles of moral reasoning in Aotearoa, New Zealand. *Medical Anthropology Quarterly* 29(3), 400–417.

Fox, R. C. (1990). The evolution of American bioethics: a sociological perspective, In Weisz, G. (ed.), *Social Science Perspectives on Medical Ethics*. Dordrecht: Kluwer Academic Publishers, pp. 201–217.

Gaines, A. D., & Juengst, E. T. (2008). Origin myths in bioethics: constructing sources, motives and reason in bioethic(s). *Culture, Medicine and Psychiatry* 32(3), 303–327.

Gbadegesin, S. (1993). Bioethics and culture: an African perspective. *Bioethics* 7(2–3), 257–262.

Ghotbi, N. (2014). The ethics of organ transplantation in the Islamic Republic of Iran. *Eubios Journal of Asian and International Bioethics* 23, 190–193.

Gottfreðsdóttir, H., & Vilhjálmur, Á. (2010). Bioethical concepts in theory and practice: an exploratory study of prenatal screening in Iceland. *Medicine, Health Care and Philosophy* **14**(1), 53–61.

Guerrero, M. (2011). International women's rights and the war of cultures: avoiding the Westernization debate. *Vienna Journal on International Constitutional Law* 5(3), 379–399.

Harper, M. G. (2006). Ethical multiculturalism: an evolutionary concept analysis. *Advances in Nursing Science* **29**(2), 110–124.

Häyry, M. (2003). European values in bioethics: why, what, and how to be used. *Theoretical Medicine and Bioethics* **24** (3), 199–214.

Holloway, K. F. C. (2011). *Private Bodies, Public Texts: Race, Gender, and a Cultural Bioethics*. Durham, NC: Duke University Press.

Howell, S. (ed.) (1997). *The Ethnography of Moralities*. London: Routledge.

Kleinman, A. (1999). Moral experience and ethical reflection: can ethnography reconcile them? A quandary for "the new bioethics." *Daedalus* **128**(4), 69–97.

Luna, F. (2006). In Herissone-Kelly, P., & Pakter, L. (eds.), *Bioethics and Vulnerability: A Latin American View*. Amsterdam: Rodopi.

Macer, D. (2014). AUSN Conference on Bioethics, Public Health and Peace for Indigenous Peoples. *Eubios Journal of Asian and International Bioethics* **24**, 106–113.

Macklin, R. (1999). *Against Relativism*. Oxford, UK: Oxford University Press.

Marshall, P., & Koenig, B. (2004). Accounting for culture in a globalized bioethics. *Journal of Law, Medicine and Ethics* **3**, 252–266.

Matsuoka, E. (2007). The issue of particulars and universals in bioethics: some ideas from cultural anthropology. *Journal of Philosophy and Ethics in Health Care and Medicine* **2**, 44–65.

McGrath, P., & Phillips, E. (2008). Western notions of informed consent and indigenous cultures: Australian findings at the interface. *Journal of Bioethical Inquiry* **5**(1), 21–31.

McMillan, J. (2018). *Methods in Bioethics*. Oxford, UK: Oxford University Press.

Meskus, M. (2012). Personalized ethics: the emergence and the effects in prenatal testing. *BioSocieties* **7**(4), 373–392.

Nie, J.-B. (2005). *Behind the Silence: Chinese Voices on Abortion*. Oxford, UK: Rowman & Littlefield.

Nie, J.-B. (2007). The specious idea of an Asian bioethics: beyond dichotomizing East and West, in Ashcroft, R. E., et al. (eds.), *Principles of Heath Care Ethics*, 2nd ed. London: Wiley, pp. 143–149.

Nie, J.-B. (2011). *Medical Ethics in China: A Transcultural Interpretation*. London: Routledge.

Nie, J.-B., & Fitzgerald, R. (2016). Special Issue on "Transcultural and Transglobal Bioethics: A Search for New Methodologies." *Kennedy Institute of Ethics Journal* **26** 3).

Nie, J.-B., & Jones, G. (2019). Confucianism and organ donation: moral duties from *xiao* (filial piety) to *ren* (humaneness). *Medicine, Health Care and Philosophy*. doi.org/10.1007/s11019-019–09893-8.

Nie, J.-B., & Kleinman, A. (2018). Special Issue on "Rebuilding Patient-Physician Trust in China, Developing a Trust-Oriented Bioethics." *Developing World Bioethics* **18**(1).

Pessini, L., de Barchifontaine, C. P., & Stepke, F. L. (eds.) (2010). *Ibero-American Bioethics: History and Perspectives*, trans. J. Bulcock, A. Sobral, & M. S. Gonçalves. New York: Springer.

Pickering, N., & Nie, J.-B. (2016). Trans-Cultural ADHD and bioethics: reformulating a dichotomized debate. *Kennedy Institute of Ethics Journal* **26**(3), 249–275.

Prinz, J. (2007). *The Emotional Construction of Morals*. Oxford, UK: Oxford University Press.

Rafique, Z. (2015). Ethical issues of clinical ethics and research ethics in the developing world and Pakistan: is there any solution? *Eubios Journal of Asian and International Bioethics* **25**, 81–82.

Raja, A. J., & Wikler, D. (2001). Developing bioethics in developing countries. *Journal of Health Population and Nutrition* **19**(1), 4–5.

Rehman-Sutter, C. (2010). "It is her problem, not ours": contributions of feminist bioethics to the mainstream, in Scully, J. L., Baldwin-Ragaven, L. E., & Fitzpatrick, P. (eds.), *Feminist Bioethics: At the Center, on the Margins*. Baltimore: Johns Hopkins University Press, pp. 23–44.

Roetz, H. (1993). *Confucian Ethics of the Axial Age*. Albany: State University of New York Press.

Salles, A. L. F., & Bertomeu, M. J. (2002). *Bioethics: Latin American Perspectives*. Amsterdam: Rodopi.

Scully, J. L. (2008). *Disability Bioethics: Moral Bodies, Moral Difference*. Lanham, UK: Rowman & Littlefield.

Shankman, S., & Lollini, M. (ed.) (2002). *Who, Exactly, Is the Other? Western and Transcultural Perspectives*. Eugene: University of Oregon Books.

Shildrick, M. (1997). *Leaky Bodies and Boundaries: Feminism, Postmodernism, and (Bio)Ethics*. London: Routledge.

Sleeboom, M. (2004). *Academic Nations in China and Japan: Framing in Concepts of Nature, Culture and the Universal*. London: Routledge Curzon.

Sleeboom-Faulkner, M. (2016). "(East) Asia" as a platform for debate: grouping and bioethics. *Kennedy Institute of Ethics Journal* **26**(3), 277–302.

Sugarman, J., & Sulmasy, D. (2010). *Methods in Medical Ethics*, 2nd ed. Washington, DC: Georgetown University Press.

Tangwa, G. B. (1996). Bioethics: an African perspective. *Bioethics* **10**(3), 183–200.

Tipene-Matua, B., & Wakefield, B. (2007). Establishing a Maori ethical framework for genetic research with Maori, in Henaghan, M. (ed.), *Genes, Society and the Future*. Dunedin, NZ: Human Genome Research Project.

Tong, R. (2001). *Globalizing Feminist Bioethics: Crosscultural Perspectives*. Boulder, CO: Westview.

Tong, R., Donchin, A., & Dodds, S. (2004). *Linking Visions: Feminist Bioethics, Human Rights, and the Developing World*. Lanham, UK: Rowman & Littlefield.

Turner, L. (2003). Zones of consensus and zones of conflict: questioning the "common morality" presumption in bioethics. *Kennedy Institute of Ethics Journal* **13**(3), 193–218.

Ujewe, S. (2016). Just healthcare in Nigeria: the foundation for an African ethical framework. PhD thesis, University of Central Lancashire, UK.

Veatch, R. (2000). *Cross-Cultural Perspectives in Medical Ethics*, 2nd ed. Boston: Jones & Bartlett.

Wallace, K. A. (2009). Common morality and moral reform. *Theoretical Medicine and Bioethics* **30**(1), 55–68.

Giving Voice to African Thought in Medical Research Ethics[*]

Godfrey B. Tangwa

Introduction

In this chapter, I consider the virtual absence of an African voice and perspective in global discourses of medical research ethics against the backdrop of the high burden of diseases and epidemics on the continent and the fact that the continent is actually the scene of numerous and sundry medical research studies. I consider some reasons for this state of affairs as well as how the situation might be redressed. Using examples from the HIV/AIDS and Ebola epidemics, I attempt to show that the marginalization of Africa in medical research and medical research ethics is deliberate rather than accidental. It is causally related, in general terms, to a Eurocentric hegemony derived from colonialism and colonial indoctrination cum proselytization. I end by proposing seven theses for the critical reflection and appraisal of the reader.

The idea of "giving voice to African thought in medical research ethics" recalls the "African philosophy" debate that raged for decades, particularly in the 1970s and 1980s (Bodunrin, 1985; Hountondji, 1996; Oruka, 1990; Tangwa, 1992). The debate was sparked by the following provocative question: given the absence of written texts and identifiable individual philosophers in the traditional past, how can there be traditional African philosophy? The debate arose among African scholars and academics formally trained in Western pedagogic institutions, where they had been exposed to the various branches of Western academic philosophy.

In the face of this question, some African scholars, exemplified by Paulin Hountondji (1996), argued that the claim that there is philosophy in the absence of written texts and identifiable philosophers is at best

a claim about the existence of a collective philosophy, a folk philosophy, an ethnophilosophy, a consensual philosophy common to all members of a group. The scholars considered such a claim to be a fallacy and a myth. Others conceded that there is "African thought" and even "African philosophical thought" but denied that there is anything like "African philosophy." However, many others felt that denying the existence of African philosophy was akin to denying the humanity of Africans and the existence of a distinctive African culture.

The entire problematic seems to revolve around two senses of philosophy (Tangwa, 1992):

1. A system or set of fundamental beliefs and convictions, usually reflected in actions ("philosophy at the second moment of vision") Tangwa, 1992 or

2. A consciously articulate critical discourse (verbal or written) that is necessarily individual in origin or a corpus or system of such discourses with the supporting structures in which they are symbolically encoded.

The purpose of philosophy in the second sense is arguably to convert critical discourses into philosophy in the first sense. Philosophizing is not an end in itself, a purposeless exercise, a prize in a vacuum, a purely aimless intellectual pastime. Its aim is or should be to discover or demonstrate the good, the true, and the beautiful with a view to making use of them in human living. Human thought and action are dialectical – earnest thought necessarily manifests in action, and actions provide the agenda for reflection. African philosophy is therefore any work or discourse, any reflective critical thought that arises mainly from, is rooted in, or that in some other sense concerns the historical, cultural, social, or political experience of Africa or is particularly relevant to Africa.

A further important question is whether relevant work by either an African or non-African philosopher

[*] Reprinted with minor modifications from Godfrey B. Tangwa (2017). Giving voice to African thought in medical research ethics. *Theoretical Medicine and Bioethics* 38,101–110. Used by permission of Palgrave Macmillan Springer.

is classifiable as African philosophy. The answer is yes, if and only if the discourse is about Africa or is relevant to the African contemporary, historical, socio-cultural, or politico-economic experience or context. A single work can, of course, be relevant to several contexts, to varying degrees, all at once. It is quite possible for the work of a non-African to be justifiably classed as African philosophy and for the work of an African to fail to meet the conditions of such classification. But, in general, a good reason is called for in classifying either the work of a non-African as African philosophy or the work of an African as non-African philosophy.

It can therefore be concluded that if there is African philosophy or an African philosopher in the preceding sense, then, *a fortiori*, there is African thought. And if there is African thought, we can legitimately talk about giving voice to African thought in medical research ethics. This thought, though marginalized in the current global state of affairs, is important because reality and human experience are too vast and too diverse to be captured by any one cultural or conceptual paradigm, be it globally dominant or not. Medical research ethics is coextensive with and has evolved directly from medical ethics in general, through healthcare ethics, and there is no human culture that has not been preoccupied with healthcare and therefore healthcare ethics. Western proselytizing and colonial mentality might lead one to dismiss African philosophy or healthcare ethics lightly in the same manner as some African and non-African Christians and Islamists dismiss African Traditional Religion as being nothing but a form of paganism or heathenism and of no consequence or religious value.

Why Give Voice to African Thought in Medical Research Ethics?

The idea of giving voice to African thought in medical research ethics is compelling not only because reality and human experience are vast and diverse and cannot be adequately captured by one paradigm or from one perspective but also on the consideration that the continent of Africa has, historically, been colonized, exploited, indoctrinated, proselytized, mentored, marginalized, and excluded. The cumulative result of these historical experiences has been to turn many Africans into more or less mute and mimetic beings

or disciples and catechists of received foreign systems on the world stage. Yet the continent, because of its high burden of disease and epidemics, is the scene of numerous medical research studies by all and sundry researchers from all over the globe for all and sundry motives and motivating factors.

There is a crying need for conceptual decolonization for both Africans and non-Africans having to do with Africa (Nyamnjoh, 2012). The exploitative agendas and greediness of erstwhile colonizers of Africa and the so-called developed world and its determination to maintain global hegemonic dominance is complemented by inducement and proselytization of elite Africans, especially experts, to subvert the emergence of Africa as an equal partner on the global stage. An African scientist or other expert who decides to stay and work in Africa on local problems faces a huge dilemma. African governments and non-governmental agencies do not yet seem aware of the importance of funding research for development. The scientist or expert is left with only the option of applying for funding to Western governmental or non-governmental agencies. But these funders are not philanthropists. Funding comes usually with strong strings attached, including the compulsion to work within a rigid procedural framework, including even the ethics rules to be followed.

African scientists and experts working with Western funding are very comfortable and can rapidly achieve high professional standards and status, but they are at the service of Western global dominance and hegemony. This is why there has been little change in Africa and the lives of Africans in spite of the high-level African scientists and experts working for Western institutions and agencies both in and out of Africa.

Culture, Context, and Healthcare

Culture is the way of life of a group of people, underpinned by adaptation to a particular environment, worldview, similar ways of thinking and acting and doing, and similar attitudes, expectations, and practices (Tangwa, 2010). There is great variety and diversity between the different African ethnicities, but they are all united by commonalities that give them a remarkable family resemblance analogous to the family resemblance of groupings that are in some ways remarkably different from one another but all justifiably bracketed under the term 'Western' (Tangwa, 2004). In Western culture, in which literacy, science, technology, and individualism predominate, health is understood mainly as the absence of disease, particularly of bacteria and viruses – hence evidence-based medicine and evidence-based allopathic medical research. In African culture, in which orality and aurality, communalism, and relatedness predominate (London et al., 2014; Tutu, 1999), health is a much more complex concept, and healing from affliction or misfortune is more than a technique for eliminating a scourge or contagion (Tangwa, 2015).

Different cultural contexts offer opportunities for discovering and appreciating different perspectives, paradigms, and frameworks. Western culture, as the most successful human culture (materially), understandably (though not acceptably) has a big mouth but small ears. This posture may be the result of its practices of colonization, proselytization, and domination. But it must not be forgotten that other cultures also have holistic perspectives on life and the universe that need to be listened to and appreciated, even if they speak only in whispers. In the World Federation of Cultures (Mazrui, 1976), it is evident that just as one hand cannot tie a bundle by itself, one culture cannot alone fix the world. Cultures are like dancing masquerades, to recall a metaphor popularized by African novelist Chinua Achebe. None of the masked dancers can be ignored, and none can adequately be viewed from a single or static position. In comparing and contrasting industrialized Western culture with African traditional culture, it can be said that Western culture is predominantly an anthropocentric, literate culture, technologically advanced, epistemologically and morally driven by an obsession with certainty and a Manichean syndrome that strictly distinguishes good from evil. It embodies an attitude that leaves the impression of knowing all that is knowable and is shaped in many ways by free-market forces and profit motives; it is outward-looking, dominant, and domineering of other cultures, which it tries to assimilate or at least proselytize into its ever-expanding universal vision and operations. By contrast, traditional African culture is a "live and let live" culture, predominantly oral rather than literate, and marked by great variety and diversity. Traditional African culture is, in essence, eco-bio-communitarian (Tangwa, 1996), tolerant, cautious, eco-bio-communitarian, non-proselytizing, and inward-looking.

Culture, Disease, and Medical Research

Every individual human being lives within a particular cultural framework, which may involve overlapping and intersecting cultural perspectives, whether or not the individual is aware of it. Cultures form intersecting concentric circles (Tangwa, 2004). A particular disease (physical or mental) may have the same or similar "causes." Understanding a disease, its perceived causes and possible remedies, is culturally anchored. Within African culture, it may not be enough to identify the physical cause of an ailment or illness because there is a tendency to search for the cause of the cause in a regressive chain that can terminate only in God or else become interminable. The ontology of the African cultural universe recognizes non-material beings and presences, including dead-living ancestors, sundry spirits, divinities, gods, and God.

Cultural context is therefore all important in healthcare, and treatment of illness needs to be culture congruent to be effective and satisfactory. Industrialized world medical research is not only based on physicalism and materialism but also generally on market-oriented and profit-driven motives and tends to be susceptible to morally blind economic forces. As a consequence, it engages to a high degree in ad hoc rationalizations and justifications. For these reasons, the ethical challenges of industrialized world research, especially in non-Western contexts, are many and varied. Is it possible to combine commercial motives with philanthropic altruism or ethical imperatives in general? Can high-tech medical research avoid harming the vulnerable or exploiting the desperately weak, poor, and ill? Can it avoid undue inducement or the application of double standards (Tangwa, 2002)? Can it apply convincingly the imperative of respect for the autonomy of others, their culture, and their way of life? These questions indicate high ethical hurdles that cannot easily be surmounted.

Nevertheless, the attraction to do medical research in the so-called developing world, particularly in Africa, is nothing if not overwhelming for myriad reasons: altruistic philanthropy, abundant availability of suitable research subjects given a high burden of diseases and epidemics of all descriptions, poverty, illiteracy, and weak regulatory frameworks, and so on. In the wake of the HIV/AIDS and Ebola epidemics, for instance, most vaccine trials and hopeful but unproven therapy trials are concentrated in Africa. The question as to whether such trials can, even in principle, be carried out ethically is an important and unanswered one.

The WHO and the Ebola Epidemic

Take, for example, the recent Ebola epidemic, which broke out in West Africa during the first quarter of 2014 (WHO, 2016). By August 12, 2014, the WHO released a short statement captioned, "Ethical Considerations for Use of Unregistered Interventions for Ebola Virus Disease (EVD): Summary of a Panel Discussion" (WHO, 2014), which generally was well received and appreciated around the world. The statement in effect endorsed a procedure that is justifiable from the point of view of ordinary commonsense intuition; namely, in the face of certain death and absence of any proven remedy, it is ethically acceptable to try a hopeful unproven remedy in an attempt to save life. On September 29–30, 2014, the WHO organized a "consultation to assess the state of the art work to test and eventually license candidate Ebola vaccines," in which more than 70 experts, including many from affected countries in West Africa, are supposed to have taken part. This panel considered and apparently approved urgently carrying out clinical tests on humans of some candidate Ebola vaccines in the development pipeline, including chimpanzee adenovirus serotype 3 (Chad 3) by Glaxo Smith Kline and others and recombinant vesicular stomatitis virus (rVSV) vaccine by a consortium involving Canadian Public Health plus others.

On July 31, 2015, a ground-breaking publication, "Efficacy and Effectiveness of an rVSV-Vectored Vaccine Expressing Ebola Surface Glycoprotein: Interim Results from the Guinea Ring Vaccination Cluster-Randomised Trial" (Henao-Restrepo et al., 2015), was published in the very influential journal *Lancet*. The paper was copyrighted by the WHO, with some of its high officials as co-principal investigators and co-authors. The announcement of this publication in newspapers and on radio and television was accompanied by hyperbole quite uncharacteristic of the scientific domain: the results of the clinical test were variously described as "spectacular," "first time ever," "100% effective," "game changer," and so on.

The successful molecule, hurriedly tested on Africans in Guinea, had originally been developed not against the Ebola virus but as an anti-bioterrorism product for North Americans, and while it had been subjected to non-human animal tests, it had not been tested in humans. The following preliminary questions thus naturally arise:

- Was the WHO statement on clinical trials for Ebola of September 2014 tailor-made to ensure tests in humans of this particular candidate vaccine?
- Was this not an opportunistic trial reminiscent of the Trovan trials for meningitis during an epidemic in northern Nigeria in 1996?
- As an agency of the United Nations with oversight for global health, is it right for the WHO itself to engage directly in commercial drug discovery, development, and clinical tests while at the same time issuing guidelines and directives for all and sundry research competitors on how these should properly and ethically be done? Can the WHO avoid conflicts of interest or favoritism and discrimination in such situations?

The HIV/AIDS Epidemic and VANHIVAX

When the HIV/AIDS epidemic broke out in the early 1980s, one of the African scientists who tackled it in a serious and determined manner by researching toward a possible vaccine was Professor Victor Anomah Ngu of the Faculty of Medicine and Biomedical Sciences, University of Yaounde 1, Cameroon. Anomah Ngu, an oncologist and professor of surgery, had won the Lasker Prize for Cancer Research in 1972 and was therefore no neophyte in this domain. But his work on HIV/AIDS did not receive any recognition, let alone support, from either the local authorities or the powerful developed world, and he eventually passed on to eternity (2011) without having had the opportunity to confirm or disconfirm his candidate vaccine, VANHIVAX (Ngu & Ambe, 2001; Ngu et al., 2002; Ngu et al., 2007). His idea of an immunotherapeutic vaccine, which seems to have gained scientific currency today, was dismissed by some as an impossible and contradictory concept.

In 2000, Ngu and I made a joint presentation, "Effective Vaccine Against and Immunotherapy of HIV: Scientific Report and Ethical Considerations from Cameroon," at the Fifth World Congress of Bioethics on September 21–24 in London (Ngu & Tangwa, 2000, 2015). The gist of our presentation was that Victor Anomah Ngu had, through his research and clinical practice, discovered a candidate HIV/AIDS vaccine, VANHIVAX, already tested on a limited scale with remarkably promising results and now needing to be tested more carefully and systematically on a wider scale under the sponsorship of a body such as the WHO.

Our conclusion was that the promise of this preliminary report would be fully realized only after its confirmation in a study involving a better and bigger sample of patients and a collaborative effort with adequate logistic support. We were confident that after such confirmation, effective and cheap vaccines could confidently be proposed for trial to the public with a high probability of acceptance because the vaccine would have shown its effectiveness in patients in the therapeutic context.

We hoped that the WHO and other interested partners could then lead the production of vaccines on a regional or sub-regional basis using the type or subtype of the virus prevalent in each region. Nothing of what we expected came to pass. Although a number of research teams from Europe and the United States did come to see Ngu in Yaounde, pretending that they wanted to collaborate with him on his candidate vaccine project, they, as it turned out, only wanted to have the scientific details of his protocol. Having acquired it, they departed, and Ngu never heard from them again. On October 17–19, 2005, the African AIDS Vaccine Programme (AAVP) was organizing a conference in Yaounde, Cameroon, to which I was invited as an ethicist. I noticed from the program and list of participants that Victor Anomah Ngu was not invited to this meeting, which was by invitation only. I immediately sent the following email on September 21, 2005, to the organizers of the conference:

> I suggest that you find space in the programme to invite Professor Victor Anomah Ngu to make a presentation of his claims to have a candidate AIDS Vaccine, VANHIVAX. Although his claims may not be scientifically uncontroversial, this is no good reason for not hearing him out but rather a very good reason for letting him present his idea so that other scientists might assess it in all scientific rigor and objectivity. If the adjective "African" in the African AIDS Vaccine Programme has any real significance, it would surely be a little surprising to hold such a conference in Cameroon while completely ignoring Anomah Ngu and his claims.

He was eventually invited to the meeting as an observer.

During the recent Ebola epidemic in West Africa (2014–2015), some African medical scientists and allied experts decided to do something unprecedented. They came together and urgently created the Global Emerging Pathogens Treatment Consortium (GET; www.getafrica.org/), aimed at coordinating an effective response not only to the Ebola epidemic but also to any future similar deadly pathogen that may emerge. They created several workgroups and launched many capacity-building initiatives to harness indigenous knowledge and experience, with the view to using culturally appropriate methods and procedures. Scientifically, they initiated research on the use of blood plasma (plasmapheresis) of Ebola survivors for the treatment of Ebola patients. The GET got some collaborators from the developed world but otherwise very little particular encouragement, let alone support.

Of the African physicians and other medical personnel who were victims of the deadly Ebola infection – Sheik Umar Khan, Obi Justina Ejelonu, Ameyo Adadevoh, John Combey, John Taban Dada, Patrick Shamndzee, Eric Thomas Duncan, and Martin Salia – none were offered any of the unproven experimental substances (such as ZMapp), which at least saved the lives of some of their Western counterparts, such as Kent Brantly and Nancy Writebol.

In this situation, it is hard to know what attitude to recommend to an observant African. But given the moral equality of all human beings and their epistemological and moral limitations, a strong case can be made for an attitude at once of self-reliance and cautious optimism, an attitude that avoids pessimism and extremism of all types but that maintains a healthy skepticism at all times.

Some Theses for Reflection and Critical Consideration

Before concluding, I propose seven theses for reflection and critical consideration.

1. Some populations (not to say races) seem particularly suitable as subjects of medical experimentation given their disease burden, genetic configuration, poverty, illiteracy, and perceived dispensability.
2. Exploitability tends naturally (and perhaps necessarily) to simulate philanthropy.
3. It seems very difficult for the privileged anywhere – the rich, knowledgeable, and powerful – to refrain from exploiting the exploitable.
4. In all cases of human exploitation of humans, the exploited are, at least partly, accomplices of their own exploitation.
5. Among all exploited populations, there are individuals who reap enormous benefits and

343

advantages as apostles, disciples, interpreters, catechists, and propagandists of the exploiter's dogmas and agendas.

6. Those who elaborate the most articulate rules of procedure for the ethics of medical research are the same people who are also complicit in medical research scandals.

7. The impulse of the industrialized Western world for power and control is nicely complemented by the strong belief among some Africans that African problems require external solutions.

Conclusion

In spite of the numerous biomedical research studies that have been carried out and continue to be carried out all over the African continent, the thinking, views, and perspectives of Africans are not evident in the global bioethics discourse; indeed, their voice can be said to be almost completely absent. In this chapter, I have attempted to highlight this situation, to hazard an explanation, and to hint at a general framework that is needed for redressing the situation. The main objective of this chapter has been to provoke further critical thinking on the marginalization of Africa, especially in the biomedical domain, despite its potentialities and available human and material resources.

References

Bodunrin, P. O. (1985). *Philosophy in Africa: Trends and perspectives.* Ile-Ife: University of Ife Press.

Henao-Restrepo, A. M., Longini, I. R., Egger, M., et al. (2015). Efficacy and effectiveness of an rVSVvectored vaccine expressing Ebola surface glycoprotein: interim results from the Guinea ring vaccination cluster-randomised trial. *Lancet* **386**(9996), 857–866.

Hountondji, P. J. (1996). *African Philosophy: Myth and Reality*, 2nd ed. Bloomington: Indiana University Press.

London, L., Tangwa, G., Matchaba-Hove, R., et al. (2014). Ethics in occupational health: deliberations of an international workgroup addressing challenges in an African context. *BMC Medical Ethics* **15**:48.

Mazrui, A. A. A. (1976). *A World Federation of Cultures: An African Perspective.* New York: Free Press.

Ngu, V. A., & Ambe, F. A. (2001). Effective vaccines against and immunotherapy of the HIV: a preliminary report. Journal of the Cameroon Academy of Science 1(1), 2–8.

Ngu, V. A., & Tangwa, G. B. (2000). Effective vaccine against and immunotherapy of the HIV: scientific report and ethical considerations from Cameroon. Paper presented at the Fifth World Congress of Bioethics, Imperial College, London.

Ngu, V. A., & Tangwa, G. B. (2015). Effective vaccine against and immunotherapy of the HIV: scientific report and ethical considerations from Cameroon. *Journal of the Cameroon Academy of Sciences* **12**(2), 76–83.

Ngu, V. A., Ambe, F. A., & Boma, G. A. (2002). Significant reduction of HIV loads in the sera of patients treated with VANHIVAX. *Journal of the Cameroon Academy of Science* **2**(1), 7–12.

Ngu, V. A., Besong-Egbe, B. H., Ambe, F., et al. (2007). The conversion of HIV seropositive to seronegative following VANHIVAX. *Journal of the Cameroon Academy of Science* **7**(1), 17–20.

Nyamnjoh, F. B. (2012). "Potted plants in greenhouses": a critical reflection on the resilience of colonial education in Africa. *Journal of Asian and African Studies* **47**(2), 129–154.

Oruka, H. O. (1990). *Sage Philosophy: Indigenous Thinkers and Modern Debate on African Philosophy.* Nairobi: Acts Press, African Center for Technology Studies.

Tangwa, G. 1992. African philosophy: appraisal of a recurrent problematic, part 1: the sources of traditional African philosophy. *Cogito* **6**(2), 78–84.

Tangwa, G. (1992). African philosophy: appraisal of a recurrent problematic, part 2: what is African philosophy and who is an African philosopher? *Cogito* **6**(3), 138–143.

Tangwa, G. B. (1996). Bioethics: an African perspective. *Bioethics* **10**(3), 183–200

Tangwa, G. B. (2002). International regulations and medical research in developing countries: double standards or differing standards? *Notizie di Politeia* **18**(67), 46–50

Tangwa, G. B. (2004). Bioethics, biotechnology and culture: a voice from the margins. *Developing World Bioethics* **4**(2), 125–138.

Tangwa, G. B. (2010). *Elements of African Bioethics in a Western Frame.* Mankon: Langaa RPCIG.

Tangwa, G. B. (2015). Traditional medicine, in ten Have, H. (ed.), *Encyclopedia of Global Bioethics.* Berlin: Springer, pp. 1–8.

Tutu, D. (1999). *No Future Without Forgiveness.* New York: Doubleday.

World Health Organization (WHO) (2016). Ebola virus disease (Fact sheet No. 103). Available at www.who.int/mediacentre/factsheets/fs103/en/ (accessed March 2, 2017).

World Health Organization (WHO) (2014). Ethical considerations for use of unregistered interventions for Ebola virus disease (EVD): Summary of the panel discussion. Available at www.who.int/mediacentre/news/statements/2014/ebola-ethical-review-summary/en/ (accessed March 2, 2017).

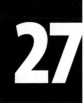

Chapter 27

Interphilosophies Dialogue
Creating a Paradigm for Global Health Ethics[*]

Solomon Benatar, Ibrahim Daibes, and Sandra Tomsons

The progress of history rests on the battle for supremacy of competing ideas. . . .
The power and wealth of western countries give them a dominant role in shaping the international public discourse. This is a privileged position . . . [an] imbalance of voice in the international discourse [that] has built up a dangerous sense of resentment by the silent majority of the world's people.
(Thakur, 2007)

Introduction

The dominant bioethical paradigm that provides the context for research ethics discourse has evolved within Western philosophy's powerful normative framework and is built on a relationship model that explains and underpins the obligations doctors have to their patients. In this one-to-one relationship, the doctor is claimed to have primary duties to do no harm to patients and to respect patients' rights. Employing the values of liberal individualism currently dominant in Western civilization, this model provides the starting point for understanding ethical research practice. Hence, researchers, like doctors, have obligations to do no harm to subjects and to respect their rights within the dominant conception of what these rights are or should be.

Global health researchers generally accept the values and moral principles of the dominant bioethical paradigm; however, some have expressed ethical concerns that point to problems with this paradigm (Pratt & Loff, 2013). For example, in many instances, parsimonious practical application of these values in impoverished countries has resulted in minimal respect for the rights of the participants in research, minimal commitment to do no harm, and inadequate attention to the sharing of benefits flowing from research (Benatar, 1998). In the late 1990s and early 2000s, when a hotly contested debate was raging on the standard of care in HIV clinical trials in low- and middle-income countries (LMICs), "A New Look at International Research Ethics" was advocated (Benatar & Singer, 2000). This call to enlarge the context for research ethics, to include considerations of inequities in health and capacity and of the social, economic, and political conditions where research was being conducted, was buttressed by critical challenges to the ethics of research in LMICs – including accusations of exploitation (Benatar, 2000, 2002). Although initially contested, the need for a new look at international research ethics gradually gained ground (Shapiro & Benatar, 2005). By 2010, some progress had been made both in acceptance of the proposed extended ethical reasoning for international research and in putting new values into practice, with inclusion of considerations of fairness in the distribution of burdens and benefits (Benatar & Singer, 2010). Whereas many of these extensions to the values of the dominant bioethical paradigm are incorporated in a draft of updated Council for the International Organization of Medical Sciences (CIOMS) guidelines (CIOMS, 2015), it is arguable that the penumbra of change was shaped by the dominant paradigm.

Hand in hand with the development of the paradigm's ethical values, there have been supporting developments in researchers' methods. For example, the initially resisted participatory research methodology has been strongly advocated in global health research and could become the norm. Communities are now to a lesser extent merely the subjects of research and are increasingly participating in determining research questions, designing the methodology, collecting and analyzing the data, and using results of research to change conditions within communities to better support community health (Lavery et al., 2010).

Though early advances in understanding and implementing improvements in ethical values and standards in research are laudable, inadequate attention is being paid to ethical challenges in global health and to addressing the broader practical challenges associated with cross-cultural global health research partnerships (Pang, 2011). Faced by the theoretical and practical obstacles to interacting across cultures, we are using global health research as an example of the need for broadening our whole approach to enhance consensus regarding definitions and goals of global health work (Benatar & Upshur, 2011). The moral starting points for such work are clear: (1) the reality of unjust inequalities in the global distribution of conditions necessary for human health and well-being and (2) the reality that unjust inequalities arise from deliberately structuring the global political economy to advantage the wealthy (Benatar, 2003). Yet the dominant paradigm glosses over these injustices and indeed impoverishes concern for rectifying them by overemphasizing minor improvements – for example, in reducing poverty without consideration for the breadth and depth of poverty and its implications (Kochhar, 2015; Benatar, 2016).

In 2010, to better understand the ethical challenges encountered by the North-South research partnerships of the Teasdale-Corti grant program, the Canadian Global Health Research Partnership of the Global Health Research Initiative (GHRI) supported two ethical research projects. One of the teams, a North-South interdisciplinary team, integrated the methods of philosophical inquiry with the quantitative and qualitative methods of the social sciences. Seeking the sources of the ethical challenges and ways to resolve them, this team found that North-South global health researchers faced issues such as (1) power imbalances in partnerships, (2) potential for exploitation of vulnerable populations, (3) fulfillment of obligations toward research participants, (4) conflicting moral and cultural values, and (5) the responsibilities of researchers from wealthy countries toward institutions and partners from poorer countries (Tomsons et al., 2013). GHRI research teams found policy statements, research ethics board guidelines, and procedures to be silent regarding the situations in which their research was implemented. Furthermore, the study's analysis identified significant inadequacies in the dominant bioethics paradigm, which explained why it was proving to be an inadequate basis for understanding

and implementing ethical global health research and practice. The paradigm's inadequacies pointed to some necessary changes and also provided direction regarding how to proceed to remedy them. Whereas it was clear that there was a need to challenge and address the inadequacy of the prevailing bioethical paradigm, it was equally clear that those addressing its problems also had to address broader challenges faced by cross-cultural global health partnerships (Benatar, 2004). In particular, fixing the dominant paradigm required acknowledging that it is a specific product that does not include fundamental values from within other worldviews and hence disadvantages partners (e.g., researchers, participants, and ethics review board members) who may hold alternative or traditional worldviews. Consequently, the study argued that exclusion of such values means that it is essential that the voices of the disadvantaged should be heard and protected in the process of expanding the bioethical paradigm.

This call for change in the bioethical paradigm is supported by global health bioethics researchers who, seeing inequities in human well-being, call for wealthy countries to acknowledge their (1) central role in creating and sustaining the social, economic, and political inequalities resulting in inequalities in conditions for human well-being (Benatar, 2005a) and (2) their obligations to address these inequalities (Pogge, 2008). Researchers often seem confident about the obligations of wealthy countries, but this confidence cannot be justified within the narrow confines of the dominant bioethics paradigm. In the real world, research takes place in many contexts with varying impacts on different people in circumstances of unjust distributions of the world's resources. If, as many global health researchers now agree, wealthy nations have responsibilities to poor nations, given the manner in which they have enriched themselves and continue to do so, and if the dominant bioethical paradigm can neither explain nor justify these obligations, the paradigm is a problem. Within the paradigm, weighty justice-based obligations – for example, the obligation to ensure that the poor benefit equally from research and knowledge – are characterized by weak benevolence-based obligations. Because the core obligations guiding global health research are grounded in justice principles (human rights more broadly understood and social justice) that are outside the paradigm, there is an obligation to address the weaknesses in the dominant paradigm (Gill & Benatar, 2016).

Some global health researchers are keenly aware that the weak political and economic powers of LMICs result in a weak voice in global ethical/justice discourse, which, in turn, allows the strong voice to dominate in such discourse (Benatar, 2003). The result is that the moral and justice values of poor nations and their understanding of these are not represented in the dominant "ethical" paradigm for global health work. This absence impacts discourse, researchers, and decision making, allowing dominant decision makers to be unaware of (or neglect/deny) the full extent of their justice-based obligations to rectify unjust inequalities and unequal conditions for human flourishing. The strong-weak voice problem complicates the obligation to address weaknesses in the dominant paradigm because the process for critiquing and revising the paradigm must now be structured to correct for this imbalance and resulting injustice.

To address the inadequacies of the dominant paradigm, to support justice in global health discourse and decision making, and to strengthen suppressed voices, we propose developing an innovative cross-cultural methodology. We call this collaborative, interdisciplinary, worldview-inclusive methodology an *interphilosophies dialogue*. Interphilosophies dialogue creates a power-balanced space for critical engagement with the dominant paradigm and the many, varied ethical and justice concerns of global health researchers.

Comparing Dominant and Alternative/Traditional Philosophies

Metaphysical Beliefs and Moral and Political Values

The dominant bioethical paradigm is a small component of a complex worldview that reigns supreme in Western societies, shaping their economic and political structures and resisting decision making that would address the inequities in the distribution of human well-being that concern global health researchers. Consequently, the interphilosophies dialogue must also engage the dominant metaphysical and epistemological beliefs accompanying the moral and political frameworks that support and sustain the dominant bioethical paradigm. The single reality metaphysic (materialism) of the dominant worldview conceives of persons as autonomous, unencumbered, self-interested, and rational. This individualistic

understanding of human existence attaches epistemic value to methodologies that are rational, scientific, quantitative, and reductionist. In identifying objective knowledge exclusively with science and disvaluing subjectivity, the dominant epistemology dismisses unscientific knowledge. The resulting epistemic hierarchy that is embedded in the education process in modern societies predisposes researchers to make negative judgments about all nonscientific sources of knowledge and forms of inquiry.

In *Thinking Ecologically*, Bruce Morito (2002) traces the historical development of the currently dominant worldview. His account of the dominant epistemology demonstrates the power of its ability to silence those representing alternative, dissenting epistemologies from within or outside its paradigm. Without rejecting or diminishing the value of reason and the scientific method, Morito illustrates the problematic consequences of the dominant epistemology and argues for epistemic recognition of other forms of understanding and knowing. Aiming for a paradigm shift in our understanding of our obligations to nature, Morito focuses on explaining how the dominant epistemology has resulted in our fundamental misunderstanding of the human/nature relationship. Our detachment from nature and our disvaluing of nature are rooted in this misunderstanding. Analogously, from the point of view of global health research, one could show that the dominant epistemology has resulted in our fundamental misunderstanding of the wealthy/poor relationship and how this misunderstanding creates and sustains an unjust power imbalance in this relationship. By explaining the power of the dominant epistemology and exposing its weaknesses, Morito's historical account of the dominant philosophy's paradigm enables the possibility of moving toward a meeting point.

Informed by Indigenous and Eastern worldviews and philosophies, Morito's critique of Western philosophy's dominant paradigm nonetheless is also an internal critique from *within* Western philosophy. Recognizing that alternative epistemologies and metaphysics exist within Western philosophy, as well as in non-Western societies, is important to understanding the nature, structure, and potential of the interphilosophies dialogue methodology we are recommending. The radical polar opposition between dominant Western philosophy and alternative philosophies, both explicit and implicit in Table 27.1, suggests incommensurability. The dominance of

Table 27.1 Comparing the Dominant Western Paradigm with Alternative/Traditional Philosophies/Worldviews

Dominant metaphysics
- Single reality (materialism) – reductionism
- Human nature – independent, autonomous individuals
- Focus: self-interest
- Competitive relations

Alternative/traditional metaphysics
- Multiple realities – holism
- Human nature – interdependent/group-oriented/autonomous individuals
- Focus: community interest
- Cooperative close relations to others past and present

Dominant epistemological values – knowledge sources
- Reason (abstract/conceptual thinking)
- Logic (consistency)
- Objective knowledge/disvalues subjectivity
- Scientific method
  - Hypothesis tested by manipulation and observation
  - Quantifiable, measurable "facts"
- Rejects unquestioned received knowledge
- Minimizes complexity/ambiguity/emotional realities

Alternative/traditional-valued knowledge sources
- Human memory (history)
- Imagination/creativity
- Examined emotions
- Moral intuition
- Traditional knowledge
  - Long-term; multifaceted experience of place
  - Qualitative interpretation of observed interactions
- Traditional knowledge has higher epistemic status than reason/logic
- No objective knowledge/values subjectivity
- Attends to complexity/ambiguity/emotional realities

Dominant moral and political values
- Anthropocentric
- Concept of identity – liberalism's concept of identity: "I think, therefore I am"; "self-made person," I am because I choose.
- Fundamental moral values: individual autonomy and well-being
- Conflict/tension between negative/positive human rights and between individual human rights/social justice
- Moral reasoning marginalizes virtues
- Consumerism
- Electoral democracy
- Primary values in decision making:
  - Self-interest
  - Rights/entitlements freedoms to . . .

Alternative/traditional moral and political values
- Concept of identity – individual within community: "I am because we are. I am a person through other people."
- Fundamental moral values: community autonomy and well-being
- Ecological (kincentric)
- Harmony/consistency between positive notion of human rights and social justice
- Moral reasoning assigns high priority to virtues
- Sustainability
- Participatory democracy
- Primary values in decision making:
  - Community
  - Responsibilities, needs, solidarity, living the good life: freedoms to . . . and freedoms from . . .

Western epistemology implies that dialogue is impossible and could not contribute to increased understanding or resolution of conflicts in values. Because the dominant philosophy's tendency to a pejorative hierarchy of value for human beings justified oppressing those deemed inferior, its current hierarchy of epistemic status justifies ignoring and even silencing alternative epistemologies. Therefore, this epistemic hierarchy is an obstacle to the epistemic respect presupposed by the interphilosophies dialogue.

Global health researchers educated predominantly in the natural and social sciences, where the dominant epistemology is assumed, are likely predisposed to employ it in their thinking. Hence it is important that there are philosophers such as Morito whose critique of the dominant epistemic hierarchy makes room for alternative/traditional epistemologies and thereby creates a space for interphilosophies dialogue. It is equally significant for the success of this dialogue that Morito and others critique metaphysical, moral, and political theories within the dominant philosophical paradigm. By weakening the latter, they demonstrate the potential for interphilosophies dialogue in the measure to which their critiques open the door for other voices and promise participants in this dialogue epistemic as well as moral and political respect and equality.

Morito's subsequent detailed research, titled "An Ethic of Mutual Respect: The Covenant Chain and Aboriginal-Crown Relations" (2012), which uncovers ways in which mutually respectful relations were formed and sustained between Europeans and Indigenous peoples, shows that the mutual respect we are aiming for in structuring our methodology is not an improbable ideal. Despite fundamental differences in metaphysical, epistemological, and axiological assumptions, when the parties are in a relationship characterized by mutual respect and communication, understanding and collaboration are possible. Morito and others within the dominant tradition who recommend revisions to their paradigm supply global health researchers and practitioners with justice principles in which to ground their solidarity with those suffering the unjust distributions of the world's resources and human well-being.

The different worldviews in Table 27.1 are characterized in discrete and widely opposed polar terms. Yet commonalities between dominant and alternative/traditional worldviews mean that it is problematic to unconditionally characterize these worldviews as polar opposites. However, the table is useful because contrasting the dominant Western worldview in which the dominant bioethics paradigm is embedded with an equally polar alternative First Nations framework provides the opportunity to seek common ground between less polarized versions of each of these worldviews and identify how health researchers from each could collaborate to restructure a global bioethics paradigm.

Because according to the dominant Western metaphysics human beings are independent, individualistic, self-interested, and competitive, it is not surprising that individual autonomy and well-being are its dominant moral and political values. Analysis of research policy statements such as Canada's Tri-Council Policy Statement (TCPS) establishes that these are the central values of the bioethics paradigm. The individualistic core of the paradigm favors moral discourse about research practice that is explicitly and implicitly grounded in human rights theory. Building on human dignity/value, this theory makes individual freedoms and entitlements the basis for assessing actions as right or wrong and human rights as central to explaining the notion of justice. Although human rights have been and continue to be an invaluable tool in efforts to dismantle unjust institutions and practices, arguably, the narrow, truncated notion of human rights in the dominant Western paradigm is an obstacle to the efforts of global health researchers to implement global human well-being. Focusing on individual perpetrators and individual victims of "human rights abuses" ignores the vastly greater contribution of flawed systems to the failure to achieve human rights more widely for whole populations of people (Benatar & Doyal, 2009; Benatar, 2011b). By attaching human rights to libertarian capitalism, the paradigm promotes individual economic freedoms and liberties and either protests or downplays social responsibility. Charity not justice grounds an individual's responsibilities at the level of community, nation, and the planet.

The alternative account of moral and political values in Table 27.1, because it is built on an individual-within-community metaphysic, fosters solidarity and community cohesion. Because we are fundamentally interdependent and in community, being in relationships precludes the sharp distinction between self-interest and others' interests that underlies the individualistic and competitive relations account in the dominant paradigm.

Solidarity and sense of responsibility to community generate an understanding of obligations that conflicts with and challenges the dominant paradigm's entitlement account. However, discussions of whether an alternative paradigm could contribute to the currently dominant "Western" discourse on research ethics and global health should include allies from several influential standpoints within this tradition who argue that the dominant account of human rights is misconceived and impoverished.

Respected theorists such as Henry Shue (1996), James Nickel (2007), Thomas Pogge (2007), and Martha Nussbaum (2011) maintain that basic needs or human capabilities support a broader conception of human rights and richer notions of justice. Arguably, their alternative moral and political theories have more commonalities with traditional/alternative worldviews than the dominant paradigm. In the ongoing debate about liberalism and communitarianism within the Western tradition, communitarians as diverse as Charles Taylor (1989) and Mary Ann Glendon (1991) employ aspects of alternative philosophies in their arguments against the individualism of the dominant paradigm.

In their book on relational ethics, Bergum and Dossetor (2005) illustrate how healthcare ethics provides an important context for challenging the core of the dominant paradigm. Arguing that morality is rooted in the collective life, like alternative worldviews, they reject a narrow individualistic framework that undervalues community. Ethical reasoning needs to be refocused to recognize that we are situated in families and communities where relationships are primary and solidarity within a web of relations is valued no less than autonomy. These metaphysical and ethical value revisions to the paradigm are more substantial challenges to the dominant paradigm than the shift within human rights theories to valuing needs as much as autonomy. Understanding human interconnectedness and dependency as fundamental, moves us closer to the alternative metaphysics and in the direction of the alternative philosophies' valuing of community autonomy and well-being. Both challenges to the dominant paradigm will facilitate interphilosophies dialogue and increase its potential for constructing an interphilosophies paradigm for research ethics

More recently, Bruce Jennings (2015) has also argued that civic republicanism can cater to communitarian critiques of liberalism: "liberty, membership, and solidarity are all part of a web of implication that includes a normative conception of place. Relational liberty, freedom through interdependence, is an embedded rather than an abstract form of living. To be embedded is not to be dominated or stifled, narrow-minded, or uncritical. It is to have a soil from which freedom and individuality can grow – out of a tradition, out of a civic life of shared purpose, and out of the experience of a life rooted in a sense of natural and cultural place and in a sensibility of care for others in that place."

Epistemology

Bergum and Dossetor (2005) also illustrate how ethical reasoning in the context of healthcare moves one away from the dominant epistemology's narrow understanding of knowledge. Their notion of embodiment integrates the feeling body with the thinking mind, with both scientific knowledge and human compassion being accorded equal status in ethical reasoning and action. The implied rejection of the epistemological hierarchy built on the dominant epistemology's objective/subjective distinction is crucial for the mutual respect they claim is essential in the ethical relationships they describe between medical experts and those needing their expertise. Because genuine interphilosophies dialogues presuppose a similar epistemic valuing of subjective methodologies, Bergum and Dossetor's bridge over the epistemic divide between the dominant epistemology and alternative epistemologies shows that interphilosophies dialogue is more than an impossible dream. Scholars critiquing the dominant paradigm from within are typically explicit about the fact that by opening the door to the methodologies of non-Western alternative worldviews and by rejecting the sharp line between objective and subjective knowledge, they are neither disvaluing scientific inquiry nor opting for a relativism that makes the notions of knowledge and rational discourse unintelligible. While arguing for the epistemic value of the nonscientific sources of knowledge that are part of alternative worldviews, Morito (2012) explains the value as well as the limitations of science's methods and reason's powers. Bergum and Dossetor (2005) also make it clear that value-free factual knowledge and analytical reasoning are necessary. In his account of the evolution of Western thought, Richard Tarnas (1991) has portrayed a greater breadth of thinking within this tradition than is reflected in its current dominant paradigm. He characterizes two distinct approaches to knowledge that emerged from the Renaissance that resemble the polar opposite of the epistemologies in Table 27.1.

The first is a rational, atomistic, intellectual concept of the world that is characterized by linear, focused, analytical thinking based on observations, discrimination, measurement, and categorization that produces fragmented knowledge. The second is, by contrast, a romantic, intuitive, imaginative worldview based on direct experience of reality with an expanded state of awareness that considers knowledge as relational (as in Bergum and Dossetor, it blends heart and head), synthesizing, holistic, nonlinear, and transformative.

For those presently embedded in the dominant paradigm or those challenging it, knowing that the dominant paradigm's epistemic hierarchy was not always the only part of the dominant tradition is important. However, Morito's explanation of how Tarnas' first approach became the dominant epistemology and from its position of epistemic power marginalized and silenced the second approach is equally important. Morito examines the strengths and weaknesses of this approach in a manner that highlights the value of the sources of knowledge it excludes and potentially diminishes its unjustified power. Opposing methodological monism and arguing for methodological pluralism, Morito shows that we require many sources of knowledge to understand the human/nature relationship and our moral obligations while demonstrating the disastrous consequences to human well-being and the planet of restricting knowledge in the manner of the dominant epistemology.

Isaiah Berlin was also opposed to methodological monism, and he preferred methodological pluralism that goes beyond the natural sciences. He believed that much writing about human nature and society – in philosophy, political theory, and sociology – risks simplification of the human condition. His views led him to conclude that there is a plurality of goods that often collide, with some of them being incommensurable, and that the freedom of person and the plurality of ideals preclude the achievement of a final synthesis of cultural ends. He accepted the critique that moral relativism is incoherent, but he argued that in making moral judgments, balance and toleration are required. He advocated moral pluralism and argued that "a horizon of common human values" can be found

without entailing moral relativism (Galipeau, 1994: 70).

Given these considerations, it should be possible to address perceived differences in the belief systems outlined in this chapter through a broader understanding and interpretation of liberal values that have not been distorted by excessively individualistic concepts of freedom and autonomy. Stated in another way – rather than seeking unexplored philosophical (not merely anthropological) insights that arise from alternative belief systems, it is possible for these to be uncovered through available but neglected components of the dominant discourse. This offers a more hopeful solution to resolving irreconcilable tensions. This view is supported by Margaret Somerville (1998: 301), who has argued that "our ways of knowing" go beyond reason to include "examined emotions, ethics, moral intuition, human memory (history) imagination and creativity." This makes sense within Joseph Heath's (2014) reminder that our thoughts and actions result from complex cultural influences and that excess faith is placed on our cognitive powers. Acknowledging that reasoning characterized by abstract and conceptual thinking and testing of hypotheses using empirical data has been the source of much-admired progress toward human flourishing as well as the means to our self-destruction, our methodology aims to sharpen humankind's moral reasoning tools so that decision making would more consistently support the former.

Anthropocentricism and Global Bioethics

Moral reasoning arises out of our shared experience, so if we experience the world in significantly different ways, then our moral reasoning should be expected to reflect these differences. One of the most significant differences between the dominant paradigm and alternatives in terms of experiencing the world is the former paradigm's anthropocentricism. Only human beings are in the dominant paradigm's moral community, which contrasts sharply with First Nations' "all my relations" way of being in the world and the understanding of moral community in alternative worldviews. Anthropocentricism keeps the moral community small, thereby reducing the scope of moral responsibility and increasing permissibility in the realm of human/nature interaction. Unlike the ecological/

kincentric understanding of alternative philosophies which promote ecosystem-friendly economic activity, anthropocentricism supports deregulated capitalism, unconstrained economic growth, and lavish consumerism, all of which are driven by narrow rights' claims and open-ended entitlements of free individuals. Unfortunately, the economic activity that the anthropocentric paradigm deems adequate for progress benefits as few as 20% of the world's population (Benatar, 2015a, 2005b). Increasingly, even within Western societies, it is recognized that the dominant paradigm's disvaluing of nature contains the seeds of destruction of our civilization because the economic activities it sanctions are at the core of massive increases in the use of energy, wasteful consumption patterns with consequent depletion of the planet's nonrenewable resources, and the ensuing environmental degradation and climate change that threaten the sustainability of all life (Oreskes & Conway, 2013; Waters et al., 2016). The understanding and valuing of nature and the more inclusive moral community in alternative philosophies in traditional societies provide an important standpoint from which to engage the dominant paradigm's basis for moral value and its foundation for economic activity. An increasing awareness of the extent of the environmental crisis in Western societies makes timely our call for collaboration between proponents of alternative philosophies and those from within the Western paradigm protesting the destruction of the planet and calling for sustainable living. Many decades ago, Van Rensselaer Potter's (1971) call for a global bioethics that recognizes human health and well-being as inseparable from the health and well-being of ecosystems preceded the currently dominant bioethical paradigm. Mounting an informed, prudential, and essentially anthropocentric (survival of our species) argument, he called for bioethical wisdom that combined ecological knowledge with a sense of moral responsibility for a livable world. Recognizing that a cultural change is needed if our civilization is to delay its extinction, he challenged excess consumption and demanded that we notice those who are not at the table. To know we are obliged to care for the planet in order to care for our species is to know that a global all-inclusive perspective is inescapable. To take the global perspective is to know that everyone has to be at the table. The dominant bioethical paradigm, which does not take the perspective of the whole and is silent

about either the intrinsic or significant instrumental value of ecosystems, is an important component of the cultural change necessary if we are to survive as a species (Benatar, 2005a, 2015b).

Van Rensselaer Potter and Lisa Potter (1995) have identified five virtues that could support global bioethics practitioners in their search for knowledge of the requirements of healthcare and Earth care and in the ethical decision making that makes knowledge implementation possible and just. These virtues, which are as relevant to our recommendation for interphilosophies dialogue as to any component of global bioethics practice, include two intellectual virtues, namely interdisciplinary competence and intercultural competence, and three moral virtues, namely responsibility, compassion, and humility. Given the complexity and diversity of the philosophies being examined and the extent to which the dominant paradigm has been imposed on non-Western societies, the interphilosophies dialogue's success will depend on all participants practicing these virtues.

We have previously suggested that increasing global instability, despite spectacular progress, calls for new ways of thinking and acting. "An extended public debate promoted by building capacity for this process through a multidisciplinary approach to ethics in education and daily life could be a driving force for such change … Achieving human development globally requires more than economic growth. It also requires confronting the current challenging context of global health, developing a global mind-set, basing a response on shared values, and adopting transformational approaches in governance, global political economy, and capacity strengthening. Education and the development of such human values as empathy, generosity, solidarity, civic responsibility, humility, and self-effacement require a space in which transdisciplinarity could thrive" (Benatar et al., 2003).

Interphilosophies Dialogue

Global health researchers are keenly aware of the stark inequality in the global distribution of conditions for health and well-being, and some are increasingly aware of problems inherent in the dominant paradigm that stand in the way of addressing the many injustices contributing to this inequality. Recognizing that the dominant bioethical paradigm is a component of the dominant philosophy paradigm and hence a Western construct, we see value in an interphilosophies dialogue methodology focused on constructing a shared paradigm for global health research. This methodology supports moral reasoning conducive to consensus decision making and can transform the dominant paradigm's understanding of justice, human rights, and moral responsibility.

Our comparison of alternative philosophies with challenges to the dominant paradigm coming from within the Western tradition makes us optimistic that the rational discourse we are recommending can arrive at an account of common values and develop a new model (Table 27.2). A new shared paradigm for global health ethics would increase capacity for all decision makers involved in global health research and practice by combining moral and scientific starting points for research with a more comprehensive relationship model inclusive of solidarity and social justice. The deeply embedded economic and political power imbalances between the rich and poor have long been recognized. Here we show that these power imbalances are supported by epistemic values that are obstacles to decision making and actions to address these imbalances and explain the relationship between epistemic and moral respect and the significant role of the dominant philosophical paradigm in sustaining injustices.

The only way to move away from the dominant paradigm and ensure that global health research is grounded in a shared cross-cultural understanding of the foundational values is to build voices for alternative/traditional philosophies into a new model. Full non-Western participation is essential, but so is dialogue. Replacing a Western monologue with a non-Western monologue will not accomplish the goal. Western voices are crucial in these dialogues because of the rational support they provide for challenges to the dominant paradigm and for inclusion of

Table 27.2 Making Change to Imbalances

Epistemic power imbalances
- Epistemic presumptions of bioethics paradigm:
  - The doctor is expert/authority.
  - The patient /"client" should accept the doctor as the knowledge holder.
- Epistemic presumptions of ethical research practice paradigm:
  - The researcher is expert/authority.
  - The subject /"participant" should accept the researcher as the knowledge holder.

Toward a shift in methodological values (epistemic values)
Participatory research methodology becomes a research method requirement in global health.
Old paradigm: Communities deserve moral respect, that is, ethical treatment as participants.
Evolving paradigm: Communities deserve moral respect and epistemic respect because participants add epistemic value to research outcomes

Adding epistemic value to research
Epistemic value is increased when communities help researchers:

- Determine research question(s) and design methodology.
- Collect and analyze data.
- Use research results to change conditions in communities to better support community health.

Challenges in global health research
The research ethics literature does not sufficiently address

- Injustices in social/economic/political contexts for global health research.
- Ethical challenges faced by diverse cultural global health research partnerships.
- Consensus about definitions/goals of global health work, and different perspectives provide different answers to "What should be (needs to be) done?" questions.

New perspective on the justice duties of the dominant culture
Moral starting points for global health:

- The reality of unjust inequalities in the distribution of the conditions necessary for human health and well-being.
- Unjust inequalities in distribution result from deliberately structuring the global political economy to advantage the wealthy.
- The role of power/wealth in creating unjust inequalities obligates the powerful to redress inequalities.

alternative/traditional values. By buttressing the arguments for alternative/traditional values, Western alternative philosophies establish commonalities, contribute to epistemic respect in the interphilosophies dialogue, and ensure that the paradigm is global/universal rather than cultural.

We call the methodology that we are proposing *interphilosophies dialogue* to be explicit about its normative nature. The philosophical underpinnings of the dominant paradigm and alternative philosophies are the immediate subject matter of the dialogue because it is recognized that these need to be understood in order to proceed to cross-cultural dialogue aimed at a new global health paradigm that aims to answer "What should we do?" questions and resolve particular moral conflicts. Philosophical inquiry is inescapably a component of the methodology because of the nature of the questions it is addressing. However, our methodology is multidisciplinary and transdisciplinary, incorporating the natural and social sciences, and inclusive of alternative/traditional sources of knowledge.

The potential for more widespread human well-being stimulates us to seek some middle path that could be rationally founded on common values and a desire to reduce inequity. A new model based on a cross-cultural interphilosophical dialogue could provide means to construct a shared paradigm for global health, thereby increasing capacity for all decision makers involved in global health research and practice by combining moral and scientific starting points for research with a more comprehensive relationship model inclusive of solidarity and social justice. This methodology requires careful attention to the deeply embedded power imbalances between the wealthy and the poor and to ensuring equal moral and epistemic respect for all.

Constraints needed on the power wielded in constructing/controlling the popularized paradigm of privileged lives will require understanding the limits of the old paradigm and of the extent to which some voices continue to be excluded from global structuring that profoundly affects health. There is a need to address those epistemic assumptions that consider the epistemic status of experiential knowledge and traditional knowledge as inferior and to ensure improved balance of epistemic respect through reflection about the issues arising from an epistemic hierarchy, which typically (and not entirely without justification) assigns higher

status to the scientific method and certain "values" (sadly often distorted from their real meaning) than to other sources of knowledge.

We should recognize that differences in the values held by the dominant power groups and others are nuanced rather than absolute. A dialogue at the level of the philosophical underpinnings could more clearly explicate these differences and reveal how they could be reconciled and applied to guide research and to resolve moral conflicts.

The interphilosophies methodology we are proposing will build on existing commonalities between non-Western philosophies and other philosophies within the Western tradition and work toward developing an interphilosophies global health ethics paradigm. Ethical conflicts and challenges have provided the opportunity for global health researchers to become aware of alternative moral and political values. Dialogue is vital, language becomes critical, and the requirement is for a language that is dialogical, collaborative, and interactive rather than defensive, commanding, and imposing. A moral language that is richer than "rights language" is needed, and languages of responsibility (justice) and responsiveness (care) must be included. Power is also an important consideration, and the point is well made that "power over," enabled by technology, needs to be leavened by "power with," which requires mutual respect, and "empowerment" through such processes as informed decision making.

In seeking to find a middle ground between opposing polar views without detracting from hard-won and highly prized values that have resulted in progress that has advanced the lives of many, it is arguable that our global plight is not so much due to pursuit of these values per se but rather to pursuit of *distortions* of these values in ways that advantage a small proportion of people at the expense of the vast majority (Benatar, 2011b, 2013). We suggest that a self-destructive mode of life is propagated when individualism becomes hyperindividualism; when freedom of the powerful reduces the freedom of the weak; when rights are defined as mainly civil and political with little attention to social, cultural, and economic rights as inalienable components of the Universal Declaration of Human Rights (UDHR); when economic dogma pervades all aspects of life, diluting other values such as a sense of community and solidarity with others; when we

Four Perspectives on Ethical
Dilemmas

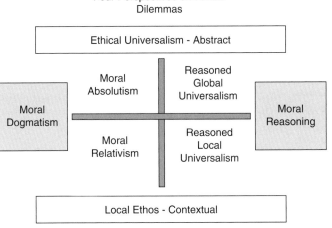

Figure 27.1. Four perspectives on ethical dilemmas.

ignore interdependence of all life within a natural world of limited resources; and when the medical research agenda is so skewed toward illnesses that afflict the wealthy.

In the field of international research ethics, prominent bioethicist Ruth Macklin (2001) argued that while there was superficial agreement on several deeply contested issues, it was not possible to obtain agreement at the level of detail. Yet the potential for finding resolutions to such seemingly intractable dilemmas (as described previously) through a reasoning process depicted graphically in Figure 27.1 provides an example for reconsidering other spheres of intractable conflict that may be resolved through reasoned dialogue between seemingly polar extremes such as idealized abstract universalism and local relativism. Such reasoned dialogue can take account of morally significant contextual factors that are ignored at the peril of inevitable ongoing conflict (Benatar, 2004).

Conclusion

In a world in which money, power, bureaucratic processes, the law, technology, and self-directed action increasingly dominate life, there is a great danger of eroding the generosity, self-effacement, sharing, love, compassion, empathy, and solidarity required to link each of us to many others – within families, small communities, nations, and the world. The capacity to imagine a better future is an integral aspect of macro ethical relationships (Benatar, 2005b).

The state of the world today, threatened by conflict, widening disparities in wealth and health, lack of access to decent living conditions, and inadequate achievement of respect for the full spectrum of human rights, calls for new paradigms of thinking and action. Maintaining the status quo or making minor changes is insufficient to reverse current trends. Relationships are important and need to be studied and improved at many levels. Although it seems obvious to those within the Western philosophical tradition to begin with relationships between individuals, alternative philosophies remind us of the complexity of real-world relationships and direct us toward moral reasoning that recognizes and supports essential ethical relationships within and between communities, institutions, and nations and with our environment. In the new paradigm's fuller understanding of ethical relationships, global health researchers will find the reasoning and motivational tools to erode the destructive individualism supported by the dominant Western paradigm. Human rights will not stand apart from or oppose solidarity, empathy, and sharing. Rather, these notions will be at the core of our understanding of human rights and at the heart of our determination to respect them.

All researchers live within a knowledge paradigm that frames their understanding of reality and the functions and nature of research, and there is a powerful tendency to see these as absolutely polarized. Our project, briefly outlined in this chapter, is designed to explore the idea that frames for rationality and intuition are dynamic rather than static and that through partnerships and the quest for equity, a middle ground can be found that respectfully embraces both perspectives (Zarowsky, 2011). We suggest that adverse power relations that sustain local and global inequalities persist not because of lack of insight, ingenuity, or resources. The problem is lack of imagination and a paradigm for decision making that has gradually constricted our understanding of the extent of local and global social, economic, physical, ecological, and moral interdependence in the face of ongoing natural, biological, and human-induced tragedies (Benatar, 2015a, 2015b). Deeper understanding of the fragility of all lives, including those of privileged and powerful people, coupled with wise cosmopolitan political, moral, and humanitarian leadership engaged in reasoning within a global paradigm, developed and evolving in interphilosophies dialogue, could enable an expanded ethical and political discourse and action. We should not ignore the potential of this methodology to ameliorate looming environmental and social tragedies that are visible writings on the wall and its power to promote a trajectory toward a more peaceful, healthy, and sustainable future.

References

Benatar, S. R. (1997). Just healthcare beyond individualism: challenges for North American bioethics. *Cambridge Quarterly of Healthcare Ethics* 6, 397–315.

Benatar, S. R. (1998). Imperialism, research ethics and global health. *Journal of Medical Ethics* 24, 221–222.

Benatar, S. R. (2000). Avoiding exploitation in clinical research. *Cambridge Quarterly of Healthcare Ethics* 9, 562–565.

Benatar, S. R. (2002). Some reflections and recommendations on research ethics in developing countries. *Social Science & Medicine* 54(7), 1131–1141.

Benatar, S. R. (2003). Bioethics, power and injustice. *Bioethics* 17, 387–398.

Benatar, S R. (2004). Towards progress in resolving dilemmas in international research ethics. *Journal of Law, Medicine and Ethics* 32(4), 574–582.

Benatar, S. R. (2005a). Moral imagination: the missing component in global health. *Public Library of Science Medicine* 2(12), e400. http://medicine.plosjournals. org/perlserv/?request=getdocument and doi=10%2E1371%2Fjournal%2Epm ed%2E0020400.

Benatar, S. R. (2005b). Forward, in Bergum, V., Dossetor, J., & (eds.), *Relational Ethics: The Full Meaning of Respect*. Hagerstown, MD: University Publishing Group.

Benatar, S. R. (2010). Responsibilities in international research: a new look revisited. *Journal of Medical Ethics* 36 (4), 194–197.

Benatar, S. R. (2011a). Global leadership, ethics and global health: the search for new paradigms, in *Global Crises and the Crisis of Global Leadership*. S Gill (ed) Cambridge University Press 127–143

Benatar, S. R. (2011b). Global health and human rights: working on the 20th century legacy. Human Rights and Social Justice Lecture, University of Alberta. Available at www.globaled.ualberta.ca/en/VisitingLectureshipinHumanRights/20102011SolomonBenatar.aspx.

Benatar, S. R. (2013). Global justice and health: re-examining our values. *Bioethics* 27(6), 297–304.

Benatar, S. R. (2015a). Health: global, in ten Have, H. (ed.), *Encyclopedia of Global Bioethics*. New York: Springer.

Benatar, S. R. (2015b). Explaining and responding to the Ebola epidemic. *Philosophy, Ethics, and Humanities in Medicine* 10, 5.

Benatar, S. R. (2016). The poverty of the concept of poverty alleviation. *South African Medical Journal* 106(1), 16–17.

Benatar, S. R., & Doyal, L. (2009). Human rights abuses: balancing two perspectives. *International Journal of Health Services* 39(1), 139–159.

Benatar, S. R., & Singer, P. A. (2000). A new look at international research ethics. *British Medical Journal* 321, 824–826.

Benatar, S. R., & Singer, P. A. (2010). Responsibilities in international research: a new look revisited. *Journal of Medical Ethics* 36(4), 194–197.

Benatar, S. R., & Upshur, R. (2011). What is global health?, in Benatar, S. R., & Brock, G. (eds.), *Global Health and Global Health Ethics*, 13–23. New York: Cambridge University Press.

Benatat, S. R., & Upshur, R. (2013). Virtue in medicine reconsidered: individual health and global health. *Perspectives in Biology and Medicine* 56(1), 126–147.

Benatar, S. R., Daar, A., & Singer, P. A. (2003). Global health ethics: the rationale for mutual caring. *International Affairs* 79, 107–138.

Bergum, V., & Dossetor, J, (eds.) (2005). *Relational Ethics: The Full Meaning of Respect*. Hagerston, MD: University Publishing Group.

Council for the International Organization of Medical Sciences (CIOMS) (2005). "CIOMS Draft Guidelines." Available at www.cioms.ch/images/stories/guidelines_demo/AllGuidelines-1-25.pdf.

Galipeau, C. J. (1994). *Isaiah Berlin's Liberalism*. Oxford, UK: Clarendon Press.

Gill, S., & Benatar, S. R. (2016). Global health governance and global power: a critical commentary on the Lancet–University of Oslo Commission Report. *International Journal of Health Services* 46(2), 346–365.

Glendon, M. A. (1991). *Rights Talk: The Impoverishment of Political Discourse*. New York: Free Press.

Heath, J. (2014). *Enlightenment 2.0*. Toronto. Harper Perennial.

Jennings, B. (2015). Relational liberty revisited: membership, solidarity and a public health ethics of place. *Public Health Ethics* **8**(1), 7–17.

Kochhar, R. (2015). A global middle class is more promise than reality. Pew Research Center Report. Available at www.pewglobal.org/2015/07/08/a-global-middle-class-is-more-promise-than-reality/.

Lavery, J. V., Tindana, P. O., Scott, T. W., & Harrington, L. C. (2010). Towards a framework for community engagement in global health research. *Trends in Parasitology* **26**(6), 279–283.

London, A. J. (2011). Justice in research in developing countries, in Benatar, S. R., & Brock, G. (eds.), *Global Health and Global Health Ethics*. New York: Cambridge University Press, pp. 293–303.

Macklin, R. (2001). After Helsinki: unresolved issues in international research. *Kennedy Institute of Ethics Journal* **11**(1), 17–36.

Morito, B. (2002). *Thinking Ecologically: Environmental Thought, Values and Policy*. Halifax: Fernwood Publishing.

Morito, B. (2012). *An Ethic of Mutual Respect: The Covenant Chain and Aboriginal-Crown Relations*. Vancouver: UBC Press.

Nickel, J. (2007). *Making Sense of Human Rights*. Malden, MA: Blackwell.

Nussbaum, M. (2011). *Creating Capabilities: The Human Development Approach*. Cambridge, MA: Harvard University Press.

Ooms, G. (2010). Why the West is perceived as being unworthy of cooperation. *Journal of Law Medicine and Ethics* **38**(3), 594–613.

Oreskes, N., & Conway, E. (2013). The collapse of Western civilization: a view from the future. *Daedalus* **142**(1), 40–58.

Pang, T. (2011). Global health research: changing the agenda, in Benatar, S. R., & Brock, G. (eds.), *Global Health and Global Health Ethics*. Cambridge, UK: Cambridge University Press, pp. 285–292.

Pogge, T. (2007). Severe poverty as a human rights violation, in Pogge, T. (ed.), *Freedom from Poverty as a Human Right: Who Owes What to the Very Poor*. Oxford, UK: Oxford University Press.

Pogge, T. (2008). *World Poverty and Human Rights*, 2nd ed. Cambridge, UK: Polity Press.

Potter, V. R. (1971). *Bioethics: A Bridge to the Future*. Englewood Cliffs, NJ: Prentice-Hall.

Potter, V.R., & Potter, L. (1995). Global bioethics: converting sustainable development to global survival. *Medicine and Global Survival* **2**(3), 185–191.

Pratt, B., & Loff, B. (2013). Linking international research to global health equity: the limited contribution of bioethics. *Bioethics* **27**(4), 208–214.

Shapiro, K., & Benatar, S. R. (2005). HIV prevention research and global inequality: steps towards improved standards of care. *Journal of Medical Ethics* **31**, 39–47.

Shue, H. (1996). *Basic Rights: Subsistence, Affluence, and U.S. Foreign Policy*, 2nd ed. Princeton, NJ: Princeton University Press.

Somerville, M. A. (1998). Making health not war: musing on global disparities in health and human rights. *American Journal of Public Health* **88**(2), 301–303.

Tarnas, R. (1991). *The Passion of the Western Mind: Understanding the Ideas that Have Shaped our World View*. New York: Crown Press.

Taylor, C. (1989). *Sources of the Self: The Making of Modern Identity*. Cambridge, UK: Cambridge University Press.

Thakur, R. (2007). Opening Western minds to international crosswinds. *The Hindu*, March 3, 2007.

Tomsons, S., Morrison, K., Gomez, A., et al. (2013). Ethical Issues Facing North-South Research Teams. Final Report to the International Development Research Centre (Grant No. 103460–093), Ottawa:, January 13. Available at https://idl-bnc.idrc.ca/dspace/bitstream/10625/52782/1/IDL-52782.pdf.

Waters, C. N., Zalasiewicz, J., Summerhayes, C., et al. (2016). The Anthropocene is functionally and stratigraphically distinct from the Holocene. *Science* **351** (6269).

Zarowsky, C. (2011). Global health research, partnership, and equity: no more business-as-usual. *BMC International Health and Human Rights* **11**(S2), S1.

Reframing Global Health Ethics Using Ecological, Indigenous, and Regenerative Lenses

Mark D. Hathaway, Blake Poland, and Angela Mashford-Pringle

We are as much alive as we keep the Earth alive.
(Tsleil-Waututh Chief Dan George, 1989: 56)

Human health is utterly dependent on the well-being of the wider Earth community (McMichael, 2014; Díaz & Brondizio, 2019). Without clean air and water, livable climatic conditions, and nutritious food, humans cannot survive, let alone thrive. Already, for many, these necessities are increasingly scarce, if not out of reach. Moreover, ecosystems – and the human communities that depend on them – are rapidly deteriorating. Several key boundaries that delineate the safe operating space for humanity have already been exceeded – particularly biodiversity loss and climate change – and the limits in other areas such as ocean acidification are rapidly being approached (Rockström et al., 2009). Ehrlich and Ehrlich (2013) conclude that human civilization may collapse unless concerted action is taken to address the problems threatening the health of the entire planet.

In this chapter, we explore some of the ethical challenges posed by the ecological crisis – a crisis in how humans relate to each other and to the wider community of life. In so doing, we consider how this crisis is the result not only of destructive practices and systems but also of a pathologic worldview rooted in a paradigm of separation, manipulation, domination, and exploitation prevalent in modern industrial capitalist societies. Western ethics, while providing needed checks and balances within the dominant system, seldom calls into question the deeper assumptions in Western thinking that have precipitated the ecological crisis by

- Emphasizing separation of the individual from community and nature,
- Perceiving living beings (human and other-than-human) as resources to be exploited rather than as subjects with intrinsic value worthy of respect and care, and

- Naturalizing competition, acquisition, and hierarchy over reciprocity, interconnectedness, and equality.

Together these orientations tend to license the exploitation of others (humans, other species, and Earth itself) in order that a minority of humanity may pursue profit and accumulate wealth.

To decolonize systems and mind-sets, we then consider alternative worldviews and ethical frameworks arising from Indigenous, Global South, and ecological perspectives. We believe that we can never move toward a more sustainable, just, and meaningful world where life flourishes if we cannot even imagine it. Therefore, the stories we tell ourselves about who we are, how we got here, and where we are headed profoundly influence what is seen as possible – and indeed what is perceived at all. Along with systemic change, decolonization challenges us to live a different story. Exploring alternative worldviews and the behaviors that align with these enables us to take the first steps toward a liberation of mind, heart, and practices – cultivating the ethic of care and humble cocreativity needed to regenerate diverse cultural and ecological communities with a view toward developing a unified community spirit that respects our fragile environment and could steward us into a safer future. Finally, we conclude by considering pathways to put these ethical frameworks into practice, including reindigenization, reconnection, and reinhabitation with the land and concrete approaches to regeneration such as the Permaculture and Transition Movements.

Ethical Challenge of Ecocide

We find ourselves ethically destitute just when, for the first time, we are faced with ultimacy, the irreversible closing down of the Earth's functioning in its major life systems. Our ethical traditions know how to deal with suicide, homicide, and even genocide; but these traditions collapse entirely when confronted with biocide, the extinction of the vulnerable life systems of the Earth, and geocide, the devastation of the Earth itself.   *(Thomas Berry, 1999: 104)*

Like Berry, we affirm that the wholesale destruction of the systems that sustain all life – what could be called *ecocide* – constitutes the key ethical challenge of our time. Approximately every eight minutes, another species – fruit of billions of years of evolution – disappears. Species are now disappearing nearly 1,000 times faster than before the evolution of humans (Vidal, 2010). Nearly one in eight of all known living species may be headed toward extinction, something that also threatens the health and well-being of humans and, ultimately, our very survival (Díaz & Brondizio, 2019). Pesticide use, the decimation of key pollinators, soil degradation, water depletion, and climate change undermine food security (Hathaway, 2016), while more severe natural disasters exact an increasing toll of death and destruction (Charron, 2012).

Over the past 50 years, global population has doubled, gross domestic product (GDP) has quadrupled (Díaz & Brondizio, 2019), and the use of nonrenewable fuels and minerals has increased threefold (Oberle et al., 2019), yet the "benefits" of economic growth have been concentrated in relatively few hands. Half of humanity lives on less than \$5.50 per day, receiving only 12% of global income, whereas the richest 1% earns 27% of income; a mere 26 individuals own more that the poorest half of humanity (Oxfam, 2019). The richest 10% is responsible for 50% of greenhouse gas (GHG) emissions compared with 10% for the poorest 50% (Oxfam, 2015), whereas the wealthiest nations have per capita ecological footprints nearly 10 times larger than the poorest nations (Global Footprint Network, 2019). Essentially, while the richest 10%–20% of humanity is reaping most of the short-term benefits from the exploitation of the biosphere, the consequences of this destruction are borne mostly by the poorest humans (more vulnerable to the increases in vector-borne diseases, food shortages, and natural disasters) as well as by future generations of humans and the myriad other living beings with whom we share this planet.

At the same time, Louv (2008: 35) affirms that humans increasingly suffer from a form of "nature-deficit disorder" resulting in a "diminished use of the senses, attention difficulties, and higher rates of physical and emotional illnesses." If we understand health as "a state of complete physical, mental and social well-being and not merely the absence of disease or infirmity" (World Health Organization, 1946:100), it is clear that we are moving away from the conditions that make health possible (Hancock et al., 2016). Indeed, human health cannot flourish unless the entire community of life on which we depend – physically, mentally, and spiritually – also flourishes (Redvers, 2018).

Ecocide is not only a technical, political, and economic challenge – albeit those factors play an important role in the crisis of the Earth. Evernden (1993: xii) notes that problems such as climate change, biodiversity loss, and their related health impacts are the "tips of icebergs, ... the visible portion of a much larger entity" that largely "lies beneath the surface, beyond our daily inspection." It is this "submerged mass" that constitutes our fundamental challenge, "the domain of unspoken assumptions" – and even perceptual habits and consciousness – which both legitimize and encourage the individual, collective, and systemic behaviors that precipitate the "environmental" crisis. These are questions of ethics and worldviews. For example, do we perceive the world that environs us as a storehouse of "raw materials" or "natural resources" that exist to satisfy our needs and desires, or do we perceive the world as a vibrant community, the breathing matrix of life to which we belong? Rather than an "environment" separate from our selves, are we not interwoven into a complex tapestry of relationships constituting the fabric of a single Earth community?

Rather than an *environmental* crisis, we are living through an *ecological* crisis, where ecology can be understood as "the study of the interrelations between organisms and their environments" (Ingold, 1992: 39). This crisis is ecological because it is precipitated in large part by failing to respect the logic of the *oikos* – the logic of our home, the Earth – following instead a perverse logic of suffering, of *pathos*, a systemic pathology. Fundamentally, this is a crisis of relationships: the relationship between humans and the greater community of life, the relationship of humans with each other, and the way our worldviews affect these relationships and how, in turn, these affect consciousness.

Eurocentric Modernity, Worldviews, and Ethics

I'm not so interested in ethics or morals. I'm interested in how we experience the world.
(Arne Naess, in an interview by Fox, 1995: 219)

Naess (1987: 40), founder of the deep ecology movement, drew on Kant's observation that morality could be motivated either by duty or out of spontaneous inclinations, suggesting that we should "primarily try to influence people towards beautiful acts" by working with "inclinations rather than morals" so that "care flows naturally" from a wider sense of the self that extends beyond the boundaries of our skin. Ethics, in this view, flows out of one's worldview – understood here as "a *way* of perceiving" the world via the senses (Naugle, 2002: 60) rather than simply an abstract set of assumptions. Indeed, we could understand worldviews as "an organic integration of dispositions, habits, feelings, and assumptions that orient the way we perceive, understand, and live in the world" (Hathaway, 2018: 70).

The ecological crisis – a crisis in the way we relate to one another and the wider biosphere – has its roots in a worldview characterized by a sense of separation from the wider community of life and indeed other humans. Ecopsychologists believe that the sense of separative autonomy that has come to characterize the consciousness of many in modern industrial cultures is "the essential context for domination" and "the root of exploitation" (Greenway, 1995: 131). Domination is often an attempt to deny the reality of interdependence. As Gomes and Kanner (1995: 115) affirm, "human dependence on the hospitality of the Earth is total" – something that threatens the separative self. "By dominating the biosphere and attempting to control natural processes," humans seek to "maintain the illusion of being radically autonomous" yet in the process destroy the relational sources of happiness and well-being. Similarly, the exploitation and domination characteristic of imperial and colonial endeavors are rooted, at least in part, in an illusory denial of community and interdependence with other humans. To facilitate exploitation, some of us have moved from a worldview that considered the entire Earth community as alive and sacred – what Berry (1999: 82) refers to as a "communion of subjects" – to a mere "collection of objects" where other beings are perceived as mere

"stuff" to be used and consumed at ever-accelerating rates. Instead of recognizing the generosity of others and the reciprocity of being, life is seen as a frenetic competition for scarce "natural resources" and wealth. The sensibilities that have been crucial to human well-being from time immemorial have been replaced by the quest for consumption in a vain attempt to fill the gaping hole left by an atrophying connection to community, the Earth, and the sacred. Ultimately, this quest for power, domination, and exploitation – this assertion of autonomy and separation – results in a parasitic relationship with the planet and ecocide – "killing off our own host" (Gomes & Kanner, 1995: 115).

The historical genesis of this parasitic relationship arguably lies in the early processes that gave rise to patriarchy, hierarchy, and empire building but appears to have accelerated during the 1400s when John Mohawk (Cajete et al., 2008) affirms that Europeans entered a period of "collective madness" – precipitated in part by traumas such as the bubonic plague, brutal wars, and witch hunts (Hathaway & Boff, 2009). This sparked a "murderous rampage" against other people and nature. Indeed, Dussel and MacEoin (1991) affirm that European modernity began not with the Cartesian *ego cogito* but rather with the will to conquer and exploit, *ego conquiro*. Traveling around the globe in search of riches using the justification of the Doctrine of Discovery – which states that if a "land" does not have a Christian government, explorers have the right to "take" the land for "civilization" and exploitation (Canning, 2018) – Europeans and settlers in the Americas usurped the land that Indigenous People had lived in harmony with for millennia. Soon the settlers began to exploit, rape, despoil, and overreap the living abundance of the Americas while killing Indigenous peoples and ignoring their teachings and warnings about how to treat the land (Armstrong, 2008; Nelson, 2008b; Canning, 2018).

Even today, though, it should be noted that not *all* humans have a parasitic relationship with the planet. Indeed, for most of human history, people have lived in relative harmony with the wider biosphere, and many people – particularly in Indigenous and traditional cultures – continue to do so today. Others are seeking to return to a more harmonious relationship. There is nothing inevitable about the path that the richest 10%–20% of humanity is following to the detriment of the greater Earth community. Pathology is not preordained or "natural." We can choose other worldviews, values, and pathways – indeed, to do so is both logical and in line with the affirmation that humans have an innate capacity and tendency to affiliate with other organisms – to form deep relational bonds that can be a source of meaning and well-being – what Wilson (1993) calls *biophilia*.

Second, as the quote often attributed to Einstein affirms, we cannot solve our problems using the same level of thinking – or even the same consciousness – that created these problems. Separative consciousness, domination, and exploitation have not only generated and perpetuated the ecological crisis; they also prevent its resolution. Humans, by ourselves, cannot heal or restore ecosystems – we can only do so by working wisely, humbly, and sensitively in concert with other beings. For example, a myriad of microorganisms is needed to generate healthy soil, while plants can sequester carbon and filter air more efficiently than any human technology. To the extent that we separate ourselves from the greater community of life, we also separate ourselves from the beings with whom we need to ally ourselves to heal and regenerate the Earth. Conversely, by moving into a consciousness of connectivity that sees humans as part of a wider community of life, we may learn the skills needed to work with other species, learning to interact cocreatively with them to facilitate authentic regeneration.

Seeking a New Story

To move toward a more just, sustainable, and humble way of living with Earth, we need to be able to envision other possibilities; we cannot hope to discover truly transformative pathways if we cannot even imagine the desired alternatives. The crisis we face is, at least in part, a historic failure of imagination. It has been said that most people can more easily imagine the end of the world than the end of capitalism (Jameson, 2003).

The stories we tell ourselves and each other, and are socialized into, say much about what we believe to be real and possible. And stories matter: we may be 70% water, but we are surely 100% storied. Indeed, many Indigenous peoples in the Pacific Northwest say that "stories make the world" (Nelson, 2008a: 5). We make sense of our lives and the world around us via stories, and they shape us in the retelling (Baldwin, 2005). Unlike discursive description, stories value synthesis, integration, and comprehensiveness over analysis, differentiation, and precision. Moreover, as

we retell these stories – often implicitly – they tend to pass from the realm of "fiction" (storytelling) into that of "truth telling," accumulating a patina of self-evident-ness in the worldviews they subtly convey, perpetuate, and embody.

The larger stories that we tell about the world – what may be understood as cosmologies – reveal the metaphors by which we live. Korten (2015: 34) notes that while "we cannot act coherently as a society without a shared framing story," we may also be influenced by stories that have been created to serve the interests of those in power to the detriment of the vast majority of humans and other creatures. Such a story is that of "money and markets," which claims that time is money and that money alone is wealth, that income and wealth are the only true measures of worth, that those who control wealth (including corporations) are the creators of what is valuable, while the poor are seen as little more than lazy parasites. Humans are perceived as individualistic and competitive by nature, and vast economic inequalities are considered the inevitable consequence of "merit" and the "freedom" to pursue individual interest. In this story, the Earth is merely a storehouse of raw materials to be consumed, whereas capital accumulation and consumption are the goals of life. This story justifies pushing species to extinction, global climate into feverish chaos, and the majority of people into poverty and desperation. As Eisenstein (2013) affirms, at the root of the story of money and markets is a deeper "Story of Separation" that licenses the exploitation of others.

In contrast, what Korten (2015: 134) calls the story of "Sacred Life and Living Earth" sees humans as being sustained physically, mentally, emotionally, and spiritually by the Earth community in which our true fulfillment can be found. In this story, our connection to others – what Eisenstein (2013: 27) calls the "Story of Interbeing" – is essential to human flourishing, and a meaningful life is one lived in cocreative partnership with other beings. At the heart of this story is an understanding that Earth is "a creative, adapting, resilient, evolving, self-organizing community of life" on which we and other species depend for our well-being (Korten, 2015: 134). In this vision, cooperation, participation, and relationships are seen as more essential to human nature than individualism and competition, while the goals of society are reoriented toward the pursuit of social justice, ecological regeneration, participation, and meaning based on interdependence and a mutuality of flourishing.

Stories also orient and embody our sense of possibilities for the future. In the Global North, three such stories are most apparent at this time (Poland et al., 2011). Business as usual (Macy & Johnstone, 2012), predominating in media, educational systems, and political discourse, is the story of technological progress that imagines – if not a wonderful new technotopia – then at least a workable muddling through looming crises based on faith in the endless wonders of science and the magic of markets. In this view, no fundamental change is necessary – money and markets will overcome all obstacles; growing social and ecological crises are disregarded, denied, or downplayed in favor of faith in technological "progress" (Hathaway, 2017).

A second – apparently quite different – story is that of the great unraveling, revered by collapsniks and survivalists, and drawing justifiable sustenance from a steady diet of news of worsening climate, social unrest, and ecosystem collapse. This is the story of immanent ecological and civilizational collapse in the face of increasingly unworkable challenges posed by rapidly deteriorating social, ecological, political, and economic conditions. This story animates the burgeoning survivalist movements in the North and the elaborate escape plans of the uber-rich (O'Connell, 2018). Like business as usual, this story does not encourage collective action for transformation and, ultimately, is also rooted in the story of separation – seeking personal survival in the face of collective ruin.

Lastly, and perhaps most rarely heard, there is the story of the "Great Turning" (Korten, 2006: 21), which recognizes the urgent crises we face but also asserts that it is still possible to bring about the transformations needed to create "a life-sustaining society" that works for the healing of the world (Macy & Johnstone, 2012: 26). Others speak in terms of *The Great Work* (Berry, 1999) or *Conscious Evolution* (Hubbard, 1998). Drawing sustenance from a broader cosmological story (Swimme, 2008), the observation that evolution and systems change is non-linear, and that evolutionary leaps are often engendered in moments of crisis, adherents of this story maintain that humanity may be on the cusp of an evolutionary leap in consciousness that will set us on a different course of history (Hubbard, 1998; Hathaway & Boff, 2009). Unlike the previous two stories, the Great Turning suggests a path toward regeneration and liberation rooted in the story of interbeing or connection, a possible way to midwife

what Eisenstein (2013) calls *The More Beautiful World Our Hearts Know Is Possible*.

Of course, these are not the only stories available to us, and it is comforting to know that as we set out to explore this storied liminal landscape at the crossroads of the possible and probable, we are not arriving at the the table empty handed. There are many ways of knowing arising from Indigenous, Global South, postcolonial, and regenerative perspectives – often systematically suppressed in the past – that offer much in the search for new stories about who we are, where we come from, and where we are headed.

Yet we must also begin our exploration humbly. With a long history of colonization, genocide, oppression, and suppression, Indigenous peoples around the world have faced major physical, social, emotional, spiritual, and mental suffering at the hands of settlers and colonizers who have desecrated and exploited Mother Earth against the wishes of the people from whom they now seek knowledge. Indigenous peoples have always known that land was connected to humans (Mohawk, 2008; Ford et al., 2010; Wildcat, 2013) and have revered Mother Earth as they attempted to live in harmony with her and her changes (Armstrong, 2008). Certainly, in seeking a new story, we cannot simply appropriate the stories of others.

At the same time, to decolonize minds, hearts, and actions, we may need to embrace a kind of "trickster consciousness" that rejects monocultures, completion, and singularities and instead embraces what are often perceived as contradictory elements or forces, playing with surprise and difference and valuing the sensuous and relational (Nelson, 2008b). Indeed, if we understand that knowledge arises from interactions within specific ecocultural communities, we may need to use many lenses to reimagine health ethics, learning to perceive the world in a wide variety of ways, particularly those which have been undervalued by Eurocentric ways of knowing.

An Ethic of Living Well

The most substantive versions of . . . Buen Vivir reject the linear idea of progress, displace the centrality of Western knowledge by privileging the diversity of knowledges, recognize the intrinsic value of nonhumans (biocentrism), and adopt a relational conception of all life.   (Arturo Escobar, 2018: 148)

Instead of seeking to accumulate possessions, power, or wealth, we may instead attend to stories and worldviews that embody nondominant ways that emphasize relationality, interconnection, reciprocity, and the sacredness of all life. This brings us beyond the purview of conventional Western ethics, particularly those that separate human from ecological health or that seek to simply minimize harm. While ceasing to do harm would be an improvement over the dangerously destructive path of ecocide, genuine transformation may be more effectively motivated by integral visions of the living well, ways of being and doing that could enable all life to thrive. Moreover, moving away from lifeways rooted in separation and acquisition to others that celebrate relationality should not be framed as "giving up" something, but rather as a form of liberation.

Many visions of living well exist within Indigenous cultures around the world. In Andean cultures, the idea of *sumak kawsay* (Quechua) or *buen vivir* (Spanish) seeks human flourishing within the context of community focusing on the quality of relationships rather than on accumulation, linear progress, or consumption. *Sumak kawsay* is understood as a continual process of becoming (verb) rather than a fixed state (noun) in which life itself is perceived as a manifestation of relationality. *Sumak kawsay* seeks to ensure the flow of energy (*cha*) within complementarity poles (*pa*) of the interconnected *pacha*, the world conceived as a living, dynamic timespace (Estermann, 2013). *Sumak kawsay* is neither anthropocentric nor androcentric; it includes all creatures as well as the ancestors, future generations, and spirit. To live well, humans are called to create the spiritual and physical conditions for a harmonious life, maintaining right relationship with other people, other creatures, and the land so that all may flourish in a vibrant community of being (Acosta, 2015).

Sumak kawsay speaks of "another reality in which human beings are part of a more harmonious whole which includes both nature and other humans, with the alterity ... that enriches us daily" (de la Cuadra, 2015: 8). Living well recognizes and values diverse knowledges, discourses, and worldviews that respect "all living beings." *Sumak kawsay* is not the possession of any one culture nor "a magic formula ... which must be adhered to religiously" but rather an "ongoing, continuous construction" that respects and celebrates a diversity of wisdoms and cultures seeking "community and cooperation with oneself, one's peers, and with all the different beings who inhabit nature" (de la Cuadra, 2015: 9). Although conflicts and disagreements may arise, living well affirms that "obstacles and disagreements can be overcome through a collective consciousness and a commitment to lay the foundation for a more sustainable life for all" (de la Cuadra, 2015: 9).

Ethically, *sumak kawsay* seeks to ensure human dignity by satisfying physical, mental, emotional, and spiritual necessities – including the need for respect and participation – while simultaneously ensuring that the wider community of living creatures – present and future – may survive and thrive (Estermann, 2013). It rejects a paradigm of linear progress, accumulation, and individual success, instead adopting an ethic of sufficiency, where it is understood that one can only live well if the entire community – humans, other creatures, water, soil, and air – are able to flourish (Hathaway & Boff, 2009). *Sumak kawsay* therefore entails a fundamental reordering of power relationships, overcoming all forms of domination and oppression, including unequal economic relationships (Estermann, 2013). Key values – learned in community – include inner strength, balanced conduct, solidarity, generosity, a reciprocity of giving and receiving, listening, wisdom, comprehension, a vision of the future, perseverance, and compassion (Acosta, 2015).

In many North American Indigenous cultures, to live wisely similarly seeks a "good life" that is the fruit of a spiritual mind-set "in which one thinks in the highest, most respectful, and most compassionate way" about one's self and others to promote a life of dynamic wholeness where community is the context for all learning (Cajete, 2000: 276). Concretely, a good life is the fruit of strong connections to one's community (human and more-than-human), understanding ecological relationships, discerning contextually appropriate actions, learning from one's own and others' experiences, and developing a sensuous, spiritual insight that cultivates respect, reverence, and consciousness of the sacred.

In Anishinaabe culture (Debassige, 2010), for example, *mino-bimaadiziwin* conveys the idea of a worthwhile, fulfilling life, a way of walking on a straight path, a life lived to the fullest including health – not only for oneself – but for one's relations. Seeking *bimaadiziwin* requires spiritual assistance and entails an ethical responsibility to right relationships between oneself and all of creation. Like *sumak kawsay*, it encompasses a vitality transcending linear time where ethical responsibilities extend to the ancestors, future beings, and all one's relations.

Le Grange (2012: 331) notes that in many Sub-Saharan African traditions, morality is also conceived in relational terms. The Zulu/Xhosa idea of *ubuntu* affirms that "our deepest moral obligation is to become more fully human and ... this requires one to enter more deeply into community with others." Exploitative, unjust, or deceptive acts are thus seen as fundamentally unethical. The Shona concept of *ukama* is broader still, signifying relatedness to the cosmos. Human social relationships are understood as a microcosm that manifests the relationality of the entire universe. Moreover, *ukama* implies an inseparable oneness with one's ancestors and future generations and calls one to live peacefully and interdependently with soil, animals, and plants. Humans are part of the greater community of life, living a relationship rooted in identity, respect, kinship, and conviviality. Humans can only be fully alive, fully themselves, by being present to and connected with other beings.

At a national level, the Himalayan kingdom of Bhutan now measures well-being – not using GDP (which, as Korten [1995] maintains, essentially gauges how quickly the living wealth of the planet is being turned into garbage) – but, instead, happiness. Informed by the ethics of Tibetan Buddhism, happiness is conceived as a "state of well-being and contentment" (Bracho, 2004: 430) that includes not only having nutritious food but also participation in its cultivation and preparation, access to the knowledge one needs to live well, work that is meaningful and satisfying, physical and psychological security, clean water, air, light, and space, and being able to create, cooperate, and share with others. While happiness could be seen as somewhat anthropocentric, Powdyel (2004) notes that the Bhutanese have traditionally understood the more-than-human world – land, rivers, valleys, mountains, plants, and animals – as a sacred landscape, the wellspring for authentic well-being. Hershock (2004) similarly maintains that Buddhist ethics is intrinsically relational, perceiving the interdependence of all reality. Happiness, then, is always a state of well-being-in-relationship – not the fruit of possessions or the accumulation of wealth and power. Although happiness cannot be continuously prolonged, it is possible to sow "the seeds of happiness" by seeking right relationships with all sentient beings (Gayleg, 2004: 544).

At a global level, the Earth Charter – fruit of an extensive civil society consultation with peoples from around the world – articulates an ethic based on ecological sustainability, social justice, peace, and participation rooted in a worldview that sees humanity as "part of a vast evolving universe" in which "Earth, our home, is alive with a unique community of life" and in which "the protection of Earth's vitality, diversity, and beauty is a sacred trust" (Earth Charter Initiative, 2000: 1). The charter speaks of living out of an ethic of deep respect, care, and reverence toward all life and affirms that once basic necessities have been satisfied, well-being is "about *being* more, not having more" (Earth Charter Initiative, 2000: 1, emphasis added).

All these lenses view living well in diverse but interrelated ways. All are rooted in stories of interconnection, reciprocity, relationality, and the sacredness of life – where water, air, soil, and Earth itself are understood to be alive. Within these visions, the health and well-being of humans are seen as inseparable from the health of the wider Earth community. All see health as having physical, emotional, mental, and spiritual dimensions and are rooted in both ancestral wisdom and a sense of responsibility to future generations of life. Moreover, each of these visions serves to orient our journey into the future, providing insights into the transformations needed to bring about the great turning.

Pathways to Integral Planetary Health

Wisdom sits in places. It's like water that never dries up. You need to drink water to stay alive, don't you? Well, you also need to drink from places. You must remember everything about them. You must learn their names. You must remember what happened at them long ago. You must think about it and keep on thinking about it. Then your mind will become smoother and smoother. Then you will see danger before it happens. You will walk a long way and live a long time. You will be wise.

(Ndee Elder Dudley Patterson [Basso, 1996: 127])

How, concretely, might humans move out of the story of separation, markets, and money – a worldview that licenses domination, injustice, exploitation, and destruction – to stories and lifeways rooted in an ethic of relationality, interconnection, respect, care, and living well? There are many pathways, unique to each place and culture, that might lead to the great turning. Each, however, entails a creative struggle with three interrelated challenges. First, how can we decolonize mind-sets, ethics, and lifeways to enable us to live in harmony with the land – to reindigenize our hearts, minds, and actions? Second, how can we reattune ourselves to the wisdom of the cultures, creatures, and land of specific places so that we can learn to cocreate with other beings? And finally, what might be some possible models for healing and regenerating specific communities and the wider planet?

Seneca scholar John Mohawk affirms that all peoples need to engage in a process of reindigenization that seeks to renew biological and cultural diversity while learning to perceive Earth as a living being. Reindigenization is rooted in "a vision of the world in a postconquest, postmodernist, postprogressive era" (Cajete et al., 2008: 254). Nelson (2008b: 290) observes that reindigenization entails learning from the millennial, time-tested practices of Indigenous peoples; we must re-mind and re-story our futures based on "place-specific 'Original Instructions' [which] are blueprints for how to live sustainably within our home ecosystems." These serve to guide our interactions with "all our relations" including "plants, animals, trees, wind, fire, clouds, rain, soils, stars, and other life-forms" as well as "people within clans, villages, tribes, nations, or other peoples of the world." Battiste & Henderson (2000: 42) note that the purpose of these guides "is to reunify the world or at least to reconcile the world to itself," cultivating "vibrant relationships between people, their ecosystems, and other living beings and spirits that share their lands." As Armstrong (2008: 72) observes, these guides are themselves dynamic: "We should always make room for newness" when novel challenges arise, seeking out creative responses, keeping in mind that we come from the land, are fed by the land, and need to love the land so that we can generate new ideas that respect the land and all creation.

Gonzales (2008: 300) sustains that reindigenization means "becoming native to this land and its relation to the decolonization of land-territory-body-mind-spirituality," but this will look different for settlers than it will for Indigenous peoples, and it will look different in diverse contexts: "We have different stories, different histories – precolonial, colonial, and neocolonial – different experiences, different pasts, different presents, and different futures." All, however, need to recover a worldview based on "sacredness, reciprocity, nurturing, and respect," renouncing exploitation and the destruction of the living world.

At the same time, protecting and recovering Indigenous identities, languages, sovereignties, and ways of knowing are key. Manuel and Posluns (1974: 157) note that for non-Indigenous peoples, the challenge may be to "carry on their quest, and discover their own relationship with the land, the water, and the animals until the Creator [gives] them their own song," meaning that settlers must not appropriate Indigenous knowledges but rather must learn for themselves how to care for the land, water, and air that they have recklessly destroyed; they must interact with all of creation to understand their relationship with the more-than-human world and discover how to be both allies and integral parts of creation.

To decolonize and reindigenize, some key questions that those of us who have lost our connection to the land and its traditional peoples might ask include

1. How can we live on this land respectfully and lovingly, acknowledging the wisdom of the peoples and creatures who have traditionally lived here?
2. How can we concretely untangle the threads of past and present wrongs, to decolonize and unsettle in mind, heart, and action?
3. How can we cease to "possess" this land and instead inhabit and heal this place that is infused with the wisdom, love, and sacredness of other beings?

These are questions that ultimately must be lived rather than simply answered, but perhaps they serve to help us begin the journey toward decolonization and reindigenization.

Decolonization and reindigenization are intimately entwined with the process of reconnecting to and learning from the land. At its heart, an ethic of respect, humility, and reciprocity is rooted in the perception that the world is *alive*. This may even be embedded in language. In Potowatomi, many nouns – for rocks, mountains, water, fire, and places – are animate; these are all *beings* rather than mere things (Borrows, 2018). Valladolid Rivera (Cajete et al, 2008: 258) speaks of how Andean Indigenous peoples have a cosmic view in which Mother Earth – the Pachamama – "is alive: the hills, the clouds, the stars, the lakes, the rocks, and all of nature ... like the mother who created them and protects them." Out of this flows a relationship of reciprocity in which people understand that they are nurtured *by*

Pachamama and that they, in turn, are expected to nurture Pachamama with respect and care.

Influenced by his experience with the Sherpa in the Himalayas, Arne Naess (1995) came to see the mountain on which he often lived – and even the stones – as alive; this influenced his belief in the intrinsic value of all life. When we experience other creatures, rivers, air, and soil as alive, we feel a deep sense of awe and reverence for the Other who is subject, not object. Abram (1997: 67) notes that this entails mutuality: "Each of us, in relation to the other, is both subject and object, sensible and sentient." This relationship of reverence and the sacred simultaneously implies communion and respect for difference and divergence. The sacred is sacred, in part, because it calls us to move beyond a narrow sense of self, drawing us into a larger reality that transforms us in the process. The unique agency of each being, its spontaneity, "affords our own body" an opportunity "to participate, to enter into relation, to feel out the divergent ways in which specific things resist our advances – the utterly unique way each entity has of torquing our assumptions, and returning us to ourselves transformed" (Abram, 2014: ix).

Ultimately, we may come to perceive the wisdom of each unique being, the wisdom that sits in specific places, each with its unique story. Perhaps once we open ourselves to apprehend this wisdom in our midst, to let it encompass, embrace, and permeate into the depths of our beings, we can learn to attune ourselves to it and harmonize our actions with it in order to live well and flourish. In so doing, we may discover that we have innumerable allies with whom we can work to heal and regenerate the Earth.

Instead of seeking sustainability – often understood in terms of ceasing to do harm rather than actively working to heal and restore – it might be better to speak in terms of regeneration, of creating healthy human cultures within resilient, adaptable, and flourishing ecosystems (Wahl, 2016). Regeneration goes beyond sustainability, endeavoring to actively heal the damage to living systems while seeking to reintegrate humans as beneficial participants in living systems – actively attuning to and cooperating with other living beings.

The Daoist idea of *wu-wei*, harmonious or non-egoistic action, may provide some insights into what this entails in practice. *Wu-wei* "is bidirectionally deferential in that it entails both the *integrity* of the particular and its *integration* in context" (Ames, 1989:

138). *Wu-wei* is both participatory *and* creative – it is a kind of "making" that is contextually (or ecologically) appropriate. The art of *wu-wei* recognizes that, alone, we (humans) do not have the wisdom, skills, or energy to heal the Earth. Yet this wisdom envelops us, present in the myriad of life forms that inhabit this planet. Our task, then, is one of *working with* the greater community of life – engaging in harmonious, contextually appropriate actions – perhaps even helping to orchestrate the many wisdoms and skills of other beings. So human wisdom plays a role – our creativity and skills can make a real, perhaps even decisive difference *if* we listen carefully – drawing on the wisdom of other beings, the diversity of human (particularly Indigenous) cultures, and the many varieties of – including traditional – scientific knowledge and apply these humbly and "care-fully." We do so, however, as *part of* a much greater community of allies who also wish to see Earth's ecosystems regenerated.

One regenerative approach that provides concrete insights into how to live out an ethic of living well is Permaculture – a design philosophy first articulated by Bill Mollison and David Holgrem in the 1970s – which has grown into a global movement promoting ecologically regenerative design (Mollison, 1979, 1988; Holmgren, 2002; Hathaway, 2007, 2015, 2016). At the heart of Permaculture is an ethic of care – expressed in three simple phrases: care for the Earth, care for people, and fair share (equitable distribution) – and they accord with an ethic of living well. Drawing on insights from ecology, systems theory, Daoism, and Indigenous knowledge, Permaculture is oriented around 12 design principles that guide human-ecological interactions, essentially constituting a set of practical precepts for living well. The first principle – to observe and interact – could be expanded to include opening to, attuning to, learning from, and reconnecting with the more-than-human world. The remaining 11 principles (see Figure 28.1) serve as a practical guide for interacting humbly, responsively, and creatively with living ecological communities – working to perceive larger patterns and then embodying them – like *wu-wei* – in a contextually appropriate manner.

In practice, Permaculture and similar land-based regenerative approaches – like the restoration of fertile land in Burkina Faso by Yacouba Sawadogo (Ericksen, 2013), the Syntropic agroforestry project in northeastern Brazil (Götsch, 2015), and the Chikukwa

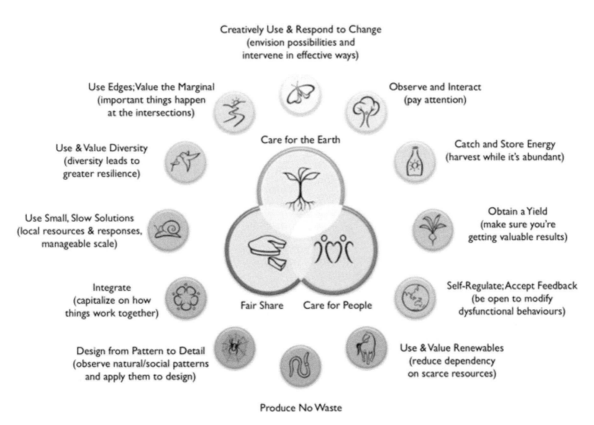

Figure 28.1. Permaculture ethics and principles.
Source: Adapted from Holmgren (2002), permacultureprinciples.com.

Permaculture Project in Zimbabwe (Leahy, 2013) – demonstrate that such cocreative interactions can unlock the regenerative capacity of living ecosystems, restoring diversity and health.

Similarly, the Transition Movement (https://transitionnetwork.org) – which originated in the United Kingdom in 2006 – uses an integrated, community-based response to regenerate human-ecological communities. Cognisant of the twin drivers of climate change and peak oil, the movement seeks a transition to a low-carbon society by building resilient communities and relocalizing the production of basic needs while emphasizing opportunities for greater connectedness and celebration (Poland et al, 2011). Citizen-led, and overlapping significantly with related relocalization, degrowth, and local food movements and based on both Permaculture principles and a distributed network model, the Transition Movement embraces the opportunity to turn crisis into an opportunity to build more resilient, convivial, and vibrant local communities, declaring that "if it's not fun, it's not sustainable"

(Hopkins, 2008) – something that echoes the idea that relational ways of living can be more fulfilling than the quest for accumulation and consumption. The Transition Movement has spread widely and rapidly and can be found in more than 50 countries throughout Europe, North America, Australia, Africa, South America, and Asia. Currently, there are more than 1,200 initiatives around the world at various stages of development (Poland et al., 2019).

Both Permaculture and Transition seek pathways to an ecologically regenerative, socially just, and fulfilling way to live well in harmony with the greater Earth community. Both are practical ways to rediscover the skills and sensibilities needed to live lovingly, responsively, and wisely with others – human and other-than-human – and create communities seeking to live well.

Conclusion

In this chapter, we have endeavored to demonstrate that to fruitfully address the challenge of ecocide, health ethics must embrace alternative ways of knowing, moving beyond hitherto mainstream formulations rooted in the dominant "Story of Separation." To do so, we include the elements of planetary health ethics articulated by Foster et al. (2019) – notably the "imagination challenges" they describe – but go beyond these to consider Indigenous, Global South, and ecologically regenerative cosmologies that offer hope and direction via their relational and animistic ontologies and the ethics of living well. We conclude by proposing a pathway to global health rooted in reindigenization, decolonization, reconnection to the land, and regenerative sustainability.

Throughout, we seek to illustrate how "another world is possible," one based on an ethic of living well that celebrates beauty, diversity, relationship, reciprocity, sufficiency, and regeneration rather than acquisition, quantitative growth, and consumption. Decentering the dominant Western worldview is a first step in decolonizing systems and mind-sets that normalize separation, competition, domination, exploitation, social inequity, and ecocide. We recognize that this great work will only be possible if it includes righting relationships with Indigenous and oppressed peoples as well as with the greater community of life. Each of us is invited into this journey. Let the work – along with the creativity, community-building, land-based reinhabitation, reciprocal learning, and celebration – begin.

References

Abram, D. (1997). *The Spell of the Sensuous: Perception and Language in a More-Than-Human World*. New York: Vintage Books.

Abram, D. (2014). On wild ethics, in Vakoch, D. A., & Castrillón, F. (eds.), *Ecopsychology, Phenomenology, and the Environment*. New York: Springer, pp. vii–ix.

Acosta, A. (2015). El Buen Vivir como alternativa al desarrollo. Algunas reflexiones económicas y no tan económicas. *Política y sociedad* **52**(2), 299–330.

Ames, R. T. (1989). Putting the te back into Taoism, in Callicott, J. B., & Ames, R. T. (eds.), *Nature in Asian Traditions and Thought: Essays in Environmental Philosophy*. Albany, NY: State University of New York Press, pp. 113–144.

Armstrong, J. (2008). An Okanagan worldview of society, in Nelson, M. K. (ed.), *Original Instructions: Indigenous Teachings for a Sustainable Future*. Rochester, VT: Bear & Company.

Basso, K. H. (1996). *Wisdom Sits in Places: Landscape and Language among the Western Apache*. Albuquerque, NM: University of New Mexico Press.

Battiste, M., & Henderson, J. Y. (2000) *Protecting Indigenous Knowledge and Heritage: A Global Challenge*. Saskatoon, Canada: Purich Publishing.

Berry, T. (1999). *The Great Work: Our Way into the Future*. New York: Bell Tower.

Bracho, F. (2004). Happiness as the greatest human wealth, in Ura, K., & Galay, K. (eds.), *Gross National Happiness and Development*. Thimphu, Bhutan: Centre for Bhutan Studies, pp. 430–449. Available at www.bhutanstudies.org.bt/public ationFiles/ConferenceProceedings/GNHandDevelopment/ 1GNH%20Conference.pdf (accessed May 15, 2019).

Cajete, G. A. (2000). *Native Science: Natural Laws of Interdependence*. Santa Fe, NM: Clear Light Publishers.

Cajete, G. A., Mohawk, J., & Valladolid Rivera, J. (2008) Reindigenization defined, in Nelson, M. K. (ed.), *Original Instructions: Indigenous Teachings for a Sustainable Future*. Rochester, VT: Bear & Company, pp. 252–264.

de la Cuadra, F. (2015). Buen vivir: ¿Una auténtica alternativa post-capitalista? *Polis: Revista Latinoamericana* **14**(40), 7–19. Available at http://polis.revues.org/10893 (accessed July 15, 2017).

Debassige, B. (2010). Re-conceptualizing Anishinaabe mino-bimaadiziwin (the good life) as research methodology: a spirit-centered way in Anishinaabe research. *Canadian Journal of Native Education* **33**(1), 11–28.

Díaz, S., Josef, S., & Brondizio, E. (2019). Summary for policymakers of the global assessment report on biodiversity and ecosystem services. The Intergovernmental Science-Policy Platform on Biodiversity and Ecosystem Services (IPBES). Available at www.ipbes.net/sites/default/ files/downloads/spm_unedited_advance_for_posting_htn .pdf (accessed May 7, 2019).

Earth Charter Initiative (2000). *The Earth Charter*. Available at www.earthcharterinaction.org/content/pages/Read-the-Charter.html (accessed May 1, 2017).

Eisenstein, C. (2013). *The More Beautiful World Our Hearts Know Is Possible*. Berkeley, CA: North Atlantic Books.

Escobar, A. (2018). *Designs for the Pluriverse: Radical Interdependence, Autonomy, and the Making of Worlds*. Durham, NC: Duke University Press.

Estermann, J. (2013). Ecosofía andina: un paradigma alternativo de convivencia cósmica y de Vivir Bien. *Revista FAIA* **2**(9), 2–21.

Evernden, N. (1993). *The Natural Alien: Humankind and Environment*. Toronto, Canada: University of Toronto Press.

Fox, W. (1995). *Toward a Transpersonal Ecology: Developing New Foundations for Environmentalism*. Albany, NY: State University of New York Press.

Gayleg, K. (2004). The characteristics and levels of happiness in the context of the Bhutanese society, in Ura, K.,

& Galay, K. (eds.), *Gross National Happiness and Development*. Thimphu, Bhutan: Centre for Bhutan Studies, pp. 541–554.

George, D. (1989). *My Spirit Soars*. Surrey, Canada: Hancock House Publishers.

Gomes, M. E., & Kanner, A. D. (1995). The rape of the well-maidens: feminist psychology and the environmental crisis, in Roszak, T., Gomes, M. E., & Kanner, A. D. (eds.), *Ecopsychology: Restoring the Earth, Healing the Mind*. San Francisco: Sierra Club Books.

Gonzales, T. (2008). Re-nativization in North and South America, in Nelson, M. K. (ed.), *Original Instructions: Indigenous Teachings for A Sustainable Future*. Rochester, VT: Bear & Company, pp. 298–303.

Greenway, R. (1995). The wilderness effect and ecopsychology, in Roszak, T., Gomes, M. E., & Kanner, A. D. (eds.), *Ecopsychology: Restoring the Earth, Healing the Mind*. San Francisco: Sierra Club Books, pp. 122–135.

Hathaway, M. (2016). Agroecology and permaculture: addressing key ecological problems by rethinking and redesigning agricultural systems. *Journal of Environmental Studies and Sciences* **6**(2), 239–250.

Hathaway, M., & Boff, L. (2009) *The Tao of Liberation: Exploring the Ecology of Transformation*. Maryknoll, NY: Orbis Books.

Korten, D. C. (2015). *Change the Story, Change the Future: A Living Economy for a Living Earth*. Oakland, CA: Berrett-Koehler Publishers.

Le Grange, L. (2012). Ubuntu, ukama, environment and moral education. *Journal of Moral Education* **41**(3), 329–340.

Louv, R. (2008). *Last Child in the Woods: Saving Our Children from Nature-Deficit Disorder*, 1st ed. Chapel Hill, NC: Algonquin Books.

Macy, J., & Johnstone, C. (2012). *Active Hope: How to Face the Mess We're in Without Going Crazy*. Novato, CA: New World Library.

Manuel, G., & Posluns, M. (1974). *The Fourth World: An Indian Reality*. New York: Free Press.

Naess, A. (1987). Self-realization: an ecological approach to being in the world. *The Trumpeter* **4**(3), 35–41.

Nelson, M. K. (2008a). Lighting the sun of our future: how these teachings can provide illumination, in Nelson, M. K. (ed.), *Original Instructions: Indigenous Teachings for a Sustainable Future*. Rochester, VT: Bear & Company, pp. 1–19.

Nelson, M. K. (2008b). Mending the split-head society with trickster consciousness, in Nelson, M. K. (ed.), *Original Instructions: Indigenous Teachings for a Sustainable Future*. Rochester, VT: Bear & Company, pp. 288–297.

Poland, B., Dooris, M., & Haluza-Delay, R. (2011). Securing "supportive environments" for health in the face of ecosystem collapse: meeting the triple threat with a sociology of creative transformation. *Health Promotion International* **26**(Suppl 2), ii202–ii215.

Global Health Research
Changing the Agenda

Tikki Pang and Gianna Gayle Herrera Amul

Background

With the launch of the United Nations' Sustainable Development Goals (SDGs), the new global compact replacing the Millennium Development Goals (MDGs), global health research remains critical in the development and implementation of inclusive, equitable, and sustainable policies and interventions. While there is a health-specific SDG 3 on good health and well-being, about 11 of the 17 SDGs have embedded and integrated health-related goals in at least 29 targets and 37 indicators (GBD 2016 SDG Collaborators, 2017). These goals reflect global priorities for global sustainable development and will attract critical funding from governments and development assistance, as was the case with the MDGs, and increasingly from philanthropies, the private sector, and public-private partnerships. Even with these global goals, there is still a need to further prioritize at the local levels, and this is increasingly critical for global health goals.

Global health financing in 2015 amounted to US$10 trillion and is projected to reach US$20 trillion in 2040 (GBD Health Financing Collaborator Network, 2018). Although there is an increasing awareness of the burden of noncommunicable diseases (NCDs) and increasing recognition of the need for further research, NCDs in low- and middle-income countries (LMICs), which in 2016 accounted for 67% of deaths, received only 2% of health funding (Ezzati et al., 2018; GBD Health Financing Collaborator Network, 2018). This highlights the continuing disconnect between global disease burden and health funding.

The burden of disease associated with NCDs is exacerbated by the continuing threat of emerging and reemerging infectious diseases and the growing threat of antimicrobial resistance coupled with growing anti-science and anti-vaccine movements and the proliferation of fake news in mass and social media that can jeopardize decades of progress in eliminating infectious diseases. At the same time, new technologies, such as gene editing with clustered regularly interspaced short palindromic repeats (CRISPR), are gaining ground with uses that will be beneficial not only for genetics research, agriculture, nutrition, antimicrobials, and global health but possibly also for planetary health (Myhrvold et al., 2018; Callaway, 2018). Global, regional, and national health policies will be needed not only to promote and support further research on these technologies but also to promote research on the application of technologies already available and prudently monitor research developments to provide the basis for sound evidence-based regulations, standards, guidelines, and policies to contribute to global development (Gutmann & Moreno, 2018).

Global Health Research System

The global health research system has grown rapidly and rather spontaneously, sacrificing efficiency in the process (Rudan & Sridhar, 2016). This can be seen primarily with the launch of at least 10 journals focused on global health in the past decade alone, including Umeå University's open-access *Global Health Action* in 2008, *Public Health Ethics* in 2008, the Royal Society of Tropical Medicine and Hygiene's *International Health* in 2009, the University of Edinburgh's *Journal of Global Health* in 2011, the Saudi Ministry of Health's *Journal of Epidemiology and Global Health* in 2011, the United States Agency for International Development (USAID) and Johns Hopkins University's *Global Health: Science and Practice* in 2013, the Lancet's *Global Health* in 2013, the renamed *Annals of Global Health* in 2014, *BMJ Global Health* in 2016, and Wuhan University's *Global Health Research and Policy* in 2016. At least 29 global health journals are being published. Table 29.1 chronicles the growth of global health research in scientific journals.

Moreover, curated global health content is growing. Some of these journals are fully online and open access, but some are subscription based or pay walled,

Table 29.1 The Phases of Growth of Global Health Research in Scientific Journals

Period 1: Early biomedical journals (1800–1950s)	Period 2: Interdisciplinary global health journals(1960s–1990s)	Period 3: Recent global health journals(2000–present)
• *New England Journal of Medicine* (1812) • *The Lancet* (1820) • *BMJ: The British Medical Journal* (1840) • *JAMA: The Journal of American Medical Association* (1883) • *American Journal of Tropical Medicine and Hygiene* (1921) • *Bulletin of the World Health Organization* (1948)	• *Social Science and Medicine* (1967) • *Health Affairs* (1981) • *Health Policy and Planning* (1986) • *Critical Public Health* (1990) • *Health and Human Rights Journal* (1994)	• *International Health and Human Rights* (2001) • *International Journal for Equity in Health* (2002) • *Health Research Policy and Systems* (2003) • *Globalization and Health* (2005) • *Global Public Health* (2006) • *Implementation Science* (2006) • *International Journal of Public Health* (2007) • *Global Health Governance* (2007) • *Global Health Action* (2008) • *Public Health Ethics* (2008) • *International Health* (2009) • *Journal of Global Health* (2011) • *Journal of Epidemiology and Global Health* (2011) • *Global Health: Science and Practice* (2013) • *Lancet Global Health* (2013) • *Annals of Global Health* (2014) • *BMJ Global Health* (2016) • *Global Health Research and Policy* (2016)

depending on whether publishers require authors to pay article processing charges (APCs). With the proliferation of social media, several global health blogs and newsletters were also launched to make global health research more accessible to scholars without institutional subscriptions in LMICs and to the general public.

State of Global Health Research: Developments, Funding, and Challenges

Since the first edition of *Global Health Ethics* in 2011, where an agenda for global health research was proposed (Pang, 2011), there have been a number of significant and important developments in global health research. This section highlights recent developments as well as challenges in global health research.

Developments

What follows are selected but not necessarily exhaustive examples of important developments in global health research.

WHO Global Observatory on Health Research and Development (R&D). In 2009, about US$240 billion was invested in health R&D, but gaps remained for LMICs that called for the need for better data "to improve priority setting and coordination for health R&D" (Røttingen et al., 2013:1286). Following the failure of efforts to establish a formal global health R&D treaty (World Health Organization [WHO], 2012), and as a response to this, the World Health Assembly requested that the WHO in 2013 establish a Global Observatory on Health R&D mainly to monitor and analyze health R&D toward identifying gaps and opportunities and defining priorities with member states (WHO, 2013). The WHO eventually launched the Global Observatory in 2017, with an aim to provide a "centralized and comprehensive source of information and analyses on global health R&D activities for human diseases" and "help identify health R&D priorities based on public health needs" decided by key stakeholders (WHO, 2020). The Global Observatory effectively took over the monitoring function of the Council on Health Research for Development's Global Forum for Health Research, which was established primarily to reduce inequities in health research, particularly in LMICs.

WHO R&D Blueprint for Action. In 2015, the WHO published a list of priority diseases under the rubric of the *WHO R&D Blueprint for Action to Prevent Epidemics* to accelerate R&D on diagnostics, vaccines, and therapeutic agents for the top 10 emerging pathogens that are likely to cause future epidemics. The diseases that were included in the initial list that need priority R&D include Crimean Congo hemorrhagic fever, Ebola, Marburg virus, Lassa fever, Middle East respiratory syndrome (MERS), severe acute respiratory syndrome–coronavirus (SARS-CoV) diseases, Nipah virus, and Rift Valley fever. In its second review in 2018, "Disease X" was included, which, according to the WHO, is an acknowledgment that a pandemic can be caused by a pathogen currently unknown to cause human disease (WHO, 2018).

World Health Report 2013. The theme for the *World Health Report* was research for universal health coverage, showing the WHO's acknowledgment of the value of research for its global health agenda. The report asserted that countries can benefit from systematic monitoring and evaluation of research programs, including investments, practices, outputs, and applications (WHO, 2013). The report highlighted that health research systems have four essential functions, including (1) setting research priorities, (2) developing research capacities, (3) defining norms and standards for research, and (4) translating evidence into practice. The report also emphasized the WHO Strategy on Research for Health, which advances the role of the WHO as a key actor in promoting and conducting research for universal health coverage with a multisectoral approach incorporating various actors and stakeholders, including governments, funding agencies, partnerships, nongovernmental and civil society organizations, philanthropies, and commercial investors.

Disease Control Priorities. The third installment of *Disease Control Priorities* (DCP) was published from 2015 to 2018 covering 21 essential packages of intersectoral policies and health sector interventions grouped into four clusters, namely age-related, infectious diseases, noncommunicable diseases and injury, and health services (Jamison et al., 2017). The third edition is a product of the DCP Network under the University of Washington's Department of Global Health and the Institute for Health Metrics and Evaluation and funded by the Bill and Melinda Gates Foundation (Gates Foundation) (University of Washington, 2018). Previous versions of the DCP were published first in 1993 and later in 2006 by the World Bank. The DCP3 introduced the concept of essential universal health coverage (EUHC) to serve as a useful model for country-specific assessments of 218 selected health system interventions that are delivered on various platforms, of which 108 interventions are considered as the highest-priority package (HPP), particularly for low-income countries (Jamison et al., 2017). The DCP3's extended cost-effectiveness analysis to estimate efficiencies for financial risk reduction is critical for assessing universal health coverage (Jamison et al., 2017). Setting priorities explicitly could help guide decisions on research funding, especially when resources are scarce, and there is lack of direct evidence that disease priorities were adequately identified.

WHO International Clinical Trials Registry Platform. Despite the evident need for transparency, only 50% of clinical trials are reported. To address this, the WHO set standards on reporting clinical trial results in May 2017 toward making the WHO International Clinical Trials Registry Platform (ICTRP) as the main repository and global database of clinical trials from the 17 different registries operating around the world. The Indian Council of Medical Research, the Norwegian Research Council, the UK Medical Research Council, Doctors Without Borders and Epicentre (its research arm), Program for Appropriate Technology in Health (PATH), the Coalition for Epidemic Preparedness Innovations (CEPI), the Pasteur Institute, the Gates Foundation, and the Wellcome Trust agreed to "develop and implement policies to require all trials they fund, co-fund, sponsor or support to be available in a public registry" and to report all results "within specified timeframes on the registry and/or by publication in a scientific journal" (WHO, 2017c). As of July 28, 2018, the ICTRP has a record of 449,596 clinical trials, of which 32% are from the Americas (AMRO), 31% from Europe (EURO), and 24% from the Western Pacific, with the other regions trailing behind. Only 13% of the ICTRP-registered clinical trials are from the Eastern Mediterranean (6%), Southeast Asia (5%), and Africa (2%) (WHO ICTRP, 2018). When clinical trials are categorized by country, 121,582 trials (27%)

are registered in the United States alone, followed by Japan (9%), Germany (7.5%), the United Kingdom (7.1%), and China (6.6%) (WHO ICTRP, 2018).

Global Antibiotic Research and Development Partnership (GARDP). The Global Antibiotic Research and Development Partnership, launched by the WHO and the Drugs for Neglected Diseases initiative (DNDi), is a virtual R&D initiative that operates through direct partnerships and inclusive collaborations involving academia, industry, international organizations, and governments as part of the WHO Global Action Plan on Antimicrobial Resistance (GARDP). GARDP was launched in 2016 to serve as the platform for new public–private partnerships for R&D on new antimicrobial agents and diagnostics. Promoting patient-needs-driven R&D, GARDP adopts the DNDi access-driven intellectual property policy in its not-for-profit R&D partnerships (DNDi, 2018).

Global Health Research Guidelines. Among the efforts to improve global health data, headway was made through the Enhancing the Quality and Transparency of Health Research (EQUATOR) Network. The network's efforts led to the *Guidelines for Accurate and Transparent Health Estimates Reporting* (GATHER), which was funded by the Gates Foundation and launched in 2016. The guidelines provide the "best reporting practices for studies that calculate health estimates for multiple populations using multiple information sources" (Stevens et al., 2016: e19). Some journals have already endorsed GATHER, including the *Lancet*, *PLOS Medicine*, the *Bulletin of the WHO*, the *Journal of Global Health*, *Revista Española de Salud Pública*, and the *International Journal of Epidemiology*.

In terms of using qualitative evidence for the development of guidelines, policies, and interventions, the international Grading of Recommendations Assessment, Development, and Evaluation (GRADE) working group with its subgroup Confidence in the Evidence from Reviews of Qualitative Research (CERQual) developed the GRADE-CERQual approach to assessing and synthesizing evidence from systematic reviews of qualitative research in 2015. In 2018, the GRADE working group published a series of papers on how to apply the GRADE-CERQual approach in the development of WHO guidelines on abortion care and maternal, newborn, and reproductive health (Lewin et al., 2018).

In addition to clinical and research guidelines promoted and recommended by the WHO, the use of research to develop rapid guidelines for international health emergencies is also critical. However, there is still a need to standardize the development of evidence-based rapid guidelines that would benefit not only national and local governments but also humanitarian organizations, nongovernmental organizations, and other front-line responders (Pang & Amul, 2018). Some proponents of the use of research evidence in developing WHO recommendations, guidelines, and policies defined a set of guiding principles toward a standardized and transparent process of rapid guidelines development (Morgan et al., 2018). The WHO and the Alliance for Health Policy and Systems Research also recently launched a practical guide for rapid reviews, highlighting the importance of engaging policymakers and health systems managers in rapid reviews (Tricco, Langlois, & Straus, 2017).

Health Policy and Systems Research. In 2017, the Alliance for Health Policy and Systems Research published the *World Report on Health Policy and Systems Research*, which traced the progress in health policy and systems research (HPSR) since 1996 when the WHO published *Health Policy and Systems Development: An Agenda for Research*. The report highlights how HPSR's growth was driven primarily by the attention to health systems strengthening (WHO, 2017d). With the SDGs in mind, the report called for increased, diversified, and long-term funding; networking mechanisms among low-income researchers; and increased links between researchers and policymakers (WHO, 2017d). The field's ability to cross disciplinary lines and link stakeholders shows promise for HPSR's capacity to further influence policy – either through the more common problem-solving models or through interactive models of health research (Peters, 2018).

Global Health R&D Funding: Multisectoral Financing and Social Impact Investments

In 2016, there were about 55 key health research funding organizations (Viergever & Hendriks, 2016). The 10 largest funders, which included the US National Institutes of Health, the European Commission (EC), the UK Medical Research Council, Wellcome Trust, USAID, and WHO, contributed about 40% (or US$37.1 billion) of all public and philanthropic health research spending (Viergever & Hendriks, 2016). By 2018, the Fogarty International Center launched the World Report mapping tool, which houses funding data on research activities supported in 2017 by several international funding organizations. As of December 2018, there were 300,000 records of funding data from 2012 to 2017. For 2017, the five largest funders remain the US National Institutes of Health (NIH; 72.9%), the UK Medical Research Council (10.2%), the European Commission (9.9%), the Wellcome Trust (6.3%), and the European and Developing Countries Clinical Trials Partnership (0.6%) (NIH, 2019).

Coalition for Epidemic Preparedness Innovations (CEPI). CEPI was launched in 2017 at the World Economic Forum. CEPI was mostly driven by the lessons from the Ebola virus outbreak from 2013 to 2016. The coalition is a multisectoral partnership composed of public, private, philanthropic, nongovernmental, intergovernmental, and civil organizations that provides an innovative funding model for vaccine development against epidemic infectious diseases, including Middle East respiratory syndrome–coronavirus (MERS-CoV), Nipah virus, Lassa fever, Rift Valley fever, and Chikungunya. CEPI's US$1 billion funding target has yet to be reached, although as of January 2019 it already had US$740 million in funding (CEPI, 2019).

Global Health Innovative Technology (GHIT) Fund. Earlier in 2012, the GHIT Fund, an international public–private R&D partnership between the Japanese government, pharmaceutical companies, the Gates Foundation, Wellcome Trust, and the United Nations Development Programme, was established in Japan. Among its objectives is to promote Japan's contribution to global health with a portfolio that includes investments in the development of new drugs, vaccines, and diagnostics for AIDS, malaria, tuberculosis, and neglected tropical diseases. It was launched with US$100 million to invest in product development from discovery through licensure (GHIT Fund, 2018). As of this writing, the GHIT Fund has invested US$132 million, the majority of which is for drug development, with about US$56 million invested in 19 projects for products at the clinical trial stage (GHIT Fund, 2018).

Global Health Investment Fund (GHIF). Managed by the nonprofit Global Health Investment

Corporation and branded as a "social impact investment fund," the GHIF is channeled to fund late-stage development of drugs, vaccines, diagnostics, and other interventions. It is supported by public, private, and philanthropic foundations, including the Gates Foundation, Grand Challenges Canada, the Swedish International Development Agency (SIDA), the UK's Children's Investment Fund Foundation, Germany's KFW Development Bank, the Federal Ministry for Economic Cooperation and Development (BMZ), pharmaceutical companies including GlaxoSmithKline, Merck, the Pfizer Foundation, and financial institutions such as the World Bank's International Finance Corporation, JP Morgan Chase, AXA, and Norway's insurance and pension fund, Storebrand. With an initial US$108 million, the GHIF has invested in at least eight projects, including treatment for onchocerciasis (river blindness) and parasitic worm infections, cheaper cholera vaccines, and improved diagnostics for various infectious diseases and vector-borne diseases (GHIF, 2018).

Public Funding. In addition to the preceding specific multisectoral funds, a substantial amount of research funding is allocated by several governments and public institutions, including the United States, the United Kingdom, and the European Commission. There are several disease-based studies on research funding. For example, the Research Investments in Global Health (ResIn) Study project estimated the United Kingdom's investment portfolio for infectious disease research from 1997 to 2010 at £2.6 billion, of which the main funders were Wellcome Trust and the Medical Research Council (ResIn, 2018; Head et al., 2013). The ResIn Study also reported on public and philanthropic investments for pneumonia research in G20 countries estimated at US$3 billion from 2000 to 2015 (Brown & Head, 2018) and global Ebola/Marburg research funding estimated at US$1.035 billion from 1997 to 2015 (Fitchett et al., 2016), among others. A separate study looked into public funding for antimicrobial resistance research in the Joint Programming Initiative on Antimicrobial Resistance, the European Commission, and related EU agencies and found that about €1.3 billion of public funding is invested in antimicrobial resistance research projects (Kelly et al., 2016).

Challenges

Capacity. In 2012, the WHO published the *WHO Strategy on Research for Health*, a product of an eight-year process that started at the 2004 Mexico Ministerial Summit on Health Research, which was meant to guide the organization's health research activities. Among the five strategies identified was capacity, with the goal to strengthen national systems for health research (WHO, 2012). In 2018, the Global R&D Observatory was able to collect data from 60 member states and reported its initial findings on the wide gaps and inequalities in global health R&D investment and the misalignment of research from the burden of disease (WHO, 2018). The observatory's finding includes (1) researcher gap (there are 40 times more health researchers in high-income countries than in low-income countries), (2) gender imbalance (women health researchers are underrepresented in low-income countries at only 27%), (3) funding imbalance ("strikingly different" levels of health official development assistance [health ODA for medical research and basic health sectors] for countries with comparable levels of poverty and health needs), and (4) funding misalignment for neglected tropical diseases (WHO, 2018).

Funding. Despite the funding mechanisms discussed earlier, funding discrepancies are still reflected, especially in neglected diseases R&D. The *Global Funding of Innovation for Neglected Diseases (G-FINDER) Report* by Policy Cures Research recorded the highest level of funding for basic research and product development for neglected diseases in 2017 at US$3.5 billion, a 7% increase from 2016. The report also highlighted how 70% of the funding goes to HIV/AIDS, malaria, and tuberculosis, with lower funding for dengue, bacterial pneumonia and meningitis, hepatitis C, and *Salmonella* infections but slightly increased funding for *Helminth* infections and diarrheal diseases (Policy Cures Research, 2018). Funding mostly came from the public sector (65%), followed by industry (16%) and philanthropic funding (19%). The United States, United Kingdom, and European Commission remain the top public funders, followed by India and Germany, while the Gates Foundation and the Wellcome Trust were the top philanthropic funders (Policy Cures Research, 2018).

Partly to address these gaps, the WHO and the DNDi launched the Global Antibiotic Research and Development Partnership in 2016. This public–private partnership aims to develop and deliver new antibiotic treatments with prices fixed to be sustainably affordable. The partnership had US$5.33 million in seed funding from Germany, the Netherlands,

South Africa, Switzerland, and the United Kingdom, as well as from Doctors Without Borders (WHO, 2017d). In addition to the observatory, the WHO also released in 2017 a global priority of pathogens list (global PPL) of antibiotic-resistant bacteria to guide R&D for new and effective antibiotic treatments. The global PPL aims "to incentivize basic science and advanced R&D by both public and private sectors investing in new antibiotics" (WHO, 2017d).

Moreover, given the similarities in health R&D priorities between governments and pharmaceutical companies, a misalignment between research priorities and burden of disease has been apparent, especially in LMIC countries (Evans et al., 2014; Yegros et al., 2018). Although pharmaceutical R&D investments grew from US$133 billion to US$150 billion from 2008 to 2015 (EvaluatePharma, 2016), public R&D funding mirrored their priorities instead of addressing the need to tackle the local burden of disease.

Ethical Dimensions of Global Health Research

Cross-Cultural Research. There is increasing debate on how to define and operationalize informed consent in different cultural contexts, especially when global health research is found to be exploitative and conducted without respect for local power relations, local knowledge and capacities, and cultural and social determinants of health (Guerrier, Sicard, & Brey 2012). Benatar, Daibes, and Tomsons (2016: 323) recently proposed a cross-cultural interphilosophies dialogue as a new "collaborative, interdisciplinary, worldview-inclusive" paradigm for global health ethics to address "unjust inequalities" in global health, including cross-cultural global health research.

"Parachutes and Parasites" in Global Health Research. This group has stimulated critical discussion in several platforms initiated by a Lancet Global Health (2018: e593) editorial explicitly titled "Closing the Door on Parachutes and Parasites." The editorial defined the parachute or parasitic researcher as "the one who drops into a country, makes use of the local infrastructure, personnel, and patients, and then goes home and writes an academic paper for a prestigious journal." The editorial highlighted that the issue applies both to primary and secondary research using open-access data. Several commentaries responded to the editorial, one of which emphasized the EU Horizon 2020–supported Global Code of Conduct for Research in Resource-Poor Settings (2018) that was born out of the TRUST Project on Equitable Research Partnerships (2018) (Merson et al., 2018). The Global Code of Conduct for Research in Resource-Poor Settings (2018) emphasizes its mission to thwart "ethics dumping," where unethical research practices are exported to resource-poor settings, through adopting values of fairness, respect, care, and honesty. Another issue raised was the context of global health research, raising the argument that parachute and parasitic research also transcends to research during health emergencies, which can lead to "conflict and confusion" not in research but among responders (Sheel & Kirk, 2018). Another commentary criticized the current debate as being "limited to the pursuit of appropriate authorship criteria," particularly the lack of recognition of how parachutes and parasites have defined and are still defining the global health discourse (Smith, 2018: e838).

Accessibility of Global Health Research. The accessibility of global health research has raised similar debates amid the proliferation of online, open-access journals. To many new scholars and researchers, open-access publishing often seems predatory (but acceptable to many high-income authors because they have publishing grants) because of the exorbitant publishing fees imposed on authors. Smith et al. (2018) looked into 3,366 global health research articles between 2010 and 2014 and found that authors paid an average of US$2,732 in article processing charges (APCs) per publication, which amounted to US$1.7 million in total APCs during that period, of which 94% went to the journals under the "oligopoly" of the 10 most prominent publication houses from high-income countries (Smith et al., 2018). Despite open-access publication, most (69%) global health research publications are still only available to subscribers (Smith et al., 2018). The implications of open-access publishing have been found to have a higher impact on citation of research articles published under the "Big Five" publishers (Springer, Sage, Elsevier, Wiley-Blackwell, and Taylor & Francis) and in journals where global health research usually falls under "biology, medicine, and science" (Li et al., 2018).

Benefit Sharing in Global Health Research. There are three key global governance instruments for benefit sharing, including the Convention on Biological Diversity, the Declaration of Helsinki, and the UNESCO Universal Declaration on Bioethics and Human Rights (Schroeder, 2014). However, in addition to these legal mechanisms, benefit sharing needs to be viewed beyond the legal benefits from "access to and utilization of biological resources" and with a broader picture of North–South international health research collaborations and justice in society as a whole (Dauda et al., 2016; Parker & Kingori, 2016). In a qualitative study done by Parker and Kingori (2016) of research collaborators, the authors found that various scientific, social, political, and ethical concerns, most of which point to values of benefit sharing, are among the various factors considered by research actors in engaging in collaborative research. They also found that beyond sharing research data, these factors include "active involvement in cutting-edge, interesting science; effective leadership; competence in and commitment to good scientific practice; capacity building; respect for the needs, interests and agendas of all partners; opportunities for discussion and disagreement; trust and confidence and; justice and fairness in collaboration" (Parker and Kingori, 2016: 1).

Research on Corporations and Global Health Governance. There is increasing interest in the commercial determinants of health: "the strategies and approaches used by the private sector to promote products and choices that are detrimental to health (Kickbusch, Allen, & Franz, 2016: e895)." Through marketing, lobbying, corporate social responsibility strategies and extensive supply chains, and driven by the "internationalization of trade and capital, the expanding outreach of corporations, and the demand for growth," corporate influence at all levels is magnified (Kickbusch, Allen, & Franz, 2016: e895). These practices have been comprehensively documented in Freudenberg's (2016) *Lethal but Legal*, which further expands the conceptual framework by defining the *corporate consumption complex*, which has far-reaching implications beyond the realm of public health. Echoing such arguments and to address the need to study the health equity impacts of transnational corporations (TNCs), several frameworks have been proposed to conduct research on the corporation's role in global health and commercial determinants of health (Baum et al., 2016; Knai et al., 2018;

Lima & Galea, 2018; McKee & Stuckler, 2018). The International Research Alliance on Public Health Governance was eventually formed out of the research agenda to analyze the involvement of "unhealthy commodity industries in public health policy" (Knai et al., 2018: 473).

Role of Corporations in Global Health Research. The private sector's role in global health research is often portrayed as a conflict of interest – profits vis-à-vis public health – as shown in the growing interest in research on the commercial determinants of health discussed earlier. For example, while pharmaceutical companies are major funders of clinical research, there is extensive documentation of sponsorship bias in clinical research (from research questions to clinical trials to publication) that impairs public trust in medical and scientific knowledge (Lexchin, 2012). Fabbri et al. (2018: e14) found in a scoping review that the industry can shift the global health research agenda by focusing research on "products, processes or activities that can be commercialized" and that can "reshape entire fields of industry through the prioritization of topics that support its policy and legal positions." This literature points to a critical need to limit corporate sponsorship of global health research. The WHO Working Group of the Global Coordination Mechanism on NCDs laid out several principles that have an impact on the management of research funding for such partnerships (Allen & Bloomfield, 2016). The argument to engage the private sector is stronger from the clinical research side given the historical sponsorship of clinical research by pharmaceutical companies. For example, the Brookings Private Sector Global Health R&D Project reported that the private sector spends about US$159.9 billion a year on health R&D, the majority of which is funded by pharmaceutical companies (US$156.7 billion) (West, Villasenor, & Schneider, 2017) .

Predatory Publishing. Whereas open access to research is strongly recommended and promoted, there is uncontrolled proliferation of online journals with questionable quality of publications and conferences. This is now known in academia as *predatory publishing*, where researchers at the start of their research careers are duped into paying exorbitant publishing and conference fees for quick acceptance for publication without peer review or editorial oversight, to keep their journal articles open-access, and mass email spamming of scholars and researchers inviting them to publish or serve on editorial boards (Stop Predatory Journals, 2018). These publishers are a serious threat to the credibility not only of scholars and researchers who are duped into publishing in predatory journals but also to science itself. Many of these predatory publishers target not only biomedical or health researchers but also other scholars in almost all disciplines (Norddeutscher Rundfunk [NDR], 2018). While exploiting the open-access model of publishing, predatory journals are "eroding the credibility of the scientific literature in the health sciences as they actually boost the propagation of errors" (Forero et al., 2018: 584). Predatory publishing creates an onus of responsibility for researchers to take cautionary steps in selecting journals for submission of their research outputs. Predatory publishing in global health research journals also puts universities in the spotlight to "discourage their researchers from submitting manuscripts to such journals or serving as members of their editorial committees," which can tarnish the reputations of both researchers and their universities (Forero et al., 2018: 584).

Waste in Research. With an estimated US$250 billion spent on biomedical research every year, there have been growing concerns about waste in research. After Chalmers and Glasziou (2009: 86) pointed out that about 85% of research funding was "avoidably wasted across the entire biomedical research range," a series of reviews was published by *The Lancet* in 2014 about reducing waste in biomedical research. The series came up with 17 recommendations ranging from research priorities; research design, conduct, and analysis; research regulation and management; accessibility; and reporting to increase the value of biomedical research for funders, regulators, journals, academic institutions, and researchers (Chalmers et al., 2014; Ioannidis et al., 2014; Al-Shahi Salman et al., 2014; Chan et al., 2014; Glasziou et al., 2014). In 2016, a review of the impact of the series was published and highlighted how the 2014 series on waste in research generated more attention from funders and researchers but little response from regulators and academic institutions (Moher et al., 2016).

Elements of a New Health Research Agenda

Using Research Evidence to Inform Advocacy and Policy. Although the originally planned *2012 World*

Health Report was delayed until 2013 and focused on research for universal health coverage instead of on the "no health without research" theme announced in 2011, the literature that grew out of the *WHO/PLOS Collection* that was intended to supplement the *2012 World Health Report* offered substantive groundwork to further promote the use of research in health policymaking, particularly in investing in the development of national health research systems in LMICs (Pang et al., 2011; PLOS Medicine Editors, 2012). A systematic review from the collection pointed out that there is a research deficiency on the role of research evidence in policies to reduce inequalities, particularly in universal healthcare systems (Orton et al., 2011). The *2013 World Health Report* was eventually published with the theme research for universal health coverage, arguing for further research to turn existing knowledge into practical applications and for all countries to produce local "research toward universal health coverage" (UHC) through increased international investment and support in research for UHC, closer collaboration between researchers and policymakers, building local research capacities, comprehensive codes of good research practice, and global and national research networks for coordination, collaboration, and information exchange (WHO, 2013). The most successful use of research evidence to inform both policy and advocacy so far is the WHO Framework Convention on Tobacco Control (FCTC). However, 10 years after implementation of the FCTC, no other health treaties have been negotiated under the auspices of the WHO.

In 2018, McLean et al. (2018) highlighted the lack of international consensus or a standard on how funders might support knowledge translation or making research useful and actionable and how approaches and mechanisms for knowledge translation vary across regions and funder types. Whereas McLean and colleagues nevertheless argued that there is no one-size-fits-all solution for knowledge translation, they recommended the need for critical evaluation of knowledge translation to enable evidence-based decision-making to become not only an objective but also a part of "how knowledge translation programmes operate and evolve (McLean et al., 2018: 13)." There is a parallel move with calls for qualitative evidence from the behavioural and social sciences to inform global health policy (Greenhalgh, 2018).

Better Data and Evidence on Return on Investment in Health Research. There is a need for further

research on the internal rate of return (IRR) on health-related research investments on health benefits. A series of papers on the return on investment of UK public R&D spending on health research showed that the IRRs for cardiovascular disease, cancer, and musculoskeletal research were 9%, 10%, and 7%, respectively (Health Economics Research Group et al., 2008; Glover et al., 2014, 2018). Further estimates from the United Kingdom on the economic spillover effects of the complementary relationship between public and private biomedical R&D expenditure showed that the real annual rate of return in terms of economic impact of public biomedical R&D in the United Kingdom ranges from 15% to 18%, and when combined with the earlier estimates of gains from cancer and cardiovascular disease research, the rate of return would range from 24% to 28% (Sussex et al., 2016). These series of papers built the foundational policy case for investments in biomedical research in a period when funding for research and science itself is being threatened by austerity measures, a growing anti-science movement, and calls for increased funding for other sectors (Grant & Buxton, 2018).

Promoting Local and National Health Research Agendas. This will be a constant part of any future global health research agenda. McKee, Stuckler, & Basu (2012) strongly argued the case for national health research strategies in 2012 by identifying countries' health research deficits and offering possible strategies that highly depend on political commitment to invest in building national capacities in health research. There is thus a need to review any effort not only in high-income countries with advanced health research systems but more so in LMICs, where the foundations of health research systems are often laid out by external, foreign research organizations and research funders with minimal engagement from actors in the local health research system. Such a review can highlight the gaps where external actors can give way to local stakeholders in both broadening and deepening the local health research agenda and can also lead to the promotion of benefit sharing and justice in global health research (London, 2012; Pratt et al., 2018).

Innovations in Research Methodology to Accelerate Implementation. There are also calls to promote implementation research that "links research and practice to accelerate the development and delivery of public health approaches" and "involves the creation and application of knowledge to improve the implementation of health policies, programmes and practices" (Theobald et al., 2018: 2214). For example, while it is definitely difficult to conduct clinical trials during outbreaks, the international consortium of research and academic institutions called Partnership for Research on Ebola Vaccinations (PREVAC) is conducting a "randomised, double-blind, placebo-controlled trial of three Ebola vaccine strategies" among 5,000 trial participants (Lévy et al., 2018: 789).

The Way Forward

Given the developments in global health research, several challenges remain to be addressed not only by the global health research community but also by research funders, governments, and the private sector. There is a need to prioritize the ethical dimensions of global health research, particularly in addressing the parachutes and parasites in global health research, cross-cultural communication issues, capacity building, predatory publishing, accessibility and benefit sharing, the role of corporations, and waste in global health research. With this in mind, the new global health research agenda needs to push for research influencing policy and advocacy, making the case for greater returns on investment in health research, promoting local and national health research systems, and innovating toward research methodologies for effective policy implementation.

References

Allen, L., & Bloomfield, A. (2016). Engaging the private sector to strengthen NCD prevention and control. *Lancet Global Health* 4, e897–e898.

Al-Shahi Salman, R., Beller, E., Kagan, J., et al. (2014). Increasing value and reducing waste in biomedical research regulation and management. *Lancet* 383, 176–85.

Baum, F.E., Sanders, D.M., Fisher, M., et al. (2016). Assessing the health impact of transnational corporations: its importance and a framework. *Globalization and Health*, 12, 27.

Benatar, S., Daibes, I., & Tomsons, S. (2016). Inter-philosophies dialogue: creating a paradigm for global health ethics. *Kennedy Institute of Ethics Journal* 26, 323–346.

Brende, B., Farrar, J., Gashumba, D., et al. (2017). CEPI: a new global R&D organisation for epidemic preparedness and response. *Lancet* 389, 233–235.

Brown, R. J., & Head, M. G. (2018). *Sizing Up Pneumonia Research: Assessing Global Investments in Pneumonia Research, 2000–2015*. Southampton, UK: ResIn.

Callaway, E. (2018). CRISPR plants now subject to tough GM laws in European Union. *Nature* 560, 16.

Chalmers, I., & Glasziou, P. (2009). Avoidable waste in the production and reporting of research evidence. *Lancet* 374, 86–89.

Chalmers, I., Bracken, M. B., Djulbegovic, B., et al. (2014). How to increase value and reduce waste when research priorities are set. *Lancet* 383, 156–165.

Chan, A. W., Song, F., Vickers, A., et al. (2014). Increasing value and reducing waste: addressing inaccessible research. *Lancet* 383: 257–266.

Coalition for Epidemic Preparedness Innovation (CEPI) (2019). *Progress*. Available at https://cepi.net/get_involved/support-cepi/ (accessed February 11, 2019).

Dauda, B., Denier, Y., & Dierickx, K. (2016). What do the various principles of justice mean within the concept of benefit sharing? *Journal of Bioethical Inquiry* 13, 281–293.

Drugs for Neglected Diseases Initiative (DNDi) (2018). Global Antibiotic Research and Development Partnership. Available at www.gardp.org/about/ (accessed September 21, 2018).

EvaluatePharma (2016). *EvaluatePharma World Preview 2016, Outlook to 2022*. London: Evaluate, Ltd. Available at http://info.evaluategroup.com/rs/607-YGS-364/images/wp16.pdf (accessed July 31, 2018).

Evans, J. A., Shim, J. M., & Ionnidis, J. P. A. (2014). Attention to local health burden and the global disparity of health research. *PLoS ONE* 9, e90147.

Ezzati, M., Pearson-Stuttard. J., Bennett, J. E., & Mathers, C. D. (2018). Acting on non-communicable diseases in low- and middle-income tropical countries. *Nature* 559, 507–516.

Fabbri, A., Lai, A., Grundy, Q., & Bero, L. A. (2018). The influence of industry sponsorship on the research agenda: a scoping review. *American Journal of Public Health* 108, e9–e16.

Fitchett, J. R. A., Lichtman, A., Soyode, D. T., et al. (2016). Ebola research funding: a systematic analysis, 1997–2015. *Journal of Global Health* 6, 020703.

Forero, D. A., Oermann, M. H., Manca, A., et al. (2018). Negative effects of "predatory" journals on global health research. *Annals of Global Health* 84, 584–589.

Freudenberg, N. (2016). *Lethal but Legal: Corporations, Consumption, and Protecting Public Health*. New York: Oxford University Press.

GBD 2016 SDG Collaborators (2017). Measuring progress and projecting attainment on the basis of past trends of the health-related Sustainable Development Goals in 188 countries: an analysis from the Global Burden of Disease Study 2016. *Lancet* 390, 1423–1459.

GBD Health Financing Collaborator Network (2018). Trends in future health financing and coverage: future health spending and universal health coverage in 188 countries, 2016–2040. *Lancet* **391**, 1783–1798.

Global Code of Conduct for Research in Resource-Poor Settings (2018). *Global Code of Conduct for Research in Resource-Poor Settings.* Available at www .globalcodeofconduct.org/wp-content/uploads/2018/05/Gl obal-Code-of-Conduct-Brochure.pdf (accessed September 24, 2018).

Global Health Innovative Technology (GHIT) Fund (2018). Portfolio analysis. Available at www.ghitfund.org/invest ment/portfolioanalysis (accessed September 7, 2018).

Global Health Investment Fund (GHIF) (2018). Current GHIF portfolio investments. Available at www.ghif.com/p ortfolio/ (accessed September 7, 2018).

Glover, M., Buxton, M., Guthrie, S., et al. (2014). Estimating the returns to UK publicly funded cancer-related research in terms of the net value of improved health outcomes. *BMC Medicine* **12**, 99.

Glover, M., Montague, E., Pollitt, A., et al. (2018). Estimating the returns to United Kingdom publicly funded musculoskeletal disease research in terms of net value of improved health outcomes. *Health Research Policy and Systems* **16**, 1–24.

Glasziou, P., Altman, D. G., Bossuyt, P., et al. (2014). Reducing waste from incomplete or unusable reports of biomedical research. *Lancet* **383**, 267–276.

Grant, J., & Buxton, M. J. (2018). Economic returns to medical research funding. *BMJ Open* **8**, e022131.

Greenhalgh, T. (2018). What have the social sciences ever done for equity in health policy and health systems? *International Journal for Equity in Health* **17**, 124–127.

Guerrier, G., Sicard, D., & Brey, P. T. (2012). Informed consent: cultural differences. *Nature* **483**, 36.

Gutmann, A., & Moreno, J. D. (2018). Keep CRISPR safe: regulating a genetic revolution. *Foreign Affairs* **97**, 3, 171–176.

Head, M. G., Fitchett, J. R., Cooke, M. K., et al. (2013). UK investments in global infectious disease research 1997–2010: a case study. *Lancet Infectious Diseases* **13**, 55–64.

Health Economics Research Group, Office of Health Economics, RAND Europe (2008). *Medical Research: What's It Worth? Estimating the Economic Benefits from Medical Research in the UK.* London: UK Evaluation Forum.

Ioannidis, J. P., Greenland, S., Hlatky, M. A., et al. (2014). Increasing value and reducing waste in research design, conduct, and analysis. *Lancet* **383**, 166–175.

Jamison, D. T., Alwan, A., Mock, C. N., et al. (2017). Universal health coverage and intersectoral action for health: key messages from *Disease Control Priorities*, 3rd edition. *Lancet* **391**, 1108–1120.

Kelly, R., Zoubiane, G., Walsh, D., et al. (2016). Public funding for research on antibacterial resistance in the JPIAMR countries, the European Commission, and related

European Union agencies: a systematic observational analysis. *Lancet Infectious Diseases* **16**, 431–440.

Kickbusch, I., Allen, L., & Franz, C. (2016). The commercial determinants of health. *Lancet Global Health* **4**, e895–e896.

Knai, C., Petticrew, M., Mays, N., et al. (2018). Systems thinking as a framework for analyzing commercial determinants of health. *Milbank Quarterly* **96**, 472–498.

Lancet Global Health (2018). Closing the door on parachutes and parasites. *Lancet Glob Health* **6,6**, e593.

Lewin, S., Booth, A., Glenton, C., et al. (2018). Applying GRADE-CERQual to qualitative evidence synthesis findings: introduction to the series. *Implementation Science* **13**(Suppl 1), 1–70.

Lévy, Y., Lane, C., Piot, P., et al. (2018). Prevention of Ebola virus disease through vaccination: where we are in 2018. *Lancet* **392**, 787–790.

Lexchin, J. (2012). Sponsorship bias in clinical research. *International Journal of Risk and Safety in Medicine* **24**, 233–242.

Li, Y., Wu, C., Yan, E., & Li, K. (2018). Will open access increase journal CiteScores? An empirical investigation over multiple disciplines. *PLoS ONE* **13**, e0201885.

Lima, J.M. and Galea, S. (2018). Corporate practices and health: a framework and mechanisms. *Globalization and Health* **14**, 21.

London, A. J. (2012). Justice and the human development approach to international research. *Hastings Center Report* **35**, 24–37.

McKee, M., Stuckler, D., & Basu, S. (2012). Where there is no health research: what can be done to fill the global gaps in health research? *PLoS Medicine* **9**, 4, e1001209.

McKee, M., & Stuckler, D. (2018). Revisiting the corporate and commercial determinants of health. *American Journal of Public Health* **108**, 1167–1170.

McLean, R. K. D., Graham, I. D., Tetroe, J. M., & Volmink, J. A. (2018). Translating research into action: an international study of the role of research funders. *Health Research Policy and Systems* **16**, 44.

Merson, L., Guérin, P. J., Barnes, K. I., et al. (2018). Secondary analysis and participation of those at the data source. *Lancet Global Health* **6**, 9, e965.

Moher, D., Glasziou, P., Chalmers, I., et al. (2016). Increasing value and reducing waste in biomedical research: who's listening? *Lancet* **387**, 1573–1586.

Morgan, R. L., Florez, I., Falavigna, M., et al. (2018). Development of rapid guidelines: 3. GIN-McMaster Guideline Development Checklist extension for rapid recommendations. *Health Research Policy and Systems* **16**, 63.

Myhrvold. C., Freije, C. A., Gootenberg, J. S., et al. (2018). Field-deployable viral diagnostics using CRISPR-Cas13. *Science* **360**, 6387, 444–448.

Norddeutscher Rundfunk (NDR) (2018). More than 5,000 German scientists have published papers in pseudo-scientific journals. Available at www.ndr.de/der_ndr/press e/More-than-5000-German-scientists-have-published-papers-in-pseudo-scientific-journals,fakescience178.html (accessed September 24, 2018).

National Institutes of Health (NIH) (2019). *World Report* (last updated September 24, 2018). Available at https://worldreport.nih.gov/app/#!/#!%2F (accessed January 18, 2019).

Orton, L., Lloyd-Williams, F., Taylor-Robinson, D., et al. (2011). The use of research evidence in public health decision making processes: systematic review. *PloS ONE* **6**, 7, e21704.

Pang, T. (2011). Global health research: changing the agenda, in Benatar, S., & Brock, G. (eds.), *Global Health and Global Health Ethics*, 1st ed. New York: Cambridge University Press.

Parker, M., & Kingori, P. (2016). Good and bad research collaborations: researchers' views on science and ethics in global health research. *PloS ONE* **11**, 10, e0163579.

Pang, T., Terry, R. F., & PLOS Medicine Editors (2011). WHO/PLoS Collection "No health without research": a call for papers. *PLoS Medicine* **8**, 1, e1001008.

Pang, T., & Amul, G. G. H. (2018). Rapid guidelines: timely and important guidance needed for setting standards and best practices. *Health Research Policy and Systems* **16**, 56.

Peters, D. H. (2018). Health policy and systems research: the future of the field. *Health Research Policy and Systems* **16**, 84.

PLOS Medicine Editors (2012). The World Health Report 2012 that wasn't. *PLoS Medicine* **9**, 9, e1001317.

Policy Cures Research (2018). *Neglected Disease Research and Development: Reaching New Heights, G-FINDER.* Available at www.policycuresresearch.org/wp-content/uploads/2019/01/Y11_G-FINDER_Full_report_Reaching_new_heights.pdf (accessed February 12, 2019).

Pratt, B., Sheehan, M., Barsdorf, N., & Hyder, A.A. (2018). Exploring the ethics of global health research priority-setting. *BMC Medical Ethics* **19**, 94.

Research Investments in Global Health (ResIn) (2018). About the study. Available at http://researchinvestments.org/about-the-study/ (accessed September 21, 2018).

Røttingen, J. A., Regmi, S., Eide, M., et al. (2013). Mapping of available health research and development data: what's there, what's missing, and what role is there for a global observatory? *Lancet* **382**, 1286–1307.

Rudan, I., & Sridhar, D. (2016) Structure, function and five basic needs of the global health research system. *Journal of Global Health* **6**, 1,010505.

Schroeder, D. (2014). Sharing of benefits, in ten Have, H. A. M. J., & Gordijn, B. (eds.), *Handbook of Global Bioethics*. New York: Springer, pp.203–223.

Sheel, M., & Kirk, M. D. (2018). Parasitic and parachute research in global health. *Lancet Global Health* **6**, 8, e839.

Smith, E., Haustein, S., Mongeon, P., et al. (2017). Knowledge sharing in global health research: the impact, uptake and cost of open access to scholarly literature. *Health Research Policy and Systems* **15**, 73.

Smith, J. (2018). Parasitic and parachute research in global health. *Lancet Global Health* **6**, 8, e838.

Stevens, G. A., Alkema, L., Black, R. E., et al. (2016). Guidelines for accurate and transparent health estimates reporting: the GATHER statement. *Lancet* **388**, e19–e23.

Stop Predatory Journals (2018). About Stop Predatory Journals. Available at https://predatoryjournals.com/about/ (accessed September 27, 2018).

Sussex, J., Feng, Y., Mestre-Ferrandiz, J., et al. (2016). Quantifying the economic impact of government and charity funding of medical research on private research and development funding in the United Kingdom. *BMC Medicine* **14**, 32.

Theobald, S., Brandes, N., Gyapong, M., et al. (2018). Implementation research: new imperatives and opportunities in global health. *Lancet* **392**, 2214–2228.

Tricco, A. C., Langlois, E. V., & Straus, S.E. (eds.) (2017). *Rapid Reviews to Strengthen Health Policy and Systems: A Practical Guide*. Geneva: WHO.

University of Washington (2018). DCP3: Disease Control Priorities, About the Project. Available at http://dcp-3.org/about-project (accessed September 7, 2018).

Viergever, R. F., & Hendriks, T. C. C. (2016). The 10 largest public and philanthropic funders of health research in the world: what they fund and how they distribute their funds. *Health Research Policy and Systems* **14**, 12.

West, D. M., Villasenor, J., & Schneider, J. (2017). *Private Sector Investment in Global Health R&D: Spending Levels, Barriers and Opportunities*. Washington, DC: Brookings Institution, Center for Technology Innovation.

WHO ICTRP (2018). ICTRP Search Portal: List by Regions/Countries, as of July 28, 2018. Available at http://apps.who.int/trialsearch/ListBy.aspx?TypeListing=2 (accessed August 1, 2018).

World Health Organization (WHO) (2012). *The WHO Strategy on Research for Health*. Geneva: WHO.

World Health Organization (WHO) (2012). Research and development to meet health needs in developing countries: strengthening global financing and coordination. Available at www.who.int/phi/CEWG_Report_5_April_2012.pdf (accessed July 31, 2018).

World Health Organization (WHO) (2013). WHA Resolution 66.22: Follow-up of the report of the Consultative Expert Working Group on Research and Development – Financing and Coordination. Geneva:

WHO. Available at www.who.int/phi/resolution_WHA-66
.22.pdf (accessed July 31, 2018).

World Health Organization (WHO) (2017a). *World Report on Health Policy and Systems Research*. Geneva: WHO.

World Health Organization (WHO) (2017b). Global Priority List of Antibiotic-Resistant Bacteria to Guide Research, Discovery and Development of New Antibiotics. Geneva: WHO. Available at www.who.int/medicines/publi cations/WHO-PPL-Short_Summary_25Feb-ET_NM_WHO.pdf (accessed July 31, 2018).

World Health Organization (WHO) (2017c). Major research funders and international NGOs to implement WHO standards on reporting clinical trial results. WHO news release. Available at www.who.int/en/news-room/det ail/18-05-2017-major-research-funders-and-international-ngos-to-implement-who-standards-on-reporting-clinical-trial-results (accessed May 20, 2017).

World Health Organization (WHO) (2017d). *Ten Years in Public Health, 2007–2017: Report by Dr Margaret Chan, Director-General, World Health Organization*. Geneva: WHO.

World Health Organization (WHO) (2018). One year on, Global Observatory on Health R&D identifies striking gaps and inequalities. *WHO: Features*. Available at: http://www .who.int/features/2018/health-research-and-development/e n/ (Accessed 28 February 2018).

World Health Organization (WHO) (2020). About the Global Health Observatory on Health R&D. Available at www.who.int/research-observatory/why_what_how/en/ind ex3.html.

WHO Research and Development Blueprint. (2018). 2018 Annual review of diseases prioritized under the Research and Development Blueprint, Meeting Report. Available at www.who.int/emergencies/diseases/2018prioritization-report.pdf (accessed July 31, 2018).

Yegros, A., Tijssen, R., Abad-Garcia, M. F., & Ràfols, I. (2018). Drug research priorities at odds with global disease toll. *Nature Index*, March 16. Available at www.natureindex.com/news-blog/drug-research-priorities -at-odds-with-global-disease-toll (accessed March 25, 2018).

Chapter 30

Justice and Research in Developing Countries[*]

Alex John London

Introduction

Clinical research is a morally complex activity. When properly conducted, it represents a powerful tool for generating information and knowledge that often cannot be obtained by other means. When properly oriented, this knowledge represents the key to advancing the standard of care and creating the policies, practices, and interventions that can be used to improve the health of large populations of people.

For almost two decades now, clinical research has become an increasingly global enterprise. With the outsourcing or off-shoring of research, new ethical complexities have arisen that are not easily accommodated within frameworks that are primarily oriented toward protecting research participants in a domestic context. In part, this is because profound conditions of social, economic, and political deprivation and inequality play a fundamental, and sometimes unique, role in cross-national research. Because of such deprivation and inequality, for instance, what is an unreasonable risk for someone in a high-income country (HIC) may represent a valuable opportunity for someone in a low- or middle-income country (LMIC). Similarly, information that has the potential to generate significant social benefits in HICs may be of little relevance to host communities that struggle with poverty and underdeveloped medical, public health, and scientific infrastructures.

Although there is widespread agreement that international research should not take unfair advantage of the disease and deprivation in LMICs, there is significant disagreement about what conditions need to be met in order to ensure that research is fair and consistent with fundamental principles of justice (Angell, 1997; Lurie & Wolfe, 1997; Crouch & Arras, 1998; Glantz et al., 1998). In the discussion that follows, I argue that a desire to remain agnostic about controversial issues of justice and to rely instead on the values that constitute the traditional pillars of research ethics result in a way of framing central issues in international research that is essentially biased in favor of what Brian Barry calls "justice as mutual advantage" (Barry, 1982: 10). As a result, someone who approaches this topic wanting to remain agnostic about controversial issues in global justice may find himself or herself formulating the basic problem in a way that tacitly presupposes a particularly anemic theory of justice.

I begin by outlining how issues of justice or fairness may arise at a variety of levels in the process of international research. I then discuss a case that dramatizes a limited subset of these issues in order to illustrate the powerful intuitions and principled commitments that make justice as mutual advantage an attractive framework in this context.

After criticizing justice as mutual advantage, I outline what I call the *human development approach* to international research. This view highlights the respect in which clinical research is a unique social good whose power to advance the health needs of large populations of people is predicated on its fitting into a particular social division of labor. This view also articulates the terms on which internationally sponsored research can satisfy claims that host community members have against one another to ensure that their basic social institutions advance the interests of all community members. It also sets out the conditions on which international research can contribute to a process of human development. This, in turn, establishes conditions under which the conduct of research represents a means of discharging a duty to aid. Finally, this approach is more likely to sustain widespread support for international research because it fosters collaborations between HICs and LMICs on terms of mutual respect and moral equality.

---

[*] An earlier version of this work appeared as: London, A. J. (2005). Justice and the human development approach to international research. *Hastings Center Report* **34**(1), 24–37.

Foci of Concern in International Research

It is often noted that the health problems of populations in HICs receive a disproportionate share of scientific attention. The so-called 10/90 research gap refers to the fact that 90% of the world's medical research dollars are spent on diseases that affect just 10% of the world's population (Commission on Health Research for Development, 1990; World Health Organization [WHO], 1996). This imbalance in research priorities raises concerns of fairness about the extent to which the scientific enterprise is systematically focusing on the health of populations that are already comparatively well off, to the exclusion of populations that bear the heaviest burdens of sickness and disease (Attaran, 1999).

Although the amount of international research has grown significantly over roughly the last decade, research priorities are still largely set by external sponsors. Because the priority health problems of LMICs differ from those of HICs, this creates the potential for a mismatch between the focus of specific initiatives and the health needs and priorities of the populations in which the research is carried out.

Additionally, many LMICs lack a robust infrastructure related to clinical research. As a result, there may not be an established system of research oversight and human/subjects protection at the local and regional levels. Additionally, LMICs frequently lack key elements in the social division of labor that operates in HICs to translate research findings into interventions, methods, or policies and to disseminate these through the medical and public health system so that they can ultimately be used to enhance the standard of care. As a result, even when research generates information or interventions that are relevant to the health needs of the host community, it can be difficult to ensure that these are integrated into or provided within the health infrastructure in the host community.

Finally, these concerns arise out of the range of social, economic, and health inequalities that often divide HICs and LMICs. People in LMICs who live in poverty and toil under some of the world's poorest social conditions also bear some of the heaviest burdens of sickness and disease. Of the 3.5 million deaths from pneumonia each year, 99% take place in LMICs, where pneumonia claims the lives of more children than any other infectious disease. To some degree, people in LMICs are more likely to die from pneumonia because they cannot afford the low-cost antibiotics that are widely available in HICs. Twenty-seven (US) cents for a five-day regimen of antibiotics is more than a day's income for roughly 1 billion people. Also, in rural communities and other places where the healthcare infrastructure is not well entrenched, hospitals and clinics may be too far away to reach.

Poverty and poor social conditions also make those in LMICs more susceptible to a wider array of illnesses. Pneumonia is more common in LMICs, for example, because children are more likely to be malnourished and suffer from medical conditions that weaken their immune systems. Where sanitation is poor and the drinking water is unsafe, diarrhea-related diseases such as cholera, dysentery, typhoid fever, and rotavirus claim the lives of nearly 2 million children under the age of five. In HICs, in contrast, such infections are much less common and more easily treated when they occur. Similarly, of the roughly 1,600 children infected with HIV every day, approximately 90% live in LMICs. Africa alone is home to some 70% of the world's HIV-positive individuals, even though the continent contains only about 10% of the world's population.

These dramatic differences between HICs and LMICs, and the toll that such social, economic, and health burdens take on the welfare and opportunities of LMIC populations, provide the context for international research. To give a concrete illustration of some of these facets, consider what I will refer to as the *Surfaxin case*.

Extremely premature infants frequently suffer from a potentially life-threatening condition known as *respiratory distress syndrome* (RDS). Respiratory distress syndrome can be successfully treated with the use of surfactant-replacement therapy. Surfactants are substances produced in the lungs that are essential to the lungs' ability to absorb oxygen and maintain proper airflow through the respiratory system. During the 1990s, several natural and artificial surfactant agents received Food and Drug Administration (FDA) approval and were in widespread use in the United States and other HICs.

In 2001, the pharmaceutical firm Discovery Laboratories proposed a large-scale placebo-controlled clinical trial of its new surfactant drug Surfaxin. The trials would be carried out in impoverished Latin American communities where neonatal intensive care units were poorly equipped and where children did not at the time have access to surfactants. Discovery Laboratories would upgrade and modernize the intensive care units that participated in the clinical trial so that all the children included in the research would receive improved medical care, including ventilator support. Half the children in the trial would then receive Surfaxin, and the other half, roughly 325 dangerously ill children, would receive a placebo.

Critics of this study argued that a placebo control would not have been permissible in the United States and that its use in an LMIC constituted an unfair double standard (Lurie & Wolfe, 2007). They argued that participants in the control arm were entitled to receive the established standard of care for treating RDS, namely surfactant-replacement therapy, and that the use of a placebo would result in roughly 17 preventable deaths. Moreover, they claimed that the relevant scientific question was whether Surfaxin was equivalent or superior to currently available therapy, not whether it was better than nothing. This claim was bolstered by the fact that Surfaxin did not have properties that made it especially well suited for use in LMICs and that it would be marketed primarily in HICs. Finally, some argued that it was unfair to conduct this study without plans to make Surfaxin available more broadly in the host community at the completion of the trial. To such critics, Discovery Laboratories was in effect leveraging the poverty and disease of LMIC communities as a mechanism to increase its profit margins.

Proponents of this study, such as Robert Temple of the FDA, argued that "[i]f they did the trial, half of the people would get surfactant and better perinatal care, and the other half would get better perinatal care. It seems to me that all the people in the trial would have been better off" (Shah, 2002: 28). They also argued that providing roughly 325 dangerously ill newborns with a placebo does not violate the standard of care because newborns in these communities do not otherwise have access to surfactants.

Others have argued that requiring the provision of surfactant-replacement therapy in the control group would eliminate the advantages associated with conducting the trial in an LMIC context. If the study were relocated to the United States, then approximately 17 infants whose lives might be saved by receiving Surfaxin would be consigned to death. Even though poverty and deprivation may have created the background conditions for this trial, those conditions alone do not make it the case that the trial was taking unfair advantage of participants. As such, proponents argued that the trial should be permitted to go forward as designed.

Justice as Mutual Advantage

Powerful intuitions, as well as a desire not to hold pressing practical problems hostage to broad theoretical disputes about the requirements of social justice, support a variety of approaches that fall under the heading of *justice as mutual advantage*. In this view, the terms of a research collaboration are just if they are mutually beneficial, and each of the parties freely accepts them without the interference of force, fraud, or coercion and with an adequate understanding of the relevant information.

Although some people may hold this view explicitly and defend it on substantive grounds, others who wish to remain agnostic about substantive issues of global justice may nevertheless find themselves committed to this view. In part, this view fits very nicely within the existing regulatory structures in HICs. For instance, the relevant unit of concern in this view is the dyadic relationship between researchers and host communities. Issues of justice or fairness are a property of the relationship between researchers and the host communities with whom they interact.

Similarly, the central focus of this view accords nicely with values that stand as the traditional pillars of research ethics: nonmaleficence, beneficence, and respect for autonomy. It seems to satisfy a requirement of *nonmaleficence* by prohibiting research agreements that would leave host communities worse off than they otherwise would have been. It seems to satisfy a requirement of *beneficence* because just agreements must provide a meaningful benefit to each of the parties. Finally, it seeks to respect the *autonomy* of host communities by leaving it to them to determine in light of their own values how much of which kinds of benefits represent a sufficient return for hosting a particular research project.

If one views issues of justice in this context as primarily a property of the way that researchers treat host community members, and if one uses these traditional pillars of research ethics to provide the content for the value of justice, then any voluntary agreement that is mutually beneficial and grounded in an adequate understanding of the relevant information will be regarded as fair or morally permissible.

Perhaps the most explicit articulation of this position has come from proponents of the *fair benefits* approach to international research (Participants, 2002, 2004). The central focus of this view is avoiding exploitation, and its proponents follow Wertheimer in holding that party A exploits party B if party A receives "an unfair level of benefits as a result of B's interactions with A" (Participants, 2004: 19). They thus hold that the crucial issue is not "what" benefits host communities receive but "how much" and that host communities should be free to choose from a wide range of possible benefits – such as receiving access to vaccinations or other public health measures.

This approach is critical of the requirement, enshrined in the Declaration of Helsinki and elsewhere, that researchers must ensure that members of the host community can obtain interventions proven to be effective by a clinical trial. From the standpoint of the fair benefits approach, the *reasonable availability* requirement is overly restrictive both of important international research and of the ability of LMIC populations to receive a wide range of potential benefits that can come from hosting a research initiative.

Similarly, if the host community is not interested in the information or the interventions that the study is designed to generate, and if it is not obligatory to provide posttrial access to the study intervention, then it would seem to follow that international research initiatives would not need to target or be aligned with the urgent health needs or priorities of the host community.

In order to ensure that host communities receive a fair level of benefits, researchers and community members are supposed to engage in a process of *collaborative partnership* in which the parties negotiate an agreement under conditions that approximate those of an ideal market. Because this view holds that "a fair distribution of benefits at the micro-level is based on the level of benefits that would occur in a market transaction devoid of fraud, deception, or force, in which the parties have full information," the outcomes of this process are regarded as fair as long as the transaction is free from the enumerated defects (Participants, 2004: 20). In order to ensure that these conditions are met, the proponents of this approach also propose a *principle of transparency* that would provide all parties with the information they need to properly value participation in a clinical trial.

Shortcomings of Justice as Mutual Advantage

One problem with justice as mutual advantage is that it is too parochial and conservative to capture the full range of concerns that are relevant in the context of international research. The charge of parochialism relates to its narrow focus on the obligations of researchers and community members. For example, proponents of the fair benefits approach are explicit that as Wertheimer explicates the concept, exploitation is a micro-level concern that deals with the fairness of discrete exchanges between identifiable parties. Even if one assumes that Wertheimer is correct in his view of exploitation, one might legitimately question whether the most relevant and important ethical issues in this context occur at the micro-level. In particular, if there are issues of justice or fairness associated with the degree to which scientific inquiry targets the needs of those who are already comparatively well off, to the neglect of those who bear the most significant burdens of disease and disability, then those concerns could not be easily accommodated within a framework exclusively focused on the researcher-participant relationship.

Similarly, it may be true that researchers have special obligations in this context, but it is questionable whether they should be seen as the primary, or even the most important, duty bearers. Other stakeholders play a powerful role in shaping the research agenda. As such, governments, nongovernmental organizations (NGOs), and the public and private entities that fund and support the research enterprise may have equal, if not more important, duties in this context.

Because Wertheimer's account of exploitation only applies to micro-level transactions between individual parties, it does not apply directly to the operation of social systems that shape and coordinate the behavior of large numbers of people, often dispersed geographically and temporally. Concerns about whether the *social systems* of international clinical research make unfair use of the sick and the vulnerable would have to be articulated in a different framework.

Justice as mutual advantage may be regarded as too conservative because it only applies once some cooperative endeavor has been initiated; it cannot ground or generate an obligation to engage in cooperation where none exists. As Brian Barry notes, it does not "say that it is unfair for a practice that would, if it existed, be mutually beneficial, not to exist" (Barry, 1982: 231).

This is a conservative approach, therefore, to the extent that it presupposes that there are not broader moral obligations or requirements that should factor into how funding for research programs is allocated, which research programs receive key social and economic support, how host communities are identified and selected, or how research should relate to the existing health-related social structures or infrastructure of the host community. These are substantive questions, and if, in fact, researchers and their sponsors have complete discretion over these issues – if there are no larger moral obligations or requirements that must be reflected in their decisions about these issues – then the conservatism of justice as mutual advantage would be entirely justified. If, in contrast, there are larger moral obligations that are relevant to the determination of these issues, then the conservatism of justice as mutual advantage would be morally objectionable.

Those who think that there is a moral imperative to address the staggering health needs of LMIC populations can object to justice as mutual advantage on a number of grounds. In particular, it encourages a piecemeal and ad hoc approach to the needs of those in LMICs for two reasons. First, it allows decisions about which research should be carried out, and where it should be conducted, to be determined primarily by interests in HICs rather than by the health needs of LMICs. Second, without focusing on host community health needs and the social environment in which they arise, justice as mutual advantage does not differentiate health needs that require new advances in understanding from those that could be met through the application of existing knowledge or interventions. Nor does it give priority to addressing the root causes of disease in LMICs over symptomatic manifestations of deeper problems.

Finally, those who think that there are broader obligations to aid LMIC populations are likely to find the bargaining model embraced by the fair benefits approach to be both detrimental and demeaning to members of LMICs. The use of a bargaining model in this context is likely to work to the disadvantage of LMIC communities because, whereas their needs are urgent and often time sensitive, sponsors can usually find alternative locations for a trial, and they have less at stake if negotiations drag out. Whatever their

individual preferences, researchers are also under pressure from funding agencies to use scarce resources only for research purposes, narrowly construed, which puts a cap on the kinds of benefits that researchers can offer a host population even if they want to offer more. Given this significant imbalance in bargaining power, agreements may satisfy the requirement that each party receives a net benefit, but the distribution of those benefits is likely to be hugely disproportionate (London & Zollman, 2010).

This approach may be seen to be disrespectful of the moral status of people in LMICs because it effectively treats the toll that morally problematic social structures exact from individuals in LMICs as a boon for research that addresses HIC health needs. In many LMICs, medical problems are often widespread, and potential research participants frequently have few treatment alternatives. Such populations can be easily recruited, at considerable cost savings to sponsors, who can use their considerable influence and bargaining power to further advance their interests. Disease and lack of access to medical care come to function as valuable commodities whose use-value gives people a place at the bargaining table.

Those who lack the "good fortune" to suffer from a condition interesting to science are consigned to die in silence because the power differential in their case is so great that they cannot either help or harm potential collaborators. The result is a system in which, as Hobbes put it, "the value or worth of a man is, as for all other things, his price, that is to say, so much as would be given for the use of his power; and therefore is not absolute, but a thing dependent on the need and judgment of another" (Hobbes, 1985, chapter X, section 16). Within such a system, there may be individuals and groups in LMICs who benefit from access to clinical trials. Although they may willingly accept succor where they can find it, this does not mean that they could not also feel disrespected and even resentful of a system that wields tremendous knowledge resources and confers the benefits of life and health not out of a concern to improve the lives of specific individuals or enhance the capacities of local communities but as a necessary means of advancing the profit motives of those who are already comparatively well off (Benatar, 2002).

Whether these objections hold, and how forceful they are, depends on the prior question of whether there are compelling reasons to believe that researchers, sponsors, or other stakeholders in the research enterprise have duties or obligations to individuals in LMICs that are broader than, or that arise prior to, those recognized by justice as mutual advantage. In the next three sections I consider several possible grounds for such obligations.

Obligations Within Host Communities

Whether members of a community have a justified claim on one another to something beyond the status quo depends crucially on whether they can endorse the terms of social cooperation set by their community's social structures as basically fair. As a minimal condition of fairness, it must be possible to see the fundamental structures of the community as organized around, and functioning in the service of, the common good of its members (London, 2003). In other words, a morally permissible division of labor must strive to secure for individuals what Rawls calls the *fair value* of their basic capacities for welfare and human agency – meaning that the division of social labor should be designed to give each person an effective opportunity to cultivate and use their basic intellectual, affective, and social capacities to pursue a meaningful life plan (Rawls, 1971; Korsgaard, 1993). Social structures that do not meet this minimal requirement create conditions in which some are denied effective opportunities to develop their basic capacities, whereas others enjoy a rich array of opportunities and benefits. In the most extreme cases, these are the social conditions in which starvation, sickness, and disease flourish.

Consider some parallels between Amartya Sen's groundbreaking work on famine and the health needs of LMIC populations (Sen, 1981; Sen & Dreze, 1989). Famines are commonly viewed as natural disasters caused principally by a combination of poverty and poor food production. Sen showed, however, that these factors alone do not account for the occurrence of famines. For example, in 1979–1981 and 1983–1984, Sudan and Ethiopia experienced declines in food production of 11% or 12% and, like a number of other countries in Sub-Saharan Africa, suffered massive famines. During the same period, however, food production declined by 17% in Botswana and by a precipitous 38% in Zimbabwe, yet these countries did not suffer the ravages of famine (Sen, 1999: 178–180). According to Sen, the reason for this difference in outcomes can be traced to differences in the social and political structures of these countries.

Botswana and Zimbabwe had rudimentary democratic social institutions that enabled them to stave off famine. They implemented a series of social support programs targeted at enhancing the economic purchasing power of affected groups while also supplementing food supplies. Mass starvation occurred in Sudan and Ethiopia because the dictatorial regimes in those nations failed to take such relatively simple social and economic steps to safeguard their citizens' interests.

These lessons should inform our view of sickness and disease in LMICs (Benatar, 1998, 2001). For example, HIV/AIDS is devastating many populations in Sub-Saharan Africa. In some nations, as much as 30% of the population is HIV positive, and infection rates continue to climb. In sharp contrast, Senegal has been able to limit both the prevalence of HIV/AIDS and the rate of new infections to about 1% of the population. The principal cause of Senegal's success lies not in advanced technology or great wealth but in the government's long-standing grass-roots investment in its human resources. In Senegal, information about HIV/AIDS, and many other sexually transmitted diseases, has been disseminated through an assortment of educational programs. Empowering individuals with information and opportunities for activism enhances the public's capacities for communal interaction, free expression, and political participation and so creates a social context in which people can more effectively safeguard and secure their welfare.

This focus on education and activism has been further enhanced by the judicious use of scarce resources. Senegal closely monitors its blood supply and distributes millions of condoms free of charge. It invests in monitoring and treating many sexually transmitted diseases, especially in target populations such as commercial sex workers, young people, truck drivers, and the spouses of migrant workers. Additionally, as part of a program of perinatal care, it has recently begun to offer antiretroviral drugs to pregnant women, although on a very limited basis. There remains room for improvement in Senegal. Still, the country's multisectoral approach to HIV/AIDS, and to public health in general, illustrates the positive health effects of policies that strive to protect citizens' basic capacities for agency and welfare.

These examples illustrate the profound impact that the basic political, legal, social, and economic institutions of a community have on the health of community members. Because they determine the distribution of basic rights and liberties within a society, these structures set the terms on which individuals may access basic goods and resources such as food, shelter, education, and productive employment, as well as more specialized healthcare resources. They therefore determine the opportunities available to individuals to develop and exercise their basic human capacities.

When individuals lack access to the basic building blocks of social and economic opportunity and healthy living, the harms that result cannot be dismissed as accidents of nature or justified by reference to the common good. They represent a failure to use the state's monopoly on force and control over basic social structures to advance the interests of community members. Those who suffer in these cases can legitimately claim, as a strict obligation of justice, an entitlement to relief from such hardships.

In such cases, resources that domestic authorities may be willing to make available for research purposes may not be "available" in a more fundamental moral sense: those who control them may have a prior moral obligation to deploy them in the service of other ends. Moreover, although the use of monetary and material resources may be particularly important in this regard, there are other social resources that matter as well. For example, regimes can fail to serve the common good by neglecting basic social institutions altogether, by misappropriating or misdirecting the time and energies of their personnel, or by inappropriately restricting or occupying important institutional spaces. These failures can generate prior moral claims that community members have against their own authorities, and such claims might constrain the ways in which important social institutions can use or allocate social resources as well as the kinds of agreements or cooperative activities that it might foster and support.

This might affect the liberties and duties of researchers in several ways. The right of community members to a social division of labor that advances their basic interests may entail that community members have a claim on their own leaders and social institutions to foster research that targets the priority health needs of their community. In the face of this claim, and the pressing needs of community members, community leaders and important social institutions may have a duty not to facilitate or cooperate in research that does not focus on or align with the priority health needs of that community. Because the rights, welfare, and opportunities of community members are profoundly influenced by the way that their basic social institutions function, researchers may thus have a duty not to propose research projects to communities that would conflict with the claims of community members and the duties of their leaders and institutions.

Duties of Rectification

If researchers, their sponsors, or other stakeholders have acted in ways that have contributed to the conditions of deprivation and disease in LMICs, then they may have a special duty to aid those populations, grounded in a duty of rectification (Benatar, 1998; Crouch & Arras, 1998). At the most general level, duties of rectification may attach to all citizens of democratic nations whose policies and international activities have contributed to the plight of those in LMICs. In a series of recent articles, Thomas Pogge has argued that Western democratic nations have contributed greatly to the poverty and poor health of the global poor simply by recognizing and supporting two international privileges, namely the *international resource privilege* and the *international borrowing privilege*. Any group that succeeds in wresting control of the national government in an LMIC is recognized as having the legitimate authority to dispose of a country's resources (the international resource privilege) and "to borrow in the name of its people and to confer legal ownership rights for the country's resources" (the international borrowing privilege; Pogge, 2002b: 73). Both these privileges provide powerful incentives for the unscrupulous to seize power and convenient mechanisms for consolidating power and then wielding it for the enrichment of a privileged few (Pogge, 2002a, chapters 4 and 6). Employing power in this way can saddle an LMIC with disastrous long-term debt and prevent most of the population from sharing in the benefits generated by their country's natural resources. Instead, the benefits are enjoyed primarily by a ruling elite and by governments and corporations of HICs.

A duty to aid grounded in this kind of preexisting relationship would apply to medical researchers insofar as they are citizens of the basically democratic nations that have contributed to and benefited from such policies. Such obligations may be strengthened if researchers are employed or funded by governments or private entities that have actively supported such policies. For example, one reason drugs are so scarce in LMICs is their cost. Many pharmaceutical companies played an active role in the negotiation of the Trade Related Aspects of Intellectual Property Rights (TRIPS) Agreement at the World Trade Organization (WTO), and the pharmaceutical lobby has used its considerable influence on US and EU trade representatives to enforce the companies' patent rights. The TRIPS Agreement allows countries to produce or import generic versions of beneficial medications in cases of national emergency, but the Western pharmaceutical industry has aggressively pressed for trade sanctions or taken active legal action against countries that have tried to implement this emergency clause (Barry & Raworth, 2002; Schüklenk & Ashcroft, 2002). In doing so, it has blocked legitimate efforts to provide medicines to some of the populations that need them most.

Taking Basic Interests Seriously

It is a fact of the contemporary world that even moderately affluent individuals and social entities have the ability to affect the lives of distant people. It is also a fact of the contemporary world that whether people are able to cultivate their most basic capacities for agency and welfare and live a life in which they find meaning and value is too often determined by their place of birth rather than by any features of their individual character. These facts have led a variety of moral theorists to argue from within diverse and even competing conceptual frameworks that claims of justice cannot be limited to the boundaries of the contemporary nation-state (Beitz, 1979; Cullity, 1994; Pogge, 1994; Ashford, 2003). Although these theorists' arguments may be controversial, they are both coherent and compelling. We should therefore be cautious of begging the question against such views by accepting, without defense, the assumption of justice as mutual advantage that no such duties exist.

When we approach the problem of assessing potential collaborative research initiatives, therefore, we must at the very least leave conceptual room to consider whether the interests that are frustrated or defeated by less-than-decent social structures are so fundamental as to generate a duty on the part of others to assist them. This point is of special importance not only for welfare consequentialist theories but also for any theory of rights that grounds the moral force of a right in the significance of the interest that it

either protects or advances. For example, Raz (1984: 166) argues that "'X has a right' if and only if x can have rights, and other things being equal, an aspect of x's well-being (his interest) is a sufficient reason for holding some other person(s) to be under a duty." Such concerns will also be salient for theories of human rights that ground rights claims in the basic capabilities of agents (Nussbaum, 1999: 236).

The Human Development Approach

The human development approach is a framework for evaluating international clinical and public health research that begins from a premise that has deep roots in liberal political theory – the idea that justice is properly *about* the basic social structures of society and the state and whether they work to advance the interests of community members. It uses this idea to define a particular vision of human development, to define a target for international aid, and to specify the conditions under which clinical or public health research represents a permissible means of discharging that duty.

In this view, *human development* is understood as the project of establishing and fostering basic social structures that guarantee to community members the fair value of their basic human capacities. Perhaps the most important determinant of health within a community is the extent to which its basic social structures guarantee its members opportunities for education, access to productive employment, control over their person and their personal environment, access to the political process, and the protection of their basic human rights (Sen, 1981, 1999; Sen & Dreze, 1989). More important than the sheer economic wealth of a community is whether the community directs the available resources to creating and sustaining the right social conditions (Sen, 1999).

The human development approach holds that governments of HICs and the individuals they represent have a duty to aid people in LMICs and that this should be understood as a duty to engage our energies and resources in this project of human development. That is, the target of the duty to aid is helping LMICs to create and sustain basic social structures that secure individuals' capacities for welfare and human agency. This focus reflects the idea that because the duty to aid is owed equally to all with an equal claim, efforts to provide aid must give priority to responses that strive for what Henry Shue refers to as "full coverage" (Shue, 1998: 690).

Decent social institutions play an essential role in providing full coverage to all with a claim to assistance because they involve a division of labor in which particular duties are assigned to individual agents or groups of agents who are given special resources, permissions, and authority to discharge those duties. Social institutions provide a mechanism through which duty bearers can pool and magnify their efforts in order to accomplish more than can be achieved by individuals alone.

What is required of different stakeholders to discharge the duty to aid depends on their ability to influence either social structures in LMICs or those social structures in HICs that influence LMIC social structures. For example, the citizens of HICs have a duty to support efforts to make better use of existing knowledge, resources, and interventions that could have a significant impact on the lives of those in LMICs.

The efforts of individuals and entities from HICs to advance the health of LMIC populations should therefore focus on what Prabhat Jha and colleagues refer to as the "close-to-client" health system in these countries (Jha et al., 2002: 2036). Because 90% of the avoidable mortality in LMICs stems from a handful of causes for which effective interventions already exist, even a relatively modest increase in international aid targeted at expanding the physical, material, and human capacities of local clinics, hospitals, and the fundamental institutions of public health would transform the health needs of LMIC populations (Jha et al., 2002; Pogge, 2002b: 79).

The human development approach recognizes, however, that even if a greater share of existing resources is directed toward providing LMICs with access to existing clinical and public health knowledge and interventions, scientific research still has an important role to play in the development process. This is because clinical and public health research plays an invaluable role in an important social division of labor when they use scientific and statistical methods to generate information that will advance the ability of the health systems of a community to better meet the health needs of that community's members.

The human development approach thus holds that stakeholders who shape the direction and focus of scientific research have a duty to ensure that research targets the priority health needs of LMIC populations and that it is carried out in a way that is responsive to and aligned with those needs. The research enterprise represents a permissible use of a community's scarce public resources and is a permissible target of social support when it functions to expand the capacity of the basic social structures of that community to better serve the fundamental interests of that community's members. *Therefore, if clinical research is to be permissible, it must function in the host community as a part of a division of labor in which the distinctive scientific and statistical methods of the research enterprise target and investigate the means of filling the gaps between the most important health needs in a community and the capacity of its social structures to meet them.*

Once this necessary condition has been satisfied, the imperative to make the results of successful research available within the host community increases in inverse proportion to the capacity of that community's basic social structures to translate those results into sustainable benefits for community members. To the extent that the host community cannot translate the results into sustainable benefits for its population on its own, there is an imperative either to build partnerships with groups that are willing to augment the community's capacity to do so or to locate the research within a community with similar health priorities and more appropriate health infrastructure.

Research such as the Surfaxin study would not be permitted in the human development approach. In this regard, those who would have enrolled in this trial would be better off under the framework of fair benefits than under the human development approach. But the point of the human development approach is not to prohibit research – it is to foster more research that targets the health needs and priorities of LMICs. It is intended to provide a framework that informs the deliberations of researchers, research sponsors, and governmental and private entities as they make decisions about what scientific questions should be explored, which research initiatives should be funded, where research should be carried out, and how research can benefit those who most need aid. A much larger population of people, therefore, stands to benefit from the application of the human development approach.

At the institutional level, the human development approach requires changes in how international research is evaluated. Mechanisms need to be developed to facilitate reflection by various stakeholders, at various stages of research development, on how research might promote human development. This will require a proactive model in which issues of justice are considered much earlier in the research process.

For example, enhancing the basic capabilities and social opportunities of women is an important goal of development (Sen, 1999: 189–203; Ash & Jasny, 2002). Roughly half the global burden of HIV/AIDS is borne by women, and in southern Africa, more than one in five pregnant women are HIV positive. The complications of HIV/AIDS are increasing maternal death rates during labor, and vertical or maternal-fetal transmission of HIV still accounts for roughly 90% of new pediatric HIV infections – 600,000 annually – the vast majority of which occur in LMICs. When used properly and consistently, condoms are good at preventing horizontal or partner-to-partner transmission of HIV. But condoms are often not used consistently because men dislike them. As a result, the range of options available to women – who are already a disadvantaged social group and who are 1.2–2.5 times more likely to contract HIV from heterosexual intercourse than men (WHO, 2003: 7) – may be further restricted by men's preferences and behaviors.

International research aimed at developing a safe, effective, and affordable vaginal microbicide would thus contribute to several important developmental goals. A microbicide is an agent delivered in gel form that would reduce the odds of HIV transmission, and perhaps secondary sexually transmitted disease (STI) transmission, during heterosexual vaginal intercourse (Stone, 2002). It would provide an intervention that expands the range of options available to women to safeguard their own health. Given the influence of gender inequalities on condom use, this positive effect would not necessarily be achieved just by emphasizing condom usage more strongly. Also, because it could help reduce the frequency of HIV transmission to women, it could contribute to a reduction in transmission to children. Finally, by targeting the needs of an often-disadvantaged subpopulation, such research would contribute to social equity.

Similar arguments could be mounted on behalf of vaccine research and more effective treatments for a variety of tropical diseases (Flory & Kitcher, 2004). They cannot be marshaled in support of initiatives such as the Surfaxin trial. Several effective surfactant agents are widely used in HICs, and there is nothing about Surfaxin that would make it particularly attractive to LMIC communities. Many Latin American countries need improved neonatal care, but that need could be more effectively and efficiently addressed, for larger numbers of people and on a more sustainable basis, with existing medical knowledge and resources.

From the standpoint of justice as mutual advantage, this conclusion looks inefficient because it prevents Discovery Laboratories from expeditiously pursuing its research agenda and along the way benefiting people in LMICs. From the standpoint of the human development approach, justice as mutual advantage represents an inefficient means of trying to assist LMIC communities in meeting their priority health needs. Providing ad hoc benefits in exchange for participating in trials that are targeted at the health needs of HIC populations will not close the 10/90 gap or address the most pressing health priorities of communities that suffer the heaviest burdens of disease and deprivation.

Acknowledgment

This is a condensed version of London, A. J. (2005). Justice and the human development approach to international research. *Hastings Center Report* **35**(1), 24–37.

References

Angell, M. (1997). The ethics of clinical research in the Third World. *New England Journal of Medicine* **337**, 847–849.

Ash, C., & Jasny, B. (2002). Unmet needs in public health. *Science* **295**, 235.

Ashford, E. (2003). The demandingness of Scanlon's contractualism. *Ethics* **113**, 273–302.

Attaran, A. (1999). Human rights and biomedical research funding for the developing world: discovering state obligations under the right to health. *Health and Human Rights* **4**(1), 27–58.

Barry, B. (1982). Humanity and justice in global perspective, in Pennock, J. R., & Chapman, J. W. (eds.), *NOMOS XXIV: Ethics, Economics, and the Law*. New York: New York University Press, pp. 219–252.

Barry, C., & Raworth K. (2002). Access to medicines and the rhetoric of responsibility. *Ethics and International Affairs* **16**(2), 57–70.

Beitz, C. (1979). *Political Theory and International Relations*. Princeton, NJ: Princeton University Press.

Benatar, S. R. (1998). Global disparities in health and human rights: a critical commentary. *American Journal of Public Health* **88**(2), 295–300.

Benatar, S. R. (2001). Justice and medical research: a global perspective. *Bioethics* **15**(4), 333–340.

Benatar, S. R. (2002). Reflections and recommendations on research ethics in developing countries. *Social Science and Medicine* **54**, 1131–1141.

Commission on Health Research for Development (1990). *Health Research: Essential Link to Equity in Development*. New York: Oxford University Press.

Crouch, R. A., & Arras, J. D. (1998). AZT trials and tribulations. *Hastings Center Report* **28**(6), 26–34.

Cullity, G. (1994). International aid and the scope of kindness. *Ethics* **105**(1), 99–127.

Flory, J. H., & Kitcher, P. (2004). Global health and the scientific research agenda. *Philosophy and Public Affairs* **32**, 36–65.

Glantz, L. H., Annas, G. J., Grodin, M. A., & Mariner, W. K. (1998). Research in developing countries: taking "benefit" seriously. *Hastings Center Report* **28**(6), 38–42.

Hobbes, T. (1985). *Leviathan*, C. B. Macpherson (ed.). New York: Penguin Books.

Jha, P., Mills, A., Hanson, K., et al. (2002). Improving the health of the global poor. *Science* **295**, 2036–2039.

Korsgaard, C. M. (1993). Commentary: G. A. Cohen: Equality of what? On welfare, goods and capabilities, in Nussbaum, M. C., & Sen, A. (eds.), *The Quality of Life*. Oxford, UK: Oxford University Press, pp. 54–61.

London, A. J. (2003). Threats to the common good: biochemical weapons and human subjects research. *Hastings Center Report* **33**(5), 17–25.

London, A. J., & Zollman, K. J. S. (2010). Research at the auction block: problems for the fair benefits approach to international research. *Hastings Center Report* **40**, 34–45.

Lurie, P., & Wolfe, S. M. (1997). Unethical trials of interventions to reduce perinatal transmission of the human immunodeficiency virus in developing countries. *New England Journal of Medicine* **337**, 853–856.

Lurie, P., & Wolfe, S. M. (2007). The developing world as the "answer" to the dreams of pharmaceutical companies: the Surfaxin story, in Lavery, J. V., Grady, C., Wahl, E. R., & Emanuel, E. J. (eds.), *Ethical Issues in International Biomedical Research: A Casebook*. New York: Oxford University Press, pp. 159–170.

Nussbaum, M. C. (1999). Women and equality: the capabilities approach. *International Labour Review* **138**(3), 227–245.

Participants in the 2001 Conference on Ethical Aspects of Research in Developing Countries (2002). Fair benefits for research in developing countries. *Science* **298**, 2133–2134.

Participants in the 2001 Conference on Ethical Aspects of Research in Developing Countries (2004). Moral standards for research in developing countries: from "reasonable availability" to "fair benefits." *Hastings Center Report* **34**(3), 17–27.

Pogge, T. W. (1994). An egalitarian law of peoples. *Philosophy and Public Affairs* **23**(3), 195–224.

Pogge, T. W. (2002a). *World Poverty and Human Rights*. Cambridge, UK: Polity Press.

Pogge, T. W. (2002b). Responsibilities for poverty-related ill health. *Ethics and International Affairs* **16**(2), 71–79.

Rawls, J. (1971). *A Theory of Justice*. Cambridge, MA: Harvard University Press.

Raz, J. (1984). On the nature of rights. *Mind* **93**(370), 194–214.

Schüklenk, U., & Ashcroft, R. E. (2002). Affordable access to essential medications in developing countries: conflicts between ethical and economic imperatives. *Journal of Medicine and Philosophy* **27**(2), 179–195.

Sen, A. (1981). *Poverty and Famines*. Oxford, UK: Clarendon Press.

Sen, A. (1999). *Development as Freedom*. New York: Anchor Books.

Sen, A., & Dreze, J. (1989). *Hunger and Public Action*. Oxford, UK: Clarendon Press.

Shah, S. (2002). Globalizing clinical research. *The Nation*, July **1**, 23–28.

Shue, H. (1998). Mediating duties. *Ethics* **98**(4), 687–704.

Stone, A. (2002). Microbicides: a new approach to preventing HIV and other sexually transmitted infections. *Nature Review Drug Discovery* **1**(12), 977–985.

World Health Organization (WHO) (1996). *Investing in Health Research and Development: Report of the Ad Hoc Committee on Health Research Relating to Future Intervention Options*. Geneva: WHO.

World Health Organization (WHO) (2003). *AIDS Epidemic Update: December 2003*. Geneva: WHO.

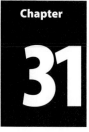

Chapter

31

The Health Impact Fund
How to Make New Medicines Accessible to All

Thomas Pogge

Introduction: Severe Poverty Persists on a Massive Scale and Could Be Greatly Reduced at Low Cost

Some 500 million people, including 260 million children under the age of five, have died from hunger and remediable diseases in peacetime in the 30 years since the end of the Cold War.[1] This is vastly more than have perished from wars, civil wars, and government repression over the entire twentieth century. And poverty continues unabated, as the official statistics amply confirm: of the 7.6 billion people alive today, 821 million are officially counted as undernourished,[2] 150 million are homeless and about 1.6 billion lack adequate shelter,[3] 2.1 billion have no safe drinking water at home, and 4.5 billion lack safe sanitation,[4] 1.2 billion lack electricity,[5] 2 billion are lacking access to essential medicines,[6] 750 million adults are illiterate,[7] and 152 million children (aged 5–17) are victims of child labor – often under slavery-like and

hazardous conditions as soldiers, prostitutes, or domestic servants or in agriculture, construction, or textile or carpet production.[8]

With the poorest half of humanity reduced to 6% of global household income as compared with 24% for the richest 1% (Alvaredo et al., 2018: 56), it is clear that we could eradicate most severe poverty worldwide if we chose to try – in fact, we could have done so decades ago. Citizens of the rich countries are, however, conditioned to downplay the severity and persistence of world poverty and to think of it as an occasion for minor charitable assistance.

Those who begin to pay attention often easily content themselves with the thought that we simply cannot avoid world poverty, at least not at a reasonable cost. In this vein, many think of the millions of poverty deaths each year as necessary to avoid an overpopulated, impoverished, and ecologically unsustainable future for humanity. Whereas this view once had prominent academic defenders (Hardin, 1974), it is now discredited by abundant empirical evidence across regions and cultures showing that when poverty declines, fertility rates also decline sharply (Sen, 1994). Wherever people have won access to contraceptives and associated knowledge and have gained some assurance that their children will survive into adulthood and that their own livelihood in old age will be secure, they have substantially reduced their rate of reproduction. We can see this in the dramatic declines in total fertility rates (children per woman) in areas where poverty has declined. In the last 70 years, this rate has dropped from 6.5 to 2.6 in Botswana, from 6.1 to 1.7 in Brazil, from 5.7 to 1.7 in Costa Rica, for instance, and from 5.6 to 1.6 in Eastern Asia and from 3.1 to 1.2 in Portugal. In economically stagnant poor countries, by contrast, there has been little change over the

---

[1] See https://vizhub.healthdata.org/gbd-compare (accessed March 31, 2019), and for child deaths, see https://ourworldindata.org/grapher/child-deaths-un-data?time=1990..2017 (accessed March 31, 2019).

[2] FAO et al. (2018). For an argument that undernourishment worldwide is far worse than reported by the international agencies, see Pogge (2016).

[3] See https://yaleglobal.yale.edu/content/cities-grow-worldwide-so-do-numbers-homeless (accessed March 31, 2019).

[4] See http://www.who.int/news-room/detail/12-07-2017-2-1-billion-people-lack-safe-drinking-water-at-home-more-than-twice-as-many-lack-safe-sanitation (accessed March 31, 2019).

[5] See https://www.wri.org/blog/2017/03/12-billion-people-lack-electricity-increasing-supply-alone-wont-fix-problem (accessed March 31, 2019).

[6] See http://www.who.int/publications/10-year-review/medicines/en (accessed March 31, 2019).

[7] See http://uis.unesco.org/en/news/international-literacy-day-2017 (accessed March 31, 2019).

[8] See http://www.un.org/en/events/childlabourday/background.shtml (accessed March 31, 2019).

same period: total fertility rates went from 6.1 to 5.8 in Chad, from 6.0 to 6.0 in the Democratic Republic of the Congo, from 4.0 to 3.7 in Gabon, from 5.3 to 5.3 in The Gambia, from 5.7 to 4.6 in Equatorial Guinea, from 7.0 to 5.9 in Mali, and from 7.3 to 7.2 in Niger.[9] The correlation is further confirmed by synchronic comparisons. Currently, the total fertility rate is 4.62 for the low-income and 2.74 for the lower-middle-income countries versus 1.72 for the high-income and 1.84 for the upper-middle-income countries.[10] The complete list of national total fertility rates also confirms a strong correlation with poverty and shows that already some 100 of the more affluent countries have reached total fertility rates below 2,[11] foreshadowing future declines in population. Taken together, these data provide overwhelming evidence that poverty reduction is associated with large fertility declines.

These data also discredit the claim that we should accept world poverty for the sake of the environment, which would be gravely damaged if billions of presently poor people began consuming at the rate that we do. Any short-term ecological harm from eradicating world poverty would be dwarfed by its long-term ecological benefit through a lower human population. Quickly eradicating poverty would make a huge contribution to an early peaking of the human population that would bring enormous ecological benefits for the rest of the third millennium. At current projections, massive eradication of severe poverty can achieve, by 2100, a declining population of 7 billion compared with a still-rising population of 12–17 billion otherwise.[12] Moreover, the short-term harm from poverty eradication is often overstated. Indeed, if the poorest half of humankind had more income, then their ecological footprint would be larger. But it is also true that the rich would then have less income with a consequently smaller ecological footprint. It is not clear that the rich, with their yachts and private planes, have a smaller ecological footprint per unit of income. But even if they did, any net harm to the environment of a more equal economic distribution would be quite small compared with the long-term ecological benefit of poverty eradication through lower population growth.

---

[9] See http://data.un.org/Data.aspx?d=PopDiv&f=variable ID%3A54 (accessed March 31, 2019).
[10] Ibid. [11] Ibid.
[12] See https://ourworldindata.org/future-population-growth (accessed March 31, 2019).

What Do We Owe the World's Poor, and What Are the Grounds of These Obligations?

Having disposed of the claim that world poverty is a necessary evil, we more affluent confront the question what, and how much, we are duty bound to "sacrifice" toward reducing severe poverty worldwide. Most of us believe that these duties are feeble, that it is not very wrong to give no help at all. Against this view, some philosophers have argued that the affluent have positive duties that are quite stringent and quite demanding: if people can prevent much hunger, disease, and premature death at little cost to themselves, then they ought to do so even if those in need are distant strangers. Peter Singer (1972) famously argued for this conclusion by likening the global poor to a drowning child: affluent people who give no aid to the hungry behave no better than a passer-by who fails to save a drowning child from a shallow pond in order not to muddy his or her pants.

One problem with Singer's view is to work out how much an affluent person is required to give when there are always yet further urgent needs he or she might help meet. On reflection, the assumption of such a cutoff point seems odd. It seems more plausible to assume that as an affluent person expands his or her assistance, the moral reason to give even more becomes less stringent. We tend to talk in binary terms, to be sure, about whether some effort is morally required or else beyond the call of duty. But there is no plausible formula that would allow us to compute, from data about a person's financial situation, exactly how much he or she is required to give toward helping those to whom an extra dollar would bring much greater benefit.

Still, as the person keeps giving, the moral reasons for giving yet more do become weaker, less duty-like, and more discretionary. The strength of these moral reasons may fade in this way on account of three factors. First, the needs of the poor may become less urgent. Second, giving an extra dollar becomes more of a burden as the donor's income declines. Third, what the donor has given continuously builds a case that he or she has already done a lot. These three factors are not in precise harmony. The relevance of the third factor is sensitive to whether the donor's current financial situation reflects the fact that he or she has already given a lot. Singer and his followers have no algorithm for assessing the relevance of these factors or for determining with any precision whether someone has done his or her duty or not. Nonetheless, Singer and his followers have a plausible case for concluding that we ought to relieve life-threatening poverty as long as we can do so without giving up anything really significant.

Other philosophers have challenged the terms of this debate and, in particular, the shared suggestion that people in affluent countries are as innocent in regard to world poverty as Singer's passerby is in regard to the drowning child. This challenge can be formulated in different ways (Pogge, 2008b: 205–210). One can question the legitimacy of the existing highly uneven global distribution of income and wealth, which has emerged from a historical process that was pervaded by grievous wrongs (genocide, colonialism, slavery) and has left many of our contemporaries without a fair share of the world's natural resources or an adequate equivalent. One can criticize the negative externalities affluent populations are imposing on the world's poor: greenhouse gas emissions that are spreading desertification and tropical diseases, for example, or highly efficient European fishing fleets that are decimating fish stocks in African waters.[13]

One can also critique the increasingly dense and influential web of global institutional arrangements that foreseeably and avoidably perpetuates massive poverty. It does so, for instance, by permitting affluent states to protect their markets through tariffs and antidumping duties and through export credits and huge subsidies to domestic producers that amount to some $736 billion annually in agriculture alone (Organisation for Economic Co-operation and Development [OECD], 2016). It does so by requiring all World Trade Organization (WTO) members to grant 20-year product patents (Trade-Related Aspects of Intellectual Property Rights [TRIPS] Agreement, 1994), thereby causing important and cheaply mass-producible new medicines to be priced out of reach of a majority of the world's population. The existing international institutional order also fosters corrupt and oppressive governments in the poorer countries by recognizing any person or group holding effective power – regardless of how they

acquired or exercise it – as entitled to sell the country's resources and to dispose of the proceeds of such sales, to borrow in the country's name and thereby to impose debt service obligations on it, to sign treaties on the country's behalf and thus to bind its present and future population, and to use state revenues to buy the means of internal repression. This practice of recognition is beneficial to many putschists and oppressive rulers, who can gain and keep political power even against a large majority of their compatriots and thereby greatly enrich themselves at their expense. This practice is also beneficial to affluent countries, which can, for instance, buy natural resources from a strongman regardless of how he came to power and regardless of how badly he rules. But this practice is devastating for the populations of such countries by strengthening their oppressors and also the incentives toward civil war, coup attempts, and dictatorial rule. Bad governance in so many poor countries (especially those rich in natural resources) is a foreseeable effect of the privileges our international order bestows on any person or group that manages to bring a country under its control.

The common conclusion suggested by these various considerations is that the moral challenge world poverty poses to the affluent is not merely to help more but also to harm less. They are not merely failing to fulfill their positive duties to assist and protect but are also violating negative duties: the duty not to uphold or take advantage of an unjust distribution of holdings or the duty not to contribute to or take advantage of unjust international practices and institutional arrangements that foreseeably and avoidably keep billions trapped in life-threatening poverty.

This assertion presupposes that it is reasonably possible for the affluent collectively to shape the international practices and institutional arrangements they design and uphold to be more poverty avoiding. This presupposition is supported by the examples just provided: it is reasonably possible for us *not* to deplete African fish stocks, *not* to distort world markets through massive subsidies and other protectionist measures that hamper exports from poor countries, *not* to insist that poor countries grant pharmaceutical monopolies that deprive the poor of access to cheap generic versions of advanced medicines, and *not* to recognize and arm rulers who oppress their poor compatriots and steal their resources. Insofar as alternative, more

---

[13] See https://qz.com/africa/1075063/eu-nations-authorized-their-vessels-to-fish-unlawfully-in-african-waters/ (accessed March 31, 2019).

poverty-avoiding practices and rules are reasonably available, the existing international practices and global institutional order must count as unjust and their continued imposition as a harm done to the world's poor. That much of today's severe poverty is institutionally avoidable is also supported by the spectacular level of global inequality: the richest 1% of humanity has four times as much income as the poorer half (Alvaredo et al., 2018), and the wealth of just the richest 42 individuals suffices to match all the wealth of the poorer half.[14]

There is no agreement on how much inequality and poverty just international practices and institutional arrangements may maximally engender. But no precise cutoff is required to conclude that existing levels of poverty and inequality are excessive. When the basic human rights of a large proportion of humanity are avoidably unfulfilled, then international practices and institutional arrangements must count as unjust insofar as they contribute to this human rights deficit. Especially the more powerful countries then have a responsibility to reform these practices and institutional arrangements so as to make them more human rights compliant – a responsibility that falls, in the last analysis, on those countries' citizens. None of us can reform international practices and institutions single-handedly to be sure, but we can work politically toward such reform and can also make individual efforts to protect poor people from the effects of the unjust arrangements imposed on them. Such efforts, though active, are required by our negative duty not to harm: insofar as one contributes to and benefits from the imposition of unjust arrangements, one is responsible for a share of the harm these arrangements cause unless one takes compensating action that prevents this share of the harm from materializing (Pogge, 2005: 60–62, 68–75).

Focusing Directly on Global Health

How, then, might affluent countries go about reforming the global institutional architecture? I noted at the outset that poverty is a major contributor to disease and early death. Average life expectancy is 35 years lower in a poor country like Chad (50.6) than in a rich

one like Japan (85.3)[15] and also varies substantially by socioeconomic class, as illustrated by the stunning 13-year gap between the lowest- and highest-income quintiles in the United States (Isaacs & Choudhuri, 2017). Life among the poor is also much more blighted by disease, as the global burden of disease (GBD) statistics developed by the Institute for Health Metrics and Evaluation amply attest.[16]

This huge burden of disease and premature death would be much lower if global poverty were reduced. But it is also possible to make substantial progress against the GBD directly: existing huge mortality and morbidity rates can be dramatically lowered by reforming our system of funding research and development (R&D) of new medical treatments. I will sketch a concrete, feasible, and politically realistic reform plan that would give medical innovators stable and reliable financial incentives to address the diseases of the poor. If adopted, this plan would not add much to the overall cost of global healthcare spending. In fact, on any plausible accounting, which would take note of the huge economic losses caused by the present GBD, the reform would actually save money. Moreover, it would distribute the cost of global healthcare spending more fairly across countries, across generations, and between those lucky enough to enjoy good health and the unlucky ones suffering from serious medical conditions.

Medical progress has traditionally been fueled from two main sources: government funding and sales revenues. The former – given to universities, corporations, other research centers, and governmental research facilities such as the US National Institutes of Health – has typically been *push* funding, focused on basic research. Sales revenues, by their nature, constitute *pull* funding: innovator firms fund applied research that develops particular new drugs to the point of marketing approval and then reap rewards through earnings from sales.

With medicines, the fixed cost of developing a new product is extremely high for two main reasons. It is very expensive to research and fine-tune a new medicine and then to take it through elaborate clinical trials and national approval processes, and most promising research ideas fail somewhere along the way, thus never resulting in a marketable product.

---

[14] See https://www.oxfam.org/en/pressroom/pressreleases/2018-01-22/richest-1-percent-bagged-82-percent-wealth-created-last-year (accessed March 31, 2019).

[15] See https://www.cia.gov/library/publications/the-world-factbook/rankorder/2102rank.html (accessed March 31, 2019).

[16] See http://ghdx.healthdata.org/gbd-results-tool (accessed April 3, 2019).

Both reasons combine to raise the R&D cost per new marketable medicine to somewhere near $1 billion. Commencing manufacture of a new medicine once it has been invented and approved is cheap by comparison. Because of this fixed-cost imbalance, pharmaceutical innovation is not sustainable in a free-market system: competition among manufacturers would quickly drive down the price of a new medicine toward its long-term marginal cost of production, and the innovator would get nowhere near recovering its investment.

The conventional way of correcting this market failure of undersupply is to enable innovators to apply for patents that entitle them to prevent others from producing or distributing the innovative product and to waive this entitlement in exchange for a licensing fee. The result of such market exclusivity is an artificially elevated sales price that, on average, enables innovators to earn a competitive return on their initial investment by selling products that, even at prices far above marginal cost, are in high demand.

Monopolies are widely denounced by economists as inefficient and by ethicists as an immoral interference in people's freedom to produce and exchange. In regard to patents, however, many believe that the curtailment of individual freedom is justified by the benefit, provided that the patent rules are carefully designed. One important design feature is that patents confer only temporary market exclusivity. Once a patent expires, competitors can enter the market with copies of the original innovation, and consumers need then no longer pay so large a markup over marginal cost. Temporal limits make sense because additional years add progressively less strength to innovation incentives: even at a low discount rate of 8% per annum, the value of the first 12 years of patent protection is over 60% of that of a patent in perpetuity.[17] It makes no sense to impose monopoly prices on all future generations for the sake of so modest a gain in innovation incentives.

During a patent's life, everyone is legally deprived of the freedom to produce, sell, or buy a patented medicine without license from the patent holder. This restraint hurts generic producers, and it also hurts consumers by depriving them of the chance to buy such medicines at competitive market prices. But consumers also benefit from any important medicines whose development is motivated by the prospect of patent-protected markups.

When all have access to vital new medicines as needed, the loss may seem to be dwarfed by the benefit. But billions are too poor to afford medicines at monopoly prices and thus cannot share the benefits of a patent regime. These benefits can therefore not be used to justify *to them* that they should be cut off from medicines at competitive market prices.

This moral point was largely respected as long as expansive patent protections were mostly confined to the affluent states, and the poorer countries were allowed to have weaker ones or none at all. This changed in 1994, when a powerful alliance of industries (software, entertainment, pharmaceuticals, and agribusinesses) pressured the governments of the richest states to impose globally uniform intellectual property rules through the WTO treaty (TRIPS, 1994). The poorer states agreed to institute TRIPS-compliant intellectual property regimes in order to qualify for membership in the WTO, which – as they were then promised – would allow them to reap large benefits from free trade.[18]

The global poor have a powerful objection to the pharmaceutical patent regime that governments have imposed. The argument might go as follows:

> If the freedom to produce, sell, and buy advanced medicines were not curtailed in our countries, then the affluent would need to find other (for them perhaps less convenient) ways of funding pharmaceutical research. Advanced medicines would then be available at competitive market prices, and we would have a much better chance of getting access to them through our own funds or with the help of national or international government agencies or nongovernmental organizations. The loss of freedom imposed through product patents thus inflicts on us a huge loss in terms of disease and premature death.

---

[17] Patent life is counted from the time the patent application is filed. Effective patent life is the time from receiving market clearance to the time the patent expires. My calculation in the text assumes constant nominal profit each year. In reality, annual profit may rise (because of increasing market penetration, rising disease incidence, or population growth) or fall (through reduced incidence of the disease or competition from competing products). For most drugs, sales decline after they have been on the market for six years or so, which strengthens the reasons for limiting patent life.

[18] The promise was not fully kept. High-income countries continue to sabotage the export opportunities of poor countries through protectionist tariffs and antidumping duties, as well as through huge subsidies and export credits to their domestic producers.

This loss cannot possibly be justified by any gain such patents may bring to the affluent.

However morally compelling, this objection is ignored by the more affluent states, which have relentlessly pursued the globalization of uniform intellectual property rights – with devastating effects, for instance, on the course of the AIDS epidemic. First introduced in 1996, combination antiretroviral therapies, which can free AIDS patients of symptoms and make them noninfectious, are still inaccessible to some 39% of patients.[19]

The world responds to the catastrophic health crisis among the poor in diverse ways: with the usual declarations, working papers, conferences, summits, and working groups, of course, but also with efforts to fund delivery of medicines through *intergovernmental initiatives* such as 3 by 5,[20] through *governmental programs* such as the US President's Emergency Plan for AIDS Relief (PEPFAR), through *public–private partnerships* like the Global Alliance for Vaccines and Immunization and the Global Fund to Fight AIDS, Tuberculosis and Malaria, and through medicine donations from pharmaceutical companies, and with various efforts to foster the development of new medicines for the diseases of the poor, such as the Drugs for Neglected Diseases Initiative, the Institute for One World Health, the Novartis Institute for Tropical Diseases, and various prizes.[21]

Such a busy diversity of initiatives looks good, communicating that a lot is being done to solve the problem. And most of these efforts are really doing good by improving the situation relative to what it would be under TRIPS unmitigated. Still, these efforts are not nearly sufficient to protect the poor. It is unrealistic to hope that enough billions of dollars will be collected year after year to neutralize the cost imposed on the world's poor by the globalization of pharmaceutical product patents. Thus, we should look for a more systemic solution that addresses the global health crisis at its root. Involving institutional reform, such a solution is politically more difficult to achieve, but once achieved, it is also politically much easier to maintain. And it preempts most of the huge and collectively inefficient mobilizations currently required to produce the many stop-gap measures, which at best only mitigate the effects of structural problems they leave untouched.

Seven Failings of the Present Pharmaceutical Patent Regime

The quest for such a systemic solution can start from an analysis of the main drawbacks of the newly globalized monopoly patent regime.

High Prices. While a medicine is under patent, it will be sold near the profit-maximizing monopoly price, which is largely determined by the demand curve of the affluent. When there are plenty of affluent or well-insured people who strongly desire a drug, then its price can be raised very high above the cost of production before increased gains from enlarging the markup are outweighed by losses from reduced sales volume. With patented medicines, markups in excess of 100,000% are not exceptional.[22] When such exorbitant markups are charged, few of the poor have access through the charity of others.

Neglect of Diseases Concentrated Among the Poor. When innovators are rewarded with patent-protected markups, diseases concentrated among the poor – even if widespread and severe – are not attractive targets for pharmaceutical research because the demand for such a medicine drops off very steeply as the patent holder enlarges the markup. There is no prospect, then, of achieving high sales volume and a large markup. Moreover, there is the further risk that a successful research effort will be greeted with loud demands to make the medicine available cheaply or even for free, which would force the innovator to write off its initial

---

[19] See https://www.kff.org/global-health-policy/fact-sheet/the-global-hivaids-epidemic/ (accessed July 9, 2020).

[20] Announced in 2003, this joint WHO/UNAIDS program was meant to provide, by 2005, antiretroviral treatment to 3 million (out of what were then estimated to be 40.3 million) AIDS patients in the less developed countries. In fact, it extended such treatment to about 900,000.

[21] A prize is a specific reward offered for the development of a new medicine that meets certain specifications. It need not take the form of a cash payment. The successful innovator may also be rewarded by subsidizing the sale of (advance market commitment) or by buying at a preset high price (advance purchase commitment) a certain large number of doses of a new medicine that meets certain specifications. Or the successful innovator may be granted an extension on any of its other patents.

[22] Harvoni entered the US market at $1,125 per pill ($94,500 per course of treatment) and can probably be mass produced for well under a dollar per pill. See https://www.generichepatitiscdrugs.com/harvoni-price/ (accessed April 5, 2019).

investment. In view of such prospects, biotech and pharma companies predictably prefer even the trivial ailments of the affluent, such as hair loss and acne, over tuberculosis and sleeping sickness. Only a tiny fraction of pharmaceutical research is devoted to the diseases of the poor despite their large presence in the GBD (Utzinger & Keiser, 2013).

Bias Toward Me-Too and Maintenance Drugs. Medicines can be sorted into three categories: curative drugs remove the disease from the patient's body, maintenance drugs improve well-being and functioning without removing the disease, and preventative drugs reduce the likelihood of contracting the disease in the first place. Under the existing innovation regime, maintenance drugs are by far the most profitable – the most desirable patients being ones who are not cured and do not die (until after patent expiration). Such patients keep buying the medicine, thereby delivering vastly more profit than if they derived the same health benefit from a cure or vaccine. Vaccines are least lucrative because they are typically bought by governments, which can command large volume discounts. This is highly regrettable because vaccines tend to confer exceptionally large health benefits by protecting from infection or contagion not merely each vaccinated person but also their contacts.

The existing patent regime also hugely overrewards me-too drugs, which supply a new molecule to tackle a problem for which other molecules are already available. Billions are spent on bringing such drugs to market, yet patients barely benefit because new product entries typically don't even lead to lower prices. In these two ways, then, the present regime once more guides pharmaceutical research in the wrong direction – and here to the detriment of poor and affluent alike.

Wastefulness. Under the present regime, innovators must bear the cost of filing for patents in dozens of national jurisdictions and of monitoring those jurisdictions for possible infringements of their patents. Huge amounts are spent on costly litigation that pits generic companies, with strong incentives to challenge any patent on a profitable medicine, against patent holders, whose earnings depend on their ability to defend, extend, and prolong their patent-protected markups (Baker, 2016: 85–89). Even greater costs are due to the deadweight losses in the hundreds of billions that arise from blocked sales to buyers who are willing and able to pay

some price between marginal cost and the much higher monopoly price.[23]

Counterfeiting. Large markups also encourage the illegal manufacture of fake products that are diluted, adulterated, inert, or even toxic. Such counterfeits often endanger patient health. They also contribute to the emergence of drug-specific resistance, when patients ingest too little of the active ingredient of a diluted drug to kill off the more resilient pathogenic agents. The emergence of highly drug-resistant disease strains – of tuberculosis, for instance – poses dangers to us all.

Excessive Marketing. When a pharmaceutical company maintains a very large markup, it has reason to make massive efforts to increase sales volume, often by scaring patients or by rewarding doctors. This produces pointless battles over market share among similar drugs as well as perks to induce doctors to prescribe medicines even when they are not indicated or when competing medicines are likely to be more suitable. With a large markup, it also pays to fund direct-to-consumer advertising to persuade people to take medicines they don't really need for diseases they don't really have – and sometimes for invented pseudodiseases (Moynihan & Henry, 2006).

The Last-Mile Problem. While the present regime provides strong incentives to sell even unneeded patented medicines to those who can pay or have insurance, it provides no incentives to ensure that poor people benefit from medicines they urgently need. Even in affluent countries, pharmaceutical companies have incentives only to sell products, not to ensure that they are actually used, optimally, by patients whom they can benefit. This problem is compounded in poor countries, which often lack the infrastructure to distribute medicines as well as the medical personnel to prescribe them and to ensure their proper use. In fact, the present regime even gives pharmaceutical companies incentives to disregard the medical needs of the poor.

---

[23] Deadweight losses are notoriously hard to estimate because they depend on how much more product would have been bought at lower prices. Baker (2016: 97, table 5-2) suggests that annual deadweight losses amount to at least $60 billion to $476 billion in the United States alone. The global figure is much higher because in many countries there is little drug insurance and hence much greater price sensitivity of consumption than in the United States.

To profit under this regime, a company needs not merely a patent on a medicine that is effective in protecting paying patients from a disease or its detrimental symptoms, but it also needs this target disease to thrive and spread because, as a disease waxes or wanes, so does market demand for the remedy. A pharmaceutical company helping poor patients to benefit from its patented medicine would be undermining its own profitability in three ways: by paying for the effort to make its drug competently available to them, by suppressing a disease on which its profits depend, and by losing affluent customers who find ways of buying, on the cheap, medicines intended for the poor.

A Structural Reform: The Health Impact Fund

All seven drawbacks can be greatly mitigated by supplementing the pharmaceutical patent regime with a complementary source of incentives and rewards for developing new medicines. With an international interdisciplinary team, I have been detailing such a pay-for-performance mechanism in the form of the Health Impact Fund (HIF).[24] The HIF is a proposed publicly financed global agency that would give pharmaceutical innovators the option to register any new product. They would guarantee to make it available, wherever it is needed, at the lowest feasible cost of production and distribution. In exchange, each registered product would, during its first 10 years on the market, participate in the HIF's annual reward pools, receiving a share equal to its share of the assessed health impact of all HIF-registered products.[25]

---

[24] See www.healthimpactfund.org for details about the team and its work, which have been generously funded by the Australian Research Council, the BUPA Foundation, the European Commission, the Canadian Social Science and Humanities Research Council, and the European Research Council. Much critical discussion of the proposal by Gorik Ooms and Rachel Hammonds, Thomas Faunce and Hitoshi Nasu, Devi Sridhar, Michael Selgelid, Aidan Hollis, and Michael Ravvin can be found in Pogge (2008a).

[25] Ten years corresponds roughly to the profitable period of a patent: under TRIPS, WTO members must offer patents lasting at least 20 years from the patent filing date, which is typically many years before the medicine receives marketing approval after clinical trials. Because some patents may outlast the reward period, HIF registration requires the registrant to offer a royalty-free open license for generic versions of the product following the end of the reward period.

The requisite health impact assessment could be conducted in terms of some version of quality-adjusted life-years (QALYs), a metric that has been deployed for some 30 years by academic researchers, insurers, nongovernmental organizations (NGOs), government agencies, and, most thoroughly, by the Institute for Health Metrics and Evaluation in its regular analyses of the GBD. Assessment would rely on clinical and pragmatic trials of the product, on tracing (facilitated by serial numbers) of random samples of the product to end users, and on statistical analysis of correlations between sales data (including time and place of sale) and variations in the incidence of the target disease. Participating firms would have to pay a fixed annual registration fee to cover the HIF's costs of assessment and administration. This fee would ensure that only effective products are registered: medicines that would achieve substantial health gains competitive with those achieved by other registered drugs. The company's net gain (health impact rewards minus fees) is meant to cover its R&D investment in the product as well as general overhead and profit.

To work well, the HIF would need to be large enough to support about 10 medicines, which implies that, each year on average, one new drug would be registered and one would exit after reaching the end of its 10-year reward period. With a substantially smaller number of drugs, the reward rate would be too strongly affected by entries and exits, making risk-averse innovators reluctant to register. A small number of drugs would also result in higher assessment costs per drug, entailing higher registration fees.

In order to support roughly 10 drugs worldwide, a global HIF would require funding of about $3.24 billion annually.[26] This is a minuscule fraction of the $1.2 trillion currently spent each year on medicines worldwide.[27] Registered drugs would then receive $324 million annually, on average, while paying about $16 million for assessment ($12 million) and administration ($4 million). Over its full reward period, the average product would earn about $3.08 billion, which should cover the cost of R&D, patenting, obtaining marketing approval, appropriate detailing, general and administrative expenses, and a decent return on the

---

[26] These estimates were developed with economist Aidan Hollis and are available from the author on request.
[27] See https://pharmaceuticalcommerce.com/business-and-finance/global-drug-spending-was-1-135-trillion-in-2017-says-iqvia/ (accessed April 7, 2019).

capital tied up during the various phases of the product cycle.

This estimate of how much of a reward would be necessary to get pharmaceutical innovators to bring new medicines to market may be too high or too low. If so, the envisioned HIF with annual reward pools of $3.24 billion might support 11 drugs, on average, or 9. Here the reward rate is self-adjusting: when innovators perceive it as unattractive, registrations slow down, the number of registered products declines, and the reward rate improves. When innovators perceive it as attractive, registrations accelerate, the number of registered products rises, and the reward rate falls. The HIF is designed to assure innovators and funders alike that the reward rate will equilibrate to a reasonable level, one that provides decent profits – but not windfalls – to innovators.

A medicine will be registered on the HIF track only if (1) its expected earnings on this track constitute an attractive return on capital and (2) these expected earnings are at least as high as the product's expected earnings on the monopoly track. Consequently, the HIF is likely – at least initially – to attract drugs that have a high impact (*large* effect against a *serious* disease that affects *many* patients) and yet low earnings prospects on the monopoly track (because the patients they can help are mostly poor and uninsured). Among them might be mosquito-borne diseases (malaria, dengue, and chikungunya), tuberculosis, hepatitis, pneumococcal diseases (pneumonia and meningitis), Chagas' disease (American trypanosomiasis), intestinal nematode infections, zoonotic parasitic diseases (echinococcosis and cysticercosis), food-borne trematodiases, soil-transmitted helminthiases (intestinal worms), onchocerciasis (river blindness), schistosomiasis (snail fever or bilharzia), chromoblastomycosis (chromomycosis), leishmaniasis, rabies, trachoma, skin diseases (Buruli ulcer, leprosy, lymphatic filariasis, scabies, yaws), and other diarrheal and neglected tropical diseases.

A simple way of financing the HIF would have countries contribute a fixed proportion of their gross national incomes (GNI). The low-income countries, accounting for only 0.7% of worldwide GNI, could be exempt.[28] Should some high- and middle-income countries decide not to contribute to the HIF, participating innovators would be allowed to sell their HIF-registered products in those countries with high patent-protected markups. Innovators would then earn some monopoly profits in those nonparticipating countries, and less of a reward would therefore be required to induce them to register. This beneficial effect might, however, initially be relatively weak in the case of noncontributing high-income countries in which the neglected diseases of the poor are rare. Consequently, it is likely that the HIF would need a higher contribution rate than 0.004% to sustain 10 products if it fails to win support from a substantial portion of the high-income countries.[29]

Nonetheless, the HIF could commence with quite a small coalition of countries. Consider a coalition of China, India, Germany, France, and the United Kingdom, representing just under 30% of worldwide GNI. Such a narrow HIF would find it much cheaper to attract product registrations because registrants could get some substantial return on their investment from noncontributing high- and middle-income countries. If it could support a stock of 10 medicines on an annual budget of $1.5 billion, then the five contributors would each need to commit some 0.0063% of their GNIs. The HIF could then grow from there through the accession of additional countries as well as through gradual growth in GNI. As more high-income countries joined, this HIF would become able to support more products, up to 16 according to the preceding stipulations.

To provide stable incentives, the HIF would need guaranteed financing some 15 years into the future to assure pharmaceutical innovators that if they fund expensive clinical trials now, they can claim a full decade of health impact rewards on marketing approval. Such a solid guarantee is also in the interest of the funders, who would not want the incentive power of their contributions to be diluted through skeptical discounting by potential registrants. The guarantee might take the form of a treaty under which each contributing country commits to the HIF a fixed fraction of its future GNI. Backed by such a treaty, the HIF would automatically adjust the contributions of the various partner countries to their variable economic fortunes, would avoid protracted struggles over contribution proportions, and would assure each country that any extra cost it agreed to bear through an increase in the

---

[28] International taxes – on air travel or financial transactions – would be another possibility, and an endowment would be a third.

[29] The contribution rate of 0.004% of GNI is derived by dividing the HIF's annual cost of $3.24 billion by the current worldwide GNI of $80 trillion.

contribution schedule would be matched by a corresponding increase in the contributions of all other partner countries.[30]

The HIF has five main advantages over conventional innovation prizes, including advance market commitments and advance purchase commitments. First, it is a structural reform, establishing an enduring source of high-impact pharmaceutical innovations. Second, it is not disease specific and therefore much less vulnerable to lobbying by firms and patient groups and much more efficient by encouraging R&D in exactly those disease areas where the greatest health gains can be achieved. Third, conventional prizes must define a precise finish line, specifying at least which disease the new medicine must attack, how effective and convenient it must minimally be, and how bad its side effects may be. Such specificity is problematic because it presupposes the very knowledge whose acquisition is yet to be encouraged. Because sponsors lack this knowledge ahead of time, their specifications are likely to be seriously suboptimal: they may be too demanding, so firms give up the effort even though something close to the sought medicine is within their reach, or they may be insufficiently demanding, so firms, to save time and expense, deliver a medicine that is just barely good enough to win even when they could have done much better at little extra cost (Hollis, 2007: 15–16). The HIF avoids this problem of the finish line by flexibly rewarding any new registered medicine in proportion to its global health impact. Fourth, formulated to avoid failure and in ignorance of the true cost of innovation, specific prizes are often much too large and thus overpay for innovation. The HIF solves this problem by letting its health impact reward rate adjust itself through competition: a high reward rate corrects itself by attracting additional registrations (raising the stock of registered medicines), and an unattractively low reward rate corrects by deterring new registrations (shrinking the stock of registered products). Fifth, the HIF gives each registrant powerful incentives to promote the optimal end use of its product: to seek its wide and effective use by any patients who can benefit from it.

There is no space here to discuss the design of the HIF in full detail (see Hollis & Pogge, forthcoming). Let me conclude then by sketching how it would, without revision of the TRIPS Agreement, provide systemic relief for the above-outlined seven failings of the existing pharmaceutical innovation regime.

High prices would not exist for HIF-registered medicines. Innovators would typically not even want a higher price because this would reduce their health impact rewards by impeding access to their product by much of the world's population. The HIF counts health gains for the poorest of patients equally with health gains for the richest.

Diseases concentrated among the poor, insofar as they contribute substantially to the GBD, would no longer be neglected. In fact, the more destructive among them would come to afford some of the most lucrative research opportunities for biotechnology and pharmaceutical companies.

Bias toward me-too and maintenance drugs would be absent from HIF-encouraged research. The HIF assesses each registered medicine's health impact in terms of how its use reduces mortality and morbidity worldwide – without regard to whether it achieves this reduction through cure, symptom relief, or prevention. This would guide firms to deliberate about potential research projects in a way that is also optimal for global public health, namely in terms of the expected global health impact of the new medicine relative to the cost of developing it. The profitability of research projects would be aligned with their cost-effectiveness in terms of global public health.

Moreover, the HIF would reward new medicines according to their *incremental* health impact. To achieve health gains, a drug must make patients better off than they would have been otherwise. This does not happen when a patient is merely switched from one drug to its functional equivalent.

Wastefulness would be dramatically lower for HIF-registered products. There would be no deadweight losses from large markups. There would be little costly litigation because generic competitors would lack incentives to compete, and innovators would have no incentive to suppress generic products (because they enhance the innovator's health impact reward). Innovators might therefore often not even bother to obtain, police, and defend patents in many national jurisdictions. To register

---

[30] Participating countries would, of course, have the option to exit. But this option should provide for a phased withdrawal in 10 equal steps in order to avoid disappointment of legitimate innovator expectations. In this way, products that had been HIF registered before the withdrawal decision would still be fully rewarded by the withdrawing country.

a medicine with the HIF, innovators need show only once that they have an effective and innovative product.

Counterfeiting of HIF-registered products would be unattractive. With the genuine item widely available near or even below the marginal cost of production, there is little to be gained from producing and selling fakes.

Excessive marketing would also be much reduced for HIF-registered medicines. Innovators would have incentives to urge an HIF-registered drug on doctors and patients only insofar as such marketing results in measurable therapeutic benefits for which the innovator would then be rewarded.

The last-mile problem would be mitigated because each HIF-registered innovator would have strong incentives to ensure that patients are fully instructed and properly provisioned so that they make optimal use (dosage, compliance, etc.) of its medicines, which will then, through wide and effective deployment, have their optimal public health impact. Rather than ignore poor countries as unprofitable markets, pharmaceutical companies would, moreover, have incentives to work with one another and with national health ministries, international agencies, and NGOs toward improving the health systems of these countries in order to enhance the impact of their HIF-registered medicines there.

Conclusion

This chapter has shown that thinking morally about global health in a constructive way, we must bear in mind three important points. First, in parallel with the institutional order of a country, global institutional arrangements have a profound effect on the lives of people everywhere. Second, the present rules governing the world economy, designed and imposed to serve powerful corporate and political interests, could be adjusted in minor but highly effective ways to better serve the interests of all. Third, small changes to the rules incentivizing pharmaceutical R&D would produce large health gains in poor and affluent countries – gains that, over time, would easily cover the economic cost of the scheme.

Acknowledgment

The author thanks Matt Peterson for substantial research and editorial assistance.

References

Alvaredo, F., Chancel, L., Piketty, T., et al. (2018). *World Inequality Report 2018*. Paris: World Inequality Lab. Available at https://wir2018.wid.world/files/download/wir2018-full-report-english.pdf (accessed March 31, 2019).

Baker, D. (2016). *Rigged: How Globalization and the Rules of the Modern Economy Were Structured to Make the Rich Richer*. Washington, DC: Center for Economic and Policy Research. Available at https://deanbaker.net/books/rigged.htm (accessed April 7, 2019).

FAO, IFAD, UNICEF, WFP and WHO (2018). *The State of Food Security and Nutrition in the World 2018: Building Climate Resilience for Food Security and Nutrition*. Rome, Food and Agriculture Organization.

Hardin, G. (1974). Lifeboat ethics: the case against helping the poor. *Psychology Today* **8**, 38–43, 123–26.

Hollis, A. (2005). An efficient reward system for pharmaceutical innovation. Working paper, Department of Economics, University of Calgary, Calgary, Canada. Available at econ.ucalgary.ca/fac-files/ah/drugprizes.pdf (accessed December 21, 2009).

Hollis, A. (2007). Incentive mechanisms for innovation. IAPR Technical Paper. Available at www.iapr.ca/iapr/files/iapr/iapr-tp-07005_0.pdf (accessed December 21, 2009).

Hollis, A., & Pogge, T. (forthcoming). *The Health Impact Fund: Making New Medicines Accessible for All*. Oxford, UK: Oxford University Press.

Isaacs, K., & Choudhury, S. (2017). *The Growing Gap in Life Expectancy by Income: Recent Evidence and Implications for the Social Security Retirement Age*. Washington, DC: Congressional Research Service.

Moynihan, R., & Henry, D. (eds.) (2006). Disease mongering. *PLoS Medicine* **3**, 425–465. Available at https://collections.plos.org/disease-mongering (accessed April 7, 2019).

Organisation for Economic Co-operation and Development (OECD) (2016). Background note for meeting of agriculture ministers. Available at www.oecd.org/agriculture/ministerial/background/notes/3_background_note.pdf (accessed March 31, 2019).

Pogge, T. (2005). Severe poverty as a violation of negative duties. *Ethics and International Affairs* **19**, 55–84.

Pogge, T. (ed.) (2008a). Access to medicines. *Public Health Ethics* **1**, 73–192. Available at http://phe.oxfordjournals.org/content/1/2.toc (accessed April 7, 2019).

Pogge, T. (2008b). *World Poverty and Human Rights*, 2nd ed. Cambridge, UK: Polity Press.

Pogge, T. (2016). The hunger games. *Food Ethics* **1**(1), 9–27. Available at http://link.springer.com/article/10.1007/s41055-016-0006-9?view=classic (accessed March 31, 2019).

Sen, A. (1994). Population: delusion and reality. *New York Review of Books* **41**, 62–71.

Singer, P. (1972). Famine, affluence, and morality. *Philosophy & Public Affairs* **1**, 229–243.

Trade-Related Aspects of Intellectual Property Rights (TRIPS) Agreement (1994). Available at www.wto.org/english/docs_e/legal_e/27-trips.pdf.

United Nations Development Programme (UNDP) (2003). *Human Development Report 2003*. New York: Oxford University Press.

Utzinger, J., & Keiser, J. (2013). Research and development for neglected diseases: more is still needed, and faster. *Lancet Global Health* **1**, 317–318. Available at www.thelancet.com/action/showPdf?pii=S2214-109X%2813%2970148-7 (accessed April 5, 2019).

Chapter 32

Evaluating Global Health Impact and Increasing Access to Essential Medicines [*]

Nicole Hassoun

Advancing the Sustainable Development Goals and Human Right to Health

Evaluating Global Health Impact and Increasing Access to Essential Medicines

Imagine a world where people everywhere have access to the lifesaving drugs they need to fight diseases such as tuberculosis, malaria, and HIV/AIDS. To help extend access to essential medicines, we have to understand the problem. Understanding the impact of key technologies on the global burden of disease is essential for policymakers to extend access to important medicines, to achieve Sustainable Development Goal (SDG) 3, and to fulfill everyone's human right to health. The Global Health Impact (GHI) Index opens the door to positive change by considering how essential medicines for some of the world's worst diseases are affecting global health. It provides new models measuring the effect of key HIV/AIDS, malaria, tuberculosis (TB), and neglected tropical diseases (NTDs) medicines on death and disability over time.

Comprehensive and accurate models of the global health impact of medicines are important for evaluating performance, setting targets, guiding the distribution of scarce health resources, and advancing access to affordable medicines. The new GHI Index models (described in the section "Implementation, Evidence, and Innovation") measure health impact over time and examine different parts of the pharmaceutical supply chain.[1] They can help advance our understanding of

the impact of pharmaceuticals and promote everyone's human right to health (Berman, 2015; Gorenstein, 2015; Prakash, 2015; Silverman, 2015). Making the new models and data on the impact of medicines on global health available to researchers, policymakers, consumers, companies, and other key stakeholders increases their abilities to fulfill individual human rights to health.

Helping to Achieve Sustainable Development and Fulfill the Human Right to Health

Impact on Public Health and Policy Coherence

The new GHI models can provide states, nongovernmental organizations (NGOs), and companies with the means to promote new market strategies and innovative health policies that can help achieve SDG 3 and fulfill individual human rights to health (Hassoun, 2016a). They create a common framework for judging health impact across a wide variety of interventions for multiple actors, including private companies and international health organizations. They can thus help advance universal access to quality essential healthcare services as well as effective and affordable essential technologies. In particular, the GHI models can help address the epidemics of HIV/AIDS, malaria, TB, and NTDs. In the future, the Global Health Impact team – a collaboration of scholars and members of civil society from around the world – plans to expand the models to help address additional

---

[*] This chapter is based on my contribution to the UN Secretary-General's High-Level Panel on Access to Medicines and was subsequently revised for the relaunch event at Princeton University, October 5, 2019 (see Acknowledgments).
[1] The original GHI models evaluated the global impact of medicines for HIV/AIDS, malaria, and TB and aggregated

---

this information by company, drug, and disease, as well as country. They estimated disease impact using data on drug effectiveness (or, barring that, efficacy), disease incidence, patient treatment coverage, and the global burden of disease that remains after treatment. Here we look at NTDs as well.

neglected tropical diseases as well as other communicable and noncommunicable diseases.

One way our models help address the epidemics of the diseases they evaluate is by highlighting the importance of paying attention not just to the burden of disease but also to the extent of its alleviation.

Consider the need versus impact graphs for HIV/AIDS from a preliminary version of the new HIV/AIDS model for 2010 (the methodology for the new model is described briefly in the Appendix). In Figures 32.1 and 32.2, we use disability-adjusted life-years (DALYs) as the basis for measuring "Need" and

Estimated Disability Adjusted Life Years Lost in the Absence of Treatment

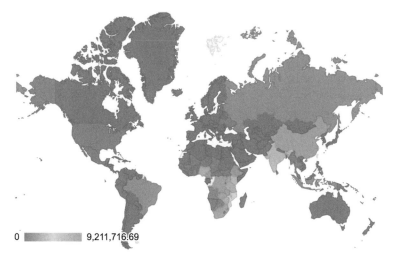

Figure 32.1. Estimated disability-adjusted life-years lost in the absence of treatment.

2015 | Country **Impact**

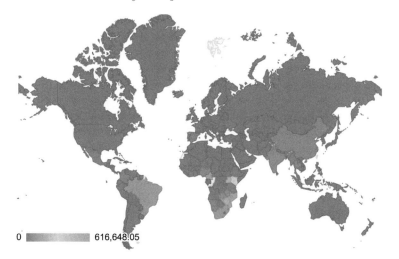

Figure 32.2. Country impact, 2015.

"Impact." Lighter colors indicate greater need and impact – the need graph is much lighter than the impact graph. Globally, the data show that there is a great amount of unmet need in the HIV/AIDS epidemic. Identifying current shortcomings is one step in identifying what can be done differently in order to advance access to essential medicines.

Although inadequate access to medicines for diseases such as HIV/AIDS receives significant media attention, understanding of the access-to-medicines issue is hampered without a systematic way to quantify efforts to address this problem. Without the ability to objectively, and accurately, measure and understand access inequality and efforts to improve it, this issue is difficult to prioritize from both the policy and innovation perspectives. By expanding and utilizing the GHI models, we can evaluate the impact of various policies for promoting access to essential medicines. Our GHI Index generates both data and a methodology for rating efforts to extend access to essential medicines that quantify the effectiveness and impact of investments. This involves using an analytical framework that can be applied to a broad array of other contexts where there are significant positive externalities of industry innovation and a "public goods" component to discovery. This framework stimulates the access movement in three critical arenas: the market (allowing consumers to easily identify companies whose products are having a large global health impact), policy creation (providing policymakers with the evidence-base needed to measure, understand, and respond to this issue), and industry (the metrics recognize and encourage investments that address the access problem).

Consider how the GHI models might stimulate the access movement through the market. It is possible for socially responsible investors to rely on our index in evaluating companies' access policy impacts. The GHI Index might also provide a basis for a label that ethically oriented consumers could rely on in deciding from which firms to purchase products. Highly rated companies might use a GHI label on everything they make from pet vitamins to pain relievers, and if ethical consumption initiatives capture 1% of the over-the-counter market in pharmaceutical products, this could give companies a US$3 billion incentive to do whatever gets them highly rated (VisionGain, 2010).

In any case, the new models illustrate the impact of attempts to fulfill the human right to health and advance the SDGs. The data provide some transparency into efforts to extend access to essential medicines, allowing policymakers to better target resources (Global Health Impact, 2014). Consider, for instance, health spending versus impact on some different diseases in the model in Figure 32.3.

Despite receiving the lion's share of research and development funding and aid money (25%), drugs for HIV/AIDS do not have a proportionate impact in our model in any given year (though their impact over time is larger because treatment can extend over decades). The GHI models also provide useful information for customers (caregivers and patients), investors, pharmaceutical companies, and researchers interested in pharmaceutical research and development (R&D) and promoting global health. The new models can, for instance, help researchers to identify conditions that potentially influence drug impact so as to promote scientific progress through a new monitoring tool. Using the data provided on the GHI website (available on request from the Global Health Impact Organization: global-health-impact.org/new), researchers might evaluate different investments' or policy instruments' effectiveness in terms of global health impact. Using regression analysis, they might, for instance, consider the impact of the patent status of medicines (on or off patent) on global health. Alternately, they can consider whether open-access licensing was used. They can also study the processes and structures that generate innovation and so achieve good health outcomes.

Consider how the models can help set targets and monitor countries' performance in utilizing the flexibilities to protect public health and provide access to medicines for all, allowed by the Doha Declaration on the World Trade Organization's Agreement on Trade Related Aspects of Intellectual Property Rights (TRIPS). Researchers can evaluate the impact of countries' efforts to take advantage of these flexibilities and expand access to important health technologies for these diseases. Researchers might conduct regression analyses to see whether countries increase treatment impact when they issue compulsory licenses for essential medicines in the model. Insofar as the licensing efforts are successful, these technologies' impacts should increase in the models helping achieve universal access to quality essential healthcare services and access to safe, effective, quality and affordable essential technologies for these diseases. Insofar as the models help us isolate promising policies or investment opportunities, they can help set

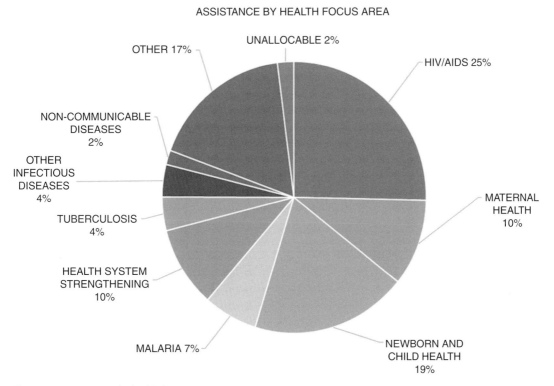

Figure 32.3. Assistance by health focus area.

targets and measure performance in fulfilling the human right to health and advancing the Sustainable Development Goals.

In summary, and as I hope will become clearer below, this groundbreaking research shows that it is possible to collect and analyze new and important data on access to essential medicines. It spurs knowledge generation by evaluating the health returns on investments in pharmaceutical research and development. The resulting models provide useful information for evaluating the structures and processes that help create new knowledge and innovation. They also show how such structures impact an important social outcome – in particular, global health. Although data alone will not solve any of the health problems people face, it can help many people secure essential medicines that save millions of lives every year.

Implementation, Evidence, and Innovation

The original GHI models are currently the "gold standard" for evaluating the impact of key medicines

for HIV/AIDS, malaria, and TB on disease burden in poor countries around the world (Hassoun, 2012a, 2012b, 2014, 2016a, 2016b, 2016c). Our methodology is significantly different from that embodied in other models because our models estimate in a simple, transparent, and consistent way the health consequences of drugs for several leading diseases in global poverty areas (Komatsu et al., 2010; Bao, 2012; Eisele et al., 2012; Bhatt et al., 2015; Galaktionova et al., 2015). Gathering data by company, drug, disease, and country into a single index, the original GHI models are able to estimate disease burden for any one or all conditions.

Whereas the original GHI models are an excellent first step to understanding the impact of major pharmaceuticals on these diseases, they fail to estimate the burden of disease that occurs in the absence of treatment, the impact of drugs on this burden over time, or the contribution of generic firms to alleviating the burden. Figure 32.4 illustrates the conceptual basis for the new GHI models.

Our models assume that the global burden of disease remaining after treatment (in DALYs lost)

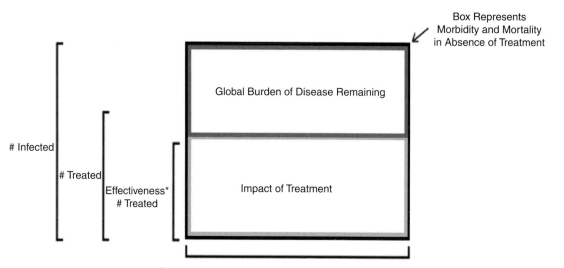

Figure 32.4. The new conceptual GHI model.

comes from people who are either untreated or for whom treatment is ineffective. Using data on disease incidence, treatment access, and effectiveness, we estimate the number of people who are not treated and the number for whom treatment is ineffective (as well as the number treated effectively). This is the height of the global burden of disease remaining box. Data on this burden come from the Institute for Health Metrics and Evaluation, so the area of that box is known. Thus, we can estimate the length – which is the average impact of an ineffectively treated case. We assume that, on average, a case of effective treatment alleviates the average impact of an untreated or ineffectively treated case. So the models can estimate treatment impact by multiplying the number of people who are treated effectively by the average impact of an untreated or ineffectively treated case (see the Appendix for a more formal presentation of the basic structure of the model). Mathematically, the impact score is calculated using the simplified formula

$$I = -\frac{D}{1 - \theta e}\theta e$$

where I indicates the impact of treatment, D indicates the DALYS lost to the relevant disease, θ indicates treatment percentage, and e indicates drug efficacy. Much of these data are available from global databases and reports, but we also do a systematic review of the academic literature to gather efficacy data (e.g., World Health Organization [WHO], 2006, 2010a, 2010b,

2011a, 2011b, 2013b, 2014, 2018, 2019; Demographic and Health Surveys, 2019). (For a complete list of data sources used in the original model, see Hassoun [2016a].)

Let's use an example to illustrate how we calculate the impact score of a drug for one country. Consider artemether lumefantrine (AL) in Bangladesh. For Bangladesh, 191,646 DALYs were lost to malaria in 2010 (Institute for Health Metrics and Evaluation [IHME], 2019). About 92% of malaria in Bangladesh is *Plasmodium falciparum* malaria (World Health Organization [WHO], 2011b). So the DALYs lost to *P. falciparum* malaria was 92% of 191,646, or 176,314. AL is used as the first-line drug for *P. falciparum* malaria in Bangladesh (WHO, 2011b). The treatment coverage for AL is 4.63% (UNICEF, 2015), and AL is efficacious in about 97.43% of cases (WHO, 2010a). For Bangladesh, the DALYs saved by AL as a first-line drug are 176,314 × 4.63% × 97.43%/ (1 − 4.63% × 97.43%) = 8,329.27.

Of course, in practice, things are often much more complicated than this because we must often estimate for missing data and look at the impacts of medicines in different subgroups of the population differently. To provide one example, we look at drug-susceptible TB in HIV$^+$ and HIV$^-$ patients separately as well as multidrug-resistant (MDR) and extremely drug-resistant (XDR) TB. We lack data on the proportion of people receiving treatment with different MDR TB regimens, so we use data on resistance rates along with treatment guidelines to estimate use.

The GHI team draws on the expertise of health outcomes researchers, pharmacologists, biostatisticians, and econometricians to construct, analyze, and validate our more sophisticated models that measure health in the presence and absence of treatment over time. The new models provide data on worldwide access to essential medicines that can be used to generate strategies for providing more equal access to these medicines and scientific innovations to address important global health problems. More generally, this information can help fulfill individuals' human right to health and achieve SDG 3.

For further information about the original models and the principles on which the contribution is based, see Hassoun (2012a, 2012b, 2014, 2016a, 2016b, 2016c) and OSF Registries (2011). These contributions also detail important limitations of the models. Our analysis does not, for instance, perfectly capture the volume of each product used in each country. Where data are lacking, an estimate is provided based on the extent to which products are listed as first-line drugs for treating a disease. If 100 patients are treated in a country and there are two first-line drugs, each drug is given credit for its potential impact on 50 patients. Our approach has the merit of allocating credit for being recognized as a first-line therapy for a given disease. Similarly, we do not attempt to determine what the incremental benefit of a drug is relative to the next-best therapy. Our analysis, in effect, indicates the impact of treatment including drugs in place of no treatment. Even with the inaccuracies that inevitably arise in this exercise, we believe that it is important to understand and illustrate what impact pharmaceuticals are having on global health and that this project can create incentives for promoting sustainable development and the human right to health (Sanofi, 2015). Sensitivity analysis of the preliminary version suggests that many of the assumptions have little impact on the model (Hassoun, 2016b).

The GHI models' methodology is significantly different from that of many other models of treatment impact (Stover & USAID, 2009; Komatsu et al., 2010; Bao, 2012; Eisele et al., 2012; Bhatt et al., 2015; Galactionova et al., 2015; Palladium Group, 2015). Several of these models are dynamic and disease specific. Most models do not use DALYs but focus on mortality rates, so they leave out a large component of intervention impacts. Dynamic (epidemiologic) models try to estimate how effective treatment will affect the future course of infectious disease epidemics. In so doing, they rely on different kinds of information and make different assumptions than the new GHI models. Avenir Health's AIDS Impact Model, for instance, assumes information "about the past and future course of adult HIV incidence and treatment coverage" as well as "the survival period from HIV infection to AIDS death, the age and sex distribution of new infections, and the perinatal transmission rate" (Stover & USAID, 2009: 4).

The GHI models have several advantages over alternative models. None of the other models combine – in a simple, transparent, and consistent way – estimates of the death and disability saved by medicines for HIV/AIDS, malaria, TB, and NTDs (Stover and USAID, 2009; Komatsu et al., 2010; Bao, 2012; Eisele et al., 2012; Bhatt et al., 2015; Galactionova et al., 2015; Palladium Group, 2015). The new GHI models provide comparable estimates of the impacts of interventions on disability and death across several diseases and include many more interventions than most models. Finally, the models aggregate this information by drug, disease, and company as well as country.

High-quality data on health impact will improve global governance for health, making it more transparent and accountable (Komatsu et al., 2010; Bao, 2012; Eisele et al., 2012; Gostin et al., 2014Bhatt et al., 2015; Galactionova et al., 2015). The AIDS crisis revealed problems with global health structures that posed barriers to reducing infections. To address these problems, recent conceptions of development expressed, for instance, in the Paris Principles have emphasized the importance of achieving *measurable health improvements*. This aim is embodied in relatively recent global public/private partnerships advancing the global health agenda by employing performance-based mechanisms for allocating assistance. The Global Fund reports that it has helped save 17 million lives, and the GAVI Alliance reports that it helped save 5.5 million (GAVI Alliance, 2012; Global Fund, 2015). Comparative evaluation facilitates learning across programs and countries and induces change: governments are much more likely to improve programs when the shortfalls are known and there are demonstrably better approaches. Other organizations can also use these data to expand access to essential medicines around the world. Several things are necessary to ensure that the project promotes sustainable health outcomes. A sustainable funding stream would allow us to scale up the model even further and improve the scientific analysis behind the project. Expanding our network to partner with international institutions and governmental and nongovernmental agencies working on promoting access to essential medicines ensures that the data are presented in a way that is most useful for efforts to expand access.

Conclusion

The Sustainable Development Goals, in setting the post-2015 development agenda, are refocusing efforts on universal health coverage and access to essential medicines. As in other areas, information is the key to success in improving health outcomes and fulfilling individuals' right to health. A broad, accurate picture of what we have achieved in extending access to essential medicines is necessary to guide national and international organizations. The Global Burden of Disease project has, over the past 20 years, been immensely valuable in illuminating areas of need, and it has had an undeniable influence on health spending. There is no similarly comprehensive effort to evaluate the impact of funding and interventions to improve global health. According to the WHO–World Bank framework for measuring universal healthcare, "the post-2015 agenda should address the unfinished agenda of the health-related MDGs as well as the emerging burden of noncommunicable diseases, and this evaluation should eventually be extended to address the global priorities embodied in the Sustainable Development Goals. Ideally, the evaluation would include preventative and diagnostic technologies as well as treatments for SDG priority health conditions (Boerma et al., 2014; World Health Organization & World Bank, 2014).

There are, moreover, many important uses for such data among numerous stakeholders – ranging from international institutions such as the WHO to bilateral or multilateral health assistance organizations such as the President's Emergency Program on AIDS Relief and philanthropies such as the Gates Foundation to national governments. Good data about effectiveness can help international and multilateral institutions (and other stakeholders) prioritize funding across countries, diseases, and interventions. Country-level health systems similarly aim to allocate their resources, and secure new resources, to have a greater impact. Comprehensive data are important

for evaluating performance, setting targets, and guiding the distribution of resources. The expanded model complements existing work by global development agencies using tools such as AIM to assess the impact of important health interventions (Walker et al., 2013). If countries can see how drug impacts would change as they are made more accessible, this would help them decide whether to invest in efforts to lower prices or extend access more broadly in other ways. Moreover, impact assessments help shape policies linked to broader macroeconomic and trade liberalization aspects of globalization and improve global health governance (Gostin & Friedman, 2013).

The High-Level Panel on the Post-2015 Development Agenda called for "a data revolution" to "help guide decision making, update priorities and ensure accountability" (High-Level Panel of Eminent Persons on the Post-2015 Development Agenda, 2013: 3). Similarly, the High-Level Panel on Access to Medicines stated that "[t]he 2030 Agenda stresses the need for 'quality, accessible, timely, and reliable disaggregated data' to measure progress, inform decision-making and ensure that no one is left behind" (High-Level Panel on Access to Essential Medicines, 2016: 30). The panel notes that "[t]here is a wide agreement on the importance of comprehensive and accurate models" (High-Level Panel on Access to Essential Medicines, 2016: 30) and echoes our call for "metrics for evaluating performance, setting targets, guiding the distribution of scarce health resources and advancing access to affordable medicines" (High-Level Panel on Access to Essential Medicines, 2016: 30, citing Hassoun, 2016a: 45). Moreover, in her commentary included in the High-Level Panel on Access to Medicines Report (High-Level Panel on Access to Essential Medicines, 2016: 59), Ruth Okediji suggested

> requiring all pharmaceutical firms to achieve, within a specified timeframe, a designated time-score on a "social-responsibility index." This index would be a fraction, the numerator of which would be an objective measure of the firm's contributions to public health (in the developing world); and the denominator of which would be a similarly objective measure of the firm's profits. Ideas like this give important flexibility to pharmaceutical firms that embrace social welfare objectives, enhancing opportunities for realistic "win-win" outcomes.

However we use the data, I believe that good information systems are as important in fulfilling individuals' human rights to health as diagnostic tests are for identifying and treating disease. As the world sets its sights on achieving the Sustainable Development Goals, it is important to collect new data that can guide these efforts. Millions of lives hang in the balance.

Acknowledgments

I would like to thank the GHI team and advisory board and all the people and organizations that have contributed to the project. I am especially thankful to Nicholas Hall, Aidan Hollis, Leon Cosler, Mark Zhang, Jake Friedman, Zeke Factor, Chatham Borsch, and Denise Teo for their contributions. I am also thankful for discussions about the project at the WHO, Global Fund, Princeton University, Cornell University, the Edmund J. Safra Center for Ethics at Harvard University, the University of Manchester, the American Philosophical Association, Yale University, Binghamton University, the University of Delaware, London School of Economics, William and Lee College, Goethe University, University College London, Santa Clara University; the Universidad De Antioquia, Carnegie Mellon University, the American Society for Bioethics and Humanities, the Philosophy of Science Association, Stanford University, Dickinson College, the University of California, San Diego, and the University of Newcastle on the Tyne. I also thank the many researchers at UNAIDS, the WHO, TB Alliance, International AIDS Vaccine Initiative, the Medicines Patent Pool, and Doctors Without Borders for their help, along with countless others. I am especially grateful for support from Academics Stand Against Poverty; Stanford University's Center for Ethics in Society; Justitia Amplificata and the Center for Advanced Studies in Frankfurt, Germany; Binghamton University's Harpur College and Interdisciplinary, DeFleur, and Citizenship, Rights, and Belonging Transdisciplinary Area of Excellence collaborative grant programs; the Swedish-Franco Program in Philosophy and Economics in Paris; the Center for Poverty Research in Salzburg, Austria; the World Institute for Development Economics Research in Helsinki; and the Berkman and Falk Foundations at Carnegie Mellon University. I ask for forgiveness in leaving this list vastly incomplete because there is not sufficient space to list by name all of those who have so generously contributed to the development of this project even in very significant ways.

Appendix

More formally, consider a patient group identified by the IHME's GBD data (IHME, 2019), for example, patients affected by a given disease indexed by j in a given country indexed by k, for this group, defined as the average impact per untreated patient of the disease in terms of DALYs lost. Similarly, define the treatment impact as

$$(1 - e_{jk})\, u_{jk}$$

where

$$0 \le e_{jk} \le 1$$

In effect, e_{jk} is the effectiveness of the treatment relative to the baseline of no treatment. For example, a drug that reduces DALYs lost by 95% would have

$$e_{jk} = 0.95$$

The DALYs observed within the patient group by the IHME's GBD study are given by

$$D = n(1 - \theta)u + n\theta(1 - e)u \qquad (A.1)$$

where θ represents the proportion of infected persons who received treatment, and n represents the number of infected persons (i.e., the prevalence of disease times the population; I have suppressed subscripts). Assuming that treated and untreated individuals are similar, except for treatment, the DALYs that would occur in the absence of treatment are simply

$$D' = nu \qquad (A.2)$$

Therefore, the impact of treatment is given by

$$I = n(1 - \theta)u + n\theta(1 - e)u - nu = -n\theta eu \qquad (A.3)$$

where this negative number represents a reduction in DALYs. Rearranging (A.1), we obtain

$$\frac{D}{(1 - \theta)u + \theta(1 - e)u} = n \qquad (A.1*)$$

Substituting (A.1*) into (A.3), we can write the impact of treatment as

$$I = -\frac{D}{1 - \theta e}\theta e \qquad (A.4)$$

The contribution of drug m to treatment regimen i with drugs is assumed to be an equal share of the regimen, and the impact of the drug is therefore simply given by

$$I_{jkim} = I_{jki} \frac{1}{M_i} \qquad (A.5)$$

In effect, using this approach, we can identify the impact of treatment with a given regimen using (1) data from the IHME's GBD study, (2) information on coverage of the patient population with a given regimen, and (3) the effectiveness of the regimen compared with no treatment.

Coverage θ is written as a stock, but in many cases, treatment takes time, so coverage should reflect the proportion of the patient population that is *completing* treatment. We therefore adjust coverage by dividing it by the average duration of treatment if this number exceeds one year.

Here is the overall impact score:

$$I_{jki} = - \frac{D_{jk}}{1 - \Sigma_i \; \theta_{jki} \; e_{jki}} \; \theta_{jki} \; e_{jki} \qquad (A.6)$$

References

Bao, L. (2012). A new infectious disease model for estimating and projecting HIV/AIDS epidemics. *Sex Transmitted Infect* **88**, i58–i64.

Bhatt, S., Weiss, D. J., Cameron, E., et al. (2015). The effect of malaria control on *Plasmodium falciparum* in Africa between 2000 and 2015. *Nature* **526**, 207–211.

Berman, J. (2015). Web tool tracks locations of vital drugs' biggest impact. *Voice of America*, December 15. Available at www.voanews.com/science-health/web-tool-tracks-locations-vital-drugs-biggest-impact (accessed December 29, 2015).

Boerma, T., Eozenou, P., Evans, D., et al. (2014). Monitoring progress towards universal health coverage at country and global levels. *PLOS Medicine* **11**, e1001731.

Demographic and Health Surveys (DHS) Program (2019). Demographic and health surveys. Available at https://dhsprogram.com/what-we-do/survey-Types/dHs.cfm (accessed June 21, 2019).

Eisele, T. P., Larsen, D. A., Walker, N., et al. (2012). Estimates of child deaths prevented from malaria prevention scale-up in Africa 2001–2010. *Malaria Journal* **11**, 93.

Galactionova, K., Tediosi, F., De Savigny, D., et al. (2015). Effective coverage and systems effectiveness for malaria case management in Sub-Saharan African countries. *PLoS One* **10**, e0127818.

GAVI Alliance (2012). Investing in immunization through the GAVI Alliance, the evidence base. Available at www

.gavi.org/sites/default/files/document/2019/GAVI_Alliance_Evidence_Base.pdf (accessed June 21, 2019).

Global Fund (2015). Results Report 2015. Available at www.theglobalfund.org/media/8253/corporate_2015resultsreport_report_en.pdf?u=637278307900000000 (accessed June 21, 2019).

Global Health Impact (2014). The Indexes. Available at https://global-health-impact.org/ (accessed December 29, 2013).

Gostin, L. O., Friedman, E. A., Buse, K., et al. (2013). Towards a framework convention on global health. *Bulletin of the World Health Organization* **91**, 790–793.

Gostin, L. O., & Sridhar, D. (2014). Global health and the law. *New England Journal of Medicine*, **370**, 1732–1740.

Gorenstein, D. (2015). New effort ranks drug makers by impact. *Marketplace*, January 23. Available at www.marketplace.org/2015/01/23/new-effort-ranks-drugmakers-impact/ (accessed December 29, 2015).

Hassoun, N. (2012a). Global Health Impact: a basis for labeling and licensing campaigns? *Developing World Bioethics* **12**, 121–134.

Hassoun, N. (2012b). Measuring Global Health Impact: incentivizing research and development of drugs for neglected diseases. *Developing World Bioethics* **12**, 121–134.

Hassoun, N. (2014). Globalization, global justice, and global health impact. *Public Affairs Quarterly* **28**, 231–258.

Hassoun, N. (2016a). Advancing the Sustainable Development Goals and human rights to health: evaluating global health impact and increasing access to essential medicines. United Nations Secretary-General's High-Level Panel on Access to Medicines. Available at www.unsgaccessmeds.org/inbox/2016/2/16/contributionn-hassoun?rq=Hassoun (accessed June 19, 2019).

Hassoun, N. (2016b). The Global Health Impact Index: promoting global health. *PLOS One* **11**, e0148946.

Hassoun, N. (2016c). Modeling key malaria drugs' impact on global health: a reason to invest in the global health impact index. *American Journal of Tropical Medicine and Hygiene* **94**, 942–946.

High-Level Panel of Eminent Persons on the Post-2015 Development Agenda (2013). Bali Communiqué, March 28. Available at www.un.org/sg/sites/www.un.org.sg/files/documents/management/Final%20Communique%20Bali.pdf (accessed June 16, 2020).

High-Level Panel on Access to Medicines (2016). Report of the United Nations Secretary-General. Available at https://static1.squarespace.com/static/562094dee4b0d00c1a3ef761/t/57d9c6ebf5e231b2f02cd3d4/1473890031320/UNSG+HLP+Report+FINAL+12+Sept+2016.pdf%20citation (accessed June 21, 2019).

Institute for Health Metrics and Evaluation (IHME) (2019). GBD results tool. IHME, Seattle. Available at http://ghdx.healthdata.org/gbd-results-tool (accessed December 29, 2015).

Komatsu, R., Korenromp, E. L., Low-Beer, D., et al. (2010). Lives saved by global fund-supported HIV/AIDS, tuberculosis and malaria programs: estimation approach and results between 2003 and end-2007. *BMC Infectious Diseases* **10**, 109.

OSF (2011). GHI spreadsheet ORS v63. OSF Registries. Available at https://osf.io/zghvy (accessed January 1, 2016).

Palladium Group. (2015). Palladium delivers positive impact solutions: international development, strategy execution and impact investment. Available at http://thepalladiumgroup.com/ (accessed December 29, 2015).

Prakash, N. (2015). SUNY professor indexes pharma companies' impact. Politico PRO, January 23. Available at www.politico.com/states/new-york/albany/story/2016/05/suny-professor-indexes-pharma-companies-impact-052709 (accessed December 29, 2015).

Sanofi (2015). Awards and recognitions. Available at www.sanofi.us/en/about-us/awards-and-recognitions (accessed December 29, 2019).

Silverman, E. (2015). A new index measures impact pharma has on infectious diseases. *Wall Street Journal*, January 23. Available at https://blogs.wsj.com/pharmalot/2015/01/23/a-new-index-measures-impact-pharma-has-on-infectious-diseases/ (accessed December 29, 2015).

Stover, J., & USAID (2009). AIM: A computer program for making HIV/AIDS projections and examining the demographic and social impacts of AIDS. Futures Group International, United States Agency of International Development Health Policy Initiative (UNAIDS), Washington, DC, 4. Available at http://data.unaids.org/pub/manual/2009/20090414_aim_manual_2009_en.pdf (accessed December 29, 2015).

UNICEF (2015). About UNICEF data and analytics. Available at https://data.unicef.org/about-us/ (accessed December 29, 2019).

United Nations Sustainable Development (n.d.). About the Sustainable Development Goals. Available at www.un.org/sustainabledevelopment/sustainable-development-goals/ (accessed June 19, 2019).

VisionGain (2010). The global OTC pharmaceutical market, 2010–2025. Available at www.visiongain.com/Report/500/The-Global-OTC-Pharmaceutical-Market-2010-2025 (accessed June 19, 2019).

Walker, N., Tam, Y., & Friberg, I. (2013). Overview of the lives saved tool (LiST). *BMC Public Health* **13**, 1–6.

World Health Organization (WHO) (2006). Preventive chemotherapy in human helminthiasis. Available at www.cabdirect.org/cabdirect/abstract/20073104734 (accessed December 29, 2015).

World Health Organization (WHO) (2010a). Global report on antimalarial efficacy and drug resistance: 2000–2010. Available at www.who.int/malaria/publications/atoz/9789241500470/en/ (accessed December 29, 2013).

World Health Organization (WHO) (2010b). World health statistics 2010. Available at www.who.int/whosis/whostat/EN_WHS10_Full.pdf?ua=1 (accessed December 29, 2013).

World Health Organization (WHO) (2011a). Global price reporting mechanism for HIV, tuberculosis and malaria. Available at www.who.int/hiv/amds/gprm/en/ (accessed January 14, 2013).

World Health Organization (WHO) (2011b). World malaria report 2011. Available at www.who.int/malaria/world_malaria_report_2011/en/ (accessed December 29, 2015).

Organization (WHO) (2013b). Global tuberculosis report 2013. Available at https://apps.who.int/iris/bitstream/handle/10665/91355/9789241564656_eng.pdf?sequence=1 (accessed December 29, 2015).

World Health Organization (WHO) (2014). Access to antiretroviral drugs in low- and middle-income countries. Available at www.who.int/hiv/pub/amds/access-arv-2014/en/ (accessed January 1, 2016).

World Health Organization (WHO) (2018). World malaria report 2018. Available at www.who.int/malaria/publications/world-malaria-report-2018/en/ (accessed June 21, 2019).

World Health Organization (WHO) (2019). PCT databank. Available at www.who.int/neglected_diseases/preventive_chemotherapy/lf/en/ (accessed June 21, 2019).

World Health Organization & World Bank (2014). Monitoring progress towards universal health coverage at country and global levels: a framework. Geneva: WHO, pp. 1–10.

Chapter 333

Philanthrocapitalism and Global Health

James Wilson

Introduction

Philanthropy is usually taken to involve private individuals donating their resources – whether time, money, or property – voluntarily for the public good (Payton, 1988). Philanthropy has a history that stretches back thousands of years, but both the scale and manner of philanthropic giving have changed significantly since the turn of the millennium. CNN founder Ted Turner's 1997 decision to donate $1 billion to the United Nations and his widely publicized criticisms of other billionaires for not doing more are often thought to have incited changes that led to Bill Gates and others committing to massive programs of giving to promote global health (Callahan, 2017).

The term *philanthrocapitalism* was coined by Bishop (2006), drawing attention to a significant new departure beyond the sheer increased scale of philanthropic giving, namely that individuals who had become massively wealthy in capitalist systems were now applying the very same skills and techniques that they used to create their wealth to the project of giving their fortunes away. The spirit of philanthrocapitalism, Bishop and Green (2008: 30) argued, is "successful entrepreneurs trying to solve big social problems because they believe they can, and because they believe they should."

The Bill & Melinda Gates Foundation (BMGF) is emblematic of philanthrocapitalism, and given the sheer scale of its influence in global health, the foundation will be a central focus of this chapter. The BMGF was launched in 2000 from a merger of several other Gates-run foundations and funds projects in global health and global development as well as public education in the United States. In 2006, Bill Gates announced that he would transition out of his day-to-day role at Microsoft to concentrate on the BMGF. Up to the end of 2017, Bill and Melinda Gates had donated $35.8 billion to the Bill & Melinda Gates

Trust (BMGT).[1] Their friend, investor Warren Buffett, has also contributed over $30 billion to the BMGT since 2006. The BMGT manages investments to return a profit and transfers proceeds to the BMGF. By the end of 2017, the BMGT had $50.7 billion in assets. The BMGF distributed $4.7 billion in grants in 2017, of which $3 billion was devoted to global health and global development. By the end of 2017, the BMGF had distributed $45.5 billion total (Bill & Melinda Gates Foundation, 2019).

Bill and Melinda Gates joined with Warren Buffett in 2010 to launch the Giving Pledge. This organization encourages billionaires worldwide to "publicly dedicate the majority of their wealth to philanthropy" and thereby to "help shift the social norms of philanthropy toward giving more, giving sooner, and giving smarter" (Giving Pledge, 2019). Giving Pledge also runs an influential yearly conference for billionaires to discuss how best to give. By 2019, 204 billionaires had publicly signed up to the pledge (Giving Pledge, 2019; Callahan, 2017: 19–28).

Other notable philanthrocapitalist projects set up by some of the world's wealthiest individuals, each of whom is also a signatory of the Giving Pledge, include the Chan Zuckerberg Initiative (founded by Facebook founder Mark Zuckerberg and his wife, Priscilla Chan, which focuses on science, education, and opportunity for all), the Jack Ma Foundation (set up by Jack Ma, founder of Alibaba, to focus on education in rural China), and Bloomberg Philanthropies (set up by Michael Bloomberg to focus, among other interests, on global health and US public health).

---

[1] Owing to a series of canny investments, the Gates' private wealth continued to increase despite this largesse, with Bill Gates being rated as either the wealthiest or second wealthiest person in the world for 18 of the last 19 years, with a net worth of $96.5 billion at the time of this writing (Forbes.com, 2019).

Bishop and Green (2008) argue that the core feature that distinguishes philanthrocapitalism from earlier forms of philanthropy is the role of leverage. Philanthrocapitalists seek to use their foundations to leverage resources that are much larger than their initial donations from either the public sector or other private individuals in order to maximize the effectiveness of their giving. This contrasts with more passive approaches to philanthropy, in which wealthy foundations provide grants directed toward specified goals but without any special attempt to enlist other resource holders to the cause.[2]

Philanthrocapitalists are in a vastly stronger position to leverage funds and to change the direction of public policy than other actors. First, and most obviously, the sheer fact of their enormous wealth – especially when combined with global fame as the public face of one the wealthiest and most powerful corporations on the planet – gives them a depth of networks and influence among other social and political elites. Because of this potential for outsized influence, Bishop and Green (2015) describe philanthrocapitalists as *hyperagents,* and it is this feature that is central to their optimistic vision of the potentially transformative effects of philanthrocapitalists: "they do not face elections every few years, like politicians, or suffer the tyranny of shareholder demands for ever-increasing quarterly profits, like CEOs of most public companies. Nor do they have to devote vast amounts of time and resources to raising money, like most heads of NGOs. That frees them to think long-term, to go against conventional wisdom, to take up ideas too risky for government, to deploy substantial resources quickly when the situation demands it – above all, to try something new" (Bishop & Green, 2008: 12).

Thus Bishop and Green's basic case for philanthrocapitalism is that people who are extremely wealthy, powerful, and well connected will use their

power and contacts to leverage far greater resources from elsewhere in order to maximize the success of their goals.

It is important to note that the very features that Bishop and Green celebrate – the philanthrocapitalists' unusual skill in leveraging resources and their lack of accountability to others – are precisely what many others find objectionable. To say that some have an oversized ability to influence the way that broader societal decisions are made implies by the same token that the vast majority have far less power.

It is useful to distinguish the two elements of *outsize influence* and *leveraging of public resources.* Where there is outsized influence without a significant leveraging of public resources, then what the philanthropist does will be in addition to what the state does. This may well allow the philanthropist to take risks, such as paying for basic research that could lead to a new vaccine, which could pay off handsomely but would be too speculative for the state to support. Where this is the case, the philanthrocapitalist's funding may bring significant additional value. However, if the philanthrocapitalist's plans involve extensive leveraging of public resources, then those plans will be in competition with other uses of public resources. The opportunity cost of the success of the philanthrocapitalist's leverage will be the sidelining of some other policies.

If the philanthrocapitalist's goals are well chosen and coincide with those that would have been chosen by citizens through a well-ordered deliberative process, then this unaccountable leveraging of public resources might seem relatively benign. But it is important not to forget that the philanthrocapitalist's goals could also be rather distant from those that most citizens would support. For example, there are a significant number of billionaires and a large network of foundations that are supported by them that purport to be philanthropic while acting to undermine goals such as universal health coverage and reductions in carbon emissions (Mayer, 2016; Callahan, 2017). To the extent that public resources are diverted toward goals that are distant from those that would be chosen through a well-functioning deliberative process, this is deeply ethically problematic. In such a case, the deployment of oversized networks of power and influence to steer public choices could be described as cooption or institutional capture – and arguably corruption (Beetham, 2015).

[2] Considered in this way, there are strong continuities between philanthrocapitalism and the kind of philanthropy practiced in the early twentieth century by Andrew Carnegie and the Rockefeller Foundation. For example, Carnegie's library-building program would pay for a library for a community only on the condition that the local authorities would pay for staffing and upkeep in perpetuity. Birn and Richter (2018) argue that there are striking parallels between the mode of operation of the BMGF and the Rockefeller Foundation, which was active at the beginnings of international health, but argue that the BMGF, if anything, is even less accountable than the Rockefeller Foundation was.

Philanthropy on the kind of scale pursued by the BMGF is possible only in circumstances of extreme global wealth inequality. By 2017, the wealthiest 1% of individuals globally owned 33% of global wealth – up from 28% in 1980. The poorest 50% of the global population owned "almost no wealth," with its share of the global total remaining fixed at around 2% over this period (Alvaredo et al., 2018: 200). Even focusing on the larger group of the bottom 75%, this group owned only around 10% of global wealth during this period (Alvaredo et al., 2018: 200). Wealth inequalities are even more eye-watering at the level of those rich enough to sign the Giving Pledge. The charity Oxfam estimated that as of 2019, the richest 26 people on the planet had the same wealth as the poorest 3.8 billion (Oxfam International, 2019). This inequality has also accelerated rapidly: in 2010, it would have taken the combined wealth of the richest 388 people to have the same as the poorest 50%. It is sobering to reflect that a single individual such as Bill Gates or Warren Buffett has more than the combined wealth of more than 100 million of the world's poorest people.

In thinking about the ethical challenges posed by extreme wealth, it is helpful to distinguish between injustices in the way that fortunes are amassed and injustices that arise from extreme inequalities in wealth regardless of how those inequalities were amassed. In a classic thought experiment Nozick (1974: 161–162) imagines how a sports star such as the then-famous basketball player Wilt Chamberlain could, through a combination of talent and sheer hard work, come to extreme wealth as a result of a series of voluntary transactions of those who wished to pay to see him play.

Nozick assumes that any distribution of wealth that arises from an initially just starting point and that proceeds by just steps will itself be just. However, as Cohen (1995: chapter 1) argues, there are a reasons for thinking that inequalities can be ethically objectionable, even if those who become wealthy have played according to the rules in obtaining their wealth. Centrally objectionable features of unequal societies include inequalities in power, social status, and ability to exercise political liberties. A just society will require at least a reasonable degree of equality of power and wealth between citizens.

Although the causes of the rise in global inequality are complex, and the comments made here can only be programmatic, there are strong reasons to think that the sharp rise in inequality and the correlative rise

in the number of individuals who are wealthy enough to do philanthropy on a grand scale are explained by institutional changes to the global economy rather than features for which individual members of the superrich could plausibly take credit. This will be significant if, as Scanlon (2018: 138) argues, wealth inequality "is objectionable, and unfair, when the institutional mechanisms generating it cannot be justified in the right way."

During the period of the Bretton Woods system (1945–1971), there were stringent capital controls on the world's major economies that severely restricted capital flows across borders. For example, in 1963, the top marginal rate of income tax was 91% in the United States and 89% in the United Kingdom. The decline of the Bretton Woods system saw an end to capital controls, and in the wake of this came international tax competition – and a growing belief among policymakers that income and corporation taxes needed to be reduced in order to avoid capital flight. By 1989, the top marginal rate of income tax had fallen to 28% in the United States and 40% in the United Kingdom, before rising slightly to 35% (US) and 45% (UK) at the time of this writing. Corporate tax rates also declined sharply during the same time period (see Piketty [2014] for data and analysis). The decline of capital controls also made possible aggressive tax avoidance through tax havens and the use of complex international ownership regimes, which have allowed the superrich to further reduce their tax liabilities.

During the same time period, the global economy transitioned from one in which the predominant source of wealth was physical goods to one in which the predominant source of wealth is intangible goods such as intellectual property, brands, and media platforms. Markets for intangible goods exhibit features such as network effects, high up-front costs but low marginal costs, and customers getting used to particular services and products, which together make for what Arthur (1989) describes as an economy of increasing returns – namely one in which companies that get ahead will tend to increase their lead. Where there are increasing returns, there are significant path dependencies, and markets will tend toward monopoly or at best oligopoly without firm governance. Oligopolistic and monopolistic markets generate excess profits for producers at the expense of consumers: this is why antitrust and competition law exists. Though the details of the cases are beyond the scope of this chapter, it is important to note that Microsoft was judged guilty of anticompetitive practices in major cases in the United States (*United States v. Microsoft Corporation*, 253 F.3d 34 [D.C. Cir. 2001]) and the European Union (*Microsoft Corp. v. Commission of the European Communities*, T-201/04). Thus, a proportion of the wealth now being funneled into the BMGF arose as a result of attempts to unlawfully stifle competition.

To say the least, the sheer scale of inequality and the nature of the institutional mechanisms that have exacerbated it complicate and render controversial the work of large-scale philanthropists – with some commentators choosing to focus solely on the good done by foundations, whereas others are more inclined to assess the apparent benevolence in the context of what they judge to be the systemically unjust system that allowed the accumulation of wealth and power in the first place. This can at times give debates within the area a polarized feel, which one prominent writer described as a feeling of being "whiplashed between hope and fear" (Callahan, 2017: 33).

Duty, Supererogation, and the Ends of Charitable Giving

Commonsense morality distinguishes between obligatory actions (those for which there is a duty to do), permissible actions (those for which an agent may or may not do as he or she chooses), and impermissible actions (those for which an agent has a duty not to do). Supererogatory actions are actions that are good or praiseworthy for an agent to perform but where doing so is permissible rather than obligatory. Acts of heroism are usually taken to be paradigm cases of such acts.

Large-scale philanthropy by the ultrarich is often addressed as if it were a matter of supererogation rather than duty. For example, Bill Gates is commonly praised for being generous in making such large donations to the BMGT.[3] The view of large-scale philanthropy as supererogation presupposes something like the following picture: As long as any legally required taxation has been paid, then the residual money belongs to the philanthropist, and it is his or her right to decide how to spend it. It is morally permissible for an ultrarich person to spend his or her money

on whatever he or she chooses; if the philanthropist prefers to spend it on conspicuous consumption – private jets and Fabergé eggs, say – no one is entitled to require him or her to do otherwise.

Acceptance of this worldview would explain why large-scale philanthropy is thought to be morally praiseworthy, in that the philanthropist is doing much more to help others than duty would require. It would also explain why philanthropy by the ultrarich is usually thought praiseworthy, even when it produces a lot less good than other things that the philanthropist could have done with the same sum.[4] Framing philanthropy as optional but praiseworthy might also go some way toward explaining the advantageous tax arrangements that accompany philanthropy in many countries – with tax relief on donations by philanthropists to charitable foundations and philanthropic foundations being tax exempt – a set of tax subsidies that cost the US Treasury at least $50 billion per year[5] (Reich, 2018: 9).

The picture of philanthropy as supererogation – and hence as something that should be praised and, in addition, incentivized via the taxation system – can be challenged in various ways. The first is by reflecting more deeply on the fact of very large inequalities in wealth and power and how this should lead us to frame the fact of extraordinary wealth. Perhaps, rather than thinking of great wealth merely as providing opportunities for the ultrarich to benefit others, it would be better to think of such wealth as wronging or actively harming the other 99.99% through the ways that great wealth undermines the central value

---

[3] Those who sign the Giving Pledge often explain their choices in terms of the ability to make an impact or other broader values (Sadeh, Tonin, & Vlassopoulos, 2017), but it is also clear that they tend to interpret any relevant duties as imperfect ones that allow them significant leeway in determining how and when to give.

[4] While some signatories of the Giving Pledge are active in global health and take great pains to use their resources effectively, many do little for the worst off and may, if anything, widen structural inequalities, for example, donating heavily to whichever of the world's wealthiest universities they studied at or funding extravagant schemes such as the $250 million given by Barry Diller and Diane von Furstenberg to build Pier 55, a new floating 2.4-acre park in Manhattan (Kilgannon, 2018).

[5] While philanthropists have standardly set up not-for-profit foundations to take advantage of the improved tax status, doing so comes with a set of requirements (different from county to country) about financial reporting and disbursal of funds. A recent trend – which received much publicity when the Chan Zuckerberg Initiative took up this option – has been for philanthropists to set up limited-liability companies (LLCs) rather than foundations in order to reduce their public accountability. For a detailed analysis of how LLCs are likely to exacerbate some of the problems that philanthrocapitalism creates, see Amarante (2018).

of social equality (Robeyns, 2016). The circumstances that allow the philanthrocapitalist to function so effectively may be judged seriously unjust, even if the philanthrocapitalist uses his or her power and resources in a way that brings significant health benefits to many who are badly off. Second, and separate from the idea that massive wealth by itself wrongs, it could be questioned whether there is an ethical entitlement to keep hold of massive amounts of surplus resources in the first place when many are in dire and urgent need. If either of these ethical arguments is correct, it would entail that it is *not* permissible for the ultrarich to hang on to the majority of their riches; it would also (as I shall discuss further later) have implications for who should decide how the riches that are devoted to philanthropy should be used.

The ethically questionable nature of extreme wealth means that there are two levels at which the ethics of large-scale philanthropy could be discussed. First, philanthrocapitalism could be examined at the level of ideal theory, in which a world with the high levels of inequality necessary for large-scale philanthropy to be possible is compared against a rather more equal world in which there is little need for philanthropy. To the extent that the unequal world that contains effective philanthropy is more unjust than a less unequal world in which no one individual has a private wealth greater than the combined wealth of millions, then perhaps the best that could be said for philanthropy is that it is "commendable, but it must not cause the philanthropist to overlook the circumstances of economic injustice which make philanthropy necessary" (King, 2010: 25).

Second, philanthrocapitalism could be examined through the lens of a real-world approach to philosophy: given that there are individuals who are extremely wealthy (even if in a just world no one would be that wealthy), what are the ethical principles by which these individuals should approach spending their resources, and to what extent should global health be a key priority for them? I address philanthrocapitalism at the level of ideal theory in the next section, before moving on to it as a real-world approach in subsequent sections.

Philanthrocapitalism and Ideal Theory: Carnegie and "The Gospel of Wealth"

In his famous essay "The Gospel of Wealth," Andrew Carnegie (1889), the superwealthy steel magnate and philanthropist, provides an early and ambitious defense of great wealth inequality as a necessary component of philanthropy at scale. He argues for four main propositions. First, the existing economic system that gives rise to massive inequalities should continue because it is an engine of growth. Second, those who become wealthy should give away most of their fortunes within their own lifetimes: "The man who dies thus rich dies disgraced." Third, it is much better for society if a few rich people distribute their resources philanthropically than it would have been if the money had been redistributed through the taxation system:

> Under its [i.e., philanthropy's] sway we shall have an ideal state, in which the surplus wealth of the few will become, in the best sense, the property of the many, because administered for the common good; and this wealth, passing through the hands of the few, can be made a much more potent force for the elevation of our race than if it had been distributed in small sums to the people themselves. *(Carnegie, 1889: 9–10)*

Fourth, the objects of the philanthropist's munificence should not be the worst off but those who are industrious and upwardly mobile:

> It is not the irreclaimably destitute, shiftless, and worthless that it is truly beneficial or truly benevolent to attempt to reach and improve. For these there exists the refuge provided by the city or the state, where they can be sheltered, fed, clothed, and kept in comfortable existence, and – most important of all where they can be isolated from the well doing and industrious poor, who are liable to be demoralized by contact with these unfortunates.
> *(Carnegie, 1889: 21–22)*

It seems unlikely that any aspiring philanthrocapitalist today would make such an argument so baldly and unreflexively – but the very tendentiousness of Carnegie's claims is useful in drawing out some of the key ethical challenges that would have to be met by any attempt to defend the combination of large-scale inequality and large-scale philanthropy as an ideal over the alternative of a well-ordered egalitarian state.

First, whatever the merits of the claim that economic inequality is helpful for economic growth in terms of gross domestic product (GDP) per capita might be, the idea that increasing wealth inequality is good for health is a nonstarter. The lack of correlation between GDP per capita and improved life expectancy in middle- and high-income countries is well known, and there is a wealth of evidence on the social determinants of health that point to the harmful effects of income and wealth inequalities on health outcomes such as life expectancy (Commission on the Social Determinants of Health, 2008; Wilkinson & Pickett, 2009).

Second, any attempt to interfere in individuals' lives faces the challenge of legitimacy. Carnegie argues that things will go better if the philanthropist, rather than the state, decides how to spend large amounts of resources. In assessing the merits of this claim, it is important to compare like with like: it would not be fair to compare an ideal philanthrocapitalist against the supposed deficiencies of actual states any more than it would be to compare the fruits of a zealous and pigheaded philanthrocapitalist ideologue against an idealized egalitarian democracy.

There are strong reasons to think that, other things being equal, functional democratic institutions will be both more legitimate and more accountable than philanthropically funded arrangements. Decisions about social goals and the direction of social policy are inherently contestable because of what Rawls (2001: 35–36) called the burdens of judgment. Although there is expertise that is relevant to setting goals in global health and domestic social policy, such expertise does not uniquely determine what should be done. Moreover, expertise in making money through software development or oil exploration does not imply expertise in solving major global health challenges such as air pollution and antimicrobial resistance or strengthening health systems. Thus, the crucial question is how to proceed legitimately given a range of reasonable disagreement about fundamental questions such as the nature of the good life or how to reconcile best overall outcomes with giving some priority to the worst off.[6]

Any legitimate approach needs to take account of the basic democratic idea that citizens – regardless of their level of wealth – are in Rawls's words (1993: 72) "self-authenticating sources of valid claims" and have a right to codetermine the conditions in which they live. Functioning democratic institutions meet this requirement through democratic political control and accountability. If political institutions fail to pursue the public interest, then those running the programs can be replaced and held accountable. By giving a voice to all citizens and a power to vote out politicians who are not perceived to promote the public good, it creates incentive compatibility. Sen (1981) argues that it is because of this that we do not see famines occurring in democracies, whereas they are frequent in nondemocratic regimes.

In contrast, philanthropically led approaches will find it more difficult to ensure incentive compatibility. If philanthrocapitalists do a bad job of helping those they purport to be helping, it is unlikely that this will lead to serious consequences for the philanthrocapitalists. The people who are the beneficiaries of the giving have no power to vote out or sanction the philanthrocapitalists if the solutions they impose fail to work, so it could very easily happen that the benefits provided by the philanthrocapitalists are not those that individuals would have chosen and may not be beneficial for them.

Putting all these features together – the need for legitimacy, the lack of expertise of philanthropists, and the requirement for incentive compatibility – and considering them also in the light of the variety of reasons there are for objecting ethically to gross disparities of wealth and power (Scanlon, 2018), then there would seem to be a good reason to favor democratically controlled approaches over philanthropic ones at an ideal level.

However, perhaps the most salient starting point in thinking about global health ethics is the fact that the world is very far from ideal. What should be the role of philanthropy be, given a much less than ideal world? I will address this question by examining the goals that philanthrocapitalists should have and the extent to which those goals should be a matter of discretion for them. The chapter then concludes by examining some of the effects of the BMGF in practice.

---

[6] The need for tradeoffs between efficiency and helping the worst off has often been noted in the parallel literature on government aid: "If the over-riding objective is to make as much aid as possible work as well as it can, then aid would be given to countries characterised by good governance; with democratically elected, accountable governments and strong parliamentary systems capable of scrutinising public finances and officials; a free press and a vibrant civil society. . . . In contrast, those countries and communities most in need of aid will be those most likely to be deficient in many, if not most, of the core characteristics that are likely to be quite crucial in ensuring the delivery of effective aid. . . . If aid is to be channelled predominantly to those who need it, then a degree of 'failure' must be expected" (Riddell, 2014: 29).

Effective Altruism and the Goals of Philanthrocapitalism

Even if the claim that wealth inequality is per se ethically problematic is left to one side, there are reasons to think that it is difficult to justify having large amounts of surplus resources when others lack the resources to meet even their basic needs. Peter Singer famously argues that even moderately wealthy people should give a sizable proportion of their income to charity based on the claim that "if it is in our power to prevent something very bad from happening, without thereby sacrificing anything morally significant, we ought, morally, to do it" (Singer, 1972: 231). Clearly, many of the evils that global health policy aims to ameliorate – such as suffering and death from avoidable illnesses – would count as very bad occurrences on any plausible reading of the term.

If Singer is correct about this principle (which he thinks should appeal not just to consequentialists but also to a wide range of those who believe that there is a duty to perform "easy rescues"), then giving to meet the basic needs of others without losing anything morally significant is not a matter of supererogation but of duty: "we ought to give the money away, and it is wrong not to do so" (Singer, 1972: 235). Singer intended this argument to have implications for the obligations of people on middle incomes and higher within wealthy countries. But if the argument establishes a duty and a direction in which to donate for those with middle incomes, it would, *a fortiori*, establish such a duty for the ultrarich.

Although there is some room for dispute about how much individuals with different degrees of wealth and income could give away without sacrificing anything morally significant, it seems clear that anyone whose wealth runs into billions could give away more than 95% of their assets without reaching this threshold. Philanthropist Ed Scott, who made his fortune in information technology middleware, explained how he got into philanthropy as follows: "I realized that unless you're a very greedy person, you can't actually spend more than ten or fifteen million dollars on yourself" (Callahan, 2017: 39). Of course, there are some projects that are impossible to pursue without hundreds of millions, if not billions – for example, owning a painting by Leonardo da Vinci. I have a couple of things to say about cases like this. First, it is far from clear that forgoing owning an artwork, while still being able to see it in a public gallery, involves a sacrifice of something morally important. Second, the extremely high prices such items command are a product of absolute scarcity of supply and extreme wealth inequality. Given the vanishingly small number of works by sought-after artists such as Leonardo or Vermeer that remain in private hands

and could potentially be bought, the project of owning such a painting may well be unfeasible even for someone who hangs on to their billions.

Singer also takes away a broader message from his argument: not only is there a requirement to give but a requirement to give *effectively*. Effectiveness is important because the ethical justification for giving does not (or should not) consist of the "warm glow" that givers gain but of the benefits that accrue to others. Givers need to discipline their giving with an impartial standard of effectiveness:

> if an uncle dies of cancer, you might naturally want to raise money for cancer research. Responding to bereavement by trying to make a difference is certainly admirable. But it seems arbitrary to raise money for one specific cause of death rather than any other. . . . By all means, we should harness the sadness we feel at the loss of a loved one in order to make the world a better place. But we should focus that motivation on preventing death and improving lives rather than preventing death and improving lives in one very specific way. Any other decision would be unfair to those whom we could have helped more.
> *(Macaskill, 2015: 42)*

This line of argument raises two important questions. First, is there a duty to give effectively to the extent that one is giving at all, and second, if so, would the duty prevent philanthrocapitalists from making a free choice among the different projects and goals they support in their giving?

Would-be philanthropists might attempt to resist the requirement for effectiveness by falling back on the claim that it is *their money*, so they should have free discretion in deciding whether and, if so, how to give it away. In doing so, they could deny that there is a duty of easy rescue at all. Alternatively, they could argue that while there are *some* duties of easy rescue, what would be required to meet those duties would be much less than the amount they are in fact giving, and anything they give above this threshold is supererogatory. Either way, the key premise would be that *if* an act of philanthropy is supererogatory, then the giver's discretion between what to fund with those resources should be absolute. To put this thought more precisely, the claim is that if someone could have permissibly funded neither A nor B, then it must be permissible for that person to choose to fund A (which creates much less good) over B (which would create much more good). Recent work within the effective altruism literature denies the legitimacy of this inference: Pummer (2016) argues that even if it would be permissible to choose neither A nor B, it does not follow that it would be permissible to choose A over B. On this argument, once one has committed to act in some way (say by donating), and where both options would entail the same personal cost or inconvenience to you, it is not permissible to make the choice that would to do less rather than more good.

To the extent that it is accepted that the ethical justification for giving is benefits to others, then there are strong reasons to think that any such giving needs to be effective if only in the minimal sense that of "using evidence and reason to figure out how to benefit others as much as possible" (Centre for Effective Altruism, 2019). Some within the movement (such as Macaskill [2015]) argue that this commitment should require in addition the more specific requirements that the broad areas chosen for giving should themselves be decided on the basis of reason and evidence, and there should be an overall measure of effectiveness (for a discussion, see Gabriel [2017]). This thicker conception of effective altruism conflicts significantly with the kind of liberty that many philanthrocapitalists would want to have in how they approach their work.[7]

Would a requirement to give effectively entail that philanthrocapitalists behave unethically if they, for example, fund something that they are passionate about – say improved palliative care within their own wealthy country – rather than a much more cost-effective intervention such as vaccine delivery in a much poorer country? It would be too hasty to assume that the philanthropists' priorities and approach have no legitimate role to play within a philanthropic approach that takes effectiveness seriously. What counts as an ethically justifiable use of resources will differ according to one's underlying ethical theory. Some reasonable moral perspectives allow for agent-relative duties and prerogatives; and on this basis, it could be justifiable to devote more resources to improving one's own community or to furthering a particular health cause, even if other potential causes could have created more good. As Lim (2018) argues, this ends up greatly complicating the idea of effectiveness in philanthropy. Perhaps the most that can definitely be required is that

philanthropic foundations should make public the ethical principles on the basis of which they allocate grants so that others can scrutinize and critique both the ethical cogency of the principles and the extent to which their decisions are congruent with those principles.

Philanthrocapitalism in Practice in Global Health

Analysis of the effects of philanthrocapitalism in global health has tended to be fairly polarized between a heroic narrative of millions of lives saved and a darker one of institutional capture and arbitrary power. Recent empirical work suggests that both pictures are too simple. Although it is true that the BMGF set out from a technocratic and largely isolationist approach that led it to disdain international standards and cooperation with international institutions, and also that it has enormous power and influence within global health, it is important to acknowledge how much the organization has changed as it has grown. Two crucial changes, as this section explores, have been the BMGF's increased appreciation of the benefits of working in partnership with governments and other organizations and its move from narrowly targeted technologically led initiatives to an endorsement of the need for structural and social changes. So the overall picture is complex: it is one of an institution with vast power and wealth that is not in its mission and strategy legally accountable to anyone beyond its three trustees but also an organization that holds itself accountable via epidemiological standards and has frequently changed direction as it has discovered more about what has worked. It is important first of all to understand a little of the institutional context within which the BMGF's power has grown.

Changing Patterns of Global Health Governance

Faith among politicians in the public sector's ability to deliver on improving the lives of the worst off has declined as inequality has increased, though whether this reduced faith constitutes the dawning of genuine insight as opposed to acceptance of neoliberal dogma is hotly disputed. Leaving on one side whether this broad shift away from the public sector and toward the private is merited, it is clear that one corollary of it has been a decline in influence since the 1980s for

---

[7] On a practical level, if philanthrocapitalists did not get any say into the causes their foundations supported – except perhaps as a tie-breaker – then we can easily see how this would make giving on a large scale much less attractive.

international bodies such as the World Health Organization (WHO). The high point of the WHO's influence is widely thought to have been the late 1970s, when the Declaration of Alma Ata triumphantly promised Health for All by 2000 and the global smallpox eradication campaign was completed. Since then, a more complex and fragmented environment for global health governance has emerged, in which well-funded international initiatives such as GAVI, the Global Fund to Fight AIDS, Tuberculosis and Malaria, and foundations such as the BMGF operate alongside a diminished WHO (Frenk & Moon, 2013).

The WHO's budget is made up of mixture of assessed contributions, which are levied on individual member states on the basis of the state's wealth and population, as well as voluntary contributions, which come from a variety of sources such as member states, international bodies such as the World Bank, and private foundations such as the BMGF and Rotary International. A key challenge for the WHO has been a reluctance by member states to increase assessed contributions. In 1993, the World Health Assembly voted that assessed contributions should not increase even in nominal terms. Since then, the WHO's core budget thus has been steadily eroded via inflation. Over the same time period, there has been a significant rise in voluntary contributions, nearly all of which are earmarked for particular purposes. The net result has been that while in the 1960s around two-thirds of the WHO's budget came from assessed contributions, by 2017, this figure had fallen 21.4% (Clift & Røttingen, 2018). In 2017, the BMGF contributed $324 million, more than 10% of the WHO's $3.15 billion annual budget, vastly more than any nonstate actor and more than every state except the United States (WHO, 2019).

A central challenge for the WHO is that its stated priorities are significantly different from those that voluntary contributors such as the BMGF wish to support. The WHO's leadership favors structural interventions such as implementation of universal health coverage and action on social determinants of health, whereas "many large donors have given priority to infectious diseases, to the extent that the WHO's polio programme accounted for more than 20% of the programme budget in 2016–17" (Reddy, Mazhar, & Lencucha, 2018: 7). This is clearly a significant problem: as the director-general of the WHO, Dr Tedros Adhanom Ghebreyesus, put it in arguing for why the

WHO needs a budget that allows for much greater flexibility, "No organization can succeed when its budget and priorities are not aligned" (WHO, 2018).

The shift from assessed and voluntary contributions has been argued to undermine the WHO's authority within global health governance while benefiting donors:

> The current dominance of earmarked contributions in effect uses the WHO to channel donor priorities. Donors then benefit from the legitimacy and credibility of a democratic institution while circumventing the very processes that underpin and establish its legitimacy, the point being here that the WHO finds itself in an ever-crowded governance contest and this reality is often beyond the control of the WHO.
>
> *(Reddy, Mazhar, & Lencucha, 2018: 8)*

One central point of contention is whether the rise of the BMGF has, in addition to the benefits that the additional billions of funding for global health projects has brought, caused significant harm by contributing to undermining the WHO's role in global health governance. The BMGF's yearly grants for global health and global development ($3 billion) are now nearly as large as the WHO's entire budget. Separately from this, the BMGF is also the second-largest contributor to the WHO's budget. The BMGF thus wields enormous sway over the governance of global health. Birn and Richter (2018) argue that unlike other bodies that wield similar power, the BMGF has no semblance of democratic accountability because it is ultimately accountable only to its three trustees – Bill and Melinda Gates and Warren Buffett. The rise of the Global Fund, they argue, further contributes to the perception of the BMGF's gain being the WHO's loss. The Global Fund was set up in a structure deliberately parallel to and not controlled by the WHO or the United Nations and has received $2 billion from the BMGF alongside more than $42 billion in contributions from states and private actors and has funded programs in 140 countries. While the WHO and UNAIDS do not have a vote on the Global Fund's board, the BMGF does.

BMGF's Journey from Isolationism to Partnership Working

In its early years, BMGF approached its task like a venture capitalist scouting out investment opportunities – looking for areas that had been neglected, with the aim of getting an outsized return on investment. Feyerskov, who has done much to research the BMGF's history and development, quotes one BMGF senior program officer as follows about these early days: "We didn't care much for what the other guys were doing out there, and picking areas that few were interested in made sure that we could be in the driver's seat" (Feyerskov, 2015: 1104). As part of this mind-set, the BMGF (and Bill Gates in particular) was actively resistant to adopting internationally established norms such as the Millennium Development Goals (MDGs) and was deeply skeptical of the value of health systems strengthening. Bill Gates is reported to have said that he was "vehemently *against* health systems" and that he would "not see a dollar or a cent of my money go to the strengthening of health systems" (Storeng, 2014: 868). His underlying objection seemed to be based on what he saw as a lack of evidence of effectiveness for health systems strengthening and a preference for targeted interventions whose effectiveness could be more easily measured.

 Focusing on targeted interventions while leaving unaddressed the structural determinants of health was not as successful as the BMGF had hoped. Mahajan (2018) provides a useful case study of the shifts in the BMGF's approach in India. In 2002–2003, the BMGF founded Avahan, an initiative for HIV/AIDS prevention in India, with an initial commitments $200 million. Initially, Avahan was isolationist – working neither with the Indian government's National Aids Control Organization nor with the Indian government more broadly. However, as the initial strategy was rolled out and success against benchmarks measured, a need to widen focus became apparent:

> Avahan's programmes initially had worked with the assumption that incisive interventions would lead members of high-risk communities to change their behaviour. For instance, in programmes targeting sex workers, there had been the expectation that peer-led outreach that provided easy access to condoms and educational materials would lead sex workers to modify high-risk behaviour. However, quick change was not easily observed.... [T]here was a whole host of social issues that prevented sex workers from using condoms even when they were fully aware of the dangers of HIV transmission. Information, condoms and conversations, in themselves, did not change behaviour. Avahan developed new insights about high-risk behaviour which led to a focus on questions of violence.... What started out as incisive interventions grew to be more capacious programmes which attempted to address complex social interactions.
>
> *(Mahajan, 2018: 1361–1362)*

 In explanation of Avahan's initial strategy of isolation, the organization cited the urgency of the problem of HIV/AIDS and the need to avoid stifling bureaucracy. One important point of learning was that it had initially framed the problem of HIV prevention much too narrowly and that once the problem was seen broadly enough, it was obvious that it required structural solutions in which government and sex workers would be key stakeholders. Ashok Alexander (2018), who directed the program, writes powerfully about his own change of perspective and the vital contribution of leadership of the sex workers for the project's success.

 The lessons of this and similar programs seem to have hit home. In an important public confirmation of the BMGF's changed approach, Melinda Gates announced in an article in *Science* in 2014 that the foundation had shifted from a "bias toward technological solutions" and now incorporated a "greater appreciation for the social and cultural factors that influence how individuals, communities, and countries develop" (Gates, 2014: 1273). In a further shift, the article signaled that women's empowerment was now a central concern the BMGF, arguing that "we cannot achieve our goals unless we systematically address gender inequalities and meet the specific needs of women and girls in the countries where we work" (Gates, 2014: 1273). In the years since 2014, the BMGF has further increased its commitment to women's empowerment[8] (Gates, 2019).

 Early ethical critiques of the BMGF tended to focus on the combination of the ill-advisedness of taking a narrowly focused and technocratic approach to structural problems, the ways in which the BMGF's use of its power and influence to encourage other actors to adopt technocratic approaches was likely to have baleful effects overall, and also the lack of accountability

---

[8] Fejerskov (2018) examines in much more detail than I can here some of the mechanisms by which the BMGF came to adopt a perspective more similar to that of other key players in global health. One significant influence – particularly as the BMGF expanded after the Warren Buffett donation in 2006 – was what Fejerskov describes as "normative isomorphism," namely that "groups of professionals sharing similar perceptions of appropriate organizational practices gradually entered into the foundation and shaped its approach to the field" (Fejerskov, 2015: 1108).

that comes from the BMGF having only three trustees. However, as we have seen, the fuller picture is more complex. As it has matured, the BMGF has become much closer in approach to existing global health organizations and much keener to work with partners to achieve internationally agreed global health goals. For example, it now runs the Goalkeepers initiative to attempt to keep international progress toward the Sustainable Development Goals (SDGs) on track (Bill & Melinda Gates Foundation, 2018).

Reubi (2018) argues that thinking about the nature of the BMGF's accountability also needs to be more nuanced. Although the organization scores weakly on democratic accountability, it does not follow that the organization acts in a way that is arbitrary and unreasoned. Philanthrocapitalist organizations such as the BMGF and Bloomberg Philanthropies are enthusiasts for data, measurement, and audit. Indeed, the BMGF has invested over $300 million in the Institute for Health Metrics and Evaluation, which publishes yearly global burden-of-disease reports to improve the quality of global health data. Setting goals such as number of lives saved and measuring progress against those goals rigorously, and making much of these data available for others to pore over and critique, create a form of epidemiologic accountability. So while there may be little or no democratic accountability, Reubi (2018: 106) argues that the "reasoned critiques" of global health commentators "can and already have forced philanthropists to listen and change the ways they work."

Conclusion

Philanthrocapitalism has risen against a background of very great, and still rising, global wealth inequality. It is hard to believe that current levels of global wealth inequality are fair, but given the lack of institutions at a global level that will fundamentally alter this, it is reasonable to assume that significant inequalities will continue. Whether philanthrocapitalism should be welcomed depends in large part on what the relevant comparator is. If the alternative is a well-ordered world with much less wealth income inequality, then the answer must be no, but if the alternative is the continuance of great inequality but where ultrawealthy persons spend their money on nothing but conspicuous consumption, then the answer must be yes.

Beyond these obvious points, performing a rigorous ethical analysis of a large-scale philanthrocapitalist endeavor such as the BMGF is complex and challenging. Large-scale organizations not only change norms and practices elsewhere but are also acted on and change themselves, so any such analysis, in order to be convincing, needs to be systemic and diachronic. In the case of the BMGF, the unchanging commitment to data and effectiveness has led over time to a more systemic approach to change and a greater willingness to partner with other organizations, leading even some of those most initially skeptical of its endeavors to reassess its contribution. One crucial question that remains is the extent to which such epidemiologic accountability alone is a good enough substitute for a significant deficit in democratic accountability.

Acknowledgments

Thanks to Sridhar Venkatapuram, and to the editors for helpful comments on an earlier draft.

References

Alexander, A. (2018). *A Stranger Truth: Lessons in Love, Leadership and Courage from India's Sex Workers*. New Delhi: Juggernaut.

Alvaredo, F., Chancel, L., Piketty, T., et al. (2018). *World Inequality Report 2018*. Available at https://wir2018.wid.world/ (accessed April 20, 2019).

Amarante, E. (2018). The perils of philanthrocapitalism. *Maryland Law Review* **78**, 1–72.

Arthur, W. B. (1989). Competing technologies, increasing returns, and lock-in by historical events. *Economic Journal* **99**(394), 116–131.

Beetham, D. (2015). Moving beyond a narrow definition of corruption, in Whyte, D. (ed.), *How Corrupt Is Britain*. London: Pluto Press, pp. 41–46.

Bill & Melinda Gates Foundation (2018). Goalkeepers. Available at www.gatesfoundation.org/goalkeepers (accessed April 20, 2019).

Bill & Melinda Gates Foundation (2019). Foundation Fact Sheet. Available at www.gatesfoundation.org/Who-We-Are/General-Information/Foundation-Factsheet (accessed April 20, 2019).

Birn, A.-E., & Richter, J. (2018). U.S. philanthrocapitalism and the global health agenda: the Rockefeller and Gates foundations, past and present, in Waitzkin, H. (ed.), *Health Care Under the Knife: Moving Beyond Capitalism for Our Health*. New York: New York University Press, pp. 155–173.

Bishop, M. (2006). Survey: the business of giving. *Economist* **378** (8466), 3–14.

Bishop, M., & Green, M. (2008). *Philanthrocapitalism: How the Rich Can Save the World*. New York: Bloomsbury Press.

Bishop, M., & Green, M. (2015). Philanthrocapitalism rising. *Society* **52**(6), 541–548.

Bullough, O. (2018). *Moneyland: Why Thieves and Crooks Now Rule the World and How To Take It Back*. London: Profile Books.

Callahan, D. (2017). *The Givers: Wealth, Power, and Philanthropy in a New Gilded Age*. New York: Alfred A. Knopf.

Carnegie, A. (2017 (first published in 1889)). *The Gospel of Wealth*. New York: Carnegie Corporation of New York. Available at www.carnegie.org/publications/the-gospel-of-wealth (accessed April 20, 2019).

Centre for Effective Altruism (2019). Combining Empathy with Evidence. Available at www.centreforeffectivealtruism.org (accessed April 20, 2019).

Clift, C., & Røttingen, J.-A. (2018). New approaches to WHO financing: the key to better health. *British Medical Journal* **361**, k2218.

Cohen, G. A. (1995). *Self-Ownership, Freedom, and Equality*. Cambridge, UK: Cambridge University Press.

Commission on the Social Determinants of Health (2008). *Closing the Gap in a Generation: Health Equity Through Action on the Social Determinants of Health. Final Report of the Commission on Social Determinants of Health*. Geneva: WHO.

Fejerskov, A. M. (2015). From unconventional to ordinary? The Bill and Melinda Gates Foundation and the homogenizing effects of international development cooperation. *Journal of International Development* **27**(7), 1098–1112.

Fejerskov, A. M. (2018). *The Gates Foundation's Rise to Power: Private Authority in Global Politics*. New York: Routledge.

Forbes.com. (2019). Bill Gates. Available at www .forbes.com/profile/bill-gates/#3705883689f0 (accessed April 20, 2019).

Frenk, J., & Moon, S. (2013). Governance challenges in global health. *New England Journal of Medicine* **368**, 936–942.

Gabriel, I. (2017). Effective altruism and its critics. *Journal of Applied Philosophy* **34**(4), 457–473.

Gates, M. F. (2014). Putting women and girls at the center of development. *Science* **345**(6202), 1273–1275.

Gates, M. F. (2019). *The Moment of Lift: How Empowering Women Changes the World*. New York: Flatiron Books.

Giving Pledge (2019). About the Giving Pledge. Available at https://givingpledge.org/About.aspx (accessed April 20, 2019).

Kilgannon, C. (2018). What's that strange new thing rising in the Hudson River? *New York Times*, December 12. Available at www.nytimes.com/2018/12/0 7/nyregion/pier-55-park-hudson-river.html (accessed April 20, 2019).

King, M. L., Jr. (2010). *Strength to Love*. Minneapolis, MN: Fortress Press.

Lim, C.-M. (2018). Effectiveness and ecumenicity. *Journal of Moral Philosophy* **19**, 1–23.

Macaskill, W. (2015). *Doing Good Better: How Effective Altruism Can Help You Make a Difference*. New York: Gotham Books.

Mahajan, M. (2018). Philanthropy and the nation-state in global health: the Gates Foundation in India. *Global Public Health* **13**(10), 1357–1368.

Mayer, J. (2016). *Dark Money: The Hidden History of the Billionaires Behind the Rise of the Radical Right*. New York: Doubleday Books.

Nozick, R. (1974). *Anarchy, State, and Utopia*. New York: Basic Books.

Oxfam (2019). Public Good or Private Wealth? Available at www.oxfam.org/en/research/public-good-or-private-wealth (accessed April 20, 2019).

Payton, R. L. (1988). *Philanthropy: Voluntary Action for the Public Good*. New York: American Council on Education.

Piketty, T. (2014). *Capital in the Twenty-First Century*. Cambridge, MA: Harvard University Press.

Pummer, T. (2016). Whether and where to give. *Philosophy & Public Affairs* **44**(1), 77–95.

Rawls, J. (1993). *Political Liberalism*. New York: Columbia University Press.

Rawls, J. (2001). *Justice as Fairness: A Restatement*. Cambridge, MA: Harvard University Press.

Reddy, S. K., Mazhar, S., & Lencucha, R. (2018). The financial sustainability of the World Health Organization and the political economy of global health governance: a review of funding proposals. *Globalization and Health* **14**(119), 1–11.

Reich, R. (2018). *Just Giving: Why Philanthropy Is Failing Democracy and How It Can Do Better*. Princeton, NJ: Princeton University Press.

Reubi, D. (2018). Epidemiological accountability: philanthropists, global health and the audit of saving lives. *Economy and Society* **47**(1), 83–110.

Riddell, R. C. (2014). Does foreign aid really work? An updated assessment. Social Science Research Network (online). Available at https://papers.ssrn.com/sol3/papers .cfm?abstract_id=2409847 (accessed April 20, 2019).

Robeyns, I. (2016). Having too much. Social Science Research Network (online). Available at https://papers.ssrn.com/sol3/ papers.cfm?abstract_id=2736094 (accessed April 20, 2019).

Sadeh, J., Tonin, M., & Vlassopoulos, M. (2017). Why give away your wealth? An analysis of the billionaires' view, in Costa-font, J., Macis, M., & Zahn, P. (eds.), *Social Economics: Current and Emerging Avenues*. Cambridge, MA: MIT Press, pp. 61–78.

Scanlon, T. M. (2018). *Why Does Inequality Matter?* Oxford, UK: Oxford University Press.

Sen, A. (1981). *Poverty and Famines: An Essay on Entitlement and Deprivation*. Oxford, UK: Oxford University Press.

Singer, P. (1972). Famine, affluence, and morality. *Philosophy and Public Affairs* **1**(3), 229–243.

Storeng, K. T. (2014). The GAVI Alliance and the "Gates approach" to health system strengthening. *Global Public Health* **9**(8), 865–879.

Wilkinson, R., & Pickett, K. (2009). *The Spirit Level: Why Greater Equality Makes Societies Stronger*. London: Bloomsbury Publishing.

World Health Organization (WHO) (2018). Dialogue with the Director-General. Available at http://apps.who.int/gb/ebwha/pdf_files/EB142/B142_2-en.pdf (accessed April 20, 2019).

World Health Organization (WHO) (2019). WHO Financial and Programmatic Reports. Available at www.who.int/about/finances-accountability/reports/en (accessed April 20, 2019).

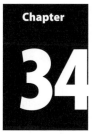

Big Data and Artificial Intelligence for Global Health
Ethical Challenges and Opportunities

Effy Vayena and Agata Ferretti

Introduction

The development of new information technologies has accelerated the pace with which data are collected, stored, and processed. As a result, the term *big data* came to life describing large and disparate data collections. Data at large scale provided a new, important resource on which powerful computational technologies and new analytical capabilities can be deployed to glean various kinds of information. More recently, a new repertoire of methods labeled *artificial intelligence* (AI) has added speed and accuracy in pattern identification and the generation of other inferences from such data. AI-based applications have been accompanied by enormous enthusiasm about the possibilities to solve a variety of problems in all aspects of life. However, most AI-based applications are currently narrow in scope: they are adopted to carry out specific tasks and to solve limited and predetermined problems (Mesko, 2017). For example, natural language processing (NLP) is used to identify keywords and phrases in unstructured texts, whereas the image- and signal-processing type of AI can analyze data produced by motions and sounds. Machine learning (ML) has been, so far, the most successful type of AI. ML is used to perform data mining and to individuate hidden data patterns (Wahl et al., 2018).

The availability of data and AI-powered technologies has ushered us into a new technological epoch. It has also promised to improve our understanding of health and disease and to transform healthcare delivery around the world. Fields such as epidemiology, precision medicine, genetics, oncology, and health-related behavioral sciences have so far made use of big data analytics with promising results (Hamet & Tremblay, 2017). The adoption of electronic health records (EHRs) has generated one main source of medical big data that includes medical records, family history, demographics, and so on. Notably, the

pervasiveness of mobile phones and the internet has enabled the collection of non–strictly biomedical data (Vayena & Gasser, 2016b) such as internet searchers, social media status and hashtags, mobile phone metadata, shopping card purchases, and geolocation information (Hagg et al., 2018). These data can also be used to infer health information. Researchers have argued that merging together data collected from various sources can help overcome the lack of accuracy occurring when using only a single source of data. The promise is that this better and more complete understanding of health and disease will allow both the delivery of more tailored care to individuals and a better picture of what underlines the continuum from health to disease (Wang et al., 2018). We should note that the potential of big data and AI has also been engulfed in hype. Although several successful examples of the immense possibilities have been presented (Bedi et al., 2015; Panch et al., 2019; Rajkomar et al., 2019), the promised transformation of healthcare is yet to come. In addition, both big data and AI uses have raised several ethical questions around privacy, consent, discrimination, and fairness that have not been sufficiently resolved (Mittelstadt & Floridi, 2016; Nuffield Council on Bioethics, 2018). Regulation of digital technologies is in its infancy, and the development of ethical frameworks to address the challenges has not yet been implemented. For example, we are still struggling to determine data access and sharing frameworks that meet ethical requirements.

Despite the many unresolved issues, the continuous growth and diffusion rate of digital health technologies are set to impact low- and middle-income countries (LMICs). In 2018, the World Health Assembly passed a digital health resolution with the aim of encouraging governments to exploit digital health technologies for the provision of better and more affordable care. The latest announcement of reforms by the World Health Organization (WHO) in March 2019 included the establishment of a new Department of Digital Health aiming to harness "the power of digital health and innovation by supporting countries to assess, integrate, regulate and maximize the opportunities of digital technology and artificial intelligence" (WHO, 2019). Other international actors have also called for the utilization of digital technologies to improve health. The United Nations considered the development and deployment of AI-based applications essential to achieve the Sustainable Development Goals (SDGs). Specifically, the UN referred to the use of AI and big data to predict the spread of infectious diseases and to improve the health and well-being of people around the world (United Nations Development Group, 2017). In 2018, the UN specialized agency for information and communication technology (ITU) promoted the "AI for GOOD" summit, which was oriented at identifying practical applications of AI and supporting strategies to reach the SDGs (International Telecommunication Union [ITU], 2018).

In response to global efforts, EHRs and online personal identifier systems have now been introduced in several LMICs. The Indian government, for example, launched in 2010 a biometric identification program that collected health and social data (including EHRs and information on health insurance) of a large-scale population. Currently, there are 1.2 billion Indian people (approximately 90% of the entire Indian population) registered within this system (Singh, 2018). The increasing penetration of mobile phones in LMICs represents a big opportunity to reach and collect data (Steinhubl et al., 2018). This is particularly true for people who, because of economic, social, and cultural barriers, cannot access formalized channels of healthcare (e.g., hospitals), where health data are usually collected (Wyber et al., 2015). The combination of mobile technology and data science and AI provides an additional opportunity to improve primary healthcare services and make them more accessible for those living in LMICs. Philanthropic foundations and corporations have already made substantial investments in this field. For example, the Bill & Melinda Gates Foundation has recently financed the Butterfly Health Network. The aim of this global health project is to create a cheap, handheld, tablet-connected, full-body ultrasound device that computes real-time data. This device is set to overcome the barriers that prevent access to medical imaging and deliver better services to patients living in rural or poor areas (Mobile Health News, 2018). Overall, new digital technologies offer the chance to better target public health intervention, maximizing the effectiveness of the interventions, while reducing healthcare expenditures. In March 2016, Google partnered with UNICEF to combat the Zika virus, providing a forecast of Zika outbreaks through the analysis of water usage and peoples' travel pattern data. More recently, IBM has initiated a collaboration with the South African government to improve healthcare access using big data and AI (IBM, 2017).

This strong state and corporate sector's interest in developing and implementing digital health solutions attests to digital technologies potential impact on global health. However, this potential has also raised a number of thorny ethical challenges around privacy, bias discrimination, benefit sharing, and trust. These issues have mostly been discussed in lay and scholarly work stemming from high-income countries and focusing on that context. There is limited academic literature focusing on the implications of these new technologies for LMICs or considering the perspectives of populations residing in them. The ethics of big data and AI for global health has received limited attention, although these are issues that will be crucial in the successful implementation of digital technologies in LMICs (Schwalbe & Wahl, 2020). In this chapter, we attempt to fill some of this gap by discussing the potential of digital technologies and AI to improve global health and by exploring the ethical challenges such applications are raising. We conclude with recommendations about how some of these challenges can be addressed to ensure the promotion of justice in global health.

Opportunities for Improving Global Health

Health Service Delivery and Clinical Care

The predictive power of AI has already been used in the field of medical imaging to detect diseases such as pneumonia and breast cancer (Wang et al., 2016; Rajpurkar et al., 2017), in the field of neurology and psychiatry to predict and prevent psychotic episodes (Kim et al., 2018), and in the field of cardiology to reveal patterns of heartbeats and diagnose coronary heart diseases (Alsharqi et al., 2018). The main advantage of predicting disease risks via new technologies is to anticipate care interventions. Early interventions can have a significant impact in LMICs by both saving lives and also reducing healthcare costs that are typically higher at advanced stages of disease (Barnett et al., 2014). In LMICs, new portable devices can leverage AI technology to help healthcare providers to accurately diagnose diseases (Mathenge, 2019). For example, in Nigeria, AI has been used in combination with signal processing and cloud computing to predict child asphyxia in newborn children. The technology installed on a portable device can recognize the patterns of asphyxiating crisis in infants from their way of crying and prevent the condition from deteriorating (Onu, 2014). Researchers working in Sub-Saharan Africa reported a new AI-based portable diagnostic system that can help physicians diagnose malaria with an accuracy of 91% (Oliveira et al., 2017). Similarly, in China, an internet health company developed a portable all-in-one diagnostic station capable of running 11 medical tests (including blood test, blood analysis, and electrocardiograph). This machine directly uploads online results and medical records to an AI-based data analysis system to generate diagnoses (Guo & Li, 2018).

Another application with potential for LMICs is in the area of cognitive computer systems that can be accessed by healthcare providers to support them in the diagnosis and treatment of disease. For example, cognitive computer systems (provided by IBM Watson) have helped physicians in India, China, and Thailand to provide diagnoses and best treatments to oncology patients (Coccoli & Maresca, 2018). In LMICs, beyond big urban centers, most healthcare is delivered by community health workers (CHWs) or pharmacists. They may lack sufficient knowledge or up-to-date training, but access to computerized systems that provide the latest knowledge or best practice in the context of the local environment can improve care delivery and health outcomes (Adepoju et al., 2017).

Socioeconomic, geographic, or cultural barriers can limit access to primary healthcare services for people living in LMICs. Mobile health (mHealth) is a tool that can extend healthcare access by providing direct care (e.g., with chatbots or telehealth) while also increasing medical literacy in the general population (Steinhubl et al., 2018). Most mHealth available today comes in the form of health apps. These apps can facilitate diagnoses and support clinical decision

making, as in the case of *ADA Health* or *Babylon Health* (ADA, 2019; Babylon, 2019). In high-income countries, these apps suggest tailored-to-the-user healthy lifestyles, track fitness progress, and offer meditation courses. Instead, in LMICs, mHealth mainly focuses on primary care assistance. For example, *Matibabu* is a smartphone app that in Uganda helps healthcare workers to diagnose malaria without a blood sample (Matibabu, 2018). And *Uamuzi Bora* is an EHR system used by hospitals in Kenya to track people with HIV and improve healthcare support (Uamuzi Bora, 2019). Medical departments in LMICs are also using mHealth to monitor and train their medical students remotely. This is the case for *VulaMobile* in South Africa. This app is used not only to train young doctors but also to connect healthcare workers in the field with on-call specialists in medical centers to discuss treatment options for patients (Vula, 2016).

Such applications can reduce demands on healthcare professionals and family caregivers while improving healthcare service delivery. Moreover, mHealth, which relies on big data – and sometimes on AI systems – can offer personalized health assessment and real-time care, even in the absence of healthcare specialists (Latif et al., 2017). This characteristic makes its adoption extremely suitable in LMICs, where there is a shortage of physicians and where self-care is often the primary form of healthcare (Wilton Park, 2018). *MedMee* is an example of a self-care mHealth device. This Pakistani mobile software not only allows searching for pharmacies near a patient's home but also permits ordering medications (which are directly delivered to the patient's home) and receiving an interacting explanation through a chatbot about how to take the medicine (MedMee, 2019). Similarly, the *Child Growth Monitor* is an Indian app that helps parents to identify malnutrition in their children through a three-dimensional scan and if necessary, automatically contact health professionals (Child Growth Monitor, 2018).

Public Health

Over the last two decades, big data and AI have been used to model, forecast, and monitor vector-borne disease outbreaks and spreading (Hornyak, 2017; O'Shea, 2017). In LMICs, big data sources outside the healthcare system have been used increasingly for health-related purposes. For example, remote sensing techniques and satellite images contributed to better identifying and fighting vector-borne diseases in metropolitan areas of Argentina. Open-source data have been used by platforms such as *ProMED-mail, Ushahidi, HealthMap*, and *EpiCore* to automatically track disease outbreaks and provide population health surveillance (Smolinski et al., 2017).

The field of digital epidemiology is growing fast (Salathe et al., 2012). AI-based applications are increasingly analyzing content posted online in the form of Twitter hashtags, Facebook messages, Amazon queries, Wikipedia searches, and so on for the purpose of public health surveillance. All the traces that internet users leave while interacting with the web shape their *digital phenotype* (Jain et al., 2015). The concept of digital phenotype presumes that not only the biological processes but also the daily interactions that people have with digital technologies describe and shape their health status. In other words, all the data – biological and not – that can be collected about or from a person can contribute to delineate his or her health profile (Vayena & Madoff, 2018). It follows that analyzing these data can help public health authorities and specialists understand disease patterns and trajectories, outbreaks, and epidemics. Since 2009, Google has used delocalized search query data as early-warning signals to predict influenza pandemics. Despite not being consistently successful (Butler, 2013), this Google program recently helped to predict a dengue fever outbreak in Venezuela (Strauss et al., 2017).

To reach public health goals, researchers and governments are increasingly deploying new available technologies, such as NLP. Researchers in Uganda used this technique to screen Facebook data to determine real-time attitudes concerning contraception and pregnancy levels among teenagers (Global Pulse, 2014a). Similarly, in Indonesia, researchers analyzed tweets to identify the public perception toward vaccines and immunization, including concerns related to religious issues, disease outbreaks, and vaccine side effects (Global Pulse, 2014b).

In *participatory disease surveillance* (Wójcik et al., 2014), digital disease detection increasingly relies on self-reported symptoms. Symptoms (e.g., headache, fever, vomiting) are provided by the users of mobile phones and are further analyzed by an algorithm. Thanks to the widespread use of mobile phones, today largely also accessible in LMICs, syndromic and case-based surveillance is also progressively guaranteed in rural and less accessible areas of the planet (Flahault et al., 2017). Some influenza-focused detective systems include *Salud Boricua* in Puerto Rico and *DoctorMe* in Thailand (Smolinski et al., 2017). *AfyaData*, a participatory event-based system in Tanzania, relies on trained volunteers in local communities to report suspected cases of dengue fever, contaminated water sources, and disease outbreaks in livestock (Karimuribo et al., 2017).

Another application of big data and AI is in health management. National governments have increasingly introduced data science techniques to better allocate available resources and target useful public health interventions. Currently, AI-based management technologies can identify high-cost patients, adverse drugs events, treatment optimizations, and possible hospital readmissions, therefore allowing for better and more cost-efficiency planning (Cinaroglu, 2019). Cost efficiency is a crucial factor, particularly in LMICs. For this reason, countries such as Pakistan and Malaysia have introduced EHRs in public hospitals. Their objective is to simplify the provision of patient monitoring services (e.g., immunization procedures and referral systems), which heavily rely on patient historical data (Khan et al., 2012; Ariffin et al., 2018). Time is another scarce resource for healthcare providers in LMICs. To allow public health improvements and extend access to healthcare, LMICs need to optimize CHW scheduling. Because of the shortage of practicing physicians, CHWs are tasked with visiting several patients per day to deliver the treatments (despite the long distance that might separate them). Therefore, CHWs often face the issue of how to prioritize patients while providing cost-effective services in the limited time available. Big data analytics and AI can contribute to overcome this problem (Wahl et al., 2018). For example, AI technology can manage a triage system that automatically favors acute cases of illness (Kim et al., 2018).

Challenges in Harnessing the Potential of Big Data and AI in Global Health

Digital Divide

One major challenge in the development and implementation of digital tools in LMICs remains the so-called digital divide. While internet connectivity is improving around the world, technical infrastructures, data storage, and computational power are not equitably distributed. LMICs still face difficulties in securing stable access to electricity and internet connectivity, as well as in providing information technology (IT) services, online platforms, and data storage systems (Wahl et al., 2018). This state of affairs poses challenges for all aspects of digital health, including data collection and analysis. Even mHealth applications that can work offline and synchronize with online databases when the bandwidth connection is strong enough require stable IT infrastructures if they are to function reliably (Cinaroglu, 2019). Although progress has been made over the years, so has the dependence of digital devices on connectivity. Connectivity still remains a problem for many countries, limiting what services users can access. If such infrastructural problems remain unresolved, the potential of digital health cannot be harnessed.

Another aspect of the same problem relates to the actual data collected in some LMICs. Often data are poor in quality and not interoperable, which make them less reliable and usable (Carrell et al., 2017). Curation of not-optimized data requires a significant standardization effort. Preparing data to be computed is a costly activity, in particular when the data are merged from different sources. Although many countries are slowly introducing EHRs, many hospitals in LMICs still maintain hand-written medical records (in local dialects), and they do not refer to standardized medical dictionaries (Wahl et al., 2018). These practices make the implementation of AI technologies that rely on big data extremely challenging (Muinga et al., 2018).

The lack of harmonized approaches to data collection and standardization is also associated with low digital literacy. In LMICs, healthcare providers usually have limited exposure to digital health systems and lack training. Research shows that misinformation concerning data processing is a notable barrier to the implementation and use of digital technologies for healthcare (Olayinka et al., 2017). Therefore, to implement AI-based applications might be expensive if not disadvantageous in contexts where there is lack of storage and computational capacity, as well as limited technical literacy among healthcare providers.

Privacy and Data Security

Health data are sensitive and in need of privacy protections. Securing privacy, however, is a wicked problem (Ienca et al., 2018). First, for the purposes of big data analytics, health-related data could be accessed by multiple users (e.g., health practitioners, hospital staff, researchers, service providers, and nonstate actors), which increases the risk of data leakage or potential misuse (Vayena & Madoff, 2018). Second, the computational power of AI allows for the merging and analysis of data for various purposes that are not foreseen when data were obtained, and patients may have consented only to specific uses of their data (Altman et al., 2018). Therefore, traditional consent processes might not be an adequate tool to inform patients about the risks and benefits that arise from future data uses (Vayena & Gasser, 2016a). Third, big data analytics link disparate data, increasing the risk of reidentification, despite privacy protection measures applied on single data types (Lacroix, 2019). Among middle-income countries, Mexico, the Philippines, and South Africa have already introduced data monitoring mechanisms to protect privacy and grant legal redress to their citizens. Nevertheless, the majority of LMICs still lack advanced privacy regulation and guidance about data anonymization. In these countries, privacy and data management issues arise particularly in relation to the implementation and use of EHRs. To secure EHRs, a robust software for password protection might not be sufficient, and servers must also be physically secured by trained staff. In the absence of strong governance that guarantees the protection of data and minimizes the risk to privacy, breaches that threaten the privacy of health data persist. We should note that even in high-income countries, the issue of data privacy remains a hard problem to tackle. There are frequent reports about misuses of health data and their unauthorized access, and health data in big hospitals not only have been hacked but also have become subject to ransomware (Gordon et al., 2017; Smith et al., 2016).

Privacy loss can have severe implications for individuals and communities anywhere in world. In the sensitive area of health, privacy loss entails revelations about one's health status (e.g., HIV status, mental health status). Many diseases are still a source of stigmatization and discrimination in many parts of the world, leaving those who suffer from them vulnerable to repercussion such as unemployment, social exclusion, and even violence (Hosein & Martin, 2010). Therefore, access to care through digital technology or use of big data to improve healthcare systems can result in serious and tangible harms if effective privacy protection and antidiscrimination legislation are not in place. What is more, if people are concerned about their privacy on matters of health, they might hesitate using digital health or might not seek care altogether to avoid the collection of their data. Mistrust of healthcare delivery is detrimental to improving public health and can have catastrophic effects on communities.

Bias

Big data analytics and AI require large quantities of good-quality and easy-to-digitize data sources. In many LMICs, where even collecting data about births and deaths is still not routine, it is all the more burdensome to collect a broad spectrum of health-related data (Guo & Li, 2018). Often environmental, social, and economic barriers make it difficult to reach the most vulnerable groups. Such groups may not be seeking care in places where data are collected. The paucity of data sources available in LMICs might indirectly affect the digital tools that were built on such limited data sets. First, the scarce representativeness of collected data may render the results of data analysis not generalizable. Second, in the case of ML-enabled tools, lack of training data sets from the context in which the digital tools will be used can lead to the development of biased tools. It is very likely for these tools to produce incorrect outputs if they have not captured the context-specific physical, cultural, or socioeconomic factors (Rajkomar et al., 2019). Using AI-based applications that have been developed with data from other populations and healthcare systems will be generally less applicable to certain LMIC contexts. The data sets that are used in high-income countries are notorious for their lack of diversity, and concerns have been raised about their applicability even in their home countries. Perhaps the most well-documented case is genomic data that are almost exclusively composed from the genomes of white people, making the findings about pathogenic or harmless variants less applicable to genetically diverse populations (Bentley et al., 2017). Third, beyond genetic data, however, if poorly representative data sets (e.g., including fewer women, ethnic minorities, and low-income groups) are used to develop digital tools, there is a risk that such tools may perpetuate existing prejudices. Biased tools can lead to further exacerbation of existing disparities in healthcare (Popejoy & Fullerton, 2016). Consider, for example, that very disadvantaged population groups may respond badly to a certain healthcare intervention because of poor access to care, low literacy, and so on. If an algorithm does not account for such reasons

and simply associates this group with a bad response, it might suggest avoiding offering such an intervention to people of this group in the first place (Blasimme & Vayena, 2019). This type of bias risks worsening health disparities instead of improving the health of those most in need.

Some AI systems that are based on ML technology are opaque, making it hard to detect embedded biases (Ferretti et al., 2018). Opacity also adds difficulty in the validation of such algorithms. This has led to concerns about the clinical validation of algorithms that are to be used in the clinical setting and some hesitation on the part of clinicians about the extent to which they can trust such systems (Verghese et al., 2018). While this might be partly motivated by uncertainty about liability in high-income countries, the point remains relevant for LMICs too. The question is whether AI-enabled systems that are used in patient care can be trusted to deliver on the promise of providing better and more affordable care. For these reasons, it is paramount that evidence is generated to show that bias and discrimination are not built into the data sets used to train AI models (Mathenge, 2019). Furthermore, it is important to consider thoroughly the applicability of data and AI-enabled technologies across countries. Technical and clinical validations are crucial issues in AI for global health, and context-adapted standards are a necessary condition for the responsible clinical innovation.

Fair Distribution of Benefits

The advancement and progress of digital tools are predicated on access to data. As a result, there is ongoing interest in the generation and acquisition of data. The current models of health research include not only health data from hospitals and healthcare centers but also data from a variety of sources, which means that a number of actors are in possession of those data. For example, mobile devices and apps that record daily behaviors are an important source of data. Companies such as Facebook, Google, Amazon, and the like possess tremendous amounts of data that can be mined for health-related purposes. For example, in the United States, Facebook has released an algorithm for suicide prevention on its platform that mines text posted by users to detect alarming signals (Coppersmith et al., 2018). Once these signals are picked up, messages with helpful content are sent to the user at risk or, in some cases, law enforcement services are alerted. This example is emblematic of the new roles gradually being taken on by actors who were not part of the health ecosystem. In LMICs, especially in those with serious limitations in the delivery of healthcare, these new, powerful actors can play important roles. The fact that technology companies can continuously collect data allows them to develop digital tools (e.g., digital health tools) from which they are likely to benefit. This raises the question of what kinds of obligations they may have to groups and populations in need of such technology and from whom the data were derived in the first place.

If there is benefit to be gained from access to data, the question is how this benefit ought to be distributed (Vayena et al., 2018). Does the benefit belong only to those collecting the data and refining their technology so that they can monetize them? Or should those from whom the data have been sourced share the benefit, for example, in the form of a benefit that is meaningful to them, such as free use of a validated digital health tool? If companies are able to freely mine resources, in this case the resources of data from a country's population, what does the company owe to the population of the country? When similar issues were raised in the context of collecting and mining genetic data from populations around the world, a debate emerged on genetic sovereignty and the rights of nations and population groups to control the uses of their genetics. We have not yet had a discussion on digital sovereignty. So far the concept of digital sovereignty has been used with reference to an individual's sovereignty over his or her personal data (Sachverständigenrat für Verbraucherfragen, 2017). However, we should entertain the question of the digital sovereignty of nations. And if we are in favor of digital sovereignty, what is the role of the state in protecting the data of its nationals? To what extent must the state negotiate fair access to data and distribution of benefits when such a resource is used? The current model of negotiating benefits with data-collecting companies is between the companies and the individual. This is essentially the all-or-nothing option, where data are collected, some service may or may not be provided to individual users, and the perpetual use of data is authorized.

The emergence of mHealth and other digital technologies has been accompanied by a rhetoric of empowerment of individuals. It is true that if people are given the opportunity to use safe and effective digital health technologies, they can improve their health. However, this model of empowerment is often predicated on individuals being constantly under surveillance and actively contributing their data. If this is the condition of empowerment, one should consider two further issues. First, as people are tasked with increased responsibility for their own health, one should be concerned about whether this trend may also enable healthcare systems to limit their responsibilities toward the community. Second, one should be concerned about whether the increased individual responsibility will leave behind vulnerable groups or those who are ill-equipped to use technological solutions to improve their health because of poor digital literacy or old age (Vayena & Madoff, 2018). This matter is relevant irrespective of the country, but we consider it to be more significant for countries where larger population segments may fall into the preceding categories of vulnerability.

Accountability and Governance

The nature of the ethical issues raised by big data and AI is complex and multifaceted. Regulation on privacy, health research, and market authorization of medical devices has mostly been designed for analogue applications. Attempts to develop digital governance frameworks, however, are in the works, with the aim of addressing some of the complex issues that we discussed. For example, the recently implemented General Data Protection Regulation (GDPR) in the European Union entails provisions attempting to give individuals greater control over EU data and increasing the accountability and responsibility of data collectors and processors (Information Commissioner's Office, 2018). In the United States, the Food and Drug Administration (FDA) has introduced a number of programs with the aim of reviewing and authorizing the use of digital medical devices. In the near future, we will likely see more regulatory developments that will attempt to strike a good balance between promoting safe and effective digital health innovation and protecting the rights of individuals and communities. Emerging regulation and ethical frameworks highlight the importance of accountability in ensuring that this balance can be achieved. The complexity of the data systems we develop, coupled with the immense possibilities they allow and inevitably with the many interests to which they cater, might create opaque structures. Clear accountability mechanisms and processes will be crucial in enabling the many actors of these complex systems to act responsibly to meet ethical requirements. It should be noted, however, amid these growing digital opportunities that appropriate ethical frameworks for responsible data processing and responsible AI are still in development. Data governance models based on ethical principles are necessary for the right kind of progress in digital health.

At this point, most of the effort in developing ethical principles and governance approaches comes from high-income countries potentially also only focusing on what concerns high-income settings. Furthermore, there is still no concerted global effort devoted to data governance for global health. The closest initiative that is applicable to global health is the nine principles for digital development (Principles for Digital Development, 2017) issued by a group of institutions, namely the Bill & Melinda Gates Foundation, the Swedish International Development Agency (SIDA), the UN's Children's Fund (UNICEF), the UN Development Program (UNDP), the World Bank, the US Agency for International Development (USAID), and the WHO. These principles are a mix of ethical requirements (e.g., sustainability and respect for privacy) and broader good practice requirements (e.g., use of open standards, open source, codesign with users, etc.). Another global effort in terms of data, but only confined to genomic data and focused on data sharing, is the Global Alliance for Genomics and Health ethical framework. This framework is guided explicitly by the human rights to privacy, nondiscrimination, and procedural fairness (Knoppers, 2014).

Conclusion

Big data and digital technologies hold great promise to improve global health. In this chapter, we have given some examples of the potential, and we have discussed the ethical challenges that the development and implementation of such technologies are raising. Future developments should ensure that these ethical challenges are addressed. The overall goal of health technology is not the technology itself but the achievement of just global health. Any technology has to be developed and used in ways that contribute to the main global health goals, for example, achievement of universal healthcare. The major contribution of the digital revolution is not going to be in the improvement of services among those who already enjoy good healthcare. The real need for justice lies in improving the conditions of those who justifiably demand access to basic and fundamental healthcare services.

The enthusiasm about the digital revolution should ignite our moral imagination. In 2005, Benatar argued that the missing piece in global health action is our lack of moral imagination, and he issued a call for all to use this moral imagination to fill the many gaps in global health (Benatar, 2005). Today we have more technological and informational tools that can elicit global action. Current technologies open new possibilities that were unthinkable even 10 years ago. It is time to reissue this call and invite the many actors in the digital world to imagine and act. To do so, it is crucial to give voice to people in LMICs who have already incorporated digital technologies into their lives in ways that might differ from those in the high-income countries. Citizens of LMICs might have different expectations and possibly different needs that technology can serve. It is crucial to listen to people's concerns about new technologies. It is also of paramount importance to develop digital technologies for the priority needs in local contexts. By simply transporting technologies related to locally significant health problems to other parts of the globe might not bring about global health progress. Furthermore, It is necessary for new digital technologies to become integrated into healthcare systems in order strengthen these. Because digital technologies are distributed and individuals can use them outside standard healthcare facilities, efforts for good-quality healthcare provision should be increased. Finally, given the rapid progress in the digital space, success in global health requires the active involvement of many more stakeholders than ever before. Many powerful forces in the private sector hold data and knowledge. Their role in global health should be defined within ethical frameworks that can guide the development and success of digital technology in global health.

Ethical and governance issues have not been sufficiently addressed in the current global health literature or in practice. A global effort is urgently needed to ensure that the digital revolution can promote global health in alignment with ethical principles and by including all stakeholders.

Acknowledgment

This paper has benefited from discussions with Professor Jennifer Gibson.

References

ADA (2019). Our Global Health Initiative (online). Available at https://ada.com/global-health-initiative/ (accessed April 24, 2019).

Adepoju, I.-O. O., Albersen, B. J. A., De Brouwere, V., et al. (2017). mHealth for clinical decision-making in Sub-Saharan Africa: a scoping review. *JMIR mHealth and uHealth* **5**(3), e38.

Alsharqi, M., Woodward, W., Mumith, J., et al. (2018). Artificial intelligence and echocardiography. *Echo Research and Practice* **5**(4), R115–R125.

Altman, M., Wood, A. B., O'Brien, D., & Gasser, U. (2018). Practical approaches to big data privacy over time. *International Data Privacy Law* **8**(1), 29–51.

Ariffin, N. A., Ismail, A., Kadir, I. K. A., & Kamal, J. I. A. (2018). Implementation of electronic medical records in developing countries: challenges and barriers. *Development* **7**(3), 187–199.

Babylon (2019). Babylon Health (online). Available at www.babylonhealth.com/ (accessed April 24, 2019).

Barnett, J. H., Lewis, L., Blackwell, A. D., & Taylor, M. (2014). Early intervention in Alzheimer's disease: a health economic study of the effects of diagnostic timing. *BMC neurology* **14**(1), 101.

Bedi, G., Carrillo, F., Cecchi, G. A., et al. (2015). Automated analysis of free speech predicts psychosis onset in high-risk youths. *NPJ Schizophrenia* **1**, 15030.

Benatar, S. R. (2005). Moral imagination: the missing component in global health. *PLoS Medicine* **2**(12), e400.

Bentley, A. R., Callier, S., & Rotimi, C. N. (2017). Diversity and inclusion in genomic research: why the uneven progress? *Journal of Community Genetics* **8**(4), 255–266.

Blasimme, A., & Vayena, E. (2019). The Ethics of AI in Biomedical Research, Patient Care and Public Health (online). Available at https://papers.ssrn.com/sol3/papers.cfm?abstract_id=3368756 (accessed April 26, 2019).

Butler, D. (2013). When Google got flu wrong. *Nature News* **494**(7436), 155–156.

Carrell, D. S., Schoen, R. E., Leffler, D. A., et al. (2017). Challenges in adapting existing clinical natural language processing systems to multiple, diverse health care settings. *Journal of the American Medical Informatics Association* **24**(5), 986–991.

Child Growth Monitor (2018). Child Growth Monitor (online). Available at https://childgrowthmonitor.org/ (accessed April 24, 2019).

Cinaroglu, S. (2019). Big data to improve public health in low-and middle-income countries: big public health data in LMICs, in Evans, G. W., Biles, W. E., & Ki-Hwan, G. B. (eds.), *Analytics, Operations, and Strategic Decision Making in the Public Sector*. Hershey, PA: IGI Global, pp. 88–110.

Coccoli, M., & Maresca, P. (2018). Adopting cognitive computing solutions in healthcare. *Journal of e-Learning and Knowledge Society* **14**(1), 57–69.

Coppersmith, G., Leary, R., Crutchley, P., & Fine, A. (2018). Natural language processing of social media as screening for suicide risk. *Biomedical Informatics Insights* **10**, 1–11.

Ferretti, A., Schneider, M., & Blasimme, A. (2018). Machine learning in medicine: opening the new data protection black box. *European Data Protection Law Review* **4**(3), 320–332.

Flahault, A., Geissbuhler, A., Guessous, I., et al. (2017). Precision global health in the digital age. *Swiss Medical Weekly* **147**, w14423.

Global Pulse (2014a). Analyzing attitudes towards contraception and teenage pregnancy using social data (online). Available at www.unglobalpulse.org/projects/UN FPA-social-data (accessed March 23, 2019).

Global Pulse (2014b). Understanding public perceptions of immunizartion using social media (online). Available at www.unglobalpulse.org/projects/immunisation-parent-perceptions (accessed March 23, 2019).

Gordon, W. J., Fairhall, A., & Landman, A. (2017). Threats to information security: public health implications. *New England Journal of Medicine* **377**(8), 707–709.

Guo, J., & Li, B. (2018). The application of medical artificial intelligence technology in rural areas of developing countries. *Health Equity* **2**(1), 174–181.

Hagg, E., Dahinten, V. S., & Currie, L. M. (2018). The emerging use of social media for health-related purposes in low and middle-income countries: a scoping review. *International Journal of Medical Informatics* **115**, 92–105.

Hamet, P., & Tremblay, J. (2017). Artificial intelligence in medicine. *Metabolism* **69**, S36–S40.

Hornyak, T. (2017). Mapping dengue fever hazard with machine learning. *Eos* **98**. https://doi.org/10.1029/2017EO076019.

Hosein, G., & Martin, A. (2010). Electronic health privacy and security in developing countries and humanitarian operations. London School of Economics and Political Sciences, pp. 1–28. Available at http://personal.lse.ac.uk/martinak/eHealth.pdf.

IBM (2017). IBM's African scientists look to tackle the continent's pressing healthcare challenges with AI (online). Available at www.ibm.com/blogs/research/2017/11/ibms-african-scientists-look-tackle-continents-pressing-healthcare-challenges-ai/ (accessed April 24, 2019).

Ienca, M., Ferretti, A., Hurst, S., et al. (2018). Considerations for ethics review of big data health research: a scoping review. *PloS One* **13**(10), e0204937.

Information Commissioner's Office (2018). Guide to the General Data Protection Regulation (GDPR) (online). Available at https://ico.org.uk/media/for-organisations/gui

de-to-the-general-data-protection-regulation-gdpr-1–0.pdf (accessed April 26, 2019).

International Telecommunication Union (ITU) (2018). AI for Good: Global Summit Report (online). Available at www .itu.int/en/itu-t/ai/documents/report/ai_for_good_global_ summit_report_2017.pdf (accessed April 24, 2019).

Jain, S. H., Powers, B. W., Hawkins, J. B., & Brownstein, J. S. (2015). The digital phenotype. *Nature Biotechnology* **33**(5), 462–463.

Karimuribo, E. D., Mutagahywa, E., Sindato, C., et al. (2017). A smartphone app (AfyaData) for innovative one health disease surveillance from community to national levels in Africa: intervention in disease surveillance. *JMIR Public Health and Surveillance* **3**(4), e94.

Khan, S. Z., Shahid, Z., Hedstrom, K., & Andersson, A. (2012). Hopes and fears in implementation of electronic health records in Bangladesh. *Electronic Journal of Information Systems in Developing Countries* **54**(1), 1–18.

Kim, D., You, S., So, S., et al. (2018). A data-driven artificial intelligence model for remote triage in the prehospital environment. *PloS One* **13**(10), e0206006.

Kim, S. S., Dohler, M., & Dasgupta, P. (2018). The Internet of Skills: use of fifth-generation telecommunications, haptics and artificial intelligence in robotic surgery. *BJU International* **122**(3), 356–358.

Knoppers, B. M. (2014). Framework for responsible sharing of genomic and health-related data. *HUGO Journal* 8, 3. ht tps://doi.org/10.1186/s11568-014-0003-1.

Lacroix, P. (2019). Big data privacy and ethical challenges, in Househ, M., Kushniruk, A. W., & Borycki, E. M. (eds.), *Big Data, Big Challenges: A Healthcare Perspective.* New York: Springer, pp. 101–111.

Latif, S., Rana, R., Qadir, J., et al. (2017). Mobile health in the developing world: review of literature and lessons from a case study. *IEEE Access* 5, 11540–11556.

Mathenge, W. C. (2019). Artificial intelligence for diabetic retinopathy screening in Africa. *Lancet Digital Health* **1**(1), e6–e7.

Matibabu (2018). *Matababu* (online). Available at www .matibabu.io/ (accessed April 24, 2019).

MedMee (2019). *MedMee* (online). Available at https://me dmee.co/ (accessed April 24, 2019).

Mesko, B. (2017). The role of artificial intelligence in precision medicine. *Expert Review of Precision Medicine and Drug Development* **2**(5), 239–241. DOI:10.1080/23808993 .2017.1380516.

Mittelstadt, B. D., & Floridi, L. (2016). The ethics of big data: current and foreseeable issues in biomedical contexts. *Science and Engineering Ethics* **22**(2), 303–341.

Mobile Health News (2018). Butterfly Health Network gets $250 m for low-cost smartphone-connected ultrasound (online). Available at www.mobihealthnews.com/content/b

utterfly-health-network-gets-250m-low-cost-smartphone-connected-ultrasound (accessed April 24, 2019).

Muinga, N., Magare, S., Monda, J., et al. (2018). Implementing an open source electronic health record system in Kenyan health care facilities: case study. *JMIR Medical Informatics* **6**(2), e22.

Nuffield Council on Bioethics (2018). Artificial intelligence (AI) in healthcare and research (online). Available at http:// nuffieldbioethics.org/wp-content/uploads/Artificial-Intelligence-AI-in-healthcare-and-research.pdf (accessed April 24, 2019).

O'Shea, J. (2017). Digital disease detection: a systematic review of event-based internet biosurveillance systems. *International Journal of Medical Informatics* **101**, 15–22.

Olayinka, O., Kekeh, M., Sheth-Chandra, M., & Akpinar-Elci, M. (2017). Big data knowledge in global health education. *Annals of Global Health.* https://doi.org/10.1016 /j.aogh.2017.09.005.

Oliveira, A. D., Prats, C., Espasa, M., et al. (2017). The malaria system microApp: a new, mobile device-based tool for malaria diagnosis. *JMIR Research Protocols* **6**(4), e70.

Onu, C. C. (2014). *Harnessing Infant Cry for Swift, Cost-Effective Diagnosis of Perinatal Asphyxia in Low-Resource Settings,* trans. IEEE, pp. 1–4.

Panch, T., Pearson-Stuttard, J., Greaves, F., & Atun, R. (2019). Artificial intelligence: opportunities and risks for public health. *Lancet Digital Health* **1**(1), e13–e14.

Popejoy, A. B., & Fullerton, S. M. (2016). Genomics is failing on diversity. *Nature News* **538**(7624), 161–164.

Principles for Digital Development (2017). Principles for Digital Development (online). Available at https://digital principles.org/about/ (accessed May 3, 2019).

Rajkomar, A., Dean, J., & Kohane, I. (2019). Machine learning in medicine. *New England Journal of Medicine* **380** (14), 1347–1358.

Rajpurkar, P., Irvin, J., Zhu, K., et al. (2017). Chexnet: radiologist-level pneumonia detection on chest x-rays with deep learning. arXiv preprint arXiv:1711.05225.

Sachverständigenrat für Verbraucherfragen (2017). Digital Sovereignty (online). Available at www.svr-verbraucherfragen.de/wp-content/uploads/English-Version.pdf (accessed May 1, 2019).

Salathe, M., Bengtsson, L., Bodnar, T. J., et al. (2012). Digital epidemiology. *PLoS Computational Biology* **8**(7), e1002616.

Schwalbe, N., & Wahl, B. (2020). Artificial intelligence and the future of global health. *Lancet* **395**(10236), 1579–1586. https://doi.org/10.1016/S0140-6736(20)30226-9.

Singh, S. (2018). Understanding Aadhaar: the unique identification authority of India and its challenges. *Human Rights Defender* **27**, 21–24.

Smith, R. J., Grande, D., and Merchant, R. M. (2016). Transforming scientific inquiry: tapping into digital data by building a culture of transparency and consent. *Academic Medicine: Journal of the Association of American Medical Colleges* **91**(4), 469–472.

Smolinski, M. S., Crawley, A. W., Olsen, J. M., et al. (2017). Participatory disease surveillance: engaging communities directly in reporting, monitoring, and responding to health threats. *JMIR Public Health Surveillance* 3(4), e62.

Steinhubl, S. R., Kim, K.-i., Ajayi, T., & Topol, E. J. (2018). Virtual care for improved global health. *Lancet* **391**(10119), 419.

Strauss, R. A., Castro, J. S., Reintjes, R., & Torres, J. R. (2017). Google dengue trends: an indicator of epidemic behavior. The Venezuelan case. *International Journal of Medical Informatics* **104**, 26–30.

Uamuzi Bora (2019). Uamuzi Bora (online). Available at http://uamuzibora.github.io/uamuzi-bora/ (accessed April 26, 2019).

United Nations Development Group (2017). Data privacy, ethics and protection guidance note on big data for achievement of the 2030 agenda (online). Available at https://undg.org/wp-content/uploads/2017/11/UNDG_Big Data_final_web.pdf (accessed April 24, 2019).

Vayena, E., Dzenowagis, J., Brownstein, J. S., & Sheikh, A. (2018). Policy implications of big data in the health sector. *Bulletin of the World Health Organization* **96**(1), 66–68.

Vayena, E., & Gasser, U. (2016a). Between openness and privacy in genomics. *PLoS Medicine* **13**(1), e1001937.

Vayena, E., & Gasser, U. (2016b). Strictly biomedical? Sketching the ethics of the big data ecosystem in biomedicine, in Mittelstadt, B., & Floridi, L. (eds.), *The Ethics of Biomedical Big Data*. New York: Springer, pp. 17–39.

Vayena, E., & Madoff, L. (2019). Navigating the ethics of big data in public health, in Mastroianni, A. C., Kahn, J. P., &

Kass, N. E. (eds.), *The Oxford Handbook of Public Health Ethics*. Oxford, UK: Oxford University Press, pp. 354–367.

Verghese, A., Shah, N. H., & Harrington, R. A. (2018). What this computer needs is a physician: humanism and artificial intelligence. *Journal of the American Medical Association* **319**(1), 19–20.

Vula (2016). Vula (online). Available at www.vulamobile.com/ (accessed April 24, 2019).

Wahl, B., Cossy-Gantner, A., Germann, S., & Schwalbe, N. R. (2018). Artificial intelligence (AI) and global health: how can AI contribute to health in resource-poor settings? *BMJ Global Health* 3(4), e000798.

Wang, D., Khosla, A., Gargeya, R., et al. (2016). Deep learning for identifying metastatic breast cancer. arXiv preprint arXiv:1606.05718.

Wang, Y., Kung, L., Wang, W. Y. C., & Cegielski, C. G. (2018). An integrated big data analytics-enabled transformation model: application to health care. *Information & Management* **55**(1), 64–79.

Wilton Park (2018). Reimagining global health: self-care interventions and implications for healthcare (online). Available at www.wiltonpark.org.uk/wp-content/uploads/WP1639-Report.pdf (accessed April 24, 2019).

Wójcik, O. P., Brownstein, J. S., Chunara, R., & Johansson, M. A. (2014). Public health for the people: participatory infectious disease surveillance in the digital age. *Emerging Themes in Epidemiology* **11**(1), 1–7.

World Health Organization (WHO) (2019). WHO unveils sweeping reforms in drive towards "triple billion" targets (online). Available at www.who.int/news-room/detail/06–03-2019-who-unveils-sweeping-reforms-in-drive-towards-triple-billion-targets (accessed April 28, 2019).

Wyber, R., Vaillancourt, S., Perry, W., et al. (2015). Big data in global health: improving health in low-and middle-income countries. *Bulletin of the World Health Organization* **93**, 203–208.

Global Health Governance for Developing Sustainability

Erica Di Ruggiero

Global Policy Context

Health is an intrinsically and indisputably global endeavor. Global challenges to the health of populations and to the planet are on the rise, as are concomitant calls for innovative strategies and "solutions" that aspire to contribute to the development of sustainability (Bensimon & Benatar, 2006). Increased economic globalization; the flow of trade, capital, and labor; widening gender and health inequities; increased migration; and planetary health are among the many complex issues that challenge nation-states, global institutions, and the overall governance of the global commons (or the commonly pooled resources at global, international, and supranational levels). Health has also become highly vulnerable in a global policy context dominated by growing interests in national security and economic competitiveness (Labonte, 2014). Efforts to "depoliticize" health and the work of global institutions such as the World Health Organization (WHO) dedicated to the achievement of health for all have not necessarily succeeded, and suggestions that health is not political have been repeatedly refuted (Kickbusch & Reddy, 2015). If health is considered "critical for national and international security, domestic and global economic well-being, and economic and social development in less developed countries, and is also a major growth sector of the global economy" (Kickbusch & Reddy, 2015: 841), then what are the implications for its governance?

At its core, governance is said to be realized when a collective of individuals or of institutional arrangements come together to accomplish an agreed end, which can and should involve the participation of state and nonstate actors. It usually encompasses an identifiable authority as well as rules and mechanisms for decision making and accountability (Lee & Kamradt-Scott, 2014). It should perhaps come as no surprise that health has become by far one of the most

extensively discussed topics of governance globally, with a wide array of institutions seeking to contribute to its development or attainment (Holzscheiter et al., 2016). Scholars such as Stone have characterized the global arena as a "domain of relative disorder and uncertainty where institutions are underdeveloped and political authority unclear, and dispersed through multiplying institutions and networks" (Stone, 2008: 21). This increased attention to health, especially after the end of the Cold War, has resulted in considerable heterogeneity in approaches to global governance alongside an increase in fragmentation of global institutions and increased competition for resources and the control of agendas (Kickbusch & Reddy, 2015). This added complexity has also resulted in policy inaction and gridlock periodically disrupted by global crises. In essence, this complex global arena can be characterized by a push by state and nonstate actors for greater coherence and order, contrasted by efforts to disrupt and even dissolve this order (Holzscheiter et al., 2016). In contrast, important critiques of global health governance efforts have also challenged the neoliberal development model of global capitalism – founded in individualist and market-driven conceptualizations of development – as well as exposed its pervasive influences on the practices of global institutions. These scholars have called for an alternative model for developing sustainability, grounded in history, political economy, and ecologically responsible health ethic, in order to better address the current challenges of global health governance (Gill & Benatar, 2016).

Many policy narratives about what health means and what can be achieved in the name of health are consequently circulating in the global arena. The use of policy as an instrument to govern or to describe a pattern of governing as a whole is not a new phenomenon of study. The term *policy* comes from *polis*,[1]

---

[1] Derivatives from *polis* include *polity*, *politics*, and *police*.

meaning the "classical Greek city-state" (Colebatch, 2006). Policy is inextricably linked to governance, but the two concepts are not the same, although they are at times conflated in the literature (as discussed later). Policy can be planned and unplanned, passive and active, and operating at different levels and scales (e.g., international versus local). It is also important to identify which institutions or governing bodies are accountable for policy and its consequences. At the global level, policy takes on a distinctive character, shaped through a particularly dynamic and iterative set of transactions and processes involving diverse state and nonstate actors (Stone, 2008). The policy process is in essence a struggle for the determination of meanings. Consequently, a policy being advanced globally in the name of health can have multiple readers with different rationalities and conceptions of power, knowledge, and political influence (Yanow, 1996). There can be resistance among state and nonstate actors constructing different meanings of policy, and ongoing struggles over meanings and control of resources may inevitably arise. This contested meeting ground that is "governed" globally provides ample opportunity for policies and actions with equitable benefit to be generated, but it can also be used by certain actors as a deliberate instrument to advance agendas that are neither progressive nor just (Taylor, 2018).

Given the complexity, I examine some of the conceptual and analytical issues related to global health and its governance. I begin by reflecting on the global policy context with particular attention to the Millennium Development Goals (MDGs) and the Sustainable Development Goals (SDGs) and the implications for governance. I provide background on different conceptualizations that arise in the study of global health governance. I then explore issues of competing priorities, actor dynamics, and power that emerged from analyzing a subset of scholarly literature. I conclude by proposing some avenues requiring further attention.

Global Policy Goals

As noted earlier, several competing global health policy initiatives are afoot, with the aim of *governing* the global commons. One such global policy initiative that is receiving considerable attention is the 2030 Sustainable Development Agenda, comprised of 17 SDGs (United Nations, 2016). Adopted by the United Nations in 2015, the SDGs articulate a bold

policy vision for *all* countries to take action in the name of the people and the planet and for prosperity while professing to leave no one behind (a nod to equity). This intersectoral policy orientation builds, to some extent, on lessons learned from the MDGs, which had previously shifted the gaze and reporting burden toward low- and middle-income countries (LMICs) and primarily targeted specific diseases, conditions, and populations. The MDGs were criticized for not being sufficiently well integrated, for reinforcing fragmentation and vertical programming, and for not being explicit about addressing the social determinants of health, equity, human rights, or their monitoring (Buse & Hawkes, 2015). This difference in emphasis between the SDGs and the MDGs, where the relative value of vertical programs (e.g., disease specific) versus horizontal programs (e.g., focused on the social determinants of health and health systems strengthening) versus diagonal programs (a combination of both approaches) is contrasted, remains a point of debate among members of the international community (Bennett et al., 2018). There is also a widespread perception that developed countries primarily in the Western world (although this is also shifting with the rise in influence of countries such as China) dictate the governance of the global health commons.

The SDGs are therefore not without their critics. Some scholars have argued that the SDGs may actually undermine democracy by pushing a policy agenda designed not to upset dictators and human rights offenders (Smith, 2018). Missing from the SDG policy narrative are terms such as *anticorruption*, *separation of powers*, *free and fair elections*, and *civil society* (to some extent, although SDG 16 does attend to the role of civil society), which are all fundamental to the pursuit of democracy and human development (Smith, 2018). Whereas civil society organizations can play a critical role in advocating for the right to health for all or playing the role of watchdog, not all are progressive, nor should they be seen as substitutes for the role of the nation-states (Smith et al., 2016). Inherent in the SDGs are many competing health, economic, and/or social agendas from climate change to migration to poverty, which are also human rights crises. "Because the world adopted the SDGs, they offer [however] one of our best, contemporary global opportunities to oppose social injustices that human rights advocates can use as a tool" (Winkler & Williams, 2017: 1024). Despite advice from scholars, human rights activists, and civil society, time will tell whether the protection of human rights will run the risk of being continuously neglected (a similar critique of the MDGs).

Although the scope for addressing gender inequalities and women's empowerment has broadened under the SDG agenda, postcolonial feminist critiques of these goals have also challenged their limited attention to the systemic drivers of these inequalities (Esquivel, 2016). "Development is about power," yet a discussion about power relations and power asymmetries and the privileged role of actors, including powerful nation-states, transnational corporations, international financial institutions, and other actors who actively favor neoliberal economic arguments, is conspicuously absent from the 2030 Development Agenda (Esquivel, 2016; Struckmann, 2018). The global economic model reinforced by the SDGs consists of pro–economic growth policies, trade liberalization, and public–private partnerships. Without better safeguards to hold the most powerful to account who stand the most to benefit from this dominant economic model, the SDGs will definitely not live up to their ultimate and most aspirational goal – to leave no one behind.

That said, the "promise" that *better* global governance can contribute to sustainable development permeates several SDGs (United Nations, 2016). For instance, SDG 16 calls for just, peaceful, and inclusive societies, realized in part through the "development of strong institutions," another implicit appeal to global governance. However, individual goals and the SDGs as a set present several challenges to their governance. Within SDG 3 ("Ensure healthy lives and promote wellbeing for all at all ages"), there is an increased call for universal health coverage alongside other sub-goals related to risk factors (e.g., tobacco), diseases (e.g., injuries), and causes of mortality such as maternal mortality representing several potentially competing "health agendas" for resources. Other SDGs reflect inherent tensions, each with competing interests. For example, SDG 8 ("Promote sustained, inclusive and sustainable economic growth, full and productive employment and decent work for all") and related targets emphasize the relationship between growth and employment, said to be best achieved through technological change and increased productivity, but without really calling into question the potential perils of increased growth. A paradigm shift is required to counter the several challenges presented by the SDGs.

These include the need for improved leadership for intersectoral coherence and coordination on the structural drivers of health, shifting the focus of efforts from treatment to prevention, more effective means to tackle the commercial determinants of ill-health, further integrating rights-based approaches, and improved civic engagement and accountability (Buse & Hawkes, 2015). Several invoke or imply a governance response – for instance, increased policy coherence and global collective decision making across sectors, greater attention to the realization of human rights, and sustainable development that requires representative and accountable global governance mechanisms.

Global Health Governance

Given this complex global policy context, the meaning of global health governance merits further unpacking. I next review and analyze selected issues related to the characterization of global health governance (with full and explicit recognition of the several interpretations and variations in terminology noted later). To focus this analysis, I conducted a purposeful review of a subset of the academic literature on global health governance guided by the following questions: How is "governance" described in the peer-review literature on global health since the advent of the SDGs? What multiple meanings of governance related to global health emerge? The relative recency of the SDGs means that much of the literature does not explicitly reference or engage directly with these goals as an object of empirical study, with some exceptions.

I adapted the search strategy referenced in Lee and Kamradt-Scott (2014) to identify published articles in public health and social sciences databases (CINAHL Plus [EBSCO], International Bibliography of the Social Sciences [ProQuest], PAIS International [ProQuest], Sociological Abstracts [ProQuest], Worldwide Political Science Abstracts [ProQuest], Scopus [Elsevier], and Web of Science [Clarivate]). The broad search terms "governa*" and "global health" were derived based on the concepts of governance, global health governance, and global health. All English peer-reviewed primary research articles that discussed both governance and global health and that were published between January 1, 2014, and December 31, 2018, were included for initial screening. I chose this timeframe to account for the preperiod leading to the adoption of the SDGs in

November 2015 up to the end of December 2018. Although limited, this subset of literature aims to provide an early snapshot and analysis of some of the scholarly literature. The initial search resulted in 444 articles, and after deduplication, 413 articles were included in the first stage of screening. This stage involved a review of titles and abstracts in line with the preceding questions. Articles that narrowly pertained to a particular global health issue (e.g., antimicrobial resistance) or highlighted the implications of an issue for governance but were not sufficiently focused on governance were excluded from this more in-depth review. Fifty articles were included for full-text review in line with the preceding questions. I supplemented these articles with recurring citations within selected articles and core literature in the field.

Based on this review, I highlight some of governance issues that emerged in this literature. These include the following: competing global health priorities, actor dynamics and partnerships, and power and how they intersect with global health governance and global policy agendas, in particular the MDGs and the SDGs. Given their recent emergence, only a limited number of articles identified explicitly mentioned the SDGs or engaged with those goals as a primary object of critical interrogation. Much of the literature was conceptual, analytical, or commentary style, with some exceptions involving empirical studies. This most likely reflects disciplinary traditions and the state of the research field. When explicitly declared, several theoretical lenses were primarily derived from the fields or disciplines of international relations, political science, law, ethics, health policy, and more broadly, global public health.

Definitional Issues

Use of the term *governance* in the global health literature has grown dramatically. A 2014 review found more than 1,000 scholarly articles with reference to global health governance in use since 2002 (Lee & Kamradt-Scott, 2014). More recent reviews specific to topics such as nutrition have shown a similar exponential growth in the use of the term *governance* while also noting the lack of definitional clarity (Bump, 2018). Other scholars have reviewed the framing role of health-related policy and governance processes such as Health in All Policies and Healthy Cities on actors outside the health sector (Leeuw, 2017) or health in all (foreign) policy (Labonte, 2014). They

conclude that in the mainstream public health literature, there has been limited attention to the "existing science of governance, policy, and implementation instrumentation," leading to a blurring of concepts. Of note, "joined-up governance is not the same as integral policy, which is also not the same as intersectoral action. Governance is not policy nor is it action" (Leeuw, 2017: 344). These and other reviews signal a need to problematize what global health governance means, what problem it is trying to address or solve and therefore what it is accomplishing, and what it can or ought to realistically achieve to redress complex global health problems. They also highlight the different disciplinary interpretations of concepts, especially when imported from one field (e.g., political science) to another (e.g., public health or global health). Given the myriad public, not-for-profit, civil society, and private actors (re)defining global health agendas and the power asymmetries between them, *what* we mean by governance, *who* defines global governance, and *what* is actually being governed remain understandably contested topics in the scholarly literature.

Governance is said to be global when referring to the ensemble of governance systems across sectors and transnational borders (Lee & Kamradt-Scott, 2014). "Particular challenges arise for global governance beyond the state due to what international relations scholars call 'anarchy' or the absence of an overarching political authority above sovereign states" (Lee & Kamradt-Scott, 2014: 2). Global governance is also described as "the complex of formal and informal institutions, mechanisms, relationships, and processes between and among states, markets, citizens, and organisations, both intergovernmental and non-governmental, through which collective interests on the global plane are articulated, rights and obligations are established, and differences are mediated" (Thakur & Weiss, 2006).

Part of the definitional challenge stems from what global health governance scholars have identified as a lack of conceptual clarity regarding what the object of study interest even is. In their comprehensive review, Lee and Kamradt-Scott (2014) sought to determine how global health governance (GHG) was being discussed in the academic literature. The authors helpfully draw important conceptual distinctions between three meanings of governance arising from the literature reviewed on global health. These distinctions are derived by assessing the strengths and weaknesses of different institutional arrangements that can involve state and nonstate actors. These include the following:

- Globalization *and* health governance: refer to the collective responses taken by health-related institutions to health issues such as infectious diseases that affect populations globally.
- Global governance *and* health: refer to the impact of global governance institutions that operate outside the health sector but that have a profound influence on the social determinants of health and health equity.
- Governance *for* global health: refers to the governance arrangements in service of a specific goal (Lee & Kamradt-Scott, 2014).

Each of these meanings can understandably evoke different goals, expectations, outcomes, and principles such as human rights and social justice. A fairly frequently cited definition by Fidler characterizes global health governance as "the use of formal and informal institutions, rules, and processes by states, intergovernmental organizations, and nonstate actors to deal with challenges to health that require cross-border collective action to address effectively" (Fidler, 2010: 3). The remaining sections address how global health governance intersects with issues of competing priorities, actors and partnerships, and power and how it relates to global policy agendas (with particular reference to the SDGs).

Competing Priorities to Be "Governed"

Much of the literature focuses on how competing priorities, some more well established and/or recurring (e.g., infectious diseases) and others still emerging (e.g., noncommunicable diseases [NCDs]), are shaped by global health governance processes. The extent of interest given to a priority naturally influences its relative position and the degree of competition with other agendas. These realities are bound to be manifest with 17 SDGs with which to contend, all directly or indirectly intersecting with the pursuit of health for all while purporting to leave no one behind. As noted previously, health and the many facets it encompasses have become a focus of increased attention but also great contestation globally. A key question is how global health governance articulates the "problem" to be governed and the need to connect communities of global health governance to provide a coordinated response. For instance, Bennett et al., (2018) argue that socioeconomic interactions and community norms all contribute to how a health risk is interpreted. In an "environment of limited funds and competing priorities, it is now more important than ever for attention to be paid to what institutions global health donors are willing to pay for, for what reasons, and with what broader consequences" (Clinton & Sridhar, 2017: 331). Inherent in the shift from MDGs and SDGs are tensions arising in the continued vertical prioritization of specific diseases versus horizontal investments in health systems strengthening that continue to persist (Jönsson, 2014).

There are also useful lessons to be learned regarding the possible governance of an emerging health priority. Let us take the case of NCDs. This is an example of a priority area not explicitly addressed in the MDGs but considered until more recently to be a neglected global policy issue. "NCDs have not really benefitted from fear or empathy that can be found in the security or social justice agenda in health" (Jönsson, 2014: 308). Reasons for this limited attention include how the "NCD problem" is defined by different governance actors, the resistance to changing NCD-related risk factors (e.g., eating behaviors) because they are reinforced through social norms, practices, and culture; as well as the influence of industry and other vested interests – all considered as legitimation challenges related to the NCD issue itself. The governance of NCDs highlights the tension that exists between the need to tackle commercial determinants of health (at odds with many NCD-related risk factors such as food, alcohol, and tobacco), on the one hand, and the increased reliance on public-private partnerships to achieve global health policy outcomes, on the other hand. NCDs have to compete with other agendas, and their political prioritization is probably more likely if they can *bridge to parallel* agendas (a promise of governance), such as food and nutrition or the promise of sustainability. A major challenge in global health is thus to govern with transparent and accountable processes where potential and actual conflicts of interests are identified – if legitimacy in the eyes of the public is to remain strong (Maher & Sridhar, 2012; Hogerzeil et al., 2013). Further, complex and diffuse governance structures create challenges for increased legitimacy of an issue such as NCDs in future global health governance efforts.

Another useful consideration is the frame given to health. There are differing analyses of how effectively health can retain or expand its position in foreign policy debates (Labonte, 2014). For instance, should we invest in vaccines instead of strengthening health systems? This debate between donor countries is still ongoing, with vaccine researchers and industry largely favoring investment in vaccines (McNeill & Ingstad Sandberg, 2014). The rights- and justice-based approaches to framing health pursued by the United Nations family of institutions and global public health community at large have also been used as legitimate modes of global health governance (Jönsson, 2014), but these efforts, too, can run the risk of cooption and become diluted by other interests. For instance, some countries' disproportionate influence on transnational rule-making authority leads to the prioritization of infectious disease control at the expense of fully realizing the right to health (Ooms & Hammonds, 2016). In sum, there are many competing priorities that challenge global health governance.

Actor Dynamics and Partnerships

Over the last several decades, we have witnessed a rise in the number and influence of actors. There are many concepts and definitions in use to define these relationships and interactions between actors. Public–private partnerships (PPPs) are defined as partnerships that bring public and private interests together to achieve a common goal, network, consortium, and other constellation in the global arena, each with competing agendas and differential effects on health and health equity (note that much of this literature is about global governance and health). Global health partnerships (GHPs) are defined as the "relatively institutionalized initiatives, established to address global health problems, in which public and for-profit private sector organizations have a voice in collective decision-making" (Buse & Harmer, 2007: 259). The emergence of philanthropies and private-sector actors has resulted from deregulation and inaction by state-based actors and the hybridization of governance authority through PPPs (Youde, 2016). Critical scholars have decried this expansion and problematic logic of PPPs, which operate as "global governance tools" without sufficient oversight and accountability mechanisms by state actors (Ruckert & Labonté, 2014). PPPs have also been shown to shift the priorities of certain public goods at the expense of paying attention to other pressing issues (Andonova, 2018). For instance, they obfuscate governance structures by reconfiguring public and private realms. They can also

contribute to the normalization of the financial, informational, and technologic power wielded by the private sector (Andonova, 2018). Their agenda-setting potential in the global arena is not to be underestimated or ignored and thus should be maintained as a subject of ongoing critical inquiry. Despite these cautions, interactions between public and private spheres are likely to increase in all sectors, including health, in the name of making progress toward the SDGs.

A related theme in the literature on global governance is the lack of contestation about the "appropriateness" of reestablishing institutional order by strengthening norms that outline the individual responsibilities and competencies of actors with overlapping mandates (Andonova, 2018). Some scholars argue for further democratizing global governance and enhancing the legitimacy of international organizations. For instance, there have been numerous calls for a renewal of the WHO's role to meet twenty-first-century public health challenges. A mixed-methods qualitative research study about the WHO involving academics, policymakers, and opinion leaders from various backgrounds concluded that the dominant biomedical view of health is deeply entrenched and that the organization's departments are siloed, preventing cross-sectoral collaboration and better alignment with the SDG agenda (Gopinathan et al., 2015). Whether the recent structural changes will achieve such objectives remains to be seen.

Other scholars have studied emerging global health networks and their influence on global health governance, including how they contribute to greater fragmentation. For example, Shiffman et al. (2016) reported study findings about the emergence and effectiveness of global health networks addressing a range of health problems (e.g., tobacco use, maternal mortality). Although networks are only one of many factors influencing what is a priority, they do matter, as does their ability to develop a shared understanding of the problem and to stay focused while sustaining the network. These and other factors, in turn, shape the way the problem and its solutions are interpreted and understood as well as the networks' ability to convince different actors such as governments and international institutions to address the issue. Network membership and the broader political and historical context, including, for instance, the degree of alignment with global development goals, their past failures, and their successes in addressing the issue at hand, both play a role. These authors also highlight how network legitimacy is derived from the credibility of its members (for example) and the reasons to question it such as their "largely elite composition and the fragmentation they bring to global health governance" (Shiffman et al., 2016: i110).

Let us not forget the many civil society groups whose purpose can be to disrupt governance through social mobilization in order to call attention to neglected health and social issues and to advocate for the rights of marginalized populations. Smith et al. (2016) argue that a strong civil society in the context of SDG 3 can fulfill several essential global health functions, including, for instance, the introduction of policy alternatives, enhancing legitimacy of global health institutions, countering the commercial determinants of health, and ensuring rights-based approaches. Civil society is a global public good that merits investing in, in order to ensure meaningful progress toward the 2030 Agenda for Sustainable Development (Smith et al., 2016).

Although an actor perspective is important to global health governance, some scholars have cautioned against an undue focus on the proliferation of actors, different actor constellations, and the norms and rules that govern them. Such a focus can result in a simplistic conclusion that the global arena is messy, when in fact there are examples of "stabilising relationships and historically changing, discursively embedded instances of meta-governance that reflexively rearrange the parameters within which health international organizations interact and operate" (Holzscheiter et al., 2016: 15) (primarily related to global governance). For these reasons, the global arena is a contested space for legitimacy and power where norms and practices are continuously negotiated and debated. This leads me to interrogate the issue of power and its relationship to global health governance.

Power

There is a rich literature on the role of different forms of power that manifest in global health. Shiffman (2014) makes the distinction between different forms of power and their relationship to knowledge. Power and knowledge do not consist of independent entities, but they are inextricably related: knowledge is always an exercise of power, and power is always a function of knowledge. There are several reasons for the desire to wield influence – for example, establishing one's

legitimacy in a crowded arena with increased competition for finite resources. For some, this influence derives from control over financial resources. For others, it comes from expertise and claims to moral authority – what can be termed, respectively, *epistemic* and *normative power* (Shiffman, 2014). Much of the global health governance literature I reviewed acknowledges power, power relations between actors, and power asymmetries between actors such as global institutions, nation-states, and philanthropic foundations. Perhaps not surprising, however, is the fact that not all articles identified in this particular review theorize power or are explicit about their conception of power. There are some notable exceptions. For example, Andonova (2018) comments on the pursuit of power through partnerships, including how transnational actors play a leading role in the cocreation of up to 50% of the partnerships (i.e., governance of global health). PPPs shift the priorities of certain public goods at the expense of attention to others, the framing of priorities, and crowd out the role of global institutions such as the WHO and the influence they can have over member states (Andonova, 2018).

Other authors reflect on how power is exercised through partnerships with the private sector and major foundations. For instance, the Gates Foundation's profound influence on agenda setting and regimes of governance in global health has required other global institutions such as the World Bank and the WHO, as well as nation-states, to engage with it (Clinton & Sridhar, 2017). Mahajan's exposé (Mahajan, 2018) on the work of the Gates Foundation in India over the last decade and a half traces how the foundation initially circumvented the national government but then adopted a discourse of partnership. Ironically, after an early discounting of the role of the government, the foundation later sought to transition its programs to the state. This compelling example illustrates a more nuanced relationship between global and state-level actors in India that evolved over time. "The predicaments produced by the exigencies of philanthropic aid, the complex demands of broad-based social interventions, and the temporality required for building sustainable health systems are as relevant to a small state in Sub-Saharan Africa as they are to India" (Mahajan, 2018: 1366).

At their core, these examples speak to power as a diffuse phenomenon, expressed in different ways in the global health governance literature. There are descriptions of constructivist views of power (as relational) versus more concrete expressions of power as influence in understanding patterns of outcomes (i.e., different resources and strategies which states and other actors use to advance their objectives and influence international relations; Shiffman, 2018).

Global Health Governance and Global Policy Agendas (MDGs and SDGs)

Returning now to global policy agendas, descriptions of the MDGs or SDGs are primarily included as part of the global context rather than as an explicit "study object" related to governance or a vehicle for understanding governance processes. There are notable exceptions. As noted earlier, critiques of global health governance efforts have called for models grounded in the principles of global solidarity and the development of sustainability (Bensimon & Benatar, 2006). Van de Pas et al. (2017) carefully analyzed global health governance in the context of the SDGs, with particular attention to the right to health. These authors conclude that there is a governance gap between global health and development policies and human rights frameworks. Their analysis, which is informed by the four functions of GHG – production of global public good, management of externalities, global solidarity, and global stewardship – underscores that the SDG agenda does not represent a mode of global health governance that satisfies the demands of the right to health:

> Current representations of the right to health in the Sustainable Development Goals are insufficient and superficial, because they do not explicitly link commitments or the right to health discourse to binding treaty obligations for duty-bearing nation states or entitlements by people. If global health policy is to meaningfully contribute to the realization of the right to health and to rights based global health governance, then future iterations of global health policy must bridge this gap.
>
> *(Van de Pas et al., 2017: 47)*

As noted earlier by several authors, limited attention to the right to health, unequal power relations, and insufficient oversight and accountability mechanisms to govern them would prevent nations from fully realizing the SDGs. Without increased monitoring of SDG-related policies and their effects on the realization of the right to health, we will again not learn from the lessons of the MDGs.

Conclusion

In this chapter, I elucidate some of the conceptual and analytical issues related to global health governance (GHG), how GHG intersects with issues of competing priorities, and actor dynamics and partnerships and power within the context of global policy agendas, namely the MDGs and the SDGs. The crisis of neoliberal capitalism and persisting social and economic inequities within and between countries has placed governance on the center stage as a potential "solution" at the intersection of public, private, and political discourses and agendas. This complex governance terrain is ripe with ethical content for analysis and critique of the legitimacy and leadership of current global efforts to redress these health and social challenges (Gill, 2015). Analytical tools from ethics, law, political science, and other disciplines can surface substantive matters of significant import, including power, democracy, sustainability, and political economy, to ask questions such as *what* is being governed, for *whose* benefit, to *what* end, and *what ought to be* (see the edited book by Gill [2015] for further details).

In the absence of consensus of what global health governance should be or, more important, the different ways it is expressed and interpreted, critiques regarding its failures could be even more persuasive than they currently are (Ooms & Hammonds, 2016). Part of this more neutral and ambiguous characterization (with some notable exceptions) also stems from a growing need to find solutions to global problems by drawing from the very belief systems and cognitive biases that cannot generate sustainable solutions and cause the problems governance is purporting to fix in the first place (Benatar, 2016). "Progress is unlikely for whole populations globally without some changes to how the global political economy operates, promotion of more sustainable consumption patterns, new resource distributive mechanisms and conceptions of power such as co-operative 'power with,' instead of coercive 'power over' in order to give voice and level up" (Benatar, 2016: 602). Given this daunting global project, it may not be surprising that governance continues to be treated as a container or vehicle to "park or put aside" the "messy" dimensions of already complex global health problems in order to generate and advance more concrete and technologically oriented solutions (Bump, 2018). This tendency may result from the absence of adequate mechanisms to regulate the global commons and deal with the most pressing global health problems of our time.

For example, the migration of workers within and between regions and countries, coupled with weak protection of the rights of migrants and their families, requires increasing interdependence among nation-states but also fundamental adjustments in the global governance regime. Drawing from the literature on global constitutionalism, which seeks to surface the "legitimacy deficits of institutions," some legal scholars have proposed a Framework Convention on Global Health. The proposed framework "could create a classic division of powers" in global health governance, with the WHO as the law-making power in global health governance, a global fund for health as the executive power, and the International Court of Justice as the judiciary power (Ooms & Hammonds, 2016: 1). The WHO must, however, also become more competent in applying human rights frameworks if it is to reduce fragmentation among policy actors involved in the global health governance landscape in order to realize the highest attainable standard of health (Meier & Onzivu, 2014). Until these systemic root causes are addressed, will the efforts to pursue global health governance and the mechanisms it seeks to deploy ever be able to deliver on health effectively and equitably? This remains to be seen, but ongoing scholarly inquiry is needed to interrogate these and other drivers and ideological underpinnings of global health governance, with attention to competing priorities, actors, power, and other key issues at play in this SDG era.

Acknowledgments

I acknowledge the contributions of one of my students, Elizabeth Loftus, for her invaluable assistance with the literature search. I would also like to thank Solomon Benatar and Gillian Brock for helpful input on an earlier draft, and for the opportunity to contribute to this 2nd edition.

References

Andonova, L. B. (2018). The power of the public purse: financing of global health partnerships and agenda setting for sustainability. *Chinese Journal of Population Resources and Environment* **16**, 186–196.

Benatar, S. (2016). Politics, power, poverty and global health: systems and frames. *International Journal of Health Policy and Management* **5**, 599–604.

Bennett, B., Cohen, I. G., Davies, S. E., et al. (2018). Future-proofing global health: governance of priorities. *Global Public Health* **13**, 519–527.

Bensimon, C. M., & Benatar, S. R. (2006). Developing sustainability: a new metaphor for progress. *Theoretical Medicine and Bioethics* **27**, 59–79.

Bump, J. B. (2018). Undernutrition, obesity and governance: a unified framework for upholding the right to food. *BMJ Global Health* **3**, 1–13.

Buse, K., & Harmer, A. (2007). Seven habits of highly effective global public-private health partnerships: practice and potential. *Social Science & Medicine* **64**, 259–271.

Buse, K., & Hawkes, S. (2015). Health in the Sustainable Development Goals: ready for a paradigm shift? *Global Health* **11**, 1–8.

Clinton, C., & Sridhar, D. (2017). Who pays for cooperation in global health? A comparative analysis of WHO, the World Bank, the Global Fund to Fight HIV/AIDS, Tuberculosis and Malaria, and GAVI, the Vaccine Alliance. *Lancet* **390**, 324–332.

Colebatch, H. K. (2006). *The Work of Policy: An International Survey*, Lanham, MD: Lexington Books.

Esquivel, V. (2016). Power and the Sustainable Development Goals: a feminist analysis. *Gender & Development* **24**, 9–23.

Fidler, D. (2010). The challenges of global health governance, in *International Institutions and Global Governance Program*. New York: Council on Foreign Relations . pp. 1–33.

Gill, S. E. (2015). *Critical Perspectives on the Crisis of Global Governance: Reimagining the Future*. New York: Palgrave Macmillan.

Gill, S., & Benatar, S. (2016). Global health governance and global power: a critical commentary on the Lancet–University of Oslo Commission Report. *International Journal of Health Services* **46**, 346–365.

Gopinathan, U., Watts, N., Hougendobler, D., et al. (2015). Conceptual and institutional gaps: understanding how the WHO can become a more effective cross-sectoral collaborator. *Global Health* **11**, 1–13.

Hogerzeil, H. V., Liberman, J., Wirtz, V. J., et al. (2013). Promotion of access to essential medicines for non-communicable diseases: practical implications of the UN political declaration. *Lancet* **381**, 680–689.

Holzscheiter, A., Bahr, T., & Pantzerhielm, L. (2016). Emerging governance architectures in global health: do metagovernance norms explain inter-organisational convergence? *Politics and Governance* **4**, 1–15.

Jönsson, K. (2014). Legitimation challenges in global health governance: the case of non-communicable diseases. *Globalizations* **11**, 301–314.

Kickbusch, I., & Reddy, K. S. (2015). Global health governance: the next political revolution. *Public Health* **129**, 838–842.

Labonté, R. (2014). Health in All (Foreign) Policy: challenges in achieving coherence. *Health Promotion International* **29**(Suppl 1), i48–i58.

Lee, K., & Kamradt-Scott, A. (2014). The multiple meanings of global health governance: a call for conceptual clarity. *Globalization and Health* **10**, 1–10.

Leeuw, E. D. (2017). Engagement of sectors other than health in integrated health governance, policy, and action. *Annual Review of Public Health* **38**, 329–349.

Mahajan, M. (2018). Philanthropy and the nation-state in global health: the Gates Foundation in India. *Global Public Health* **13**, 1357–1368.

Maher, A., & Sridhar, D. (2012). Political priority in the global fight against non-communicable diseases. *Journal of Global Health* **2**, 1–10.

McNeill, D., & Ingstad Sandberg, K. (2014). Trust in global health governance: the GAVI experience. *Global Governance* **20**, 325–343.

Meier, B. M., & Onzivu, W. (2014). The evolution of human rights in World Health Organization policy and the future of human rights through global health governance. *Public Health* **128**, 179–187.

Ooms, G., & Hammonds, R. (2016). Global constitutionalism, applied to global health governance: uncovering legitimacy deficits and suggesting remedies. *Global Health* **12**, 84–98.

Ruckert, A., & Labonté, R. (2014). Public–private partnerships (PPPs) in global health: the good, the bad and the ugly. *Third World Quarterly* **35**, 1598–1614.

Shiffman, J. (2014). Knowledge, moral claims and the exercise of power in global health. *International Journal of Health Policy and Management* **3**, 297–299.

Shiffman, J. (2018). Agency, structure and the power of global health networks. *International Journal of Health Policy and Management* **7**, 879–884.

Shiffman, J., Peter Schmitz, H., Berlan, D., et al. (2016). The emergence and effectiveness of global health networks: findings and future research. *Health Policy and Planning* **31**, i110–i123.

Smith, J. (2018). How the UN Sustainable Development Goals Undermine Democracy? Available at https://qz.com/africa/1299149/how-the-uns-sustainable-development-goals-undermine-democracy/.

Smith, J., Buse, K., & Gordon, C. (2016). Civil society: the catalyst for ensuring health in the age of sustainable development. *Global Health* **12**, 40–46.

Stone, D. (2008). Global public policy, transnational policy communities, and their networks. *Policy Studies Journal* **36**, 19–38.

Struckmann, C. (2018). A postcolonial feminist critique of the 2030 Agenda for Sustainable Development: A South African application. *Agenda* **32**, 12–24.

Taylor, S. (2018). "Global health": meaning what? *BMJ Global Health* **3**, e000843.

Thakur, R., & Weiss, T. G. (2006). *The UN and Global Governance: An Idea and Its Prospects*. Bloomington, IN: Indiana University Press.

United Nations (2016). Sustainable Development Goals (online). Available at www.un.org/sustainabledevelopment/sustainable-development-goals/.

Van de Pas, R., Hill, P. S., Hammonds, R., et al. (2017). Global health governance in the sustainable development goals: is it grounded in the right to health? *Global Challenges* **1**, 47–60.

Winkler, I. T., & Williams, C. (2017). The Sustainable Development Goals and human rights: a critical early review. *International Journal of Human Rights* **21**, 1023–1028.

Yanow, D. (1996). *How Does a Policy Mean?*, Washington, DC: Georgetown University Press.

Youde, J. (2016). Private actors, global health and learning the lessons of history. *Medicine Conflict and Survival* **32**, 203–220.

Teaching Global Health Ethics

James Dwyer

Introduction

In Japan and Switzerland, the average life expectancy is about 83 years. In Sierra Leone and Chad, it is about 53 years. Within the United States, people in some social groups can expect to live 20 years longer than people in other social groups. What are we to make of a world with such unequal health prospects? What does justice demand in terms of global health? And what is our moral responsibility?

I have thought about these questions for many years. In fact, I have fallen into a pattern that is both commendable and deplorable. I grow concerned about global health, study the causes of poor population health, think about the moral implications, and take some action. Then, gradually, I slip back into my daily concerns and work. These concerns and work are not without merit, but they do not provide much space for activities that promote global health and justice.

Over the last 25 years, I have done one thing consistently: I have integrated ethical issues about global health into my teaching. In courses for medical students, I've tried to address fundamental issues about global health, justice, and responsibility. I've done the same in courses attended by students from nursing, biology, engineering, philosophy, and other fields. I've also reached out beyond the university to discuss global health ethics with high school students, professional associations, religious groups, and the general public.

Now is a good time to reflect on my experience teaching global health ethics. In this chapter, I describe how I address some key issues, comment on how students respond, and speculate about what needs to be done. To begin, I describe health prospects in the world. Then I frame those prospects in terms of justice. After a brief discussion of theories of justice, I turn to issues of responsibility. The issues of responsibility lead to questions about responsiveness – about

how to respond. To conclude the chapter, I note what needs to be done and how that work connects to education.

Health Prospects in the World

Most people are vaguely aware of the large inequalities in health that exist in the world, but they do not reflect very carefully on the extent, nature, and implications of these inequalities. So I describe in my classes some measures of population health that illustrate these inequalities. One measure is average life expectancy (World Health Organization [WHO], 2019a). This is simply the number of years that people who are born now can expect to live. In about 25 countries, people can now expect to live more than 80 years. Whereas people born in countries such as Japan, Switzerland, Australia, Sweden, South Korea, and Canada can expect to live long and relatively healthy lives, people born in other countries cannot. In about 20 countries, the average life expectancy is fewer than 60 years.

Another measure of population health is the under-five mortality rate. This is simply the number of children, per 1,000 live births, who will die before they are five years old (WHO, 2019a). In about 20 countries, the under-five mortality rate is fewer than five. In countries such as Sweden, Finland, Japan, Germany, and France, less than 0.5% of children will die before they are five years old. However, in about 25 countries, the under-five mortality rate is greater than 100. In these countries, more than 10% of all children will die before they reach their fifth birthday.

Even after studying health prospects in low-income countries, I find one statistic particularly shocking: the number of women who die of causes related to pregnancy. In about 20 countries, the maternal mortality rate is fewer than 7 per 100,000. In countries such as Greece, Italy, Austria, Norway, and Australia, pregnancy and childbirth are relatively safe experiences. In some countries, though, pregnant women face grave risks. In about 20 countries, the maternal mortality rate is greater than 500. In 2015, the WHO estimated that the maternal mortality rate in Sierra Leone was 1,360. This risk of death is repeated with each pregnancy.

In a sea of statistics, we sometimes lose sight of the human meaning of the numbers. So I give students a few comparisons. I compare the risk of live liver donation in the United States with the risk of pregnancy in some other countries. Here is a prospective donor reflecting on the risks of liver donation:

> To make things work, they need a living donor with a good liver, a recipient with a bad liver, two adjacent operating rooms, and two sets of transplant surgeons. While the surgeons in one room are cutting out half of your liver, the surgeons in the next room are cutting out the recipient's liver. Then your surgeons pass the good piece over to the other surgeons, who hook it up in the recipient. Each operation takes about 8 hr.
>
> If things go well, you recover. Slowly. When you wake up, you have a ventilator tube in your mouth, a catheter in your bladder, a feeding tube in your stomach, some kind of drain in your abdomen, and several intravenous lines stuck here and there. If there are no complications, you need 6 days in the hospital, 3 months off work, and lots of home care.
>
> If things don't go well, you die.
>
> "How often does that happen?" I asked the surgeon.
>
> "Although we have to quote a mortality rate of 1%," he told me, "we think the actual rate may be as low as 1 in 200."
>
> "As low as?" I wanted to say. Think about it. Two hundred people are sitting in a theatre watching a movie. One of them doesn't go home.
>
> *(Dwyer, 2003: 1266)*

This prospective donor accurately describes the risks and fears associated with liver donation. But the risk of death to the donor (about 1 in 200) is less than the risk that a pregnant woman faces in 20 countries!

The health prospects for many people are actually worse than I have described because national averages tend to mask inequalities within nations. The poor and marginalized within a country often have shorter life expectancies, higher mortality rates, and more illness than average. Measures of health inequalities within the United States illustrate the problem. Chris Murray and his colleagues divided Americans into eight epidemiologic groups (Murray, Kularni, & Ezzati, 2005). They found that life expectancy

among Asian-American women was almost 21 years greater than life expectancy among urban African-American men. Even if we confine comparisons within one gender, the gap is huge. Asian-American men can expect to live 15 years longer than urban African-American men. This is roughly the difference in life expectancy between Switzerland and Cambodia! Studies such as this one actually complicate the picture: should we focus more ethical attention on the inequalities between countries or the inequalities within our own country?

All the measures that I have cited are based on mortality. They ignore morbidity and the suffering, impairment, and lost opportunity that come with it. Measures that do take these factors into account suggest a grimmer picture. Rather than cite more statistics, I give my students one example. In low-income countries, pregnant women who have protracted labor sometimes survive but are left with a fistula that causes urine and feces to leak out of them. The medical consequences of an obstetrical fistula are bad, but the social consequences are often worse: loss of job, loss of spouse, and loss of social support.

A Matter of Justice

When we learn that so many people in the world have such poor health prospects, most of us react with concern. I've never had a student who was really indifferent to the suffering and ill-health of millions of people. However, our initial reactions do not take us very far. They do not lead automatically to ethical understanding and action. Without education and effort, they rarely lead to active personal habits, just social institutions, and responsive international arrangements.

Although most students react with concern, many of them see poor health prospects as a matter of misfortune. I try to show them that the poor health prospects of populations are often a matter of justice. Toward the end of his life, John Rawls wrote an account of international justice (Rawls, 1999). Because he did not want to presuppose traditional views about the sovereignty of nation-states, he referred to his work as the "Law of Peoples." He made explicit the ideas that motivate this work:

> Two main ideas motivate the Law of Peoples. One is that the great evils of human history – unjust war and oppression, religious persecution and the denial of liberty of conscience, starvation and poverty, not to mention genocide and mass murder – follow from

political injustice. . . . The other main idea, obviously connected with the first, is that, once the gravest forms of political injustice are eliminated by following just (or at least decent) social policies and establishing just (or at least decent) basic institutions, these great evils will eventually disappear.

(Rawls, 1999: 6–7)

In this work, Rawls tries to specify a conception of justice that will address these great evils.

To the list of evils that destroy lives and plague human history, I want to add two: ill-health and premature death. This seems plausible enough. I also want to suggest that these evils follow from political injustice. This seems implausible at first. Don't people die of diseases and accidents caused by microbes and mishaps? Yes and no. Health often depends on exposure to risks, susceptibility to illness, access to healthcare, the social consequences of ill-health, and other factors. Many of these factors are influenced by the social environment, structures, and conditions. Whereas the health of an individual may depend on particular exposures or susceptibilities, the health prospects of a group often depend on the justice of the social conditions. Or so I argue.

One way to shift the perspective from misfortune to injustice is to examine the root causes of poor health. I ask medical students to list the leading causes of death among children in countries with high mortality rates. Most students place AIDS at the top of their lists. In fact, in many of these countries, the leading causes of childhood death are respiratory infections and diarrhea. Some students do include these immediate causes, but few students list poor sanitation, malnutrition, lack of access to healthcare, and shortages of healthcare workers. Even fewer students list poverty, war, poor governance, and international arrangements.

To illuminate the role of social structures and conditions, it helps to examine a problem like malnutrition. I ask students to research how malnutrition contributes to poor health prospects and how much it contributes to childhood mortality. The students explain very carefully how deficiencies in minerals and vitamins cause or exacerbate a number of diseases and how malnutrition renders people more susceptible to many diseases. They estimate that malnutrition in various forms is responsible for 20%–50% of childhood deaths. The WHO estimates that malnutrition contributes to 45% of under-five mortality (WHO, 2019b).

Chronic malnutrition and outright starvation are rarely due to a lack of resources or declines in food production within a country. Amartya Sen and others have shown that famines and malnutrition are often due to the way land, food, entitlements, and power are distributed (Sen, 1981; Lappé & Collins, 1986). The real problem is that governments and privileged groups do not care enough to create systems of entitlements to supplement the food supplies that marginalized groups have.

A careful study of malnutrition shows that what looks at first to be a matter of misfortune is also a matter of justice because some of the causes of malnutrition are embedded in social and international structures. What is true of malnutrition is also true, to a greater or lesser degree, of many health problems. For example, one could look at the role that social structures and gender inequalities play in the HIV epidemic. With all health problems, it is important to consider a full range of causes: biological, behavioral, cultural, social, international, and environmental. It is too easy to focus on the biological and behavioral factors and ignore the social and international structures that form the context. Yet these structures profoundly affect health prospects and access to healthcare. Because these structures are human constructs, they are under human control and subject to ethical evaluation. They are a matter of justice.

Theories of Justice

Because poor health prospects often raise issues of justice, it is natural and important to consider theories of justice when teaching global health ethics. A theory of justice might serve many roles. It could help to focus attention on features that we come to see are morally salient. It could conceptualize problems in ways that help to guide action and change. It could provide methods to help us decide between conflicting ethical concerns. For the most part, I focus on the first two roles. I sketch very briefly three kinds of theories, noting the features they highlight and the actions they suggest.

Because many students feel that they owe more to their compatriots (whose taxes fund part of their medical education) than to other people, I begin with a political theory of justice. John Rawls' account of justice is political in two senses. First, he attaches moral significance to political boundaries. He notes how issues of justice arise at three levels: at the local level, about associations like families and civil groups; at the societal level, about basic institutions like constitutions and economies; and at the international level, about interactions like war, aid, and trade. Because the arrangements at different levels have different natures and serve somewhat different purposes, he believes that they call for different principles and duties. In his view, the duties we have to family members are different from the duties we have to fellow citizens, which, in turn, are different from the duties we have to people in other countries.

Rawls' account is also political in a deeper sense. When he wrote *A Theory of Justice*, he suggested that his account of justice is part of a comprehensive moral view (Rawls, 1971). Later he emphasized that his account of justice is a political view that appeals to the idea of public reason and that recognizes the fact that a democratic culture will be marked by a plurality of reasonable comprehensive moral views. His work on international justice continues in this vein. It recognizes a plurality of reasonably just and decent societies, gives a prominent place to political autonomy, looks for an overlapping consensus, and appeals to the idea of public reason.

In his work on justice, Rawls begins with and emphasizes the role of *societal* justice in shaping people's life prospects. He believes that poor life prospects rarely reflect an absolute lack of resources; more often they reflect problems with political traditions, rule of law, respect for rights, division of property, class structures, and the status of women. The two principles of justice that he formulates address these points. The principle of equal liberty and the difference principle are meant to secure equal liberties, ensure the fair value of political liberty, promote fair equality of opportunity, and improve the situation of the least advantaged. Those aims require background institutions that

> work to keep property and wealth evenly enough shared over time to preserve the fair value of the political liberties and fair equality of opportunity over generations. They do this by laws regulating bequest and inheritance of property, and other devices such as taxes, to prevent excessive concentrations of private power. *(Rawls, 2001: 51)*

Because concentrations of power often lead to political domination and grossly unequal opportunities, a society needs to frame and regulate economic structures and conditions in order to ensure fair value of political liberty and to promote fair equality of opportunity.

Although societal justice is crucially important, modern societies are not isolated, closed, and self-contained. They interact in many areas: the natural environment, war and peace, legitimacy and human rights, trade and finance, migration and travel, disease and public health, communication and culture, and forms of aid. Because interactions in these areas often raise questions of justice, Rawls needs to formulate an account of international justice.

In *The Law of Peoples*, he tries to articulate principles that specify just relations between societies (Rawls, 1999). These principles aim to set out basic terms for guiding cooperation and regulating conflict among peoples. To begin, he explains that peoples should respect the freedom, independence, and political autonomy of other peoples. This principle of respect recognizes a reasonable pluralism among peoples, but it does not entail that peoples or states have unlimited sovereignty. In their internal affairs, peoples may not treat their own members and minorities in any way they please. Internally, they must adhere to certain standards, such as respecting human rights and engaging in consultation with representatives from all groups. In their external affairs, peoples should recognize limits on both the right to wage war and the way war is conducted. Peoples may only go to war in self-defense or to stop very grave violations of human rights (like genocide). And in conducting war, peoples should recognize constraints that aim to protect rights and achieve a just peace.

The last principle that Rawls articulates deals with the duty to assist. He believes that societies have a duty to assist other societies when unfavorable conditions make it difficult for those societies to achieve a reasonably just social and political order (Rawls, 1999: 5, 37). The principal aim of this duty is not to directly aid individuals or small groups who are in dire straits. Nor is it to implement a principle of distributive justice that would operate between societies. In Rawls' account, the aim of the duty is to help societies to create and maintain reasonably just institutions so that the assisted societies become autonomous and good members of a just federation of peoples.

What is the best way to fulfill the duty to assist? In general, the means should be chosen to further the aims. Assistance should not aim to promote the narrow interests of the assisting country but to promote just and decent conditions in the assisted countries. Well-designed assistance would avoid the ignorance, arrogance, and narrow self-interest that so often characterize aid. And it would involve the right combination of short- and long-term projects. To do all this in practice requires knowledge of particular situations, good political judgment, and a willingness to experiment. In some situations, assistance to organizations in civil society may prove worthwhile because these organizations are often working to fight injustices and empower marginalized people.

Rawls' work on justice focuses attention on vitally important matters: societal justice, international relations, war, assistance, and the need to create a confederation of reasonably just societies. But other important matters do not receive enough attention. Following the social contract model, Rawls starts with individual units and builds up relationships, structures, and conditions. Although he notes that the economic background conditions for international justice "have a role analogous to that of the basic structure in domestic society" (Rawls, 1999: 42), he does not emphasize this point. Hence I worry that Rawls' way of proceeding does not focus enough critical attention on the background conditions and transnational structures that characterize the world in the twenty-first century. This concern has prompted some scholars to develop theories and perspectives that are more critical of the dominant forms of globalization.

Whereas Rawls develops a conception of international justice, other scholars develop a conception of transnational justice (Cohen & Sabel, 2006; Young, 2006, 2011). They begin by characterizing some of the existing and emerging features of globalization: the patterns and structures that surround trade, consumption, labor markets, capital flows, corporations, and so on. To these patterns, I would add carbon emissions and ecological footprints (Dwyer, 2008, 2009). This characterization of globalization includes the fact that organizations such as the World Trade Organization come to acquire considerable power and independence in making rules that profoundly affect people and the environment (Cohen & Sabel, 2006: 164–173). The point is not merely that people are causally linked across borders but that they are connected by transnational structures and rules.

What moral norms are appropriate for the transnational structures and associations that have emerged? Although this question is debated and contested in global civil society, it receives too little attention in accounts of justice that start with separate national units. I believe that the norms of justice appropriate for transnational structures and associations are much closer in substance to principles of societal justice than to traditional principles of international justice. By focusing our attention on important features, an account of transnational justice helps to make sense of demands for alternative forms of globalization – forms that are more inclusive and more responsive to basic needs.

Both transnational and international views of justice tend to assume that the appropriate norms of justice depend on the relations and associations that exist among people. However, this assumption may lead us to overlook some important ethical features. Peter Singer develops a cosmopolitan view that starts with the idea that ethics requires us to give equal consideration to other people's fundamental interests, quite apart from the connections between them and us (Singer, 1993, 2002). This assumption makes sense of the reaction and concern that many of us have when we learn more about health inequalities in the world.

Although Singer recognizes an increased responsibility to care for family members, he views national boundaries as morally arbitrary, and he remarks on the contingency of being born into a rich or poor country. So he argues that people in relatively affluent circumstances – most people in high-income countries – have a strong duty to assist those who are worse off. In specifying this duty, he sees no moral justification for taking into account distance, community membership, or citizenship (Singer, 2002: 150–195). He conceptualizes the problem of global health in a way that emphasizes aid to individuals in need, wherever they are.

Conceptions of Responsibility

When I first began teaching global health ethics, I devoted a lot of time to explaining, contrasting, and evaluating theories of justice. I analyzed a theory of international justice, transnational justice, and cosmopolitan justice, but I noticed that most of the students grew impatient with my detailed analysis. When I came to understand why they were impatient, an unexpected thing happened: I too grew impatient.

What the students sensed, in a somewhat inarticulate way, was that the points of agreement among various accounts of justice are more important than the points of disagreement. The theories of justice that we considered tend to focus our attention in different ways and to emphasize different features, but they all agree that our world is marked by severe and persistent injustices. They all agree that we need to reconstruct institutions and practices so as to respect basic human rights and meet basic human needs.

Once the students learned basic ideas about population health, they were able, with some help, to see how poor health prospects raise issues of justice. And once they used theories of justice to focus their attention on key features, they were quick to see some of the underlying injustices, including structural injustices. But what they really wanted to know was how they should respond, what they should do to change institutions and practices. So I focused more attention on responsibility and responsiveness. Discussions of responsibility presuppose some rough and overlapping judgments of justice, but they do not require agreement on a general and abstract theory of justice.

I began with the idea of legal responsibility. Accounts of legal responsibility try to set out the conditions under which it would be right to punish people for acts or to hold them liable for harms (Hart, 2008). Although these accounts sometimes include the idea of deterrence, they tend to be backward looking; they focus on a particular harm in the past. Then they hold an individual person liable if a clear causal chain connects that person's action to the past harm and if that person acted intentionally, recklessly, or negligently. This form of responsibility is an important feature of social life. It applies to some actors in the realm of global health: soldiers who rape women, armies who target hospitals, people who sell counterfeit drugs, doctors who accept government salaries but do not show up for work, pharmaceutical companies that conduct research without informed consent, and so on.

However, a legalistic account of responsibility does not illuminate and fit many of the underlying problems in global health. Many problems are not past harms but future risks that are spread across populations. Clear causal chains rarely link these risks to particular actions or omissions. More often the diffuse causes are social structures or background conditions. Many people may contribute to these structures and conditions, but they do not do so

intentionally. For example, high-income countries accept doctors and nurses from low-income countries, overlooking the unintended harms and risks of this practice (Dwyer, 2007).

We need an account of responsibility that focuses attention in a different way. Before her untimely death, Iris Marion Young developed an account of responsibility for structural injustices (Young, 2011). Although her examples often deal with housing and labor, her insights also apply to global health. These insights help us to address three key questions about responsibility for global health.

First, what should we take responsibility for? Social structures, background conditions, economic systems, political processes, and accepted practices have a profound effect on people's health prospects. Often these structures and conditions unfairly contribute to food insecurity and poor nutrition; exposure to pathogens, accidents, and harm; lack of access to care, doctors, and medicines; lack of social support and income; and degradation of the natural environment. Looking forward, many of us need to take more responsibility to try to change these structures and conditions so that they are more just.

Second, why should we take responsibility? As we go about our lives, many of us participate in and reinforce structures, conditions, and processes that unfairly contribute to poor health prospects. My involvement in these structures and conditions grounds my responsibility. Young writes:

> The ground of my responsibility lies in the fact that I participate in the structural processes that have unjust outcomes. These processes are ongoing and ought to be transformed so they are less unjust. Thus I share with others the responsibility to transform these processes to reduce and eliminate the injustice that they cause. My responsibility is essentially shared with others because the harms are produced by many of us acting together within accepted institutions and practices, and because it is not possible for any of us to identify just what in our own actions results in which aspects of the injustice that particular individuals suffer. *(Young, 2011: 110)*

This responsibility is grounded in my relationship to the problem. Because of how I am related to the structures and conditions that shape health prospects, I have a shared responsibility to change those structures that unfairly disadvantage people, including people in distant places and future generations. Climate change is one striking example.

Third, how should we take responsibility? To change social structures and background conditions often requires political action, in the best and broadest sense of that term. Political action includes not only action by governments but also actions that citizens take in civil society. Young notes that those "who share responsibility for structural injustice may also find ways of making social changes ... through collective action in civil society independent of or as a supplement to state policies and programs" (Young, 2011: 112). This approach is promising, but the task is enormous: to generate political will to create new structures or adapt old structures to address injustices.

The first conception of responsibility that I considered emphasizes juridical responsibility and the assignment of liabilities and costs. The second conception emphasizes political responsibility and the need to change structures and conditions. A third conception, found in many ethical and religious traditions, emphasizes human responsibility to aid those in need. Some of our responsibilities may not be based on actions we take, promises we make, or roles we assume; they may not even be based on our relationships to structures and conditions. Some responsibilities may be based on our nature as human beings. This idea may take different forms and be explicated in different ways. A contemporary form is the discourse about human rights and responsibilities. People may have some rights by virtue of their status and dignity as human beings, and we may have responsibilities to uphold and protect those rights. Another form of this idea draws on Kant's philosophy. Kant bases positive duties on our status as rational and autonomous beings. According to Kant, not to acknowledge positive duties to aid others leads to a contradiction in will (Kant, 1981: 11–12, 32–33). Simply because we are human beings with the ability to help, we may have some responsibilities to improve global health.

Discussion of conceptions of responsibility brought us closer to the question of how to respond, but it didn't get us there. The students wanted more discussion about how to combine, in practice, a responsibility to address structural injustices and a responsibility to aid. So we turned directly to the issue of responsiveness.

Responsiveness

Even when we work with others, we cannot be responsible for addressing all health injustices and health problems in the world. At some point, we simply need to *take responsibility* for addressing some of the problems of global health. This selective taking of responsibility comes closest to the idea of responsiveness. Based on our ability, situation, and relationship to problems, we need to respond appropriately. To find an appropriate response, we may need to take many factors into account: the nature of the injustice, the effectiveness of action, possible partners, our abilities, our roles, our histories, and so on. In matters such as these, appropriate moral responses will often involve creativity and discretion, but discretion in responding does not mean that responses are exempt from ethical examination and evaluation.

More and more medical students from high-income countries respond by going abroad to work in low-income countries. They go to places like Guatemala, Haiti, Mali, and South Africa to work in clinics and hospitals or to work on public health projects and campaigns. These sojourns abroad are enormously educational but morally problematic. First, consider some of the ways that these sojourns are educational. Students often learn about and see a wide range of diseases and medical conditions. They also learn to practice medicine in a way that is less reliant on tests and more reliant on clinical skills and reasoning. Sometimes the learning goes deeper. The students observe how underlying social conditions and structures affect people's health. They also learn from experience what poor health prospects mean in human terms. Sometimes the learning goes even deeper. In their work abroad, students see forms of relationships, solidarity, and community that are underdeveloped in their own society. When they return, they see troubling aspects of their own society: the hyperindividualism, the consumer mentality, the wasteful medical system, and the ecological costs.

If these experiences abroad are so educational, why are they morally problematic? They are morally problematic because they do little to remedy injustice. Indeed, in some cases, they perpetuate unjust patterns. Because many students go abroad without adequate preparation and at an early stage in their training, they require considerable supervision or end up working without adequate supervision. They stay for a short time, disrupt local systems of care, and leave no sustainable benefits. Many countries extract more benefits from the host countries than they provide: while relatively wealthy and healthy societies are sending medical students abroad to work for four weeks, they are hiring away foreign doctors and nurses to work for 40 years (Dwyer, 2007). In sum, too many experiences and projects provide little sustainable benefit, lack forms of reciprocity, and even embody elements of paternalism.

What is to be done? People need to develop projects that provide educational benefits while more adequately addressing problems of sustainability, reciprocity, respect, and justice. Although responses to problems of global health involve creativity and discretion, they are subject to ethical examination and evaluation. So, before going abroad, students might consider the following questions in order to examine and evaluate possible responses.

1. *Have I studied adequately the language of the people I will be working with?* Students should consider how much help they can provide and how much burden they will be to bilingual staff if they don't have an adequate command of the local language. They should reconsider going to Honduras without a fair grasp of Spanish or going to Mali without a fair grasp of French. If the aim is really to provide benefits, then an adequate study of the relevant language seems like a reasonable prerequisite.

2. *Have I prepared by studying the history, culture, and social structures of the society I will be working in?* Students need to learn important things about the context in which they will be working. For example, before going to Guatemala, students should learn about the treatment of the indigenous peoples, the history of American involvement in the country, the human rights movements, and so on. A study that is equivalent to a college course does not seem too much to ask.

3. *Have I committed adequate time for my work abroad?* Students need to consider how much time is needed to understand the setting, adapt their skills, and provide significant benefits. Four-week electives seem more suited to the medical students' schedules than to the needs of projects. Even short stays by experienced physicians can reinforce bad attitudes and patterns. To make a positive difference, people need to consider longer commitments.

4. *Am I going at an appropriate stage in my training?* Students need to think about the best time in their careers to go abroad. The point is not to avoid working abroad but to choose a time in their careers that would benefit others. Too many experiences abroad reflect a troubling pattern: early in their careers, students learn and develop their clinical skills on poor people and then move on to apply those skills for the benefit of rich people (Dwyer, 1993).

5. *Is the project that I am considering part of a respectful and meaningful partnership?* Students need to consider whether a particular project is based on mutual respect and meaningful collaboration. Too many projects aim to benefit people without consulting and collaborating with those people. The local people, healthcare workers, and institutions should have a leading voice in a dialogue about how to define needs, develop capacities, and provide care.

6. *Are the benefits and burdens of the project fairly distributed?* The host institution and country should benefit more than the sending institution. After all, this is the principal point of the project. To meet this requirement, experienced faculty and senior doctors, as well as medical students, should devote substantial time to the project. And the sending institution should devote enough resources to cover the true costs of its part.

7. *In addition to providing clinical care, can I work with people to remedy structural injustices?* Everyone needs to take some responsibility for working with others to remedy structural injustices. Of course, not every clinical encounter needs to address structural injustices, but all projects and work abroad should keep this aim in mind because these injustices are often the big obstacles to improving health prospects.

8. *Do I want to go abroad primarily for the adventure and feeling of altruism?* Motives will always be complex and mixed, but students should consider whether they are concerned enough about health and justice to also work in their own country to address problems that impede better global health. Everyone could learn a lot and do some good by working on campaigns to protect human rights, improve labor conditions, change the brain drain, regulate the pharmaceutical industry, reduce antibiotic use, respond to refugees, address climate change, and so on.

Reflecting on questions such as these could lead to more appropriate responses.

Conclusion

To begin, I noted some of the inequalities in health prospects that exist between and within countries. The ways these inequalities come about and the ways they might be changed raise deep issues of justice. Theories of justice have many roles, but I used them mostly to help focus attention on salient features and to guide possible actions. Because most reasonable theories, students, and people agree that the present situation is marked by serious injustices in health prospects, I then considered conceptions of responsibility. Conceptions of responsibility brought us closer to the question of how to respond, but appropriate responses to the current situation depend on many individual and particular factors. So I formulated questions to help medical students consider a number of important factors.

Although the present situation is marked by deep injustices, it also shows great potential. Developments in science, public health, and communication have the potential to improve health prospects and reduce inequalities. But much will need to change in order to realize this potential. People will need to change social structures, background conditions, and political processes. People will need to change habits of acting, feeling, and thinking. People will need to change or reinterpret ideas about justice, responsibility, and responsiveness. Changes such as these take a lot of work by many people at many levels, but changes such as these bring us closer to the deepest meaning of education and growth (Dewey, 2008).

References

Cohen, J., & Sabel, C. (2006). Extra republicam nulla justitia? *Philosophy and Public Affairs* **34**(2), 147–175.

Dewey, J. (2008). *John Dewey: The Middle Works, 1899–1924*, Vol. 9. Carbondale, IL: Southern Illinois University Press.

Dwyer, J. (1993). Case study: one more pelvic exam. *Hastings Center Report* **23**(6), 27–28.

Dwyer, J. (2003). Part of my liver. *Transplantation* **76**, 1266–1267.

Dwyer, J. (2007). What's wrong with the global migration of health care professionals? *Hastings Center Report* **37**(5), 36–43.

Dwyer, J. (2008). The century of biology: three views. *Sustainability Science* **3**(2), 283–285.

Dwyer, J. (2009). How to connect bioethics and environmental ethics: health, sustainability, and justice. *Bioethics* **23**(9), 497–502.

Hart, H. L. A. (2008). *Punishment and Responsibility: Essays in the Philosophy of Law*, 2nd ed. New York: Oxford University Press.

Kant, I. (1981). *Grounding for the Metaphysics of Morals*. Indianapolis, IN: Hackett Publishing Company.

Lappé, F., & Collins, J. (1986). *World Hunger: Twelve Myths*. New York: Grove Press.

Murray, C. J. L., Kularni, S., & Ezzati, M. (2005). Eight Americas: new perspectives on U.S. health disparities. *American Journal of Preventive Medicine* **29** (5S1), 4–10.

Rawls, J. (1971). *A Theory of Justice*. Cambridge, MA: Harvard University Press.

Rawls, J. (1999). *The Law of Peoples*. Cambridge, MA: Harvard University Press.

Rawls, J. (2001). *Justice as Fairness*. Cambridge, MA: Harvard University Press.

Sen, A. (1981). *Poverty and Famines*. Oxford, UK: Clarendon Press.

Singer, P. (1993). *Practical Ethics*. Cambridge, UK: Cambridge University Press.

Singer, P. (2002). *One World*, 2nd ed. New Haven, CT: Yale University Press.

World Health Organization (WHO) (2019a). Global Health Observatory. Available at www.who.int/gho/countries/en/ (accessed January 4, 2019)

World Health Organization (WHO) (2019b). News releases. Available at www.who.int/news-room/fact-sheets/detail/children-reducing-mortality (accessed January 5, 2019).

Young, I. M. (2006). Responsibility and global justice: a social connection model. *Social Philosophy and Policy* **23** (1), 102–130.

Young, I. M. (2011). *Responsibility for Justice*. New York: Oxford University Press.

Teaching Global Health Ethics
An Ecological Perspective

Sarah Elton and Donald C. Cole

Introduction

It's not easy to talk about global health during the Anthropocene in a university classroom in the Global North. It's confusing and upsetting to grapple with the data on rising chronic disease rates, the impact of climate change on infectious disease, the effects of toxic exposures from industry globally, and the connection between health and people's access to land, water, and clean air to breathe. Many of the challenges have been summarized in several Lancet Commission reports (e.g., Whitmee et al., 2015). In class, discussion goes something like this: "Is it really that bad? If it is, there must be someone doing something about it. Technology will save us anyway. Moreover, how do we make sure that everyone has enough food to eat and can live healthy lives if we make changes to the system? What makes us, here in the Global North, more worthy of this good life than those in the Global South, where so many of our families come from and many remain? If we can waste less food, eat less meat, throw away less, recycle more, and find technological fixes, we shall be all right."

Wading into the morass of competing ethical issues with students can reflect the state of public discourse on these topics, yet it is easier to remain confused or unengaged. The Anthropocene, a term increasingly used to describe our current era, is characterized by a changing climate, environmental degradation, mass migrations, and growing inequality (Steffen et al., 2011). The Greek root *anthro* in Anthropocene assigns responsibility to human activity for this state of affairs. Though, as scholars such as Davis and Todd (2017), Haraway (2015), and Moore (2017, 2018) have observed, only some of us *anthropos* – specifically those groups of people who have benefited most from Western European imperialistic colonialism – are responsible for these changes. This is because while some groups[1] have benefited from the economic development that began with European colonization and its extraction

economy (of both people and the Earth's ecological systems), other groups have been shut out from the spoils – for example, as evidenced by the steady flow of migrants from Sub-Saharan Africa and Latin America. A conversation about global public health ethics today must start by acknowledging this structural dynamic. The conversation also must grapple with the fact that the impacts of climate change similarly are experienced unequally – the floodwaters of the latest hurricane or monsoon typically flow through the same well-worn lines of oppression and injustice (Schlosberg & Collins, 2014).

In the last two decades, the field of global health increasingly has embraced equity among people as a goal, although in practice various perspectives jostle for ascendance (Cole et al., 2017). In the Introduction to the first edition of this book, Benatar and Brock wrote that part of working toward global health, a state defined as sustainable and healthy living for all, requires an understanding of "the value systems, modes of reasoning, and power structures that have driven and shaped the world" (p.1). This approach frames the social and societal determinants of health as a conceptual tool for scholars, policymakers, and practitioners and enables them to make connections between social conditions and health. Equity analysis tools have illustrated health inequalities and articulated some of the causes of these inequalities globally (Barreto, 2017), although Sen (2009) has argued that they need to go deeper in facing the practical circumstances of peoples' lives.

Here we argue that to push a global health equity agenda forward in the Anthropocene epoch, we must invoke an even wider perspective. When discussing global health ethics today, we must make climate change front and center and also reckon with the damage to ecological systems that societies depend on that is caused by the "developed" lifestyle and the global growth-driven economic structures that

---

[1] Wynter (2003) names this group the *ethnoclass*.

support it. This means thinking about ecology when thinking about global health, as Goldberg and Patz (2015: e37) argued when they called for a "global health ethic." This is an expansive field, ranging from conceptions of justice to governance to infectious disease and migration and so many of issues implicitly connected to environmental concerns and ecological approaches to health. This range is visible in the diversity of chapters in this book, situated in the broader Anthropocene discourse, including David Benatar's chapter, "Animals, the Environment, and Global Health" (Chapter 23), and Christine Straehle's look at migration in the Anthropocene (Chapter 22) and others.

As university instructors in global public health, we regularly tackle how to teach these topics. In the classroom, how do you broach an issue so vexing that societies around the world have failed to grapple with it, as evidenced by lack of adequate action on climate change by world leaders? How do we teach students to make the connections between environment and health without grinding them down? Instead, how might we spark what Norgaard (2018: 171) calls the "ecological imagination"? Built on *The Sociological Imagination* (Mills, 2000) and the "moral imagination" (Benatar, 2005: 1207), this imagination-awareness can permit people to see "the relationships within society that make up our environmentally damaging social structure" (Norgarard, 2018: 171). Then we ask, how might that ecological imagination be used to identify the ontological and political shifts that need to be made so that those concerned about equity and global health might respond effectively and hopefully? In the opening of her book about Indigenous ecological consciousness, *Braiding Sweetgrass*, Kimmerer (2013: 6), as a botanist and member-citizen of the Potawatomi Nation, describes how her university students – training for careers in environmental protection – were unable to name a beneficial relationship between humans and their environments when she surveyed them. She laments this lack of ability to see the good in the human–nonhuman nature relationship and asks, "How can we begin to move toward ecological and cultural sustainability if we cannot even imagine what the path feels like?" Her anecdote identifies a gap that we too have seen as university educators.

In this chapter, we propose three ecological perspectives that we have drawn on to teach the connections between people and the nonhuman world and to try to stimulate this ecological imagination. The three theoretical perspectives are rooted in social sciences scholarship. They are posthumanism, political ecology, and the ecological determinants of health framework. We recognize that there are other important approaches to teaching the connection between health and environment, specifically land-based learning from Indigenous perspectives, that scholars and traditional knowledge keepers are implementing, including at our own university (Chapter 31 of this book explores Indigenous approaches to planetary health).

Here we focus on the three perspectives with which we have experience. In the first part of this chapter, we outline these three perspectives and how they have been applied to education by other scholars. Next, we describe the courses where we attempt to put these theories into action, that is, where we explore our praxis. Then we reflect on our application of these perspectives to facilitate teaching related to global public health ethics. We also explore how we approach what we optimistically call the *challenges-barriers-opportunities* that arise. In the final part of this chapter, we reflect on what more might be done to bring ecological perspectives into teaching such that they change the conversation about global health.

Part One: Ecological Perspectives for Teaching-Learning

Political Ecology

Political ecology is a theoretical framework used by scholars in fields such as geography, political science, and public health to understand the relationships between political economy and ecology, between human societies and nonhuman nature. Work in the field of political ecology sheds light on how socioeconomic and political forces have an impact on the environment and how the environment interacts with economics, politics, and culture (see Peet & Watts, 1996; Peet et al., 2011; Bryant, 2015). Political ecology politicizes the relationship between societies and their environment by interrogating how economics and politics shape the way things are. There have been several waves of political ecology mirroring larger trends in academia, its original structuralist approach being challenged in the 1990s by poststructuralist perspectives, including feminist analyses.

Throughout these various turns in its scholarship, political ecology has provided a solid framework for scholars to unpack diverse topics such as land degradation and the role of natural systems, such as water, in the city (Swyngedouw, 1996).

In 2015, Meek's (2015: 448) assessment that there was no political ecology of education led him to define the concept. He describes a political ecology of education as being "a framework for understanding how the reciprocal relations between political economic forces influence pedagogical opportunities – from tacit to formal learning – affecting the production, dissemination, and contestation of environmental knowledge at various interconnected scales" (Meek, 2015: 448). He describes this approach to education as drawing from the theory and practice of political ecology and enabling a view of how political and economic forces shape what is typically known as nature. This, in turn, permits a better understanding of the relationships between society and nature, including providing an opportunity to understand how knowledge about nature is produced. We identify political ecology as holding particular promise in helping to ignite Norgaard's ecological imagination. By providing a lens that makes visible social structures, it is possible for one to see the factors that constrain dominant Western society's current responses to climate change. Norgaard believes that a structural understanding will make way for new perspectives on the scale of social change required to make the shifts necessary to address climate change (Norgaard, 2018: 173).

Posthumanism

Posthumanism is the term we use to group the theories[2] that challenge a dominant Western worldview that sees humans as the center of life and relegates nature to the backdrop. Scholars working in this area challenge the idea that the natural world is separate from the human sphere. They posit that the

human, for example, doesn't exist on his or her own but rather lives in a body cocreated by human and bacterial DNA, in relation to all matter and beings with which he or she interacts constantly as part of life here on planet Earth. In a posthumanist framework, it is argued that the concept of the human is in fact a political category (Lloro-Bidart, 2015) that has been used to create other categories designed to exclude and oppress, particularly in a colonial context (see Wynter, 2003). Posthumanism has been applied to many topics to identify the interdependencies that exist between humans and nonhuman nature in our personal lives and domestic spaces (Haraway, 2008), in our bodies (Lorimer, 2016), and along the food chain (Elton, 2018, 2019). Rock (2013) even proposes a posthumanist version of health promotion in a city that considers the beneficial interspecies relationships in dog ownership. Posthumanism has been identified by scholars as being increasingly relevant during the Anthropocene. Braidotti (2017: 84), a feminist philosopher and leading thinker in posthumanism, writes that the importance of these theories "is framed by the urgency of the Anthropocene condition." There is an urgency to figuring out how to live with nonhuman nature and respect the rights of water, trees, and other species (Cheater, 2018) because our health and future depend on it.

A posthumanist approach to education involves upending ideas fundamental to pedagogy, writes Kuby (2017). For example, posthumanism disrupts a mainstream understanding of what happens when one person teaches and another learns. When the human is decentered and seen in relation to other things, learning becomes a process that takes place *between* the student and the world rather than a process that happens independently, in a student's brain. Taguchi (2010) uses Barad's (2007: 409) term "ethico-onto-epistemology" to indicate that ethics cannot be parsed from ontology and epistemology – the study of what we know (ontology) and how we come to know it (epistemology). This is a weighty way of saying that the student comes to learn through living and doing.

Perhaps one of the most fruitful areas of applied posthuman research is in childhood studies (see, e.g., Malone, 2016; Pacini-Ketchabaw & Taylor, 2015) and in the field of education, specifically among scholars interested in the child-nature relationship. Scholars in both fields have looked to posthumanist theories to understand how educators might work with children to prepare them for life in the Anthropocene. They ask, how might adults educate children to "co-inhabit these

[2] The social theories we group together in posthumanism include new materialisms, more-than-human perspectives, and actor-network theory. We also note that posthumanist theory follows the lead of many other ontologies in recognizing the agency and vitality in nonhuman nature. These other long-standing ways of knowing are diverse and include Indigenous philosophies in North America, the ontologies of Australian Indigenous people (as described by Bawaka Country et al. [2016]), in addition to the views espoused for millennia in religions originating in the eastern hemisphere (see Gethmann & Ehlers, 2003).

messy, complex (post-) colonial and multispecies worlds" (Pacini-Ketchabaw & Taylor, 2015: 45). Those who think about adult education, too, are considering the potential of posthumanism because it examines what values are embedded in the approach we take to teaching others. Ferrante and Sartori (2016), for example, argue that posthumanism challenges a fundamental assumption of education and the Western humanist worldview, in which much of global health ethics is also rooted, the assumption that humans are the only species that is able to hold moral values. The idea that humans are alone in conceiving of an ethical framework, they explain, justifies the human domination of nature that put nonhuman species in such a precarious position in the first place. Applied to education, posthumanism puts front and center the question of what role education plays in reproducing, from generation to generation, the ontological dualism present in Western society that separates nature from humans (Lloro-Bidart, 2015). What it does not, or should not, do, writes Pedersen (2010: 247), is provide a "'corrective device' to reform education curricula in a more sustainable direction." The real promise of posthumanism, rather, is to challenge and even destroy the "authoritative position of human subjectivity" (Pedersen, 2010: 247). Posthumanism applied to pedagogy requires a fundamental questioning of how one comes to know what one knows and what one values as education and learning in relation to nonhuman species and the places all beings inhabit.

Ecological Determinants of Health

The *ecological determinants of health* is a concept that parallels the social determinants of health. In the same way that social determinants, such as gender and racialization, shape both individual and population health, ecological determinants are environmental factors that influence human health and well-being. The three primary ecological determinants of health are oxygen, water, and food. When the group of health scientists and public health practitioners first articulated the concept in a Canadian Public Health Association position paper (2015), they had to distill the many health-supporting acts of nonhuman nature and decide what to consider the fundamental determinants. This list includes fresh and marine water systems, including the ecosystems that detoxify water, and those that provide for foods; the soil systems in which nitrogen and phosphorus cycle, because these are important fertilizers for the plants we grow and depend on; the ozone layer; a stable climate for the planet; the materials we use for shelter and tools; and energy too. The concept's contribution to the fields of public health and global health is a clear articulation of humanity's fundamental dependence on nonhuman nature to be healthy.

Likely because the idea of the ecological determinants of health is an emerging concept in the field of public health, its utility in teaching is still being explored (Ecological Determinants Group on Education [EDGE], 2018). Williams (2017: 720) notes that health promoters interested in multilevel change – what she calls "empowerment practitioners" – require a shift in their ontoepistemology to "working with the ecological determinants of health." This requires seeing nonhuman nature as "relational participants" in socioecological systems. She sees three empowerment paradigms that can contribute to greater action on the ecological determinants of health: transformatist/critical postmodern, participatory, and Indigenous (Williams, 2017: table 1, p. 719), each of which brings opportunities for agents of change in health. The ecological determinants of health thus can work well in coordination with political ecology and posthumanism because the concept explicitly ties human health and well-being to the nonhuman world.

Part Two: Teaching Practice Applying These Frameworks

Both authors teach at the University of Toronto, centered in the Dalla Lana School of Public Health. However, we come to the question of how to teach global health ethics from two different perspectives, each informed by our divergent career stage and paths. Sarah is a senior PhD candidate in social and behavioral health sciences, which she approaches as a critical food systems scholar and from a posthumanist perspective. She teaches undergraduate courses in food studies, where she explores with her students the connections between society and the nonhuman world. Sarah comes to this work from a previous career as an environmental journalist and university journalism instructor. Donald is an occupational and environmental medicine specialist and an epidemiologist with many decades of experience teaching clinicians as well as graduate students in public health; he also has many years of experience working across cultures in Kenya and Ecuador. Donald and Sarah share an interest in food systems and a commitment to paying close attention to the connection between human health and well-being and the biosphere. They have worked together as doctoral student and committee member, as well as teaching assistant and professor.

In both the critical food studies courses that Sarah teaches and the ecological public health class that Donald leads, conversations about global public health ethics occur naturally. While neither class is explicitly focused on global health ethics – food studies less so than ecological public health – it is impossible not to engage with the topic throughout the term. In ecological public health, the syllabus includes topics such as systems thinking, ecoregional grounding of health, place-based health promotion, public health ecosystems approaches, and the Sustainable Development Goals. Students apply these to resource extraction and the global food system in the class, but they also select topics for their group projects and scholarly papers. Recent examples include the health impact legacies of resource extraction in Peru and water scarcity in Cape Town, for which global health ethics questions are regular class fodder. Global health ethics are also relevant in critical food systems studies in modules covering the global livestock industry and meat consumption, food security from a global perspective, and the *nutrition transition*, which is the term used to describe a trend taking place globally whereby populations are moving from so-called traditional diets to ultraprocessed foods and North American–style food consumption (Pan American Health Organization [PAHO], 2015). Conversations that relate to global health ethics become central given the inequalities between north and south, including access to resources for producing food. Also, because the globalized food system connects every person who eats to the many people and beings along the food chain who work to provide food, this approach to critical food systems studies raises ethical issues of complicity with an exploitative and damaging system. Further, critical food systems studies provide the opportunity for conversations about how social change might address the problems. In both classes, students are encouraged to engage in the issues of the Anthropocene, including global health.

Political Ecology in Teaching Practice

Political ecology as a theoretical framework can be a challenge for students to understand. Among undergraduate students, only the most theoretically inclined typically grasp political ecological frameworks. To engage everyone equally, regardless of their training or openness to critical social theory, Sarah draws on the notion of the sociological imagination to help students think abstractly and critically. This term was articulated in the 1950s by American sociologist C. Wright Mills (2000) and helps to uncover the ways social forces shape how we live. It has been used to consider the human–nature nexus, including in animal studies (DeMello, 2012). With her students, Sarah describes the sociological imagination as a lens – or a pair of glasses – that allows students to see the social, political, and economic structures that shape relationships in society and in ecosystems, making the bridge to the ecological (Norgaard, 2018) and moral (Benatar, 2005) imaginations (see earlier).

Similarly, Donald does not explicitly describe political ecology but draws on the theories when teaching global environmental health to postgraduate physicians. He draws on case studies to demonstrate the power of this kind of analysis. For example, in the Environmental Health Module of the Global Health Education Initiative, he and a doctoral student explored a lead poisoning outbreak in northern Nigeria (Pringle & Cole, 2012). In early 2010, an international humanitarian medical organization heard about an outbreak of child illness and deaths. Mothers of the sick children disclosed to health workers that there had been a surge in artisanal gold mining around the time of the first deaths. The price of gold had spiked after the recent global financial crisis, and men in Zamfara State turned to artisanal gold mining to supplement their incomes. They were poor subsistence farmers reeling from recent cuts to fertilizer subsidies. Farming brought in a dollar or two a day, but artisanal gold mining could bring in 20 dollars a day. New rock-grinding machines were being used in family compounds where wives could assist while still minding children and cooking meals. With special government permission, the organization had blood samples of affected children analyzed, encountering the highest blood lead levels ever recorded. It is estimated that more than 700 children below the age of five died and thousands of others remain in dire need of chelation treatment. Without proper occupational safety and public health capacity, the outbreak grew into a humanitarian emergency. In Donald's class, students analyzed how an ore of high lead content had entered an artisanal production chain, stimulated by rural poverty and a high global price for gold. This case study demonstrates how a political ecological approach to a global health issue can reveal how a crisis that may at first appear to be localized in fact is produced across multiple political and economic scales and is shaped by the intimate relationships between ecology and society.

Posthumanism in Teaching Practice

In the ecological public health class, Donald has drawn on experience with the Canadian Community of Practice in Ecosystem Health (Cole et al., 2018), using a posthumanist exercise to help students decenter the human and appreciate the perspectives of things other-than-human. The "Council of All Beings" exercise involves separating the class into six groups, with each group representing the point of view of an actor in the Toronto and region ecosystem, the geographic area where the course is held. This activity, however, has been organized in other watersheds and could easily be adapted to any location. The six actors in the Toronto context are an ash tree; a woman active in the Toronto Environmental Alliance, a nonprofit environmental and equity advocacy group in the city; a male construction worker of Caribbean origin; a female salmon in the Humber River, one of the significant watercourses in the larger Toronto area; an elder of the Mississaugas of the Credit River, one of the Indigenous nations whose traditional territory includes the current city of Toronto; and a Canadian corporate leader in international finance. Together these six perspectives represent the so-called Council of All Beings.

Students are asked to adopt the persona and perspective of the actor they have been assigned and to think through what their understanding of health might be. They are also asked to consider how their character's perspective on health might shape how they would address ecological public health challenges. Because this exercise is assigned in advance of class, students are asked to draw on scholarly research and the gray literature while developing their character's point of view. In class, students discuss their ideas first as a group with the other students who share their perspective. Then the whole class comes together to come up with a working definition of health in ecosystems across actors. The purpose of this exercise is to underline the "situatedness" of different understandings of health and to begin to

identify how the diverse socioecological positionality of different species affects how they approach health.

Ecological Determinants of Health in Teaching Practice

The topics of meat eating, the industrial livestock industry, and its alternatives has provided an accessible way to explore the ecological determinants of health and begin to think about global health ethics. In Sarah's critical food systems class, the topic of meat eating and the livestock industry was integrated into the course over several classes, with students asked to read an article by animal rights ethicist Peter Singer, as well as an article that presented the perspective that a "better beef" than what is conventionally produced by the industrial livestock industry was possible. Effort was made to expose students to different perspectives and to get at the complexity of the issues. In the lecture and discussion, the political, economic, and ecological structures and social relationships that shape meat eating were discussed, and in-class participatory activities encouraged students to make connections between the material and their own experiences. A guest speaker, who was a PhD in soil sciences and also an ecological livestock farmer, explained how on her farm she uses pigs, chickens, and only a few cows to help regenerate soil health.

Students became very engaged in the topic, making their own connections between eating and the ecological determinants of health. Because meat eating is an activity that all students are exposed to in contemporary Western society, whether they are vegan, vegetarian, or omnivore, the personal nature of the topic rendered the material salient to their lives. Several students reflected on how what previously had seemed like a natural part of eating was in fact a learned practice that had ethical and ecological repercussions. However, the class quickly divided into two camps made up of meat eaters, supporting the current meat industry, and non–meat eaters, who opposed it. The meat eaters almost uniformly expressed how their decision to eat meat was cultural; however, many of the non–meat eaters, who often cited ethical reasons for not eating animals, also had cultural ties to cuisines where meat is considered to be important. Class discussion took on the tone of a debate as opposed to a conversation. One of the meat eaters in particular was hostile to the idea that meat could have a negative side and discounted the scientific research, subsequently writing a paper about how meat eating was beyond reproach. Later, in a reflection session, the meat eaters revealed that they felt judged in the class. Learning about the ecological determinants of health, albeit easier to grasp for some students in the context of a common practice like meat eating, in fact alienated others. This revealed a challenge that educators must deal with when teaching complex topics that can implicate students in ethical dilemmas they would rather not confront.

Part Three: What We Encounter/How We Respond

Positionality: Intersectionality and Grounding

We often note that students and clinical residents struggle to locate themselves socially and ecologically. Socially, many high-income-country students have limited recognition of their privilege, though those who immigrated as children or whose parents immigrated from lower- and middle-income countries in our anecdotal experience can have a more nuanced view. Further, the often cosmopolitan students, the large proportion of women in classes, and their varied socioeconomic situations make sharing of intersectional perspectives on environmental justice feasible (Jampel, 2018). One perspective that we note most students share is an urban or suburban viewpoint. In Sarah's critical food system classes, many students never have visited a farm. So she invites students with rural or agricultural experiences, either in Canada or in other countries, to share their perspectives.

For largely urban students, connecting with a particular ecoregion is a challenge. In their education thus far, students have been taught to think about political jurisdictions and boundaries rather than ecological features. In the ecological public health course, for example, colleagues organized a field trip down Toronto's Don River watershed to teach students about its history, socially and ecologically. Walking together in the watershed, where the sounds of the running water and the calls of red-winged blackbirds can be heard over the rumble of the nearby highway, allows students to observe and then discuss the session material on site, deepening an understanding of the ecoregion concept.

Both social and ecological positionality becomes relevant when considering Indigenous peoples' contexts, particularly with global environmental changes (Ford et al., 2016). Starting from digital stories produced by youth in a small Inuit community in Nunatsiavut, ecological public health students were asked to identify relationships that people have with the land, their culture, and their health (Richmond, 2015). Many students remarked on how much more they understood about the role of the land and other species in the youth's expression of their Indigenous identity and where the points of connection were with their own experiences and locations. Such an ability to reflect iteratively on social and ecological positionality and its ethical implications is highly relevant to teaching global health ethics in keeping with transformative learning approaches (see Cole et al., 2013).

Struggling with Complexity

Students inevitably struggle with the complexity of existing socioecological relationships, their historical origins, and their future consequences (Waltner-Toews, 2017). There are ethical implications across different scales, over different time periods, and in different global locations that need to be unpacked (Brisbois et al., 2017; Buse et al., 2018). In the ecological public health course session on cumulative impacts of resource development in remote watersheds (Parkes et al., 2016), Donald asks the students not only to read the peer-reviewed papers cited but also to view videos that capture the ideas well (Berlow, 2010). Drawing on substantial experience with teaching about complexity (CoPEH-Canada, n.d.), we work with students to make complexity graspable on a few scales (not global), grounding themselves in the experience of a concrete ecoregion. For example, we ask students to map out sets of relationships between key actors (of whatever social strata, species, or ecosystem) using influence or spaghetti diagrams. These visualization tools have been used in participatory exercises to conduct joint assessments and intervention planning in lower-income countries in particular (Waltner-Toews et al., 2003), and Donald has found that they work well in university classrooms. Examples of scenarios for which students have created spaghetti diagrams include the ecological and health impacts of promotion of bottle-feeding in cyclone-prone Pacific islands and the use of pesticides impacts on biodiversity and neurotoxic impacts among small farmers in an East African highland region. In each case, ethics are scrutinized.

Affective Ecological Grief, Anger at Those in Power, Yet Active Hope

Coming to grips with the extent of biodiversity loss and climate change and associated impacts can stir strong feelings among students, including deep sadness or ecological grief (Cunsolo & Ellis, 2018), hopelessness at the enormity of the changes needed, and frustration or anger at the seeming unwillingness of people and institutions to change. We listen to the students and validate such feelings. We also point to stories of resilience, as exemplified by Indigenous peoples who move from deficit to desire, in practice and in research (Hyett et al., 2018). To speak to some students' views that "somebody has got to be taking care of the situation," we highlight mobilization efforts such as the Friday school strikes for climate ongoing in 2018–2019 around the world, through which young people are claiming their right to a future. In keeping with collective learning (Brown & Lambert, 2013) and social design approaches (Escobar, 2018), the ecological public health course group project is focused on responses to socioecological problems. Students are asked to characterize the problem, describe opportunities for change, and address governance issues (Porter et al., 2013) drawing on a combination of critical analysis and creative communications. Students have produced skits on the oil sands, petitions around toxics control, green beef campaigns, and other collective-action designs.

Part Four: Directions for Exploration

Given the potential of ecological perspectives to enrich conversations in global health ethics by recognizing our fundamental dependence on the biosphere – or in posthumanist terms, providing for a recognition that we are the biosphere and the biosphere is us – we see a number of opportunities. We group them according to the classic pedagogical triad of students, teachers, and institutions and the relationships that exist among them (Biggs & Tang, 2011).

First, we can better respond to the heterogeneous understanding and interests of our students. Some come to class barely believing that global environmental change has health implications, whereas others are passionate about injustices and are eager to campaign. With the first group of tepid believers,

we may be able to build on their positionality in ways that speak to Rumi's insights, as captured in Leonard Cohen's song "Anthem": "There's a crack in everything – that's where the light comes in." The crack may be personal vulnerabilities in their own stories, social location, or desires that may be affected by ecological determinants of health. We can support the second enthusiastic group through linking learning to contemporary outlets of expression such as Twitter and other social media where groups like Great Britain's grassroots activist group Extinction Rebellion spread word of their zealous demands for climate action. We can also encourage students who favor action to take the time needed to analyze and better articulate ethical implications of the status quo they wish to change.

Second, as teachers, we can mainstream ecological perspectives in ethics training by *glocally* drawing on the examples we have provided here as well as reports by other scholars published in journals such as *Environmental Ethics* and the *Journal of Political Ecology*. We can foster greater affective connections with outdoor places as part of outdoor education, linking to Leopold's famous land ethic, a call to moral responsibility to and caring for the natural world (Goldberg & Patz, 2015). For example, the University of Toronto Outdoors initiative has been experimenting with place-responsive teaching: convening food studies sessions on farms, leading hiking courses in India, paddling the rivers of Ontario, and other forms of immersive, embodied student engagement. From a research perspective, we can involve students in addressing ecological and environmental determinants of health globally (Lavery et al., 2003) such as doctoral research on the political ecology of health associated with pesticide use (Brisbois et al., 2018). Finally, we can critically reflect on the educational programs we develop, engaging in greater scholarship of teaching and learning, for example, CoPEH Canada's long experience with education on ecosystems, society, and health, which gradually evolved with opportunities to teach students, practitioners, and policymakers (Cole et al., 2018).

Third, we can push our educational institutions to better embrace ecological and equity perspectives in dialogue, teaching, and actions. Milder forms of this strategy would include lecture series on relevant topics or sustainability initiatives such as cataloguing the ways sustainability is addressed in courses across the university, similar to those discussed in the

International Journal of Sustainability in Higher Education. Moderate approaches include pushing for greater transparency in sources of donations, such as from extractive industries and fossil fuel corporations (Tannock, 2010), and opening discussions of their appropriateness – such as the TransCanada Pipelines Chair in Aboriginal Health and Well-Being at our own school of public health. Stronger forms of action would aim to explicitly mitigate the harms that current institutional partnering and investment have inflicted globally, such as the work of 350.org, which promotes divestment from fossil fuel corporations among universities. (Note that such combined student and faculty initiatives have been successful at many universities, though not the University of Toronto.) Without such educational institutional reorientation, it is hard to convince students of the seriousness of ecological perspectives across their educational experience.

We opened this chapter by observing that it is not easy to talk about climate change and all the topics that both confront and implicate students in the big issues that affect our society today. We conclude by repeating this observation: it's not easy, but it is necessary. As we are reminded by international report after international report, these topics are of critical importance – from the Lancet's EAT Report to the United Nation's May 2019 barn burner of a study describing "natures' dangerous decline." As university educators, we feel that it is our responsibility to engage students in what's going on in current events, if only to get them to think critically about the world around them. By teaching the way we do, our aim is to encourage students to think about their future – and reimagine it. In our collegial discussions in Donald's office, where we have shared our own ecological grief and frustrations, we have come back to the concept "to defuture" (see Escobar, 2018). This idea was coined by Tony Fry (1999), a philosopher of design, to highlight how something that is unsustainable is a threat to the future. Fry (1999) argues that the idea of defuturing challenges commonly held visions of the future as a limitless space of possibility when, in fact, the future is made by the decisions and actions taken today. Defuturing is a form of intergenerational violation that goes against our cherished notions of beneficence. For those involved in global health ethics, when considering the biosphere that supports all life, we are reminded again and again how the decisions made today limit what will be possible in the future for all species including our own. This small insight is the kernel we hope all students will take away from our courses.

References

Barad, K. (2007). *Meeting the University Halfway: Quantum Physics and the Entanglement of Matter and Meaning.* Durham, N.C.: Duke University Press.

Barreto, M. L. (2017). Health inequalities: a global perspective. *Ciênc. saúde coletiva* **22**(7), 2097–2108.

Bawaka Country, Wright, S., Suchet-Pearson, S., et al. (2016). Co-becoming Bawaka: towards a relational understanding of place/space. *Progress in Human Geography* **40**(4), 455–475.

Benatar, S. R. (2005). Moral imagination: the missing component in global health. *PLoS Medicine* **2**(12), e400, 1207–1210.

Berlow, E. (2010). How complexity leads to simplicity. TED Talk. Available at www.ted.com/talks/eric_berlow_how_complexity_leads_to_simplicity (accessed May 10, 2019).

Biggs, J. B., and Tang, C. (2011) *Teaching for Quality Learning at University.* New York: McGraw-Hill/Society for Research into Higher Education/Open University Press.

Braidotti, R. (2017). Critical posthuman knowledges. *South Atlantic Quarterly* **116**(1), 83–96.

Brisbois, B., Burgos Delgado, A., Barraza, D., et al. (2017). Ecosystem approaches to health and knowledge-to-action: towards a political ecology of applied health-environment knowledge. *Journal of Political Ecology* **24**, 692–715.

Brisbois, B. W., Harris, L., & Spiegel, J. (2018). Political ecologies of global health: pesticide exposure in southwestern Ecuador's banana industry. *Antipode* **50**(1–2), 61–81.

Brown, V. A., & Lambert, J. A. (2013). *Collective Learning for Transformational Change: A Guide to Collaborative Action.* London: Routledge.

Bryant, R. L. (2015). Reflecting on political ecology, in Bryant, R. L. (ed.), *The International Handbook of Political Ecology.* Northampton, MA: Edward Elgar Publishing.

Buse, C. G., Smith, M., & Silva, D. S. (2019). Attending to scalar ethical issues in emerging approaches to environmental health research and practice. *Monash Bioethics Review* **37**, 4–21.

Canadian Public Health Association (2015). Global change and public health: addressing the ecological determinants of health. CPHA discussion paper, Canadian Public Health Association, Ottawa. Available at www.cpha.ca/discussion-paper-ecological-determinants-health (accessed May 10, 2019).

Cheater, D. (2018). I am the river, and the river is me: legal personhood and emerging rights of nature. *Environmental Law Blog Alert*, West Coast Environmental Law, Vancouver, Canada. Available at www.wcel.org/blog/i-am-river-and-river-me-legal-personhood-and-emerging-rights-nature (accessed May 10, 2019).

Cole, D. C., Hanson, L., Rouleau, K., et al. (2013). Teaching global health ethics, in Pinto, A. D., & Upshur, R. E. G. (eds.), *An Introduction to Global Health Ethics*. Abingdon, UK: Routledge (Taylor and Francis Group), pp. 148–158.

Cole, D. C., Jackson, S., & Forman, L. (2017). What approaches can schools of public health take to engage in global health? A conceptual synthesis and reflection on implications. *Global Health Governance* **XI** (2), 71–82.

Cole, D. C., Parkes, M., Saint-Charles, J., et al. (2018). Evolution of capacity strengthening: insights from the Canadian Community of Practice in Ecosystem Approaches to Health. *Transformative Dialogues* **11**(2), 1–21.

CoPEH-Canada (n.d.). Teaching Module on Complexity. Available at www.copeh-canada.org/en/teaching-manual/module-3-complexity.html (accessed January 16, 2019).

Cunsolo, A., & Ellis, N. R. (2018) Ecological grief as a mental health response to climate change-related loss. *Nature Climate Change* **8**, 275–281.

Davis, H., & Todd, Z. (2017). On the importance of a date, or, decolonizing the Anthropocene. *ACME: An International Journal for Critical Geographies* **16**(4), 761–780.

DeMello, M. (2012). *Animals and Society: An Introduction to Human-Animal Studies*. New York: Columbia University Press.

Ecological Determinants Group on Education (EDGE) (2018). *Ecological Determinants of Health in Public Health Education in Canada: A Scan of Needs, Challenges and Assets*. Ottawa: Canadian Public Health Association. Available at www.cpha.ca/sites/default/files/uploads/about/cmte/EDGE-scan-needs-challenges-assets-2018-final.pdf (accessed May 10, 2019).

Elton, S. (2018). Reconsidering the retail foodscape from a posthumanist and ecological determinants of health perspective: wading out of the food swamp. *Critical Public Health* **29**, 370–378

Elton, S. (2019). Posthumanism invited to dinner: exploring the potential of a more-than-human perspective in food studies. *Gastronomica: Journal of Critical Food Studies*, **Summer**, 1–10.

Escobar, A. (2018). *Designs for the Pluriverse: Radical Interdependence, Autonomy, and the Making of Worlds*. Chapel Hill, NC: Duke University Press.

Ferrante, A., & Sartori, D. (2016). From anthropocentrism to post-humanism in the educational debate. *Beyond AnthropocentrismRelations* **4**(2), **175–194**. doi:10.7358/rela-2016-002-fesa.

Ford, J. D., Stephenson, E., Cunsolo Willox, A., et al. (2016). Community-based adaptation research in the Canadian Arctic. *Wiley Interdisciplinary Reviews (WIREs): Climate Change* **7**, 175–191.

Fry, T. (1999) *A New Design Philosophy: An Introduction to Defuturing*. Sydney, Australia: University of New South Wales Press.

Gethmann, C. F., & Ehlers, E. (eds.) (2003). *Environment across Cultures*. Berlin: Springer.

Goldberg, T. L., & Patz, J. A. (2015). The need for a global health ethic. *Lancet* **386**, e37–e39

Haraway, D. (2008). *When Species Meet*. Minneapolis, MN: University of Minnesota Press.

Haraway, D. (2015). Anthropocene, Capitalocene, Plantationocene, Chthulucene: making kin. *Environmental Humanities* **6**(1), 159–165.

Hyett, S., Marjerrison, S., & Gabel, C. (2018) Improving health research among Indigenous peoples in Canada. *Canadian Medical Association Journal* **190**(20), E616–E621.

Jampel C. (2018). Intersections of disability justice, racial justice and environmental justice. *Environmental Sociology* **4**(1), 122–135. DOI 10.1080/23251042.2018.1424497.

Kimmerer, R. W. (2013). *Braiding Sweetgrass: Indigenous Wisdom, Scientific Knowledge and the Teachings of Plants*. Minneapolis, MN: Milkweed Editions.

Kuby, C. R. (2017). Why a paradigm shift of "more than human ontologies" is needed: putting to work poststructural and posthuman theories in a writers' studio. *International Journal of Qualitative Studies in Education* **30** (9), 877–896.

Lavery, J. V., Upshur, R. E. G., Sharp, R. R., & Hofman, K. J. (2003) Ethical issues in international environmental health research. *International Journal of Hygiene and Environmental Health* **206**(4–5), 453–463.

Lloro-Bidart, T. (2015). A political ecology of education in/for the Anthropocene. *Environment and Society* **6**(1), 128–148.

Lorimer, J. (2016). Gut buddies: multispecies studies and the microbiome. *Environmental Humanities* **8**(1), 57–76.

Malone, K. (2016). Theorizing a child–dog encounter in the slums of La Paz using post-humanistic approaches in order to disrupt universalisms in current "child in nature" debates. *Children's Geographies* **14**(4), 390–407.

Meek, D. (2015). Towards a political ecology of education: the educational politics of scale in southern Pará, Brazil. *Environmental Education Research* **21**(3), 447–459.

Mills, C. W. (2000). *The Sociological Imagination*, 40th anniversary edition. Oxford, UK: Oxford University Press.

Moore, J. W. (2017). The Capitalocene: I. On the nature and origins of our ecological crisis. *Journal of Peasant Studies* **44** (3), 594–630.

Moore, J. W. (2018). The Capitalocene: II. Accumulation by appropriation and the centrality of unpaid work/energy. *Journal of Peasant Studies* **45**(2), 237–279.

Norgaard, K. M. (2018). The sociological imagination in a time of climate change. *Global and Planetary Change* **163**, 171–176.

Pacini-Ketchabaw, V., & Taylor, A. (2015). Unsettling pedagogies through common world encounters: grappling with (post-)colonial legacies in Canadian forests and Australian bushlands, in Pacini-Ketchabaw, V., & Taylor, A. (eds.) *Unsettling the Colonial Places and Spaces of Early Childhood Education*. New York: Routledge, chap. 2, pp. 43–62.

Pan American Health Organization (PAHO) (2015). Ultra-processed food and drink products in Latin America: trends, impact on obesity, policy implications. Available at iris.paho.org/xmlui/bitstream/handle/123456789/7699/9789275118641_eng.pdf (accessed May 10, 2019).

Parkes, M. W., Harder, H. G., Hemingway, D., et al. (2016). Cumulative determinants of health impacts in rural, remote, and resource-dependent communities, in Gillingham, M.P., et al. (eds.), *The Integration Imperative: Cumulative Environmental, Community and Health Impacts of Multiple Natural Resource Developments*. New York: Springer.

Pedersen, H. (2010). Is "the posthuman" educable? On the convergence of educational philosophy, animal studies, and posthumanist theory. *Discourse: Studies in the Cultural Politics of Education* **31**(2), 237–250.

Peet, R., & Watts, M. (1996). Liberating political ecology, in Watts, R., & Peet, M. (eds.), *Liberation Ecologies: Environmental Development, Social Movements*, 2nd ed. London: Routledge.

Peet, R., Robbins, P., & Watts, M. (2011). *Global Political Ecology*. London: Routledge.

Porter, M., Franks, D. M., & Everingham, J-A. (2013). Cultivating collaboration: lessons from initiatives to understand and manage cumulative impacts in Australian resource regions. *Resources Policy* **38**, 657–669.

Pringle, J., & Cole, D. C. (2012). The Nigerian lead poisoning epidemic: the role of neoliberal globalization and challenges for humanitarian ethics, in Abu-Sada, C. (ed.), *Dilemmas, Challenges, and Ethics of Humanitarian Action. Reflections on Medicins Sans Frontieres' Perception Project*. Montreal: McGill-Queen's University Press, pp. 48–69.

Richmond, C. (2015). The relatedness of people, land, and health, in Greenwood, M., de Leeuw, S., Beck, L., & Reading, C. (eds.), *Determinants of Indigenous Peoples' Health*. Toronto: Canadian Scholars' Press, pp. 47–63.

Rock, M. (2013). Pet bylaws and posthumanist health promotion: a case study of urban policy. *Critical Public Health* **23**(2), 201–212.

Ruby, C. R. (2017). Why a paradigm shift of 'more than human ontologies' is needed: putting to work poststructural and posthuman theories in writers' studio. *International Journal of Qualitative Studies in Education* **30**(9), 877–896.

Schlosberg, D., & Collins, L. B. (2014). From environmental to climate justice: climate change and the discourse of environmental justice. *Wiley Interdisciplinary* Reviews: *Climate Change* **5**(3), 359–374.

Sen, A. K. (2009). *The Idea of Justice*. Cambridge, MA: Harvard University Press.

Steffen, W., Persson, Å., Deutsch, L., et al. (2011). The Anthropocene: from global change to planetary stewardship. *AMBIO* **40**(7), 739–761.

Swyngedouw, E. (1996). The city as a hybrid: on nature, society and cyborg urbanization. *Capitalism Nature Socialism* **7**(2), 65–80.

Taguchi, H. L. (2010). Rethinking pedagogical practices in early childhood education: a multidimensional approach to learning and inclusion, in Yeland, N. (ed.), *Contemporary Perspectives on Early Childhood Education*. Maidenhead, UK: McGraw-Hill Education and Open University Press, pp. 14–32.

Tannock, S. (2010). Learning to plunder: global education, global inequality and the global city. *Policy Futures in Education* **8**(1), 82–98.

Waltner-Toews, D. (2017). Zoonoses, One Health and complexity: wicked problems and constructive conflict. *Philosophical Transactions of the Royal Society B Biological Sciences* **372**(1725), 1–9.

Waltner-Toews, D., Kay, J. J., Neudoerffer, C., & Gitau, T. (2003). Perspective changes everything: managing ecosystems from the inside out. *Frontiers in Ecology and the Environment* **1**, 23–30.

Whitmee, S., Haines, A., Beyrer, C., et al. (2015). Safeguarding human health in the Anthropocene epoch: report of the Rockefeller Foundation–Lancet Commission on Planetary Health. *Lancet* **386**, 1973–2028.

Williams, L. (2017). Empowerment and the ecological determinants of health: three critical capacities for practitioners. *Health Promotion International* **32**(4), 711–722.

Wynter, S. (2003). Unsettling the coloniality of being/power/truth/freedom: towards the human, after man, its overrepresentation–an argument. *New Centennial Review* **3**(3), 257–337.

Toward a New Common Sense

The Need for New Paradigms of Global Health Beyond the COVID-19 Emergency

Isabella Bakker, Stephen Gill, and Dillon Wamsley

Tax struggle is the oldest form of class struggle.
(Karl Marx, 1967, cited in O'Connor [1973: 10])

Introduction

In Chapter 18, we outlined a reading of the present global conjuncture that we characterized as one of *organic crisis*. The term was meant to invoke a paradoxical situation, one pregnant with possibilities for alternative ways in which global health might be improved, yet nevertheless a situation in which new alternatives have yet to emerge or indeed to be born.

We also noted how the broad-ranging nature of the organic crisis was characterized by a number of morbid symptoms such as deterioration in global health and global nutrition associated with the way in which capitalist social forces have come to determine increasingly not only whether we have access to useful and affordable health care but also what we eat and whether we are actually able to eat. More broadly, the deepening and extension of the power of capital – because capitalism is a system of power relations and power structures – has come to determine increasing aspects of social reproduction, our health, and indeed the very means of survival for a large proportion of the inhabitants of this planet.[1]

We noted, therefore, that the global organic crisis involves a global crisis of accumulation coupled with an economic emergency occasioned by the COVID-19 pandemic, the dominant governmental responses to this crisis that have so far been generally one-sided,

leaning in favor of financial interests and big corporations, and how capitalism in crisis and its mode of relentless accumulation intersect with deepening and long-term threats to our health and social and ecological reproduction.

To address the global organic crisis in both theory and practice, we need, in effect, a new paradigm of global political economy – one based on a new "common sense" concerning the nature and potentials of the world that can address global health challenges in a progressive way that connects to the fundamental bases of social reproduction and human security as people face them in their everyday lives. A new paradigm therefore requires new modes of thought (*epistemological perspectives*) as well as the means to be able to re-conceptualize our most fundamental objects of analysis (*ontological depth*) that help explain the deeper and broader material and political determinants of global health – issues that we initially addressed elsewhere in our earlier work (Bakker & Gill, 2003). In particular we believe that a critical feminist political economy analysis can shed light on several proposals, such as those associated with public finance, taxation, and the governance of the social commons. Such proposals, however, are only as strong as the underlying social base and political pressures necessary to advance them.

We think, therefore, that many of the well-meaning solutions proposed by liberal cosmopolitans, not withstanding the emergency economic and health measures of 2020, fail to touch the most fundamental structures and relations of power that ultimately determine questions of livelihood, life chances, and indeed life or death for billions of people. The structures of global exploitation and injustice are not simply in need of "moderate" reforms; these structures require radical surgery and transformation. As the

---

[1] As articulated in Chapter 18, social reproduction encompasses the biological reproduction of the human species, the reproduction of the labor force, and provisioning and caring needs. This is inclusive of the public provision of health and welfare needs; the socialization of risk, such as pensions, unemployment insurance, social safety nets, and kinship networks; and the structures associated with the long-term reproduction of the socioeconomic system such as education (see Bakker & Gill, 2003).

decade since 2008–2009 has demonstrated, as well as responses to the COVID-19 pandemic in 2020, even an existential threat to the global financial and economic system, the likes of which have not been experienced since the 1930s, may not be sufficient to encourage a transition to a more just and sustainable economic and social order. On the contrary, the years since 2008 have been characterized by a deepening of global inequalities. In much of the world, there has been an entrenchment of political and economic power, with wealth and power increasingly concentrated within an oligarchic class. Growing discontent and disenchantment with the prevailing neoliberal order – and a lack of progressive alternatives – has been manifested in the rise of far-right, authoritarian nationalisms across the globe. There is, nonetheless in the present context, also a clear appetite for progressive and indeed radical political reform to create a more ethical, sustainable, and just political-economic order, particularly among younger generations. Unless massive democratic pressure is placed on the dominant governments of the world, however, all that can be expected following the economic emergency is either a minor tinkering with the exploitative structures of global capitalism or a deepening of its most reactionary elements. G20 policies – with or without widely discussed Tobin or carbon taxes – will continue to be responsive to and underwrite the priorities and needs of large corporations and investors or, more broadly, what we have called the *power of capital*. We suggest that only by taming and democratizing the power of capital will it be possible to produce a different type of world economic order, one in which the right to a decent livelihood, to social justice, and to appropriate nutrition and health will become possible not just for a privileged few but for a majority, something that is an existential necessity in an era of global pandemics. Biomedical approaches to health, while crucial, are clearly insufficient. With this in mind, the rest of this short chapter outlines a few measures that would need to be made as first steps in this process – understood as practical aspects of the development of a new paradigm to adequately address global health challenges.

Measures Needed to Bolster the Social Commons

As we noted in Chapter 18, new measures are needed to provide adequate financing to rebuild and extend the social commons. These must rest on a more equitable and broad-based tax system where capital and ecologically unsustainable resource consumption are taxed more than labor. Progressive principles of taxation also suggest less reliance on value-added taxes, which are regressive and a burden on the poor (especially on basic needs such as fuel and food). Developing-world countries need help with strengthening tax administration and public financial management and many of the loopholes associated with the offshore world, and accounting innovations, such as transfer pricing, need to be closed. Feminists also point out that a more progressive and equitable tax system needs to not only be inclusive, involving tax compliance for all, but also gender sensitive, particularly because taxation regimes affect men and women across the social spectrum in very different ways.[2]

Stepping back from these exigencies, we see at least seven sets of measures, interconnected and overlapping, that are needed to both support and finance a broadening of the social commons in ways that are consistent with greater democracy, social justice, and social and ecological sustainability.

Address Our Interdependencies with Each Other and with Nature

This involves both questions of epistemology and questions of political economy and public policies. Our prevailing systems of knowledge in political economy and social science have rendered certain problems invisible, such as the ways in which mainstream public policies and systems of governance associated with market civilization have obscured issues of inequality as well as ecological and social sustainability. In other words, we need to break what has been called the "strategic silence" associated with mainstream economic and political thinking, which has rendered invisible or unknowable all these key components of social and ecological life (Bakker, 1994). This presupposes new knowledge in the fields of political economy and the social sciences in ways that are linked to:

1. A shift in the nature of agricultural and food production systems away from petroleum- and chemical-based agricultural methods toward more

---

[2] The latter requires support for expanding existing efforts to improve the collection of sex-disaggregated data and data on the gender bias in indirect taxes such as value-added (VAT), consumption, and trade taxes.

organic, localized methods of production, distribution, and provisioning and a shift away from heavily meat-based diets – here, the example of the Brazilian Landless Workers Movement, with its 1.5 million members, is instructive.

2. A transformation in existing systems of energy production and consumption and their dominant modes of governance toward "energy democracy," which denotes both a shift away from the fossil fuel economy toward renewable energy and also, more broadly, a transformation in the structures of ownership and control over sustainable energy systems. Such political transformations would be based on the principle that ecological sustainability, health, and social and economic justice are inextricably intertwined and require a revitalization of existing mechanisms of political governance.

3. A shift in thinking and practice to take more fundamental account of what feminist economists call the "care economy," which involves both paid and unpaid work relating to caring for people. The concept of the care economy recognizes that all people need, give, and receive care. Often policies assume that this work will continue no matter what, as in the case of structural adjustment and austerity responses to economic crisis and economic emergency. Indeed, policies of austerity to fund government debts often involve cuts to health spending and reductions in welfare that shift the burden of adjustment to the informal care economy and its unpaid work in households. Such work is disproportionately carried out by women in most societies. Implicit in the orthodox view of economic adjustment, therefore, women become the social safety net, by default.

4. A need for rethinking the nature of health inequities in spending and entitlements and outcomes – all of which are connected to inequalities of life chances. This is therefore not simply an issue of public policy but also a fundamental ethical question.

5. In settler colonial countries such as Canada, there is a need for the recognition and enforcement of the UN Declaration of the Rights of Indigenous People (UNDRIP), which provides an initial framework outlining the rights to Indigenous sovereignty and self-determination. Movements for a revitalization of the social commons will have to recognize and abide by such frameworks in an effort to establish a more radically democratic and egalitarian society.

6. A framework for acknowledging and seeking to remedy the unequal burden of the ecological crisis that is already disproportionately affecting the health and well-being of marginalized populations, particularly in the Global South, whose per capita contributions to climate change are minuscule compared with the West.
   A campaign for ecological reparations – or the redistribution of the burden for combating ecological devastation – thus should be at the forefront of contemporary climate justice movements.

7. A coordinated and redistributive global effort stemming from democratic pressure within each country to establish an initial regulatory regime to increase the taxation and regulation of multinational corporations, financial institutions, and the world's wealthy elite, partly to help fund much more progressive global governance institutions and practices. A range of tactics and measures might be employed to initiate this effort, which is discussed in more detail later.

Socialize the Risks of the Global Majority While Enhancing the Social Commons

One of the key characteristics of capitalism in general, and neoliberal capitalism in particular, is the way in which we are increasingly forced to become part of the so-called self-help society. In this way, however, neoliberal capitalism has involved greater human and economic insecurity for the majority of people. Progressive policies must completely overhaul the regulation of finance and in so doing protect the life savings and pensions of the vast majority of people as well as our public health systems – it should not simply be capital that receives government guarantees. This requires not only the regulation of banks and other financial firms to prevent them from taking risks with depositors' funds but also, more generally, making finance the servant, rather than the master, of production, work, and wider social purposes. One way to address this problem is through the public sector, which needs to be made much more accountable to the needs of the public as a whole, and this should be connected to policies that make private corporations more socially accountable and more willing to pay their rightful costs for the social commons and the social goods and infrastructure from which many of their activities benefit.

For this to be possible requires not only new systems of governance but also new systems of taxation, for example, to institute steeply progressive taxation on the wealth and income of the top 20% of the world's population, who have been the primary beneficiaries of neoliberal globalization. This should be coupled with measures that provide guaranteed annual income for a majority, well above existing poverty lines, as well as substantially raised minimum wages for the majority of people. Such a shift would still allow the wealthy to be able to live comfortable lives.

Within the current political and economic environment of disciplinary neoliberalism there remain a number of difficulties in terms of establishing a system of progressive taxation to fund a range of social services and provisioning needs. In particular, prevailing legal and constitutional structures – what we refer to as a process of "new constitutionalism" – established through various treaties and trade and investment deals include numerous constraints that often prohibit the taxation of corporate transactions, such as international capital transfers, and encourage the proliferation of the tax-evasion economy. In addition to these direct legal means, the broader geographic power possessed by increasingly mobile global firms – or the "structural power" of capital – allows them to engage in a system of global arbitrage, shifting investment to seek the most profitable jurisdictions, which are often characterized by lax enforcement in terms of taxation policies, labor rights, and environmental regulations (Lesage, Vermeiren, & Dierckx, 2014).

These foundational structures of neoliberalism have not been significantly challenged or ruptured in the aftermath of the global financial crisis despite the growing dissatisfaction with the widespread bailouts of banks and firms by states and the regime of austerity that has followed. Whether that will remain the case following the COVID-19 pandemic/economic emergency remains to be seen. As Lesage et al. (2014) illustrate, programs for progressive international taxation reform need to address three distinct levels of taxation enforcement in order to be effective: the financial sector, the world's wealthy individuals, and multinational firms – each of which poses its own set of difficulties and problems.

Indeed, there remain numerous practical and political barriers under neoliberal globalization for states to impose and enforce taxation structures to shift their fiscal capacities toward a more progressive basis. In particular, the capital mobility of firms and the set of incentives to establish competitive taxation regimes to attract inflows of private investment both inhibit the feasibility and political willingness of states to seriously engage in broadly progressive taxation measures in such a globally competitive environment. Failed attempts by Germany and the European Union to implement modest financial transactions taxes in the aftermath of the global financial crisis illustrate some of the immediate material and institutional constraints facing such reform movements (Lesage et al,, 2014). Indeed, multinational firms are increasingly difficult to tax, possessing enormous power and mobility within and between different national boundaries, with increasingly sophisticated global value chains and political connections in a huge number of countries that pose numerous difficulties in terms of jurisdictional tax enforcement across borders.

Moreover, numerous barriers stand in the way of targeting the vast "offshore economy" because the world's transnational corporations and billionaires continue to shield their wealth from government taxation. The scope of the offshore economy has rapidly increased over the past several decades, with recent estimates indicating that offshore wealth ranges up from US$8 trillion–US$10 trillion, or about 10% of global gross domestic product (GDP; Zucman, 2015, 2018). This represents hundreds of billions of dollars in foregone tax revenue. Government efforts to target the offshore economy have been virtually nonexistent, given the immense power of capital to debilitate national economies with threats of capital flight and currency devaluation.

Cross-national regulatory efforts buttressed by popular pressures are sorely needed to target the vast wealth held offshore. In particular, numerous reforms are needed within the realm of information exchange to begin a systematic global effort to target tax avoidance, evasion, and offshoring because, as noted, it constitutes an enormous source of potential government revenue that could be used for redistributive measures and to bolster social provisioning. This would undoubtedly require a global effort across different regions to harmonize and establish a minimum standard of regulatory and taxation enforcement by which firms and financial companies must abide.

One of the most pressing issues in the global economy, however, resides in the world of "shadow banking," although its practitioners prefer "market-based finance." It includes investment and private banks and private equity funds, some mortgage lenders, money-market funds, hedge funds, insurance firms, and even payday loan companies, forming growing sources of credit and debt in ways increasingly central to the functioning of the global economy. While conducting many of the same services as conventional banks, including short-term lending collateralized by tradable debts known as *repo markets*, they are able to operate without any prudential or effective regulation. Shadow banking is vastly understudied (Gabor & Vestergaard, 2016). No one is certain of its scope and size, though recent estimates by the Financial Stability Board (2018) suggest that it may amount to more than US$160 trillion. These shadowy elements of the global economy have wide-ranging implications for financial stability because the world of shadow banking may engage in much riskier forms of activity that may threaten the financial systems on which the world economy depends while remaining virtually entirely outside the scope of public oversight or regulation. Comprehensive efforts to study the complex role of shadow banking within the global economy, bring them into the public realm, and establish rigorous forms of macroprudential regulation are therefore necessary to ensure financial stability and unlock the enormous potential revenue within this sector for public redistributive efforts.

Although Marx may have been correct in his assertion that tax struggle is the oldest form of class struggle, and while many proposals for progressive global taxation measures have been discussed in the past, ranging from global wealth taxes to currency transaction taxes, arms sales taxes, and various taxes on global carbon emissions, each of these proposals has suffered from similar pitfalls. As Richard Bird (2018) has observed after assessing the feasibility and global appetite for such taxation policies, many barriers remain in terms of proposing – let alone adopting – such policies. A lack of feasible enforcement mechanisms on a global scale to administer such taxation programs and the need for a global government to accompany such reforms have been among the foremost barriers that have prevented any serious attempts to engage with taxation proposals on a global scale. Moreover, the differential national and regional interests that inevitably accompany such proposals in a world characterized by competitive global capital accumulation and the widespread perception of a lack of transparency and democratic representation within the international bodies tasked with superintending such proposals are among some of the impediments to implementing the global taxation policies necessary to contest the global reach of capital (Bird, 2018). Indeed, particularly at a time in which increasingly undemocratic supranational bodies such as the European Union and international financial institutions such as the International Monetary Fund have been at the forefront of enacting neoliberal policies for decades, the possibility of transferring democratic responsibilities outside national institutions into international institutions faces numerous political difficulties.

Nonetheless, many international agreements and institutions are currently financed internationally in such a way that could be built on and extended in attempting to implement globally progressive taxation initiatives. Similarly, recent international agreements, while undoubtedly limited in several ways, illustrate the possibility of working toward a more far-reaching set of initiatives. For instance, the most recent UN meeting on climate change initiatives, the Paris Agreement, though plagued by a lack of effective enforcement mechanisms within and between different countries, presents an initial framework on which future progressive taxation proposals might be developed. In order for this to be feasible, however, Bird contends that there are at minimum three conditions that need to be met: the need for tax policies and their administration to remain under national control, providing a clear linkage between taxes paid toward such initiatives and the benefits received by each country; full transparency and accountability in the payment and implementation of such initiatives; and an even playing field that includes every country in the deliberation process (Bird, 2018: 35).

To this we might add that none of these initiatives is possible without a broad base of democratic political support from below that possesses a robust yet pluralistic vision for an alternative future. There is also the need to recognize that such policies and programs will necessarily come into direct confrontation with powerfully entrenched global corporate and financial interests, such as various fossil fuel companies, whose very business models and existence may be challenged by such initiatives. Indeed, an awareness that the social, ecological, and health needs of the majority of the world's population may not be compatible with the current state of affairs – or the business plans of extractive and exploitative corporations – ought to be at the forefront of such globally democratic initiatives.

In addition, markets can be reshaped to serve more socially useful ends and to contribute to public goods and the global commons. Indeed, Albritton (2009) has argued that we should not simply accept market prices but reshape them by placing surcharges on commodities or services that generate high social costs while subsidizing those that generate social benefits. He points out that this is already done; for example, education is already subsidized, whereas cigarettes have a surtax placed on them. Building on existing practices and extending them, we can therefore radically rethink how goods and services are priced outside of market mechanisms in order to create different incentive structures across society and with respect to the effects of certain activities on the environment (e.g., by placing high taxes on carbon emissions).

However, any shift in the taxation regime needs to take full account of its redistributive consequences: Carbon taxes have to be combined with policies to redistribute wealth so that those on lower incomes are not forced into further economic difficulties because of the higher prices that result from the new taxes. One only needs to observe the aftermath of President Macron's fuel taxes imposed in 2018 as a regressive tax in France and the ongoing political uprisings that followed in order to appreciate the need to integrate socially and economically just policies with movements for ecological sustainability. Finally, with respect to government expenditures, there need to be innovations in the way in which we consider the appropriate mix of provisioning between private and public for social reproduction both now and in the future. Policies should no longer be based on a generic, ahistorical possessive individual, as with the conventional economic discourse, but instead should be based on concepts that take full account of the inequalities across social classes and across gender, as well as those caused by racialized policies.

Create a New "Common Sense" by Nurturing Alternative and Progressive Values

What we mean by the creation of a new "common sense" is a transformation in the way in which people conceive of the nature and potentials of the world in which they actually live. Market civilization has brought with it a bombardment of symbols, images, and structures associated with ever-increasing consumption and the commodification of desire. The logic of market civilization is, however, ultimately destructive of conceptions of social solidarity and social and ecological sustainability (Gill, 1995). In short, we need new paradigms from which we can gauge the potential for progress in our civilization in ways that put people before profits. One way in which we can begin to foster a new common sense is through new concepts and practices in education and media institutions.

While time and again orthodox neoclassical economics has been proven to be not only intellectually bankrupt but also increasingly detached from reality, it continues to dominate as common sense within popular culture and mainstream political discourse. Whereas many liberals and progressives predicted the shift toward a new era of Keynesian economics following the crisis of 2007–2009, after moderate bailout packages and a decade of global austerity, the neoliberal orthodoxy remains firmly entrenched, albeit with increasingly nationalist and authoritarian inflections across numerous countries. Therefore, we believe that this calls for a revolution in the way in which economics is both taught in schools and universities and discussed in political discourse and particularly in the media, in ways that encourage a variety of different viewpoints and policy prescriptions.

For this to be possible requires new means of financing so that media that are truly responsive to the diversity of public opinion begin to emerge. Indeed, the diversity of public opinion and innovations in thought itself requires a vibrant education system, one that is premised on education as a collective social good and not as a private commodity. This requires that we build on fiscal systems of the type alluded to earlier and in particular provide people with sufficient income so that they actually have the time to develop their knowledge and capacity for reflection under conditions where they do not feel insecure concerning the future. Moreover, such educational movements would undoubtedly have to confront both the possibilities and pitfalls of relying on social media technologies and the internet to substantiate educational campaigns. Whereas digital media technologies offer the unique ability to reach a broad audience in a rapidly reduced period of time, social media and digital technology companies also represent powerful corporate interests with unprecedented access to our personal data as well as promoting the commodification of identity (see Gill & Benatar, 2019).

Constructing a new set of values and discourses requires both an immanent critique of existing power structures and the dominant modes of common sense that serve to legitimize them, as well as offering a set of alternative policies and modes of thinking.

In essence, we are calling for an *epistemological revolution* in the spirit of what we call the "postmodern Prince" (Gill, 2012). The postmodern Prince is a recognition of the current set of conditions in the world and is based on the dialectical process of demystifying extant power structures and offering "alternative form[s] of intellectual and moral leadership" (Gill, 2012: 512). Such shifts in epistemology and political praxis are based on the recognition of a plurality of critical modes of political and pedagogical praxis and ought to be grounded not only within the realm of abstract theorizing by a professional class but also linked organically to political struggles and forms of "concrete cultural activity" (Gill, 2012: 519).

Current political struggles around the globe are both heterogeneous and diverse, encompassing struggles for land rights and against extractive fossil fuel projects by peasant and Indigenous groups; care labor revolts, emanating across the United States as well as South America and parts of Europe, which are led primarily by teachers and educators, the majority of whom are women; renewed labor struggles in parts of China against some of the most extreme forms of exploitation and state repression; the ongoing *gilets jaunes* ("yellow vest") movement in France, a resistance against austerity and a generalized decline in living standards; a growing movement across Europe and North America for a "Green New Deal"; and a new generation of climate activists around Europe, manifesting most recently in a UK-wide strike in which schoolchildren coordinated a country-wide walkout to demand immediate political action to resist the ecological crisis, among many more. New epistemological frameworks must both be embedded in and connected to these diverse struggles for liberation, while also grounding them in a broader theoretical worldview of how a more egalitarian, just, and sustainable world might be constructed.

While the creation of a new common sense ought to be based on a political imagination operating "according to 'horizons of desire', collectively imagining to be desirable, necessary and possible what had previously been thought to be politically impossible," such movements should not disavow the need for concrete, short-term reforms necessary to meet the immediate material, social, and economic needs of the world's population (Gill, 2012: 520). Indeed, movements to urgently establish a more progressive taxation system, extend systems of social provisioning, increase democratic regulation of financial services, increase taxes and regulation over extractive sectors, and provide mechanisms of decommodified income support to marginalized populations ought to be at the material foundation of movements for broader social and political reform. Indeed, only a set of organizations and movements capable of mobilizing around a set of realizable demands in the broader struggle for a more radically democratic political alternative will be capable of contesting the dominant disciplinary neoliberal model and reverse the deepening global organic crises that threaten the majority of people and our planetary system. This is the key political question for now and the future.

References

Albritton, R. (2009). *Let Them Eat Junk: How Capitalism Creates Hunger and Obesity*. London: Pluto Press.

Alstasaeder, A., Johannessen N., & Zucman G. (2018). Who owns the wealth in tax havens? Macro evidence and implications for global inequality. *Journal of Public Economics* **162**, 89–100.

Angel, J. (2016). *Strategies of Energy Democracy*. Berlin: Rosa Luxemburg Stiftung. Available at www.rosalux.eu/publications/strategies-of-energy-democracy-a-report/ (accessed February 11, 2019).

Bakker, I. (ed.) (1994). *The Strategic Silence: Gender and Economic Policy*. London: Zed Books.

Bakker, I., & Gill, S. (2003). *Power, Production, and Social Reproduction: Human in/Security in the Global Political Economy*. Basingstoke, UK: Palgrave Macmillan.

Bird, R. M. (2018). Are global taxes feasible? Rotman School of Management Working Paper No. 3006175, Toronto, Canada.

Campbell, A. F. (2019). A record number of US workers went on strike in 2018. *Vox*, February 13.

Financial Stability Board (2018). Global shadow banking monitoring report 2017. Available at www.fsb.org/2018/03/

global-shadow-banking-monitoring-report-2017/ (accessed May 9, 2018).

Gabor, D., & Vestergaard, J. (2016). Towards a theory of shadow money, Institute for New Economic Thinking, New York. Available at www.ineteconomics.org/research/research-papers/towards-a-theory-of-shadow-money (accessed May 8, 2019).

Gill, S. (1995). Globalisation, market civilisation, and disciplinary neoliberalism. *Millennium* **23**(3): 399–423.

Gill, S. (2012). Towards a radical concept of praxis: imperial "common sense" versus the post-modern Prince. *Millennium* **40**(3): 505–524.

Gill, S., & Benatar, S. R. (2019). Reflections on the political economy of planetary health. *Review of International Political Economy* **26**(6): 167–190.

Lesage, D., Vermeiren, M., & Dierckx, S. (2014). New constitutionalism, international taxation, and crisis, in Gill, S., & Cutler, C. (eds.), *New Constitutionalism and World Order*. Cambridge, UK: Cambridge University Press: 197–210.

Lockett, H. (2017). China labour unrest spreads to "new economy." *Financial Times*, February 1.

O'Connor, J. (1973). *The Fiscal Crisis of The State*. New York: St. Martin's Press.

Taylor, M., Laville, S., Walker, A., et al. (2019). School pupils call for radical climate action in UK-wide strike. *The Guardian*, February 15.

Zucman, G. (2015). *The Hidden Wealth of Nations: The Scourge of Tax Havens*. Chicago: University of Chicago Press.

Index